Prostate Cancer: Diagnostic and Therapeutic Strategies

Prostate Cancer: Diagnostic and Therapeutic Strategies

Editor: Olivier Douglas

FOSTER
ACADEMICS
www.fosteracademics.com

www.fosteracademics.com

FOSTER ACADEMICS

Cataloging-in-Publication Data

Prostate cancer : diagnostic and therapeutic strategies / edited by Olivier Douglas.
p. cm.
Includes bibliographical references and index.
ISBN 978-1-64646-632-0
1. Prostate--Cancer. 2. Prostate--Cancer--Diagnosis. 3. Prostate--Cancer--Treatment. I. Douglas, Olivier.
RC280.P7 P763 2023
616.994 63--dc23

Foster Academics,
118-35 Queens Blvd., Suite 400,
Forest Hills, NY 11375, USA

ISBN 978-1-64646-632-0 (Hardback)

Contents

Preface

The world is advancing at a fast pace like never before. Therefore, the need is to keep up with the latest developments. This book was an idea that came to fruition when the specialists in the area realized the need to coordinate together and document essential themes in the subject. That's when I was requested to be the editor. Editing this book has been an honour as it brings together diverse authors researching on different streams of the field. The book collates essential materials contributed by veterans in the area which can be utilized by students and researchers alike.

Males have a small walnut-shaped gland called the prostate that generates seminal fluid which nourishes and transports sperm. Prostate cancer is a type of cancer which affects the prostate gland. In the initial stages of prostate cancer, there are no symptoms or signs. However, various symptoms and signs can be observed during the progressive stage, which include blood in the sperm, erectile dysfunction, decreased force in the stream of urine, bone pain, difficulty urinating, blood in the urine, etc. There are various risk factors that contribute in the development of prostate cancer, such as family history, older age, obesity and race. The diagnosis of this type of cancer is done through prostate specific antigen (PSA), which is a serum marker. Prostate cancer is currently treated with proton beam therapy, surgery and radiation therapy. This book unravels the recent studies on prostate cancer. It strives to provide a fair idea about diagnostic and therapeutic strategies for this disease to help develop a better understanding of the latest advances in its clinical management. A number of latest researches have been included to keep the readers up-to-date with the global concepts in this medical condition.

Each chapter is a sole-standing publication that reflects each author´s interpretation. Thus, the book displays a multi-facetted picture of our current understanding of application, resources and aspects of the field. I would like to thank the contributors of this book and my family for their endless support.

Editor

1

Circular RNAs and their Linear Transcripts as Diagnostic and Prognostic Tissue Biomarkers in Prostate Cancer after Prostatectomy in Combination with Clinicopathological Factors

Hannah Rochow [1,2], Monika Jung [1], Sabine Weickmann [1], Bernhard Ralla [1], Carsten Stephan [1,2], Sefer Elezkurtaj [3], Ergin Kilic [3,4], Zhongwei Zhao [1,5], Klaus Jung [1,2,*,†], Annika Fendler [1,6,7,†] and Antonia Franz [1,†]

1 Department of Urology, Charité-Universitätsmedizin Berlin, 10117 Berlin, Germany; hannah.rochow@charite.de (H.R.); mchjung94@gmail.com (M.J.); sabine.weickmann@charite.de (S.W.); bernhard.ralla@charite.de (B.R.); carsten.stephan@charite.de (C.S.); zhaozhongweixy@163.com (Z.Z.); annika.fendler@crick.ac.uk (A.F.); antonia.franz@charite.de (A.F.)
2 Berlin Institute for Urologic Research, 10115 Berlin, Germany
3 Institute of Pathology, Charité-Universitätsmedizin Berlin, 10117 Berlin, Germany; sefer.elezkurtaj@charite.de (S.E.); e.kilic@pathologie-leverkusen.de (E.K.)
4 Institute of Pathology, Hospital Leverkusen, 51375 Leverkusen, Germany
5 Department of Urology, Qilu Hospital of Shandong University, Jinan 250012, China
6 Max Delbrueck Center for Molecular Medicine in the Helmholtz Association, Cancer Research Program, 13125 Berlin, Germany
7 Cancer Dynamics Laboratory, The Francis Crick Institute, 1 Midland Road, London NW1 1AT, UK
* Correspondence: klaus.jung@charite.de
† These authors share senior authorship.

Abstract: As new biomarkers, circular RNAs (circRNAs) have been largely unexplored in prostate cancer (PCa). Using an integrative approach, we aimed to evaluate the potential of circRNAs and their linear transcripts (linRNAs) to act as (i) diagnostic biomarkers for differentiation between normal and tumor tissue and (ii) prognostic biomarkers for the prediction of biochemical recurrence (BCR) after radical prostatectomy. In a first step, eight circRNAs (circ*ATXN10*, circ*CRIM1*, circ*CSNK1G3*, circ*GUCY1A2*, circ*LPP*, circ*NEAT1*, circ*RHOBTB3*, and circ*STIL*) were identified as differentially expressed via a genome-wide circRNA-based microarray analysis of six PCa samples. Additional bioinformatics and literature data were applied for this selection process. In total, 115 malignant PCa and 79 adjacent normal tissue samples were examined using robust RT-qPCR assays specifically established for the circRNAs and their linear counterparts. Their diagnostic and prognostic potential was evaluated using receiver operating characteristic curves, Cox regressions, decision curve analyses, and C-statistic calculations of prognostic indices. The combination of circ*ATXN10* and lin*STIL* showed a high discriminative ability between malignant and adjacent normal tissue PCa. The combination of lin*GUCY1A2*, lin*NEAT1*, and lin*STIL* proved to be the best predictive RNA-signature for BCR. The combination of this RNA signature with five established reference models based on only clinicopathological factors resulted in an improved predictive accuracy for BCR in these models. This is an encouraging study for PCa to evaluate circRNAs and their linRNAs in an integrative approach, and the results showed their clinical potential in combination with standard clinicopathological variables.

Keywords: prostate cancer; microarray; identification; validation and differential expression of circular RNAs; circular RNAs and linear counterparts; biochemical recurrence; diagnostic and prognostic tissue biomarkers; improved predictive accuracy by RNA signature

1. Introduction

Prostate cancer (PCa) is the second most common cancer type among men [1]. Following radical prostatectomy, which is used as a therapeutic curative option for patients suffering from PCa, biochemical recurrence (BCR), defined as a re-increased serum concentration of prostate-specific antigen (PSA) of >0.2 μg/L [2,3], is clinically considered to be the first sign of disease recurrence [4,5]. An evaluation of six recent studies with more than 1000 patients in each showed that approximately 15–34% of surgically treated patients suffered from BCR within 5 to 10 years after surgery [6]. Following BCR without secondary therapy, distant metastasis manifests in approximately 30% of patients and 19–27% will die within 10 years [7,8]. These data clearly show that early and reliable prediction of patients with a high risk of BCR is necessary to optimize the frequency of follow-up and thus the decision to undergo adjuvant therapy.

For BCR risk prediction, numerous scoring systems based on clinicopathological factors such as the Gleason score or the respective International Society of Urological Pathology (ISUP) grade, pathological tumor stage (pT stage), and preoperative PSA level are currently applied. Among these tools are the Cancer of the Prostate Risk Assessment Postsurgical Score (CAPRAS) [9] and those developed by D'Amico et al. [10], Stephenson et al. [7], and the National Comprehensive Cancer Network (NCCN) [11]. Although all clinicopathological factors are, to some extent, associated with patient outcome, the prognostic accuracy of these nomograms is generally unsatisfactory [12–16]. In this context, prognostic molecular biomarkers could significantly improve the predictive accuracy of tools based only on clinicopathological factors [17–21]. We recently elaborated a five-microRNA signature that outperforms the BCR scoring systems mentioned above [6]. In addition, the combined use of clinicopathological factors and molecular markers was found to significantly improve the predictive accuracy compared to the separately calculated predictive value [6]. Based on this experience using molecular markers in BCR prediction, we decided to extend this approach to circular RNAs (circRNA), which we successfully introduced as prognostic biomarkers in clear cell renal cell carcinoma [22].

Recently, circRNAs have the subject of increasing interest in medicine. These RNAs consist of a single strand of RNA in a closed loop [23,24], and are formed by alternative splicing of mostly exonic sequences. One host gene can form several different circRNAs [25,26]. The functions of circRNAs are still being investigated. Their ability to sponge microRNAs (miRNAs), a process in which circRNAs prevent the inhibitory properties of miRNA and therefore promote the expression of target mRNAs, is relatively well known [23,24,27]. Furthermore, circRNAs may regulate the expression of their parenteral genes by interacting with RNA polymerase II [28], but they can also interact with RNA-binding proteins and are therefore involved in the regulation of gene expression [29]. Some circRNAs may even be able to encode proteins [30]. CircRNAs have expression patterns that are specific to different cells or tissues and have been shown to play roles in cell regulation, including physiological as well as pathological processes [24,31–35]. It has been shown that circRNAs can act as oncogenes and tumor suppressors in the initiation and progression of different cancers, e.g., hepatocellular carcinoma, gastric carcinoma, colorectal cancer, and renal cell carcinoma [22,36–39]. All of these aspects justify a particular interest in using circRNAs as biomarkers in diagnosis, prognosis, and prediction, as well as for therapeutic targets [33,40–43].

CircRNAs in PCa are also a subject of present research. Last year, Chen et al. [44] identified a broad signature of PCa-specific circRNAs via ultra-deep rRNA-depleted RNA sequencing of localized PCa tissue samples. Moreover, specific circRNA functions were shown. Circ*CSNK1G3*, for example, seems to promote cell proliferation in PCa [44]. Furthermore, Zhang et al. [45] applied a bioinformatics approach using various PCa cells to identify numerous circRNAs, including circ*GUCY1A2*, as potential candidates for PCa progression. Other working groups using microarray platforms have reported lists of the top up- and downregulated circRNAs in PCa tissue compared with adjacent normal tissue [46,47]. Recent studies have particularly analyzed functional features and underlying molecular mechanisms of individual circRNAs [48–53]. Several publications particularly focused on androgen receptor pathway related circRNAs [54–57]. Correlations between the expression of circRNAs and relevant clinicopathological factors or survival Kaplan-Meier analyses have been reported [44,51,58–62]. However, it is astonishing that the potential of circRNAs as diagnostic and prognostic tissue biomarkers has so far only been evaluated in isolated cases [47,58,61]. As far as we know, only one study has ever conducted multivariate analyses of circRNAs in connection with clinicopathological factors [61]. Studies on the clinical validity of circRNAs in relation to BCR are still lacking.

Thus, in this study, we aimed to (i) identify differentially expressed circRNAs in six paired samples of PCa tissue and adjacent normal tissue using microarray analysis, (ii) validate the differential expression of eight chosen circRNAs and their linear counterparts via reverse-transcription quantitative real-time polymerase chain reaction (RT-qPCR), (iii) examine the differentiating potential between malignant and non-malignant prostate tissue in 194 samples of 115 PCa patients including 79 paired samples, and (iv) evaluate the potential of the chosen circRNAs and their linear counterparts as biomarkers in combination with the clinicopathological factors of PCa patients after radical prostatectomy to predict BCR.

2. Results

2.1. *Patient Characteristics and Study Design*

One hundred and fifteen untreated PCa patients who underwent radical prostatectomy between 2007 and 2014 with follow-up data until November 2019 were included in this study. Follow-up data were based on medical records and telephone contacts with the patients, their physicians, and their family members. In total, 194 tissue samples with 79 pairs of adjacent normal and malignant samples, and 36 with malignant characteristics only were investigated (Table 1). The sample size was determined using a power-adapted calculation ($\alpha = 5\%$, power = 80%; Supplementary Information S1 (Supplementary Materials)). A two-to-one selection of available samples, based on patients with BCR, was retrospectively performed with 76 patients without BCR and 39 with BCR. BCR was defined as a postoperative PSA increase above 0.2 μg/L after radical prostatectomy, as confirmed by consecutive increased values [2,3]. The workflow diagram presented in Figure 1 outlines the design of this study, which involved three phases based on the above postulated objectives for this investigation: (i) the discovery phase of identifying differentially expressed circRNAs using a microarray screening approach and the selection of circRNAs for further evaluation; (ii) analytical confirmation of the circular nature of selected circRNAs and elaboration of "fit-for-purpose" RT-qPCR assays for circRNAs and their linear transcripts; and (iii) initial clinical evaluations regarding their validity as discriminative tissue classifiers and the predictive value of these biomarkers when applied alone and in combination with conventional clinicopathological factors.

2.2. *Discovery of circRNAs in Prostate Cancer Tissue Using Microarray Analysis*

2.2.1. Identification of Differentially Expressed circRNAs

Six matched PCa tissue samples were examined using ArrayStar microarray experiment. A total of 9599 circRNAs out of 13,617 distinct probes on the array were detected (Supplementary Microarray Data File.xlsx (Supplementary Materials)). This number of circRNAs derived from 4838 host genes, since numerous host genes can form multiple circRNA isoforms [26]. Approximately 26% of all detected circRNAs were found to be from ~50% of the host genes that form only one circRNA, while the other 41% of circRNAs were found from the ~35% of the host genes that can form two or three circRNAs. Approximately 3.2% of the circRNAs were derived from only 0.6% of the host genes able to form 10 or more circRNAs (Figure 2A). Different genomic regions can be the origin of circRNAs. In this PCa microarray screening, approximately 90% of circRNAs were of exonic origin, but intronic, sense-overlapping, anti-sense, and intergenic circRNA types were also detected (Figure 2B). These data correspond with our own results in renal cell carcinoma [22] and data from studies on other tissues [25]. Regarding the differential expression between adjacent normal and malignant tissue, the array data identified

43 upregulated and 134 downregulated circRNAs with a higher than absolute 1.5-fold change ($p < 0.05$) in malignant tissue samples (Figure 2C). Using a threshold of 2-fold change, only six upregulated and 18 downregulated circRNAs were identified. Based on a principal component analysis of the microarray expression data, two separate clusters with malignant and adjacent normal tissue characteristics were ascertained (Figure 2D).

Table 1. Clinicopathological characteristics of the study group.

Characteristics	All Patients	Patients with Biochemical Recurrence	Patients without Biochemical Recurrence	*p*-Value [a]
Patients, no. (%)	115 (100)	39 (34)	76 (66)	
Age, median years, (IQR)	67 (62–70)	66 (59–71)	67 (64–70)	0.339
PSA, µg/L (IQR)	7.7 (5.4–12.2)	9.7 (6.1–19.5)	7.0 (5.4–9.5)	0.011
Prostate volume, cm^3 (IQR)	32 (25–45)	30 (23–39)	33 (26–45)	0.264
DRE, no. (%)				0.067
Non-suspicious	67 (58)	17 (44)	50 (66)	
Suspicious	32 (28)	14 (36)	18 (24)	
Unclassified	16 (14)	8 (20)	8 (10)	
pT status, no. (%)				0.005
pT1c	1 (1)	0	1 (1)	
pT2a	2 (2)	0	2 (3)	
pT2b	1 (1)	0	1 (1)	
pT2c	61 (53)	13 (33)	48 (63)	
pT3a	27 (23)	11 (28)	16 (21)	
pT3b	23 (20)	15 (39)	8 (11)	
ISUP Grade groups, no. (%)				0.0001
1	26 (23)	2 (5)	24 (31)	
2	47 (41)	13 (33)	34 (45)	
3	30 (26)	14 (36)	16 (21)	
4	4 (3	4 (11)	0 (0)	
5	8 (7)	6 (15)	2 (3)	
pN status, no. (%)				0.017
pN0/Nx	109 (95)	34 (87)	75 (99)	
pN1	6 (5)	5 (13)	1 (1)	
Surgical margin, no. (%)				
Negative	64 (56)	16 (41)	48 (63)	0.030
Positive	51 (44)	23 (59)	28 (37)	
Follow-up after surgery				<0.0001
Median months (IQR)	41 (26–72)	19.9 (9.8–41)	52 (38–80)	

Abbreviations: CI, confidence interval; DRE, digital rectal examination; IQR, interquartile range; ISUP Grade groups, histopathological grade system based on Gleason score according to the International Society of Urologic Pathology; pN, lymph node status; PSA, total prostate specific antigen before surgery; pT, pathological tumor classification. [a] *p*-Values (Mann-Whitney *U* test; Chi-square or Fisher's exact test) indicate the association of the clinicopathological variables with patients with and without biochemical recurrence.

2.2.2. Selection of circRNAs for Further Evaluation

In addition to the microarray-based expression results (absolute fold-change >1.5 with *unadjusted* $p < 0.05$ and sufficiently raw intensity on the microarray), we used interest-specific criteria to select circRNAs for further investigation. We selected six circRNAs (Table 2), for which no information on prostate carcinoma was available. Their host genes had been described in individual studies with regard to their roles in either PCa progression (e.g., *CRIM1*, *NEAT1*, and *STIL* [63–65]) or other cancers (e.g., *LPP* and *RHOBTB3* [66,67]). Some of the selected circRNAs had been partly identified in other cancers (e.g., circ*CRIM1* and circ*RHOBTB3* [22,68]). Finally, an in silico analysis of miRNA interaction with these circRNAs was performed using the algorithm provided by the CircInteractome tool and the miRDB and TargetScan databases [69–71]. In all cases, the circRNAs were found to be crucial points for potentially relevant miRNA–gene interactions (Figure S1). This also fulfilled a selection criterion for further investigations to be planned. *NEAT1* was identified as a special case because it already has miRNA-sponging functions as a long non-coding RNA (lncRNA) [65]. Thus, the relationship between the circRNA and the lncRNA transcript was of particular interest. In this circRNA panel, two additional circRNAs from the genes *CSNK1G3* and *GUCY1A2* were included as these circRNAs were recently identified in PCa tissue samples and PCa cell lines as mentioned in the introduction [44,45]. Collectively, the microarray analysis of the six paired samples in the discovery phase (Figure 1) must be considered an exploratory study for ranking deregulated circRNAs using the unadjusted *p*-values supported by the mentioned additional selection criteria. Under these conditions, an exploratory study should be preferably analyzed without *p*-value adjustment, but needs a technical replication by a different assay technique and biological validation using other clinical samples [72–74]. This was done in the two subsequent workflow phases B and C (Figure 1).

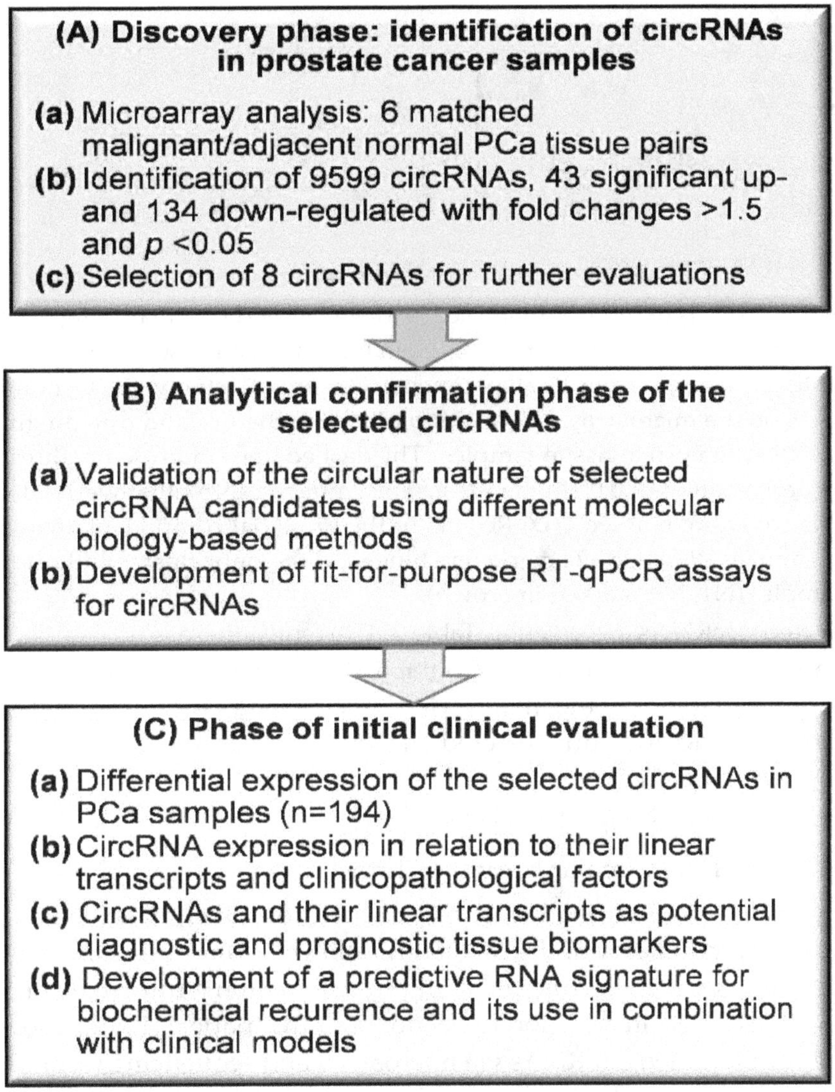

(A) Discovery phase: identification of circRNAs in prostate cancer samples
(a) Microarray analysis: 6 matched malignant/adjacent normal PCa tissue pairs
(b) Identification of 9599 circRNAs, 43 significant up- and 134 down-regulated with fold changes >1.5 and p <0.05
(c) Selection of 8 circRNAs for further evaluations
(B) Analytical confirmation phase of the selected circRNAs
(a) Validation of the circular nature of selected circRNA candidates using different molecular biology-based methods
(b) Development of fit-for-purpose RT-qPCR assays for circRNAs
(C) Phase of initial clinical evaluation
(a) Differential expression of the selected circRNAs in PCa samples (n=194)
(b) CircRNA expression in relation to their linear transcripts and clinicopathological factors
(c) CircRNAs and their linear transcripts as potential diagnostic and prognostic tissue biomarkers
(d) Development of a predictive RNA signature for biochemical recurrence and its use in combination with clinical models

Figure 1. Workflow of the study in three phases. Abbreviations: circRNA, circular RNA; PCa, prostate cancer; RT-qPCR, reverse-transcription quantitative real-time polymerase chain reaction.

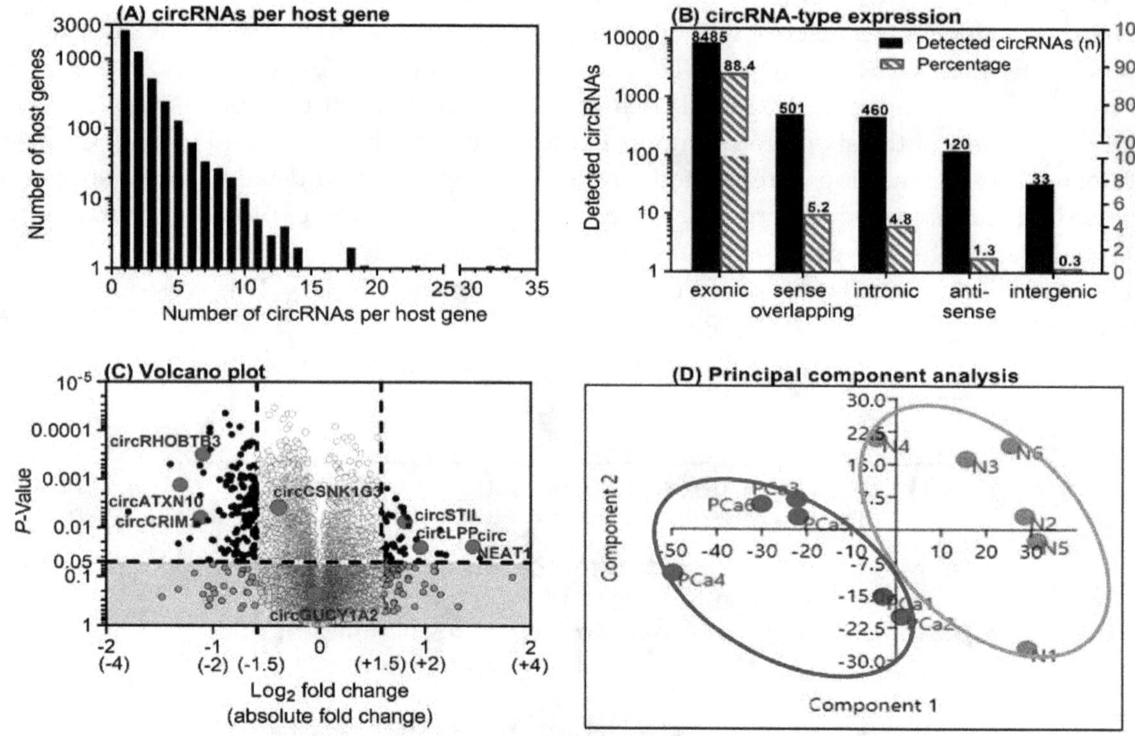

Figure 2. Microarray analysis results of six matched prostate cancer (PCa) tissue samples. (**A**) The number of circular RNAs (circRNAs) expressed per host gene in the malignant tissue samples and their matched adjacent normal tissue samples from PCa specimens after prostatectomy. (**B**) Genomic origin of the detected circRNAs on the microarray. (**C**) Volcano plot with the up- and downregulated circRNAs in malignant vs. adjacent normal tissue samples. The dashed lines indicate the thresholds: absolute 1.5-fold changes and p-values of 0.05 in the t-test. The eight circRNAs that were selected for further evaluation in this study are marked. (**D**) Results of the principal component analysis with the left cluster of tumor samples (PCa1–PCa6, marked in blue) and the right cluster with the paired adjacent normal tissue samples (N1–N6, marked in brown).

Data on the selected circRNAs are given in Table 2. Currently, there is no standardized nomenclature for circRNAs [22], and the designations of the database circBase are mainly used as a reference [75]. In order to facilitate the readability of the manuscript, official gene symbols with the prefixes "circ" and "lin" are used herein to characterize our selected circRNAs and the corresponding linear transcripts from the same host gene (Table 2).

2.3. Analytical Confirmation Phase of the Selected circRNAs

2.3.1. Experimental Proof of the Circular Nature of Transcripts

RT-qPCR assays using SYBRGreen I were established for the eight selected circRNAs and their linear counterparts, taking into account the MIQE guidelines "Minimum Information for Publication of Quantitative Real-Time PCR Experiments" [76] (Supplementary Information S3 (Supplementary Materials) with the Tables S1–S7 in addition to Section 4 of this paper). Experimental confirmation of the circular nature of the identified circRNAs via microarray and sequencing technologies was achieved using different tests to confirm the characteristics of the circRNA-specific backsplice junction [24,77,78]. Figure 3 shows that circRNAs are resitant to RNase R digestion (Figure 3A), distinctly decreased complementary DNA (cDNA) synthesis occurred when oligo(dT)$_{18}$ primers were used compared with when random hexamer primers (Figure 3B) were used, and the backsplice junction was confirmed by Sanger sequencing (Figure 3C). Melting curve analysis and electrophoresis of the amplicons were applied in order to validate the analytical specificity of the RT-qPCR products in all assays (Figures S2, S3, and Table S7).

Table 2. List of circular RNAs (circRNAs) seleceted for further evaluation in this study based on their differential expression between malignant and adjacent normal tissue samples data in the microarray discovery study phase and literature search.

circRNA in Manuscript	circRNA ID in circBase [a,b]	Absolute Fold Change on Microarray (p-Value)	Best Transcript	Official Gene Symbol (Official Gene Name)
		Upregulated circRNAs		
circ*LPP*	circ_0003759	1.94 (0.025)	NM_005578.5	*LPP* (LIM domain containing preferred translocation partner in lipoma)
circ*NEAT1*	circ_0000324	2.73 (0.0235)	NR_131012.1	*NEAT1* (Nuclear paraspeckle assembly transcript 1)
circ*STIL*	circ_0000069	1.75 (0.007)	NM_001282936.1	*STIL* (STIL centriolar assembly protein)
		Downregulated circRNAs		
circ*ATXN10*	circ_0001246	2.48 (0.001))	NM_013236.4	*ATXN10* (Ataxin 10)
circ*CRIM1*	circ_0007386	2.17 (0.006))	NM_016441.3	*CRIM1* (Cysteine rich transmembrane BMP regulator 1)
circ*RHOBTB3*	circ_0007444	2.14 (0.0003)	NM_014899.4	*RHOBTB3* (Rho related BTB domain containing 3)
		circRNAs from Literature [c]		
circ*CSNK1G3*	circ_0001522	−1.31 (0.003)	NM_001044723.2	*CSNK1G3* (Casein kinase 1 gamma 3)
circ*GUCY1A2*	circ_0008602	−1.02 (0.305)	NM_000855.3	*GUCY1A2* (Guanylate cyclase 1 soluble subunit alpha 2)

[a] The obligatory prefix *hsa_* was omitted to facilitate the readability. [b] In the separate Supplementary Microarray Data File.xlsx as part of the Supplementary Materials, detailed information is given for all detected circRNAs including source, chromosome localization, strand, circRNA type, sequences, and the circRNA IDs specific for ArrayStar Microarrays and the database circBase [75]. [c] Chen et al. [44] for circ*CSNK1G3* and Zhang et al. [45] for circ*GUCY1A2*.

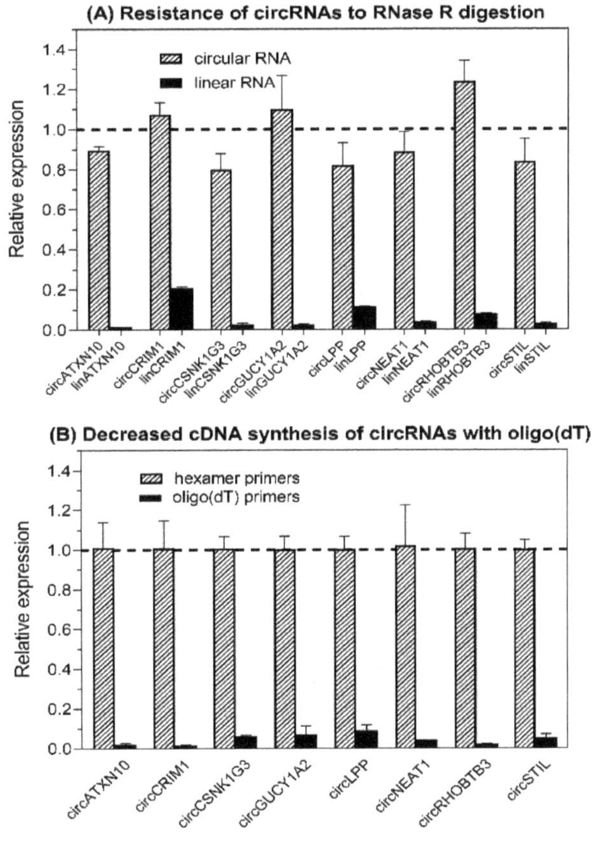

Figure 3. *Cont.*

(C) Sanger sequencing of backsplice junction

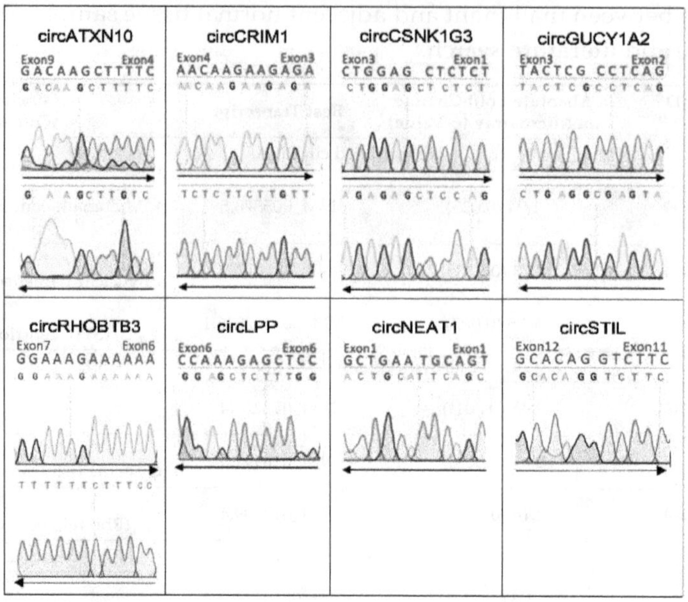

Figure 3. Experimental proof of the circular nature of the circRNAs selected in this study. (**A**) Resistance of circRNAs to RNase R digestion compared with linear RNAs. Data for triplicates (mean ± standard deviation) normalized to controls without RNase treatment are presented. (**B**) Decreased cDNA synthesis of circRNAs with oligo(dT)$_{18}$ vs. random hexamer primers. Data are given as the relative expression normalized to hexamer-primers-based cDNA synthesis. The relative expression was markedly decreased in all circRNAs (at least $n = 3$ of tissue pools) when using oligo(dT)$_{18}$ primers in comparison to random hexamer primers, indicating that the circRNAs lacked a poly(A) tail. (**C**) Base sequence of circRNA backsplice junction pictured by Sanger sequencing. Circ*LPP*, circ*NEAT1*, and circ*STIL* were only sequenced in one direction as one of the primers was junction-spanning (Table S3). The sequencing result of circ*RHOBTB3* corresponded to that in kidney carcinoma [22]. Methodical details for all experiments listed here are described in Section 4 and Supplementary Information S4 (Supplementary Materials).

2.3.2. Analytical Performance of RT-qPCR Assays

According to the MIQE guidelines [76] and also to the "Standards for Reporting of Diagnostic Accuracy Studies" (STARD) [79], the repeatability (intra-assay variation) and reproducibility (inter-assay variation) of the measurements should be used decisive criteria for the performance and robustness of RT-qPCR tests. Supported by the analytical specificity of the established assays (Figures S2 and S3) and the characteristics of the PCR standard curves (Table S7), the data shown in Table 3 proved that the assays were suitable for "fit-for-purpose" RT-qPCR measurements in clinical studies [80]. An exception was circ*NEAT1*, which had rather poor repeatability and reproducibility due to its very low expression.

2.4. Clinical Assessment

2.4.1. Differential Expression of circRNAs in Relation to Clinicopathological Variables

In the first step, we compared the circRNA expression data obtained from the six paired tumor and adjacent normal tissue samples using microarray analysis and the established RT-qPCR assays (Table 4). The expression results were in good agreement between both measurement methods for the circRNAs, with the exceptions of circ*LPP* and circ*STIL*. Circ*LPP* and circ*STIL* were found to be upregulated in the microarray analysis but downregulated in RT-qPCR measurements. Despite this clear discrepancy, we decided to include these two circRNAs together with their linear transcripts in further analyses.

Table 3. Repeatability and reproducibility of RT-qPCR measurements.

RNA	Repeatability [a]		Reproducibility [b]	
	Cq Value Mean (%RSD)	Relative Quantities Mean (%RSD)	Cq Value Mean ± SD (%RSD)	Relative Quantities Mean ± SD (%RSD)
circ*ATXN10*	24.49 (0.595)	1.345 (10.4)	24.31 ± 0.144 (0.591)	1.004 ± 0.100 (9.98)
circ*CRIM1*	24.61 (0.455)	1.299 (7.59)	24.39 ± 0.115 (0.472)	1.003 ± 0.078 (7.79)
circ*CSNK1G3*	21.47 (0.289)	1.164 (4.28)	21.34 ± 0.131 (0.613)	1.003 ± 0.093 (9.22)
circ*GUCY1A2*	24.68 (0.516)	1.461 (8.81)	24.68 ± 0.134 (0.541)	1.003 ± 0.092 (9.18)
circ*LPP*	25.71 (0.314)	1.177 (5.71)	25.76 ± 0.104 (0.406)	1.002 ± 0.070 (7.00)
circ*NEAT1*	35.56 (0.680)	1.285 (16.4)	36.80 ± 0.309 (0.838)	1.017 ± 0.214 (21.1)
circ*RHOBTB3*	23.91 (0.241)	1.055 (3.95)	24.02 ± 0.178 (0.739)	1.006 ± 0.121 (12.1)
circ*STIL*	28.51 (0.542)	1.261 (10.9)	28.47 ± 0.105 (0.369)	1.002 ± 0.0.72 (7.18)
lin*ATXN10*	20.23 (0.341)	1.250 (5.07)	20.21 ± 0.106 (0.525)	1.002 ± 0.072 (7.14)
lin*CRIM1*	21.67 (0.257)	1.305 (3.85)	21.49 ± 0.145(0.673)	1.004 ± 0.102 (10.1)
lin*CSNK1G3*	21.73 (0.275)	1.052 (4.13)	22.23 ± 0.152 (0.683)	1.003 ± 0.091 (9.08)
lin*GUCY1A2*	23.55 (0.480)	1.458 (8.22)	22.51 ± 0.134 (0.596)	1.004 ± 0.096 (9.57)
lin*LPP*	19.27 (0.472)	1.193 (6.64)	19.06 ± 0.121 (0.633)	1.003 ± 0.085 (8.46)
lin*NEAT1*	18.79 (0.231)	1.641 (2.96)	19.80 ± 0.079 (0.401)	1.001 ± 0.054 (5.38)
lin*RHOBTB3*	21.23 (0.259)	1.147 (3.73)	21.34 ± 0.170 (0.796)	1.006 ± 0.120 (11.9)
lin*STIL*	25.88 (0.411)	1.381 (5.22)	26.22 ± 0.131 (0.500)	1.003 ± 0.089 (8.94)
ALAS1	23.04 (0.305)	1.113 (4.86)	23.32 ± 0.064 (0.275)	1.001 ± 0.043 (4.33)
HPRT1	25.32 (0.411)	1.192 (7.09)	25.97 ± 0.112 (0.432)	1.002 ± 0.077 (7.75)

Abbreviations: Cq, quantification cycle; %RSD, percent relative standard deviation; SD, standard deviation; *ALAS1*, 5′-aminolevulinate synthase 1; *HPRT1*, hypoxanthine phosphoribosyltransferase 1. *ALAS1* and *HPRT1* were used as reference genes [81]. [a] $n = 20$; %RSD was calculated from duplicate measurements using the root mean square method based on Cq values and relative quantities, respectively. [b] $n = 5$ inter-assay measurements; %RSD (Cq) corresponds to the percent relative standard deviation using the Cq values. %RSD (Relative quantities) corresponds to the percent relative standard deviation using the relative quantities within the inter-assay measurements of the respective RNA variable.

Table 4. Comparison of the circRNA expression data of the six paired tumor and adjacent normal tissue samples used in the microarray and RT-qPCR analyses.

circRNA	Microarray Expression Data [a]	RT-qPCR Expression Data [b]
	Ratio of Tumor to Normal Tissue (p-Value)	Ratio of Tumor to Normal Tissue (p-Value)
circ*ATXN10*	−2.48 (0.001)	−2.09 (0.020)
circ*CRIM1*	−2.17 (0.006)	−2.45 (0.027)
circ*CSNK1G3*	−1.31 (0.003)	−1.84 (0.027)
circ*GUCY1A2*	−1.02 (0.305)	−1.07 (0.781)
circ*LPP*	**+1.94 (0.025)**	**−2.01 (0.004)**
circ*NEAT1*	+2.73 (0.024)	+4.33 (0.061)
circ*RHOBTB3*	−2.14 (0.0003)	−2.05 (0.041)
circ*STIL*	**+1.75 (0.007)**	**−1.35 (0.086)**

[a] Expression data correspond to the data shown in Table 2 (t-test of the six paired tissue samples used in microarray analyses). [b] Expression data of the paired samples used in the microarray analyses measured by the established circRNA assays in this study and normalized to the reference genes *ALAS1* and *HPRT1* (t-test of paired data).

The expression levels of the circRNAs and their linear transcripts were measured and evaluated in all samples of the studied cohort (n = 194). To examine the differential expression between adjacent normal and malignant tissue samples, only the expression results of the paired samples of adjacent normal and malignant tissue samples were compared, in order to avoid bias due to biological variations between patients (Figure 4). Significant differential expression was observed between tumor and normal tissue samples, as indicated by T/N indices (Figure 4), for both circRNAs and their corresponding linear transcripts (Figure 4 and detailed in Table S8). The expression levels of all circRNAs except circ*NEAT1* and circ*GUCY1A2* were downregulated in tumor samples; circ*NEAT1* was upregulated and the expression level of circ*GUCY1A2* did not differ between the two tissue samples. In contrast, only the linear transcripts lin*CRIM1* and lin*LPP* were downregulated in the tumor samples, while lin*STIL* and lin*NEAT1* were upregulated, and lin*ATXN10*, lin*CSNK1G3*, lin*GUCY1A2*, and lin*RHOBTB3* showed no significant differences in expression between the normal and tumor tissue samples.

Moreover, the following characteristics of the expression data were striking: (i) the upregulation of circLPP and circ*STIL* found in the microarray analysis could not be confirmed, as both circRNAs were shown to be downregulated in the RT-qPCR measurements, similarly to what was shown by the comparison of the paired samples used in the microarray analysis; (ii) all linear transcripts except circ*CSNK1G3* had significantly higher expression than their circRNAs. This can be seen on the x-axes of the corresponding panels and by the different ratios between the two tissue samples and the RNA types, as summarized in Tables S9 and S10. This was particularly remarkable for circ*NEAT1*, which showed a low expression rate, with only 45 of the 79 examined pairs having detectable expression. Although the high number of biological replicates confirmed the increased expression of this circRNA in tumor tissue, circ*NEAT1* was not included in the further multivariable prognostic BCR analysis. This was also compatible with the less reliable analytical performance data of circ*NEAT1* measurements in its low expression range, as mentioned above (Table 3), and the number of samples above the upper limit of the standard curve of this circRNA (Table S7).

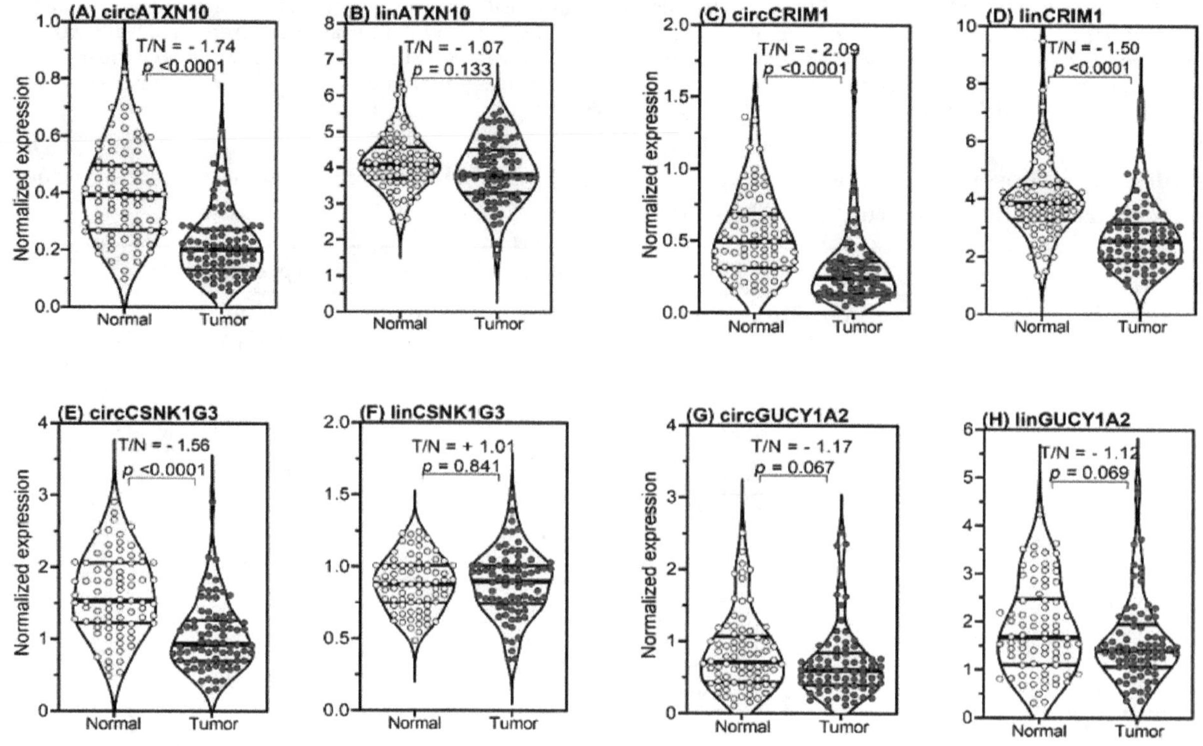

Figure 4. *Cont.*

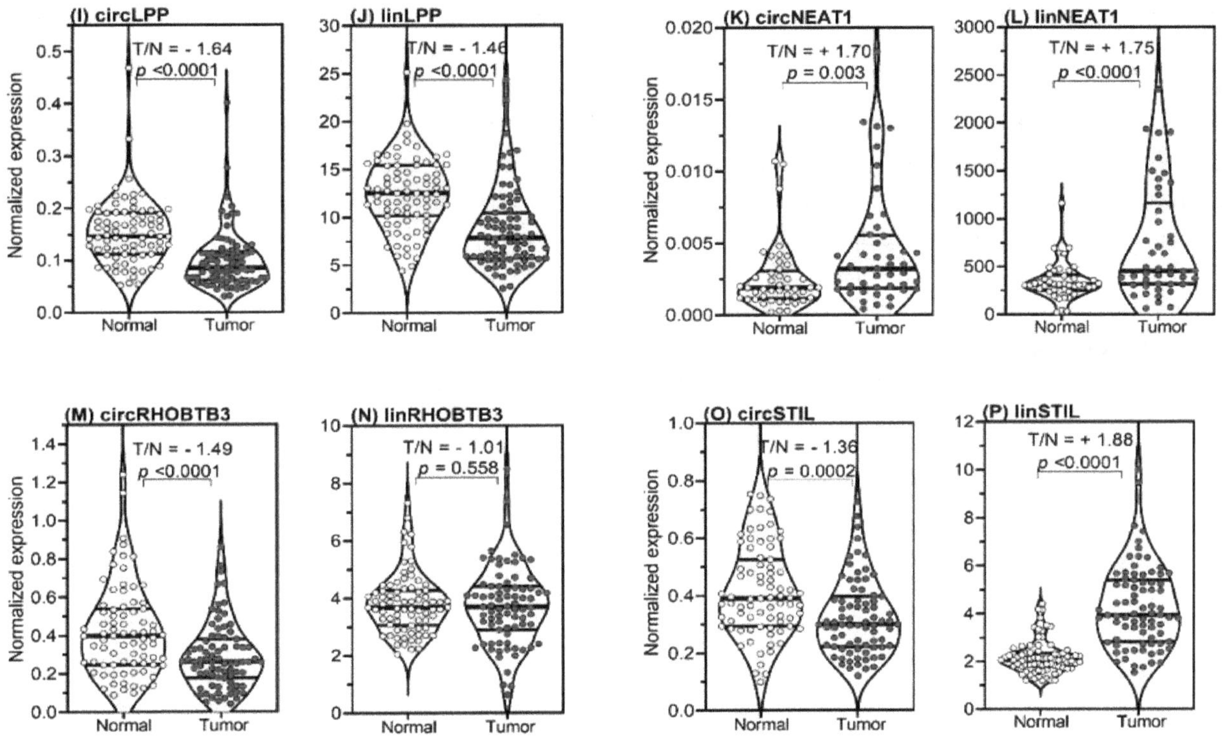

Figure 4. Expression levels of circular RNAs (circRNAs) and the linear transcripts of their host genes in tissue samples from prostate cancer (PCa) patients. The expression data of all eight circRNAs (**A**,**C**,**E**,**G**,**I**,**K**,**M**,**O**) and their corresponding linear transcripts (**B**,**D**,**F**,**H**,**J**,**L**,**N**,**P**) are shown in the matched pairs of adjacent normal tissue samples and malignant samples from PCa specimens collected by radical prostatectomy ($n = 79$, only 45 for circ*NEAT1* and lin*NEAT1*). *ALAS1* (5′-aminolevulinate synthase 1) and *HPRT1* (hypoxanthine phosphoribosyltransferase 1) mRNAs were used as stable expression normalizers of prostatic cancer [81]. Complete violin plots with the entire expression ranges, the lower and upper quartiles (dashed lines), and the medians (bold lines) are presented. Statistically significant expression differences of the malignant tissue samples compared with the adjacent normal tissue samples are given as the T/N (tumor/normal) index. To facilitate a direct comparison of the expression results of each circRNA and its corresponding linear transcript in the tumor to normal tissue, we used the term T/N index. A positive number indicates a higher expression in tumor tissue (numerator in the index) in relation to normal tissue (denominator in the index) and a negative number shows a higher expression in the normal tissue (denominator in the index) in relation to tumor tissue (numerator in the index).

The expression data of all examined circRNAs and their linear transcripts in the tumor samples were not associated with age, preoperative PSA, prostate volume, digital rectal examination, tumor stage, and surgical margin status (Table S11). However, significant associations between the ISUP grade and all circRNAs except circ*NEAT1* and circ*RHOBTB3* were found, while only lin*GUCY1A2* and lin*LPP* showed such associations for the linRNAs.

Close correlations between the expression levels of all circRNAs in both the adjacent normal and malignant tissue samples were observed, except for circ*NEAT1* and partly for circ*RHOBTB3* (Tables S12 and S13). However, these close correlations were mainly lost if data in matched normal tissue and malignant tissue samples were correlated (Table S14). Furthermore, there were several different correlation coefficients between circRNAs and the linear transcripts in malignant tissue samples in comparison to the matched adjacent normal tissue samples (Table S15).

2.4.2. CircRNAs and linRNAs as Biomarkers for Discrimination between Normal and Cancerous Tissue

The differences between the circRNAs and their linear transcripts described here support the idea, postulated in the introduction, that it makes sense to investigate circRNAs as cancer biomarkers in an integrative approach together with their linear transcripts, due to their potential differential influences in normal and cancerous tissue. From this point of view, the expression data of the circRNAs and linear transcripts were used to differentiate between adjacent normal and malignant tissue (Table 5). Data from the performed receiver operating characteristic (ROC) curve analysis revealed that circ*ATXN10* and lin*STIL* were found to be the best individual markers for this purpose, with areas under the curves (AUCs) of 0.801 and 0.841, respectively. Using a backward elimination approach of binary logistic regression with all RNAs, a combined tool using these two markers resulted (Table 5). It is of particular interest that both RNAs were differentially expressed. Circ*ATXN10* was downregulated in tumor samples, whereas lin*STIL* was upregulated. When applying the markers combined, the AUC value increased to 0.892. Both the ROC curve and the decision curve of this combination were found to run above the curves of the two individual markers (Figure 5). Thus, at least a "stabilizing" discriminative ability was achieved with the marker combination of circ*ATXN10* + lin*STIL*.

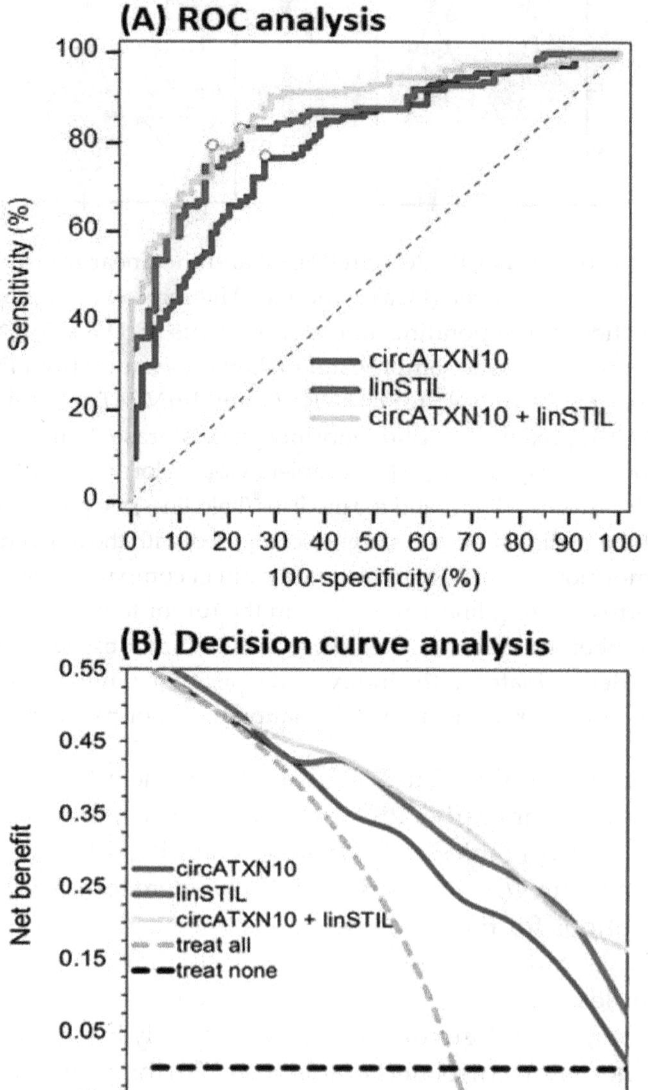

Figure 5. Receiver operating characteristic (ROC) curve and decision curve analyses of circ*ATXN10* and lin*STIL* as individual markers and in combination for discrimination between adjacent normal and malignant tissue samples. The data reflect the results shown in Table 5 for circ*ATXN10*, lin*STIL*, and their combination.

Table 5. Receiver operating characteristic (ROC) curve analyses of circRNAs and their linear transcripts for discrimination between adjacent normal ($n = 79$) and malignant ($n = 115$) tissue samples from prostate cancer specimens. For circ*NEAT1*, only 118 samples could be analyzed.

RNAs	AUC (95% CI)	*p*-Value Different to AUC = 0.5	Differentiating Ability at the Youden Index [a]		Overall Correct Classification (%)
			Sensitivity (95% CI)	Specificity (95% CI)	
Single variable					
circ*ATXN10*	0.801 (0.719–0.851)	<0.0001	77 (68–84)	72 (61–82)	74.2
lin*ATXN10* ($p < 0.0001$) [b]	0.525 (0.442–0.606)	0.534	45 (36–55)	65 (53–75)	59.3
circ*CRIM1*	0.743 (0.660–0.808)	<0.0001	74 (66–82)	66 (54–76)	67.0
lin*CRIM1* ($p = 0.143$) [b]	0.778 (0.697–0.836)	<0.0001	76 (67–83)	76 (65–85)	71.7
circ*CSNK1G3*	0.780 (0.715–0.836)	<0.0001	69 (59–77)	77 (66–86)	72.7
lin*CSNK1G3* ($p < 0.0001$) [b]	0.518 (0.436–0.602)	0.661	49 (40–59)	59 (48–70)	59.3
circ*GUCY1A2*	0.545 (0.459–0.624)	0.285	65 (56–74)	48 (37–60)	58.8
lin*GUCY1A2* ($p = 0.208$) [b]	0.583 (0.493–0.665)	0.051	70 (60–78)	49 (40–61)	58.3
circ*LPP*	0.773 (0.708–0.830)	<0.0001	71 (62–79)	75 (64–84)	72.2
lin*LPP* ($p = 0.321$) [b]	0.762 (0.696–0.820)	<0.0001	70 (61–79)	76 (65–85)	71.6
circ*NEAT1*	0.634 (0.552–0.733)	<0.013	72 (60–82)	51 (36–67)	62.5
lin*NEAT1* ($p = 0.371$) [b]	0.690 (0.608–0.760)	<0.0001	63 (53–72)	72 (61–82)	63.4
circ*RHOBTB3*	0.684 (0.613–0.749)	<0.0001	73 (64–81)	61 (49–72)	66.0
lin*RHOBTB3* ($p = 0.013$) [b]	0.520 (0.438–0.605)	0.629	45 (36–55)	67 (56–77)	59.3
circ*STIL*	0.645 (0.556–0.719)	<0.003	53 (44–62)	72 (61–82)	62.9
lin*STIL* ($p < 0.0001$) [b]	0.841 (0.804–0.912)	<0.0001	78 (70–85)	86 (77–93)	80.4
Optimized combination					
circ*ATXN10* + lin*STIL* [c]	0.892 (0.834–0.925)	<0.0001	79 (71–86)	87 (78–94)	81.4

Abbreviations: AUC, area under the receiver operating characteristic curve; CI, confidence interval. [a] The Youden index as a measure of overall diagnostic effectiveness is calculated by (sensitivity + specificity) − 1. [b] Significances between the AUC values of individual circRNAs and their linear counterparts. [c] Calculated by binary logistic regression using all RNAs in a backward elimination approach. Results are based on bias-corrected and accelerated bootstrap calculation with 2000 iterations.

2.4.3. CircRNAs and Linear Transcripts as Potential Markers for Predicting BCR

BCR, as the selected clinical outcome endpoint, was defined as the time from the radical prostatectomy until the time of the corresponding event or the last follow-up. Detailed data for the patients with and without BCR at the time of follow-up after surgery are shown in Table 1.

According to the Reporting Recommendations for Tumor Marker Prognostic Studies (REMARK) [82], we used continuous data of the normalized relative expression quantities of the RNAs in the subsequently described Cox regression analyses. This procedure of using continuous data, if possible, is strongly recommended to avoid loss of information in detecting associations between cancer markers and time-dependent events [82]. The results of the univariable Cox regression analyses in this first step, which was done to evaluate the potential predictive validity of the total RNA panel, are shown in Table 6. Those five circRNAs and three linear transcripts with p-values < 0.25 were selected for subsequent multivariable Cox regression analyses to avoid type II errors. So-called "full models", including the respective circular and linear RNAs, and "reduced models" after a backward elimination (entry: $p < 0.05$, removal: $p > 0.100$) were separately constructed for the circRNAs and linRNAs (Table 6).

Table 6. Construction of separate tools for prediction of biochemical recurrence using circRNAs and their linear counterparts.

RNA	Univariable Cox Regression [a]		Multivariable Cox Regression			
			Full Model [b]		Reduced Model after Backward Elimination [c]	
	HR (95% CI)	*p*-Value	HR (95% CI)	*p*-Value	HR (95% CI)	*p*-Value
			Circular RNAs			
circ*ATXN10*	0.39 (0.10–1.88)	0.239	0.27 (0.08–0.89)	0.032	0.31 (0.13–0.76)	0.011
circ*CRIM1*	0.69 (0.22–2.16)	0.521	-	-	-	-
circ*CSNK1G3*	2.32 (0.51–10.6)	0.240	1.96 (0.50–7.68)	0.336	-	-
circ*GUCY1A2*	1.31 (0.98–1.75)	0.065	1.32 (0.99–1.75)	0.051	1.33 (1.02–1.74)	0.037
circ*LPP*	1.86 (0.84–4.12)	0.125	1.76 (0.78–3.96)	0.169	1.89 (0.91–3.95)	0.092
circ*RHOBTB3*	0.86 (0.38–1.93)	0.705	-	-	-	-
circ*STIL*	0.53 (0.18–1.53)	0.238	0.57 (0.21–1.62)	0.293	-	-
			Linear mRNAs			
lin*ATXN10*	1.23 (0.15–10.2)	0.846	-	-	–	-
lin*CRIM1*	0.90 (0.22–3.76)	0.887	-	-	-	-
lin*CSNK1G3*	0.47 (0.09–2.60)	0.399	-	-	-	-
lin*GUCY1A2*	1.52 (0.99–2.32)	0.050	1.47 (1.09–2.00)	0.012	1.47 (1.09–2.00)	0.012
lin*LPP*	1.06 (0.23–4.76)	0.941				
lin*NEAT1*	1.41 (1.15–1.72)	0.001	1.39 (1.16–1.66)	0.0003	1.39 (1.16–1.66)	0.0003
lin*RHOBTB3*	0.78 (0.20–3.11)	0.727				
lin*STIL*	0.59 (0.32–1.08)	0.086	0.54 (0.30–0.96)	0.037	0.54 (0.30–0.96)	0.037

Abbreviations: HR, hazard ratio; CI, confidence interval. [a] As explained in chapter 2.4.1, circ*NEAT1* was excluded from Cox regression analyses. [b] The full model included all variables of the univariable Cox regression with hazard ratios of p-values < 0.250. [c] Reduced model after backward elimination with entry $p < 0.05$ and removal $p > 0.100$. All data of the univariable and final multivariable Cox regression models are calculated by the bias-corrected and accelerated bootstrap method with 2000 resamples.

For the circRNAs, only circ*ATXN10*, circ*GUCY1A2*, and circ*LPP* remained in the reduced model, while for the linRNA-based model (lin*GUCY1A2*, lin*NEAT1*, and lin*STIL*), no further variables were eliminated by the backward approach. To estimate the capacity of these models to predict BCR, the C-statistic values were compared. The C-statistic results, given as the AUC ± SE of the prognostic indices calculated in the Cox regression analyses, did not differ between the full and reduced models for the circRNA-based BCR prediction (0.676 ± 0.055 vs. 0.649 ± 0.056, $p = 0.219$; details given in Table S16). The linRNA-based C-statistic value was found to be 0.722 ± 0.053, but it was also not statistically significant compared with the circRNA-based model ($p = 0.141$; details given in Table S16). However, a Cox regression analysis with eight RNA variables from the circRNA-based and linRNA-based "full models" or the six RNAs of the "reduced models" (Table 6) and a subsequent backward elimination showed that all circRNAs were excluded from the model (Table 7). Only three linRNAs—lin*GUCY1A2*, lin*NEAT1*, and lin*STIL*—remained as independent variables in the model. This clearly shows that, compared to these linear RNAs, the circRNAs did not contribute to the BCR prediction. Thus, the model with lin*GUCY1A2*, lin*NEAT1*, and lin*STIL*, termed the "RNA signature" in the following text, was used as an additional tool for BCR prediction, together with clinicopathological factors.

Table 7. Construction of a predictive RNA signature for biochemical recurrence based on Cox regression analysis, using a combination of the separate prediction tools for circRNAs and their linear counterparts.

	Multivariable Cox Regression of the Combined Separate RNA Classifiers			
RNA Prediction Tool	**Full Model with all Separate Classifiers** [a]		**Reduced Model after Backward Elimination** [b]	
	HR (95% CI)	***p*-Value**	**HR (95% CI)**	***p*-Value**
	circRNA prediction tool			
circ*ATXN10*	0.45 (0.18–1.12)	0.086	not included	-
circ*GUCY1A2*	0.95 (0.55–1.64)	0.850	not included	-
circ*LPP*	1.37 (0.66–2.82)	0.399	not included	-
	linear RNA prediction tool			
lin*GUCY1A2*	1.77 (0.80–3.89)	0.153	1.47 (1.09–2.00)	0.012
lin*NEAT1*	1.33 (1.11–1.60)	0.002	1.39 (1.16–1.66)	0.0003
lin*STIL*	0.52 (0.29–0.94)	0.030	0.54 (0.30–0.96)	0.037

Abbreviations: HR, hazard ratio; CI, confidence interval. [a] This model included all six RNA variables indicated in Table 6 as the "Reduced model after backward elimination" of the separate circRNA and linear RNA based prediction tools. [b] Reduced model after backward elimination with entry $p < 0.05$ and removal $p > 0.100$. All data of the univariable and final multivariable Cox regression models are calculated by the bias-corrected and accelerated bootstrap method with 2000 resamples.

To assess the validity of our linear transcript data regarding the BCR prediction, we used The Cancer Genome Atlas Prostate Cancer (TCGA-PRAD) dataset, a publicly available dataset (Table S17). This dataset contains information from 427 patients and includes 89 cases of BCR, defined as a re-increase of PSA > 0.2 μg/L after prostatectomy, as in our study cohort. Univariable Cox regression analyses of the linear transcripts showed that increased expression of lin*STIL* was closely associated with BCR, as in our study, whereas statistically significant relationships of the other transcripts with BCR were not observed (Table S17).

2.4.4. BCR Prediction Models Based on Clinicopathological Variables in Combination with the RNA Signature

As briefly outlined in the introduction, different tools for predicting BCR based on the clinicopathological variables have been introduced in clinical practice. It was therefore of interest to (i) compare the predictive potential of the RNA signature elaborated above with the results of such clinical models and (ii) evaluate whether a combination of both approaches could improve the prognostic accuracy of single tools.

For this purpose, based on univariable and multivariable Cox regression analyses of the clinicopathological variables in our study cohort, we constructed full and reduced models to predict the occurrence of BCR (Table 8).

In addition, the established predictive BCR reference models CAPRAS [9] and NCCN [11] as well as those according to D'Amico et al. [10] and Stephenson et al. [7] were used. In all cases, the C-statistic values of the obtained prognostic indices were calculated using purely clinicopathological-based tools combined with the RNA signature (Table 9). As mentioned above, the C-statistic value of the RNA signature with lin*GUCY1A2*, lin*NEAT1*, and lin*STIL* was 0.722 ± 0.053 (95% CI: 0.631–0.801), which was only significantly higher than D'Amico et al.'s reference model value of 0.513 (95% CI: 0.418–0.607; $p = 0.003$). There were no statistical differences compared with the other clinicopathological tools listed in Table 9 (p-values between 0.128 and 0.640). However, the combination of the RNA signature with individual clinicopathological-based prediction tools increased the C-statistics values of all clinicopathological-based tools (Table 9). This was especially statistically significant for the tools presented by D'Amico et al. [10], CAPRAS [9], and NCCN [11]. In addition, decision curve analyses of our elaborated full model and the other four clinicopathological-based reference models were performed in combination with the RNA signature (Figure S4). The improved prediction of BCR by this inclusion of the RNA signature was confirmed, as the corresponding curves generally ran above the individual curves of the clinicopathological-based tools (Figure S4).

Table 8. Construction of a predictive classifier for biochemical recurrence using Cox regression analyses with clinicopathological variables in 115 patients.

Variable [a]	Univariable Cox Regression		Multivariable Cox Regression			
			Full Model [b]		Reduced Model after Backward Elimination [c]	
	HR (95% CI)	*p*-Value	HR (95% CI)	*p*-Value	HR (95% CI)	*p*-Value
Age	0.97 (0.93–1.02)	0.280				
PSA (> 10 <)	2.24 (1.18–4.18)	0.0130	1.59 (0.83–3.07)	0.162		
DRE	1.24 (0.83–1.95)	0.286				
Margin	2.37(1.24–4.52)	0.009	1.91 (0.98–3.72)	0.056	1.99 (1.03–3.84)	0.041
pN status	2.60 (0.92–7.35)	0.071	0.58 (0.19–1.81)	0.352		
pT stage	2.16 (1.51–3.09)	<0.0001	1.55 (1.03–2.33)	0.037	1.58 (1.05–2.40)	0.030
ISUP Group	1.66 (1.31–2.11	<0.0001	1.55 (1.14–2.10)	0.005	1.43 (1.07–1.91)	0.016

[a] Abbreviations and stratifications of the variables as indicated in Table 1; CI, confidence interval; HR, hazard ratio. [b] The full model included all variables of the univariable Cox regression with hazard ratios of $p < 0.250$. [c] Reduced model after backward elimination with entry $p < 0.05$ and removal $p > 0.100$. All data of the univariable and final multivariable Cox regression models are calculated by the bias-corrected and accelerated bootstrap method with 2000 resamples.

Table 9. Improved prediction of biochemical recurrence after radical prostatectomy using clinicopathological-based tools in combination with the RNA signature.

Prediction Tool	Clinicopathological-Based Tool	Clinicopathological-Based Tool Combined with RNA Signature	*p*-Value
	AUC (95% CI)	AUC (95% CI)	
	Present study		
Full model	0.810 (0.726–0.877)	0.841 (0.761–0.902)	0.073
Reduced model	0.804 (0.720–0.872)	0.827 (0.746–0.891)	0.104
	Reference models		
D'Amico et al. [10]	0.513 (0.418–0.607)	0.718 (0.627–0.798)	0.004
CAPRAS [9]	0.750 (0.660–0.826)	0.799 (0.714–0.868)	0.034
NCCN [11]	0.733 (0.643–0.811)	0.800 (0.715–0.869)	0.035
Stephenson et al. [7]	0.785 (0.699–0.856)	0.821 (0.738–0.886)	0.107

Abbreviations: AUC, area under the receiver operating characteristic curve as C-statistics calculated from the prognostic indices of the Cox regression analyses; CI, confidence interval; CAPRAS, Cancer of the Prostate Risk Assessment Postsurgical Score; NCCN, National Comprehensive Cancer Network; Full model, according to the Cox regression model described in Table 8 with all clinicopathological factors except of age and digital rectal examination; Reduced model, according to the Cox regression model described in Table 8 after backward elimination and finally including only the variables of pT stage, ISUP Group grade, and surgical margin status. Results are based on bias-corrected and accelerated bootstrap calculation with 2000 iterations.

3. Discussion

In this retrospective study with three working phases (Figure 1), we identified differentially expressed circRNAs in PCa tissue samples using microarray analysis, performed an analytical validation of eight selected circRNAs and their linear counterparts via RT-qPCR measurements, and successfully elaborated RNA-signatures as discriminative biomarkers to differentiate between normal and cancerous

PCa tissue and as predictive BCR biomarkers. This information was combined with clinicopathological variables to improve the prediction of BCR.

For the genome-wide identification of circRNAs in PCa tissue, we used six paired PCa tissue samples in the discovery phase in a microarray approach. Generally, microarray analysis is considered a strong and reliable tool for predicting circRNA profiles in clinically relevant tissue samples [83]. However, compared with high-throughput circRNA sequencing analysis with its discovery potential for new cirRNAs, microarray platforms have the drawback of only including a limited number of already validated circRNAs [84]. The microarray analysis identified 43 upregulated and 134 downregulated circRNAs with a higher than absolute 1.5-fold change in malignant tissue samples (Figure 2C). For further evaluation, we chose three upregulated (circ*LPP*, circ*STIL*, and circ*NEAT1*) and three downregulated (circ*ATXN10*, circ*CRIM1*, and circ*RHOBTB3*) circRNAs based on their differential expression levels identified in the microarray analysis and in an in silico circRNA-miRNA-gene interaction analysis (Supplementary Information S2 (Supplementary Materials) with Figure S1). In addition, circ*CSNK1G3* and circ*GUCY1A2* were included in this panel for control purposes, since they had already been investigated by other working groups at the start of our study [44,45]. Furthermore, in order to correlate our results with the linear products of the circRNA host genes in an integrative approach, we included the linRNA counterparts of the circRNAs in this study.

After successful experimental validation of the circular feature of the selected circRNAs and the establishment of their fit-for-purpose RT-qPCR assays (Section 2.3), a comparison of the microarray and RT-qPCR data of the eight circRNAs showed discrepant results for circ*STIL* and circ*LPP* (Table 4). For the other examined circRNAs, the results of the RT-qPCR and microarray analyses were found to be congruent. The downregulation of circ*STIL* and circ*LPP* in the malignant vs. adjacent normal PCa tissue samples was confirmed via RT-qPCR measurements of the 79 paired samples (Figure 4). Inconsistent differential expression of circRNAs in microarray or sequencing vs. in the RT-qPCR analyses has also been observed in previous studies of PCa and other cancers. Shan et al. [85] identified consistent expression between microarray and RT-qPCR analyses in four of five selected circRNAs using 90 PCa and paired non-cancerous tissue samples. Yan et al. [86] reported that three of four selected circRNAs in PCa cells analyzed by RT-qPCR showed consistent high-throughput sequencing results. Qui et al. [87] found an upregulation of circ*CASP8AP2* in hepatocellular carcinoma compared to adjacent normal tissue by sequencing, but in RT-qPCR analyses, this circRNA was downregulated. The reason for these discrepancies between microarray/sequencing data and RT-qPCR results is not clear. Since the same samples were used for the different analytical techniques, it can be assumed that there can only be analytical or post-analytical reasons for these results [31]. The use of different normalization approaches, dependence on the digestion effect of RNase R on circRNAs and linear mRNAs, and method-dependent effect of RNA integrity on the measurement results might be the reasons for these discrepancies [88–91]. Considering these aspects, the expression evaluation of circRNAs in isolated total RNA samples using RT-qPCR measurements combined with validated cancer-specific reference genes, as done in the present study, might be a practical way to minimize such discrepancies [88]. Further research is needed in this respect, but this was beyond the scope of this study. Furthermore, regarding these discrepancies, the inconsistent results reported for the same circRNAs when examined in different studies should be mentioned. For example, Kong et al. [92] found that *hsa*_circ_0006404 was upregulated in 53 paired PCa samples. In contrast, Shen et al. [48] showed that the same circRNA was downregulated in 22 low-grade and 22 high-grade PCa tissue samples in comparison with 18 normal prostate tissue samples. In addition to the above-mentioned possible analytical and post-analytical reasons, different clinicopathological characteristics of the investigated study cohorts, but also pre-analytical interferences due to the different "quality" of the tissue samples used in different studies may be responsible for these differences [88].

The comparison of the expression levels of circRNAs and linRNAs in the 79 paired PCa tissue samples revealed interesting relationships (Figure 4). Here, we found that all linRNAs except for lin*CSNK1G3* had significantly higher expression levels than the circular RNAs. This observation was concordant with results shown in earlier circRNA studies [23,24,93]. Additionally, circ*STIL* showed significantly lower expression in tumor samples than in normal tissue samples, while linSTIL was significantly higher expressed in tumor samples. Moreover, the normalized expression of lin*NEAT1* was nearly 17,000-fold higher than the expression level of circ*NEAT1* (Figure 4 and Table S10), while the ratio between tumor and normal tissue was equal for both RNAs (circ*NEAT1*: +1.70 vs. lin*NEAT1*: +1.75). A possible explanation for the high linRNA expression could be the similarly abundant expression of the lncRNA *NEAT1* (lnc*NEAT1*) in PCa, which may be an indicator of the independent expression of circRNAs and linRNAs/lncRNAs [94,95]. However, because of the limited performance data from the circ*NEAT1* RT-qPCR analyses and the incomplete detection of this analyte in all samples, we did not include this circRNAs in the multivariable analyses. Nevertheless, more analytically sensitive quantification techniques like the droplet digital polymerase chain reaction should be used to allow this circRNA to be included in future studies.

The differential expression of the malignant and adjacent normal tissue samples identified circ*ATXN10* and lin*STIL* as strong biomarkers in terms of differentiating between tumor and normal tissue. The AUC value for these two markers combined was 0.892 (95% CI: 0.834–0.925). The decision curve analysis also showed a higher discriminative ability when combining circ*ATXN10* and lin*STIL*, compared with applying them alone (Figure 5). Xia et al. [47] evaluated the diagnostic potential of the two circRNAs circ_0057558 and circ_0062019 in PCa. When applying these two circRNAs in combination, an AUC value of 0.861 was achieved. Another working group identified *hsa*_circ_0001633, *hsa*_circ_0001206, and *hsa*_circ_0009061 as possible discriminative tissue biomarkers with respective AUCs of 0.809, 0.774, and 0.711 [58]. Although these results are promising, the ability of circRNAs to differentiate between malignant and non-malignant tissue in other cancer types is much higher. In a recent study on circRNAs in clear cell renal cell carcinoma, we identified circ*EGLN3* (*hsa*_circ_0101692) as a strong marker for differentiation between normal and cancerous tissue, with an AUC of 0.98 when used alone and an AUC of 0.99 when combined with its linear counterpart [22]. Nevertheless, in the future, circRNAs might be used as components of a molecular pattern to improve diagnostic accuracy in the pathological evaluation of cancerous tissue and to provide possible helpful information on the development processes of cancer.

The associations of circRNAs and linRNAs with each other and with standard clinicopathological variables is of special interest. The following distinctive features were noteworthy: (i) the expressions of all circRNAs were found to be strongly correlated in both the adjacent normal and malignant tissue samples, except for circ*NEAT1* and partly for circ*RHOBTB3*, while this correlation feature was mainly lost between paired samples (Tables S12–S14); (ii) different correlation coefficients between circRNAs and the linear transcripts were observed in paired malignant and normal tissue samples (Table S15); and (iii) all circRNAs except circ*NEAT1* and circ*RHOBTB3* were significantly correlated with the ISUP grade but not with other relevant clinicopathological variables such as preoperative PSA, the tumor stage, and the surgical margin (Table S11). Thus, in comparison with other studies that examined other circRNAs [44,51,58–62], few associations with generally relevant clinicopathological PCa variables were identified. This is by no means a primary disadvantage with regard to their potential clinical validity as prognostic/predictive markers. In contrast, this expression of RNAs mostly independent from clinicopathological variables and the other mentioned particular correlations is a key characteristic of orthogonal biomarkers [96]. Biomarkers of this kind are a real prerequisite for gaining information additional to that derived from established variables and for improving, for example, the prediction accuracy of a clinical outcome endpoint [97].

In the introduction, we described the aim of this study as being to evaluate the clinical validity of circRNAs and their linear transcripts with regard to BCR after radical prostatectomy. The essential problems in this respect were explained and need not be repeated, but it should be stressed that data on circRNAs and BCR are lacking. It was therefore particularly important to follow the REMARK guidelines, which recommend the use of continuous expression data in Cox regression analyses as predictive variables of an endpoint and the rejection of primary dichotomized data applications [82]. This study investigated the ability of the circRNAs and linear transcripts to predict BCR occurrence alone and in combination with clinicopathological variables in a step-by-step process. Circ*ATXN10*, circ*GUCY1A*, and circ*LPP* remained after a multivariable Cox regression analysis of the examined circRNAs with backward elimination in a model of BCR prediction (Table 6). On the other hand, in combination with the linear RNAs, these circRNAs were eliminated in the multivariable Cox regression analysis and thus were found to have no role in BCR prediction in comparison to the linRNAs. Only lin*GUCY1A2*, lin*NEAT1*, and lin*STIL* were identified as relevant BCR predictor variables, and these were subsequently termed the "RNA signature" (Table 7). This result is by no means surprising. By comparing circRNA expression with the expression of linear counterparts, the independent clinical value of circRNAs and linear transcripts has already been reported in other studies [44,98]. Therefore, it makes sense to take this functional aspect into account in an integrative approach by simultaneously determining circRNAs and their linear transcripts. Loss of information could thus be avoided. However, this requires that RT-qPCR determinations, as in our study, are performed on isolated total RNA without RNase R pretreatment and that validated reference genes are used to normalize relative expression quantities. This problem was also recently highlighted when the database MiOncoCirc was introduced [39]. The authors recommended the use of a special capture exome RNA-sequencing protocol without RNase R pretreatment [99] in order to determine the actual relationship between circRNA and linRNA in the tissue [39].

Furthermore, the linRNAs were evaluated as BCR predictors in a univariable Cox regression analysis with the TCGA dataset (Table S17). Especially noteworthy was lin*STIL*, which was found to be significantly associated with the risk of BCR. In contrast, circ*CSNK1G3*, which was selected by Chen et al. [44] as an example for demonstration of its functional mechanisms, was not found to be a relevant BCR predictor in our study (Table 6) or in the TCGA dataset (Table S17).

To assess the clinical validity of this final RNA signature, we compared the C-statistic data of the prognostic indices of the RNA signature with those of four established models frequently used in clinical practice and our developed model based on using only clinicopathological variables. The C-statistic data of the RNA signature did not differ from those of established clinical models, except for the model developed by D'Amico et al. [10], which showed statistically significantly lower values. However, most importantly, when the clinical models were combined with the RNA signature, statistically significant improvements in the BCR predictive accuracy or at least corresponding tendencies were evident (Table 9). This improved predictive accuracy was confirmed by decision curve analyses (Figure S4). Decision curve analysis has been postulated as the most informative metric for an incremental predictive benefit [100]. These results support the view that there is considerable potential for improvement of the current prognostic models based only on clinicopathological factors by including molecular RNA markers [17–21]. Recently, the NCCN Prostate Cancer Guideline Panel suggested that tissue-based tests like Decipher, OncoType, Dx Prostate, Prolaris, and ProMark could be considered for initial PCa risk assessment [101].

Of the 16 RNAs examined, a total of six RNAs were represented in the combined models after ROC and multivariable Cox regression analyses (Tables 5 and 6). These were circ*ATXN10* and lin*STIL* as tissue differentiation markers and BCR predictors (Tables 5 and 6), and circ*GUCY1A2* and its linear counterpart, circ*LPP*, and lin*NEAT1* for BCR prediction. As explained above, ultimately only lin*GUCY1A2*, lin*NEAT1*, and lin*STIL* remained in the final model as the RNA signature for BCR prediction. So far, there are few data on the listed RNAs in the context of PCa and other cancers. Expression data that could be used for the differentiation of tissue samples as well as BCR markers are missing. Reference to possible biological functions has only been made in few cases, and the validity as a biomarker has only been considered for lin*NEAT1* [95]. Since our intention in this study was primarily to investigate the clinical validity of the selected RNAs as possible biomarkers, we deliberately refrained from undertaking functional investigations. Furthermore, the clinical validity of a marker and thus its applicability in a clinical setting is not primarily linked to its functional significance [102]. The development of an applicable biomarker should focus on demonstrating a benefit in comparison to the methods used to date [79]. To formulate this opinion in exaggerated terms, only proof of the meaningful use of a biomarker for a specific clinical problem should be a justified reason to characterize its possible biological background experimentally. Thus, a brief summary of the current state regarding the biological backgrounds of the relevant RNAs identified herein as potential biomarkers is given to provide directions for future work.

In detail, this is as follows:

Circ*ATXN10* has not yet been discussed in connection with cancer. Our data here represent the first results in this area.

Circ*GUCY1A2* was found to be of particular importance in PCa pathogenesis in an investigation of various PCa cells based on differential expression and bioinformatics information [45]. Experimental findings and data on human PCa tissue samples, as well as on lin*GUCY1A2*, are not yet available. In this respect, our data represent the first information in this area.

For lin*STIL*, Wu et al. [63] found increased expression in PCa tissue, similar to the results of our study. In cell experiments, these lin*STIL* changes were shown to be responsible for stimulating the proliferation of PCa cells and suppressing apoptosis through interactions with various signaling pathways. An investigation on gastric cancer confirmed these effects of upregulated lin*STIL* [103].

Circ*LPP* has not yet been investigated in PCa or other cancers regarding to its biological functions or its potential as a biomarker. Reduced expression of the host gene has been described in lung cancer, similar to the results of the present PCa study [66]. Cell culture experiments on myeloma cells showed that a loss of *LPP* leads to the upregulation of N-cadherin, subsequently promoting tumor cell invasion and metastasis through epithelial-mesenchymal transition.

Lin*NEAT1* has been described in some studies as upregulated mRNA with different oncogenic effects on PCa cells. In PCa, it promotes the expression of the oncogene *HMGA2* through the sponging of miR-98-5p, as well as leading to docetaxel resistance by sponging miR-34a-5p and miR-204-5p [65,104]. Furthermore, *NEAT1* promotes the proliferation of PCa cells in connection with the steroid receptor co-activator (*SCRC3*) through the insulin-like growth factor 1 receptor/AKT serine/threonine kinase 1 (*IGF1R/AKT*) signaling pathway [105]. As shown in the present study using BCR as the clinical endpoint, Bai et al. [95] reported increased expression of *NEAT1* mRNA as being an independent prognostic factor for overall patient survival.

Despite our efforts to make this study as comprehensive and bias-free as possible, particularly taking into account the REMARK, MIQE, and STARD guidelines, it had inherent limitations. These include the retrospective nature of this study, the lack of external validation, and the choice of BCR as an endpoint without consideration of alternative clinical endpoints such as metastasis-free survival or cancer-specific survival. On the other hand it should be emphasized that our data calculated with the bootstrapping method as preferable approach for internal validation [106] confirmed the reliability of results obtained with the constructed models in this study.

4. Materials and Methods

4.1. Patients and Tissue Samples

The Ethics Committee of the Charité-University Medicine Berlin approved the study (EA1/134/12; approval date: 22 June 2012). Informed consent was obtained from all patients. The study was performed in accordance with the Declaration of Helsinki. Corresponding study guidelines (Minimum Information for Publication of Quantitative Real-Time PCR Experiments (MIQE), Updated List of Essential Items for Reporting Diagnostic Accuracy Studies (STARD 2015), and Reporting Recommendations for Tumor Marker Prognostic Studies (REMARK)) were taken into account [76,79,82].

Tissue samples from PCa patients undergoing radical prostatectomy were snap-frozen in liquid nitrogen immediately after surgery and stored at −80 °C or were immediately transferred into RNAlater stabilization reagent (Qiagen, Hilden, Germany) and stored at −20 °C until RNA isolation as described previously [81,107,108]. Tumor staging and grading (Table 1) was reviewed by two experienced uropathologists (E.K., S.E.) according to the criteria of the International Union against Cancer (UICC TNM, 8th edition) and the World Health Organization/International Society of Urological Pathology (WHO/ISUP) [109,110], respectively.

4.2. Analytical Methods

4.2.1. Total RNA Samples and Their Characteristics

Total RNA was isolated from tissue pieces of 31 mg (median value, 95% CI: 30–32) collected from the abovementioned preserved tissue specimens using a special punch-bioptic technique as reported in our previous publications [108,111,112]. This procedure allows to obtain tumor tissue (>90%) and matched normal tissue completely free of tumor filtrates and without inflammation or atrophy. Prominent inflammatory infiltrates, lack of epithelium due to stromal hyperplasia, and prostatic intraepithelial neoplasia were used as exclusion criteria. Taking into account these criteria, a largely bias-free comparison of the expression data between the adjacent normal and malignant tissue samples can be considered. The miRNeasy Mini Kit (Qiagen, Hilden, Germany) with an on-column DNA digestion step, according to the producer's instructions, was used for total RNA isolation [107,108,112]. Spectrophotometric quantification and quality assessment of the total RNA samples were performed using the NanoDrop 1000 Spectrophotometer (NanoDrop Technologies, Wilmington, DE, USA) and the Bioanalyzer 2100 with the Agilent RNA 6000 Nano Chip Kit (Agilent Technologies, Santa Clara, CA, USA), as detailed reported in our previous publications [81,107,108]. The RNA samples, isolated with 30 µL nuclease-free water, showed the following characteristics: a median absorbance ratio at 260 to 280 nm of 2.12 (95% CI: 2.12 to 2.13), a median absorbance ratio at 260 to 230 nm of 1.99 (95% CI: 1.97 to 2.03), a median RNA integrity number (RIN) value of 7.00 (95% CI: 6.90 to 7.20), and a median RNA concentration of 1096 ng/µL (95% CI: 1001 to 1214). RNA samples were stored at −80 °C. Further details are listed in the checklist of the MIQE guidelines (Table S1).

4.2.2. Microarray Detection of circRNAs

Using isolated total RNA samples from six paired adjacent normal and malignant tissue samples of PCa specimens (1× pT3a with ISUP 2, 1× pT3b with ISUP 2, 2× pT3a with ISUP 3, 2× pT3b with ISUP 3), microarray analyses were performed as a custom order by ArrayStar Inc. (Rockville, MD, USA), as previously reported [22]. Briefly, RNA samples were digested with RNase R to destroy linear RNAs and enrich circular RNAs. Afterwards, the circRNAs were amplified, transcribed, fluorescently labeled, and hybridized on the ArrayStar Human Circular RNA Array. This array is designed to detect 13,617 circRNAs. The Agilent scanner (G2505C) and softwares (Agilent Feature Extraction software version 11.0.1.1 and Agilent GeneSpring GX) were used for imaging scanning and analysis. Quantile normalization was used to normalize the obtained probe intensities. The R Bioconductor "limma" package was applied to calculate the differential expression between the matched pairs. All data were compiled in the accompanying separate Excel file with all additional information and annotation details (Supplementary Microarray Data File.xlsx (Supplementary Materials)).

4.2.3. RT-qPCR Methodology and circRNA Validation Methods

RT-qPCR measurements were performed according to the recommendations in the MIQE guidelines [76]. The corresponding comments are listed in the abovementioned checklist of the MIQE guidelines and applied for all assays (Supplementary Information S3 with Table S1 and the additional Tables S2–S7).

Detailed validation procedures based on the general characteristics of circRNAs regarding their resistance to RNase R digestion, their lack of a poly(A) tail using separate reverse transcription with random hexamer and oligo(dT)$_{18}$ primers, and the proof of the backsplice junctions by Sanger sequencing, were described in our previous report on circRNAs in kidney cancer [22] and are briefly summarized in Supplementary Information S4 to explain the data in Figure 3. A melting curve analysis and gel electrophoresis were additionally carried out as confirmatory approaches to verify the analytical specificity of the RT-qPCR products of all circRNAs (Figures S2 and S3).

The Maxima First Strand cDNA Synthesis Kit for RT-qPCR (Thermo Fisher Scientific, Waltham, MA, USA; Cat.No. K1642) was used for cDNA synthesis of circRNAs and their linear counterparts, as this kit contains a ready-to use mixture of random hexamer and oligo(dT)$_{18}$ primers (Table S2A). For the validation of circRNAs, we addressed the issue of reliability of reverse transcription using another cDNA synthesis kit (Transcriptor First Strand cDNA Synthesis Kit, Life Science Roche, Mannheim, Germany; Cat. No. 04379012001) that allows separate priming with either random hexamer or oligo(dT)$_{18}$ primers (Table S2B).

The LightCycler 480 Instrument (Roche Molecular Diagnostics, Mannheim, Germany) with white 96-well plates (Cat.No. 04729692001) and a reaction volume of 10 μL was used for all real-time qPCR runs. The Maxima SYBR Green qPCR Master Mix (Thermo Fisher Scientific; Cat.No. K0252) was used. Primers were designed using the blasting tool provided by Primer3 [113] and synthesized by TIB MOLBIOL GmbH (Berlin, Germany). The reaction conditions with the list of primers, measurement details, setup of the assays, and performance data for all eight circRNAs and their linear counterparts as well as the reference genes *ALAS1* and *HPRT1* as a combined pair for normalizing expression data in PCa samples [81] are compiled in Table S6 with the protocols A–I. No-template controls and no-reverse transcriptase controls were always included and showed negative results. All cDNA samples were measured at least in duplicate and the resulting mean values of the quantification cycles were used for further calculations.

The software qBase+ version 3.2 (Biogazelle, Zwijnaarde, Belgium; www.qbaseplus.com) was used for Cq data evaluation [114,115]. This program is based on a generalized model of the $2^{-\Delta\Delta Cq}$ approach with correction of the amplification efficiency. Cq values were converted into relative quantities (RQs) with respect to equal amounts of total RNA for all samples used for the cDNA synthesis, and they were converted into normalized relative quantities (NRQs) based on the expression of the two cancer-specific reference genes mentioned above, *ALAS1* and *HPRT1*.

4.3. Statistics and Data Analysis

The statistical programs SPSS Version 25 (IBM Corp., Armonk, NY, USA) with the bootstrap module, GraphPad Prism version 8.4.3 (GraphPad Software, La Jolla, CA, USA), and MedCalc version 19.4. (MedCalc Software bvba, 8400 Ostend, Belgium) with bootstrapping C-statistics were used. $p < 0.05$ (two-sided) represented statistical significance. The Mann-Whitney *U*-test, Wilcoxon test, *t*-test, and Spearman rank correlation coefficients were used for continuous data and Chi-squared or Fisher's exact tests were used for categorical data. Univariable and multivariable Cox proportional hazard regression analyses were used for survival analysis of the endpoint BCR. C-statistic values based on ROC analyses with AUC calculation of prognostic indices of Cox regression analyses and corresponding decision curve analyses were determined to characterize the discrimination/prediction capacity of the different variables and models [116–119]. Sample size and power calculations were performed using the programs GPower version 3.1.9.4 [120], GraphPad StatMate version 2.0 (GraphPad Software), and MedCalc version 19.4 (MedCalc Software bvba), and the results were used to design the study. The prediction tool CircInteractome [69] was used for the in silico analysis of circRNAs to identify potential miRNA-gene interactions using the miRDB and TargetScan databases [70,71]. TCGA-PRAD RNAseq data were downloaded and analyzed with R (version 3.6) using the "TCGA2stat" library and the "survival" library for univariable Cox regression analyses of the linear counterparts of the eight circRNAs.

5. Conclusions

This study investigated the value of circRNAs and their linear counterparts as potential diagnostic and prognostic biomarkers in PCa using a genome-wide, integrative, and exploratory approach. We showed that the combination of circ*ATXN10* and lin*STIL* provides a strong marker pair that can be used to discriminate between normal and malignant PCa tissue samples. Furthermore, we identified lin*GUCY1A2*, lin*NEAT1*, and lin*STIL* as potentially useful prognostic biomarkers to increase the accuracy of BCR prediction in PCa patients in combination with standard risk prediction models based only on clinicopathological variables. These results support the thesis that there is considerable potential to improve the current clinical prognostic models by including molecular RNA markers. In future studies, it will be advantageous to include circRNAs into the clinicogenomic models in addition to the established RNA classes such as miRNA, mRNA, piwiRNA or lncRNA.

Supplementary Materials
Supplementary Microarray Data File.xlsx, Supplementary Information S1: Sample size and power calculations, Supplementary Information S2 with Supplementary Figure S1, Supplementary Information S3: RT-qPCR methodology, Supplementary Information S4: CircRNA validation methods, Supplementary Information S5: Associations between circRNAs, linear transcripts and clinicopathological variables, Supplementary Information S6: Cox regressions analyses, C-statistics, and decision curve analyses of BCR prediction tool, Figure S1: Bioinformatic analysis of circRNA–miRNA–gene interaction, Figure S2: Melting curve analysis of circular and linear qPCR products on LightCycler 480, Figure S3: Gel views of analyzed amplicons of (A) cirRNAs and (B) linear RNAs, Figure S4: Decision curve analysis of clinicopathological-based BCR prediction tools, Table S1: MIQE checklist according to Bustin et al., Table S2A: Decision curve analysis of clinicopathological-based BCR prediction tools, Table S2B: cDNA synthesis using Transcriptor First Strand cDNA Synthesis Kit, Table S3: Sequences of amplicons of circRNAs with marked backsplice junctions, primer sequences, and their locations in the host genes, Table S4: QPCR target information of the linear RNAs and the reference genes, Table S5: Primer sequences of circRNAs, linear RNAs, and normalizers, Table S6: Protocols for LightCycler 480 qPCR runs, Table S7: Characteristics of the PCR standard curves, Table S8: Expression ratios of circular and linear RNAs in 79 paired tumor tissue to adjacent normal tissue samples, Table S9: Expression of circRNAs and their linear transcripts in paired adjacent normal tissue samples and malignant tissue samples compared, Table S10: Expression ratios of linear to circular RNAs in paired adjacent normal tissue and prostate carcinoma tissue samples, Table S11: Associations of circRNAs and linear transcripts with clinicopathological variables, Table S12: Spearman rank correlation coefficients between all circRNAs in adjacent normal tissue samples, Table S13: Spearman rank correlation coefficients between all circRNAs in malignant tissue samples, Table S14: Spearman rank correlation coefficients between circRNAs in paired adjacent normal tissue samples and malignant tissue samples, Table S15: Spearman rank correlation coefficients between circRNAs and their linear counterparts in paired adjacent normal tissue and tumor samples, Table S16: C-statistics of prognostic indices of the two RNA-based prediction models, Table S17: Univariate Cox regression data of 8 linear RNAs as BCR predictors of TCGA data, References.

Author Contributions: Conceptualization, H.R., K.J., A.F. (Annika Fendler) and A.F. (Antonia Franz); data curation, H.R., M.J., S.W. and K.J.; formal analysis, H.R., M.J., S.W., C.S., Z.Z., A.F. (Annika Fendler) and A.F. (Antonia Franz); funding acquisition, H.R., C.S., K.J. and A.F. (Annika Fendler); investigation, H.R., M.J., S.W., S.E., E.K., Z.Z. and A.F. (Antonia Franz).; methodology, H.R., M.J., S.W., S.E., E.K., Z.Z. and K.J.; project administration, B.R., M.J., S.W., and K.J.; resources, B.R., C.S. and K.J.; supervision, C.S., K.J., A.F. (Annika Fendler) and A.F. (Antonia Fanz); validation, H.R., M.J. and S.W.; visualization, H.R., M.J., S.W., Z.Z., K.J., A.F. (Annika Fendler) and A.F. (Antonia Franz); writing—original draft, H.R., M.J., K.J., A.F. (Annika Fendler) and A.F. (Antonia Franz); writing—review & editing, H.R., M.J., S.W., B.R., C.S., S.E., E.K., Z.Z., K.J., A.F. (Annika Fendler) and A.F. (Antonia Franz). All authors have read and agreed to the published version of the manuscript.

Acknowledgments: The authors would like to thank Dieter Beule und Andranik Ivanov (Berlin Institute of Health, Bioinformatics Core Unit) for interpretation of the microarray data and for helpful discussions. The support of the study through the Foundation for Urologic Research, Berlin, Germany by a research fellowship to cand. med. Hannah Rochow is greatly acknowledged. The authors thank Siegrun Blauhut for her valuable technical assistance. The German Research Foundation (DFG) and the Open Access Publication Fund of Charité—Universitätsmedizin Berlin supported the Open Access publication of this article. The results here are in part based upon data generated by the TCGA Research Network: https://www.cancer.gov/tcga.

Abbreviations

%RSD	percent relative standard deviation
AKT	AKT serine/threonine kinase 1
ALAS1	5′-aminolevulinate synthase 1

ATXN10	ataxin 10
AUC	area under the ROC curve
BCR	biochemical recurrence
CAPRAS	Cancer of the Prostate Risk Assessment Postsurgical Score
cDNA	complementary DNA
CI	confidence interval
circ	circular (used in composition with gene symbols to define examined circRNAs)
circRNA	circular RNA
Cq	quantification cycle
CRIM1	cysteine rich transmembrane BMP regulator 1
CSNK1G3	casein kinase 1 gamma 3
DRE	digital rectal examination
GUCY1A2	guanylate cyclase 1 soluble subunit alpha 2
HPRT1	hypoxanthine phosphoribosyltransferase 1
HR	hazard ratio
IGF1R	insulin like growth factor 1 receptor
IQR	interquartile range
ISUP	International Society of Urologic Pathology
lin	lin (in composition with gene symbols to define examined linRNAs)
linRNA	linear RNA (mRNA)
lnc	long non-coding (used in composition with gene symbols)
LPP	LIM domain containing preferred translocation partner in lipoma
MIQE	The Minimum Information for Publication of Quantitative Real-Time PCR Experiments
NCCN	National Comprehensive Cancer Network
NEAT1	nuclear paraspeckle assembly transcript 1
NRQ	normalized relative quantity
PCa	prostate cancer
pN	pathological lymph node status
PSA	prostate-specific antigen
pT	pathological tumor classification
REMARK	Reporting Recommendations for Tumor Marker Prognostic Studies
RHOBTB3	rho related BTB domain containing 3
RIN	RNA integrity number
ROC	receiver operating characteristic
RQ	relative quantity
RT-qPCR	reverse-transcription quantitative real-time polymerase chain reaction
SCRC3	steroid receptor co-activator
STARD	Standards for Reporting of Diagnostic Accuracy Studies
STIL	STIL centriolar assembly protein
TCGA (PRAD)	The Cancer Genome Atlas Prostate Cancer
T/N	expression index of circRNA or linRNA in tumor to adjacent normal tissue
TNM	Tumor, Node, Metastases

References

1. Ferlay, J.; Colombet, M.; Soerjomataram, I.; Mathers, C.; Parkin, D.; Piñeros, M.; Znaor, A.; Bray, F. Estimating the global cancer incidence and mortality in 2018: GLOBOCAN sources and methods. *Int. J. Cancer* **2018**, *144*, 1941–1953. [CrossRef] [PubMed]
2. Cookson, M.S.; Aus, G.; Burnett, A.L.; Canby-Hagino, E.D.; D'Amico, A.V.; Dmochowski, R.R.; Eton, D.T.; Forman, J.D.; Goldenberg, S.L.; Hernandez, J.; et al. Variation in the Definition of Biochemical Recurrence in Patients Treated for Localized Prostate Cancer: The American Urological Association Prostate Guidelines for Localized Prostate Cancer Update Panel Report and Recommendations for a Standard in the Reporting of Surgical Outcomes. *J. Urol.* **2007**, *177*, 540–545. [CrossRef] [PubMed]
3. Cornford, P.; Bellmunt, J.; Bolla, M.; Briers, E.; De Santis, M.; Gross, T.; Henry, A.; Joniau, S.; Lam, T.B.; Mason, M.D.; et al. EAU-ESTRO-SIOG Guidelines on Prostate Cancer. Part II: Treatment of Relapsing, Metastatic, and Castration-Resistant Prostate Cancer. *Eur. Urol.* **2017**, *71*, 630–642. [CrossRef] [PubMed]

4. Broeck, T.V.D.; Bergh, R.C.V.D.; Arfi, N.; Gross, T.; Moris, L.; Briers, E.; Cumberbatch, M.; De Santis, M.; Tilki, D.; Fanti, S.; et al. Prognostic Value of Biochemical Recurrence Following Treatment with Curative Intent for Prostate Cancer: A Systematic Review. *Eur. Urol.* **2019**, *75*, 967–987. [CrossRef] [PubMed]
5. Pound, C.R.; Partin, A.W.; Eisenberger, M.A.; Chan, D.W.; Pearson, J.D.; Walsh, P.C. Natural history of progression after PSA elevation following radical prostatectomy. *JAMA* **1999**, *281*, 1591–1597. [CrossRef] [PubMed]
6. Zhao, Z.; Weickmann, S.; Jung, M.; Lein, M.; Kilic, E.; Stephan, C.; Erbersdobler, A.; Fendler, A.; Jung, K. A novel predictor tool of bochemical recurrence after radical prostatectomy based on a five-microRNA tissue signature. *Cancers* **2019**, *11*, 1603. [CrossRef]
7. Stephenson, A.J.; Scardino, P.T.; Eastham, J.A.; Bianco, F.J., Jr.; Dotan, Z.A.; Diblasio, C.J.; Reuther, A.; Klein, E.A.; Kattan, M.W. Postoperative Nomogram Predicting the 10-Year Probability of Prostate Cancer Recurrence After Radical Prostatectomy. *J. Clin. Oncol.* **2005**, *23*, 7005–7012. [CrossRef]
8. Brockman, J.A.; Alanee, S.; Vickers, A.J.; Scardino, P.T.; Wood, D.P.; Kibel, A.S.; Lin, D.W.; Bianco, F.J., Jr.; Rabah, D.M.; Klein, E.A.; et al. Nomogram Predicting Prostate Cancer–specific Mortality for Men with Biochemical Recurrence After Radical Prostatectomy. *Eur. Urol.* **2015**, *67*, 1160–1167. [CrossRef]
9. Cooperberg, M.R.; Pasta, D.J.; Elkin, E.P.; Litwin, M.S.; Latini, D.M.; Du Chane, J.; Carroll, P.R. The University of California, San Francisco Cancer of the Prostate Risk Assessment Score: A Straightforward and Reliable Preoperative Predictor of Disease Recurrence after Radical Prostatectomy. *J. Urol.* **2005**, *173*, 1938–1942. [CrossRef]
10. D'Amico, A.V.; Whittington, R.; Malkowicz, S.B.; Schultz, D.; Blank, K.; Broderick, G.A.; Tomaszewski, J.E.; Renshaw, A.A.; Kaplan, I.; Beard, C.J.; et al. Biochemical outcome after radical prostatectomy, external beam radiation therapy, or interstitial radiation therapy for clinically localized prostate cancer. *JAMA* **1998**, *280*, 969–974. [CrossRef]
11. Mohler, J.L. The 2010 NCCN Clinical Practice Guidelines in Oncology on Prostate Cancer. *J. Natl. Compr. Cancer Netw.* **2010**, *8*, 145. [CrossRef] [PubMed]
12. Kang, M.; Jeong, C.W.; Choi, W.S.; Park, Y.H.; Cho, S.Y.; Lee, S.; Lee, S.B.; Ku, J.H.; Hong, S.K.; Byun, S.-S.; et al. Pre- and Post-Operative Nomograms to Predict Recurrence-Free Probability in Korean Men with Clinically Localized Prostate Cancer. *PLoS ONE* **2014**, *9*, e100053. [CrossRef] [PubMed]
13. Shariat, S.F.; Karakiewicz, P.I.; Suardi, N.; Kattan, M.W. Comparison of Nomograms with Other Methods for Predicting Outcomes in Prostate Cancer: A Critical Analysis of the Literature. *Clin. Cancer Res.* **2008**, *14*, 4400–4407. [CrossRef] [PubMed]
14. Remmers, S.; Verbeek, J.F.M.; Nieboer, D.; Van Der Kwast, T.; Roobol-Bouts, M. Predicting biochemical recurrence and prostate cancer-specific mortality after radical prostatectomy: Comparison of six prediction models in a cohort of patients with screening- and clinically detected prostate cancer. *BJU Int.* **2019**, *124*, 635–642. [CrossRef] [PubMed]
15. Meurs, P.; Galvin, R.; Fanning, D.M.; Fahey, T. Prognostic value of the CAPRA clinical prediction rule: A systematic review and meta-analysis. *BJU Int.* **2012**, *111*, 427–436. [CrossRef] [PubMed]
16. Lorent, M.; Maalmi, H.; Tessier, P.; Supiot, S.; Dantan, E.; Foucher, Y. Meta-analysis of predictive models to assess the clinical validity and utility for patient-centered medical decision making: Application to the CAncer of the Prostate Risk Assessment (CAPRA). *BMC Med. Inform. Decis. Mak.* **2019**, *19*, 1–12. [CrossRef]
17. Spratt, D.E.; Zhang, J.; Santiago-Jiménez, M.; Dess, R.T.; Davis, J.W.; Den, R.B.; Dicker, A.P.; Kane, C.J.; Pollack, A.; Stoyanova, R.; et al. Development and Validation of a Novel Integrated Clinical-Genomic Risk Group Classification for Localized Prostate Cancer. *J. Clin. Oncol.* **2018**, *36*, 581–590. [CrossRef]
18. Ross, A.E.; Johnson, M.H.; Yousefi, K.; Davicioni, E.; Netto, G.J.; Marchionni, L.; Fedor, H.L.; Glavaris, S.; Choeurng, V.; Buerki, C.; et al. Tissue-based Genomics Augments Post-prostatectomy Risk Stratification in a Natural History Cohort of Intermediate- and High-Risk Men. *Eur. Urol.* **2016**, *69*, 157–165. [CrossRef]
19. Hiser, W.M.; Sangiorgio, V.; Bollito, E.; Esnakula, A.; Feely, M.; Falzarano, S.M. Tissue-based multigene expression tests for pretreatment prostate cancer risk assessment: Current status and future perspectives. *Future Oncol.* **2018**, *14*, 3073–3083. [CrossRef]
20. Fine, N.; Lapolla, F.W.Z.; Epstein, M.; Loeb, S.; Dani, H. Genomic classifiers for treatment selection in newly diagnosed prostate cancer. *BJU Int.* **2019**, *124*, 578–586. [CrossRef]
21. Alam, S.; Tortora, J.; Staff, I.; McLaughlin, T.; Wagner, J. Prostate cancer genomics: Comparing results from three molecular assays. *Can. J. Urol.* **2019**, *26*, 9758–9762. [PubMed]

22. Franz, A.; Ralla, B.; Weickmann, S.; Rochow, H.; Stephan, C.; Erbersdobler, A.; Kilic, E.; Fendler, A.; Jung, M.; Jung, K. Circular RNAs in Clear Cell Renal Cell Carcinoma: Their Microarray-Based Identification, Analytical Validation, and Potential Use in a Clinico-Genomic Model to Improve Prognostic Accuracy. *Cancers* **2019**, *11*, 1473. [CrossRef] [PubMed]
23. Jeck, W.R.; Sorrentino, J.A.; Wang, K.; Slevin, M.K.; Burd, C.E.; Liu, J.; Marzluff, W.F.; Sharpless, N.E. Circular RNAs are abundant, conserved, and associated with ALU repeats. *RNA* **2012**, *19*, 141–157. [CrossRef] [PubMed]
24. Memczak, S.; Jens, M.; Elefsinioti, A.; Torti, F.; Krueger, J.; Rybak, A.; Maier, L.; Mackowiak, S.D.; Gregersen, L.H.; Munschauer, M.; et al. Circular RNAs are a large class of animal RNAs with regulatory potency. *Nat. Cell Biol.* **2013**, *495*, 333–338. [CrossRef] [PubMed]
25. Maass, P.G.; Glažar, P.; Memczak, S.; Dittmar, G.; Hollfinger, I.; Schreyer, L.; Sauer, A.V.; Toka, O.; Aiuti, A.; Luft, F.C.; et al. A map of human circular RNAs in clinically relevant tissues. *J. Mol. Med.* **2017**, *95*, 1179–1189. [CrossRef]
26. Salzman, J.; Chen, R.E.; Olsen, M.N.; Wang, P.L.; Brown, P.O. Cell-type specific features of circular RNA expression. *PLoS Genet.* **2013**, *9*, e1003777. [CrossRef]
27. Hansen, T.B.; Jensen, T.I.; Clausen, B.H.; Bramsen, J.B.; Finsen, B.; Damgaard, C.K.; Kjems, J. Natural RNA circles function as efficient microRNA sponges. *Nat. Cell Biol.* **2013**, *495*, 384–388. [CrossRef]
28. Li, Z.; Huang, C.; Bao, C.; Chen, L.; Lin, M.; Wang, X.; Zhong, G.; Yu, B.; Hu, W.; Dai, L.; et al. Exon-intron circular RNAs regulate transcription in the nucleus. *Nat. Struct. Mol. Biol.* **2015**, *22*, 256–264. [CrossRef]
29. Abdelmohsen, K.; Panda, A.C.; Munk, R.; Grammatikakis, I.; Dudekula, D.B.; De, S.; Kim, J.; Noh, J.H.; Kim, K.M.; Martindale, J.L.; et al. Identification of HuR target circular RNAs uncovers suppression of PABPN1 translation by CircPABPN1. *RNA Biol.* **2017**, *14*, 361–369. [CrossRef]
30. Pamudurti, N.R.; Bartok, O.; Jens, M.; Ashwal-Fluss, R.; Stottmeister, C.; Ruhe, L.; Hanan, M.; Wyler, E.; Perez-Hernandez, D.; Ramberger, E.; et al. Translation of CircRNAs. *Mol. Cell* **2017**, *66*, 9–21. [CrossRef]
31. Franz, A.; Rabien, A.; Stephan, C.; Ralla, B.; Fuchs, S.; Jung, K.; Fendler, A. Circular RNAs: A new class of biomarkers as a rising interest in laboratory medicine. *Clin. Chem. Lab. Med.* **2018**, *56*, 1992–2003. [CrossRef] [PubMed]
32. Aufiero, S.; Reckman, Y.J.; Pinto, Y.M.; Creemers, E.E. Circular RNAs open a new chapter in cardiovascular biology. *Nat. Rev. Cardiol.* **2019**, *16*, 503–514. [CrossRef]
33. Guria, A.; Sharma, P.; Natesan, S.; Pandi, G. Circular RNAs—The Road Less Traveled. *Front. Mol. Biosci.* **2020**, *6*, 146. [CrossRef] [PubMed]
34. Ng, W.L.; Mohidin, T.B.M.; Shukla, K. Functional role of circular RNAs in cancer development and progression. *RNA Biol.* **2018**, *15*, 1–11. [CrossRef] [PubMed]
35. Yang, Z.; Xie, L.; Han, L.; Qu, X.; Yang, Y.; Zhang, Y.; He, Z.; Wang, Y.; Li, J. Circular RNAs: Regulators of Cancer-Related Signaling Pathways and Potential Diagnostic Biomarkers for Human Cancers. *Theranostics* **2017**, *7*, 3106–3117. [CrossRef] [PubMed]
36. Bachmayr-Heyda, A.; Reiner, A.T.; Auer, K.; Sukhbaatar, N.; Aust, S.; Bachleitner-Hofmann, T.; Mesteri, I.; Grunt, T.W.; Zeillinger, R.; Pils, D. Correlation of circular RNA abundance with proliferation—Exemplified with colorectal and ovarian cancer, idiopathic lung fibrosis and normal human tissues. *Sci. Rep.* **2015**, *5*, 8057. [CrossRef]
37. Sun, D.; Chen, L.; Lv, H.; Gao, Y.; Liu, X.; Zhang, X. Circ_0058124 Upregulates MAPK1 Expression to Promote Proliferation, Metastasis and Metabolic Abilities in Thyroid Cancer Through Sponging miR-940a. *Onco Targets Ther.* **2020**, *13*, 1569–1581. [CrossRef]
38. Wang, M.; Yu, F.; Li, P. Circular RNAs: Characteristics, Function and Clinical Significance in Hepatocellular Carcinoma. *Cancers* **2018**, *10*, 258. [CrossRef]
39. Vo, J.N.; Cieslik, M.; Zhang, Y.; Shukla, S.; Xiao, L.; Zhang, Y.; Wu, Y.-M.; Dhanasekaran, S.M.; Engelke, C.G.; Cao, X.; et al. The Landscape of Circular RNA in Cancer. *Cell* **2019**, *176*, 869–881.e13. [CrossRef]
40. Li, D.; Li, Z.; Yang, Y.; Zeng, X.; Li, Y.; Du, X.; Zhu, X. Circular RNAs as biomarkers and therapeutic targets in environmental chemical exposure-related diseases. *Environ. Res.* **2020**, *180*, 108825. [CrossRef]
41. Zhang, H.; Shen, Y.; Li, Z.; Ruan, Y.; Li, T.; Xiao, B.; Sun, W. The biogenesis and biological functions of circular RNAs and their molecular diagnostic values in cancers. *J. Clin. Lab. Anal.* **2019**, *34*, e23049. [CrossRef] [PubMed]
42. Chen, X.; Yang, T.; Wang, W.; Xi, W.; Zhang, T.; Li, Q.; Yang, A.; Wang, T. Circular RNAs in immune responses and immune diseases. *Theranostics* **2019**, *9*, 588–607. [CrossRef] [PubMed]
43. Liu, J.; Li, D.; Luo, H.; Zhu, X. Circular RNAs: The star molecules in cancer. *Mol. Asp. Med.* **2019**, *70*, 141–152. [CrossRef]

44. Chen, S.; Huang, V.; Xu, X.; Livingstone, J.; Soares, F.; Jeon, J.; Zeng, Y.; Hua, J.T.; Petricca, J.; Guo, H.; et al. Widespread and Functional RNA Circularization in Localized Prostate Cancer. *Cell* **2019**, *176*, 831–843.e22. [CrossRef] [PubMed]
45. Zhang, C.; Xiong, J.; Yang, Q.; Wang, Y.; Shi, H.; Tian, Q.; Huang, H.; Kong, D.; Lv, J.; Liu, D.; et al. Profiling and bioinformatics analyses of differential circular RNA expression in prostate cancer cells. *Futur. Sci. OA* **2018**, *4*, FSOA340. [CrossRef] [PubMed]
46. Ge, S.; Sun, C.; Hu, Q.; Guo, Y.; Xia, G.; Mi, Y.; Zhu, L. Differential expression profiles of circRNAs in human prostate cancer based on chip and bioinformatic analysis. *Int. J. Clin. Exp. Pathol.* **2020**, *13*, 1045–1052. [PubMed]
47. Xia, Q.; Ding, T.; Zhang, G.; Li, Z.; Zeng, L.; Zhu, Y.; Guo, J.; Hou, J.; Zhu, T.; Zheng, J.; et al. Circular RNA Expression Profiling Identifies Prostate Cancer—Specific circRNAs in Prostate Cancer. *Cell. Physiol. Biochem.* **2018**, *50*, 1903–1915. [CrossRef] [PubMed]
48. Shen, Z.; Zhou, L.; Zhang, C.; Xu, J. Reduction of circular RNA Foxo3 promotes prostate cancer progression and chemoresistance to docetaxel. *Cancer Lett.* **2020**, *468*, 88–101. [CrossRef]
49. Gao, Y.; Liu, J.; Huan, J.; Che, F. Downregulation of circular RNA hsa_circ_0000735 boosts prostate cancer sensitivity to docetaxel via sponging miR-7. *Cancer Cell Int.* **2020**, *20*, 1–13. [CrossRef]
50. Liu, F.; Fan, Y.; Ou, L.; Li, T.; Fan, J.; Duan, L.; Yang, J.; Luo, C.; Wu, X. CircHIPK3 facilitates the G2/M transition in prostate cancer cells by sponging miR-338-3p. *Onco Targets Ther.* **2020**, *13*, 4545–4558. [CrossRef]
51. Weng, X.-D.; Yan, T.; Liu, C.-L. Circular RNA_LARP4 inhibits cell migration and invasion of prostate cancer by targeting FOXO3A. *Eur. Rev. Med. Pharmacol. Sci.* **2020**, *24*, 5303–5309. [PubMed]
52. Dong, C.; Fan, B.; Ren, Z.; Liu, B.; Wang, Y. CircSMARCA5 Facilitates the Progression of Prostate Cancer Through miR-432/PDCD10 Axis. *Cancer Biother. Radiopharm.* **2020**. [CrossRef] [PubMed]
53. Dai, Y.; Li, N.; Chen, X.; Tan, X.; Gu, J.; Chen, M.; Zhang, X. Circular RNA Myosin Light Chain Kinase (MYLK) Promotes Prostate Cancer Progression through Modulating Mir-29a Expression. *Med. Sci. Monit.* **2018**, *24*, 3462–3471. [CrossRef] [PubMed]
54. Kong, Z.; Wan, X.; Zhang, Y.; Zhang, P.; Zhang, Y.; Zhang, X.; Qi, X.; Wu, H.; Huang, J.; Li, Y. Androgen-responsive circular RNA circSMARCA5 is up-regulated and promotes cell proliferation in prostate cancer. *Biochem. Biophys. Res. Commun.* **2017**, *493*, 1217–1223. [CrossRef] [PubMed]
55. Luo, J.; Li, Y.; Zheng, W.; Xie, N.; Shi, Y.; Long, Z.; Xie, L.; Fazli, L.; Zhang, D.; Gleave, M.; et al. Characterization of a Prostate- and Prostate Cancer-Specific Circular RNA Encoded by the Androgen Receptor Gene. *Mol. Ther.- Nucleic Acids* **2019**, *18*, 916–926. [CrossRef]
56. Cao, S.; Ma, T.; Ungerleider, N.; Roberts, C.; Kobelski, M.; Jin, L.; Concha, M.; Wang, X.; Baddoo, M.; Nguyen, H.M.; et al. Circular RNAs add diversity to androgen receptor isoform repertoire in castration-resistant prostate cancer. *Oncogene* **2019**, *38*, 7060–7072. [CrossRef]
57. Greene, J.; Baird, A.-M.; Casey, O.; Brady, L.; Blackshields, G.; Lim, M.; O'Brien, O.; Gray, S.G.; McDermott, R.; Finn, S.P. Circular RNAs are differentially expressed in prostate cancer and are potentially associated with resistance to enzalutamide. *Sci. Rep.* **2019**, *9*, 10739. [CrossRef]
58. Song, Z.; Zhuo, Z.; Ma, Z.; Hou, C.; Chen, G.; Xu, G. Hsa_Circ_0001206 is downregulated and inhibits cell proliferation, migration and invasion in prostate cancer. *Artif. Cells Nanomed. Biotechnol.* **2019**, *47*, 2449–2464. [CrossRef]
59. Umemori, M.; Kurata, M.; Yamamoto, A.; Yamamoto, K.; Ishibashi, S.; Ikeda, M.; Tashiro, K.; Kimura, T.; Sato, S.; Takahashi, H.; et al. The expression of MYC is strongly dependent on the circular PVT1 expression in pure Gleason pattern 4 of prostatic cancer. *Med. Mol. Morphol.* **2020**, *53*, 156–167. [CrossRef]
60. Wang, X.; Wang, R.; Wu, Z.; Bai, P. Circular RNA ITCH suppressed prostate cancer progression by increasing HOXB13 expression via spongy miR-17-5p. *Cancer Cell Int.* **2019**, *19*, 1–11. [CrossRef]
61. Huang, E.; Chen, X.; Yuan, Y. Downregulated circular RNA itchy E3 ubiquitin protein ligase correlates with advanced pathologic T stage, high lymph node metastasis risk and poor survivals in prostate cancer patients. *Cancer Biomark.* **2019**, *26*, 41–50. [CrossRef] [PubMed]
62. Huang, C.; Deng, H.; Wang, Y.; Jiang, H.; Xu, R.; Zhu, X.; Huang, Z.; Zhao, X. Circular RNA circABCC4 as the ceRNA of miR-1182 facilitates prostate cancer progression by promoting FOXP4 expression. *J. Cell. Mol. Med.* **2019**, *23*, 6112–6119. [CrossRef] [PubMed]
63. Wu, X.; Xiao, Y.; Yan, W.; Ji, Z.; Zheng, G. The human oncogene SCL/TAL1 interrupting locus (STIL) promotes tumor growth through MAPK/ERK, PI3K/Akt and AMPK pathways in prostate cancer. *Gene* **2019**, *686*, 220–227. [CrossRef] [PubMed]

64. Hudson, B.D.; Hum, N.R.; Thomas, C.B.; Kohlgruber, A.; Sebastian, A.; Collette, N.M.; Coleman, M.; Christiansen, B.A.; Loots, G.G. SOST Inhibits Prostate Cancer Invasion. *PLoS ONE* **2015**, *10*, e0142058. [CrossRef] [PubMed]
65. Guo, Z.; He, C.; Yang, F.; Qin, L.; Lu, X.; Wu, J. Long non-coding RNA-NEAT1, a sponge for miR-98-5p, promotes expression of oncogene HMGA2 in prostate cancer. *Biosci. Rep.* **2019**, *39*, BSR20190635. [CrossRef] [PubMed]
66. Kuriyama, S.; Yoshida, M.; Yano, S.; Aiba, N.; Kohno, T.; Minamiya, Y.; Goto, A.; Tanaka, M. LPP inhibits collective cell migration during lung cancer dissemination. *Oncogene* **2015**, *35*, 952–964. [CrossRef]
67. Zhang, C.-S.; Liu, Q.; Li, M.; Lin, S.-Y.; Peng, Y.; Wu, D.; Li, T.Y.; Fu, Q.; Jia, W.; Wang, X.; et al. RHOBTB3 promotes proteasomal degradation of HIFα through facilitating hydroxylation and suppresses the Warburg effect. *Cell Res.* **2015**, *25*, 1025–1042. [CrossRef]
68. Wang, L.; Liang, Y.; Mao, Q.; Xia, W.; Chen, B.; Shen, H.; Xu, L.; Jiang, F.; Dong, G. Circular RNA circCRIM1 inhibits invasion and metastasis in lung adenocarcinoma through the microRNA (miR)-182/miR-93-leukemia inhibitory factor receptor pathway. *Cancer Sci.* **2019**, *110*, 2960–2972. [CrossRef]
69. Dudekula, D.B.; Panda, A.C.; Grammatikakis, I.; De, S.; Abdelmohsen, K.; Gorospe, M. CircInteractome: A web tool for exploring circular RNAs and their interacting proteins and microRNAs. *RNA Biol.* **2015**, *13*, 34–42. [CrossRef]
70. Wong, N.; Wang, X. miRDB: An online resource for microRNA target prediction and functional annotations. *Nucleic Acids Res.* **2014**, *43*, D146–D152. [CrossRef]
71. Agarwal, V.; Bell, G.W.; Nam, J.-W.; Bartel, D.P. Predicting effective microRNA target sites in mammalian mRNAs. *eLife* **2015**, *4*, e05005. [CrossRef] [PubMed]
72. Bender, R.; Lange, S. Adjusting for multiple testing—When and how? *J. Clin. Epidemiol.* **2001**, *54*, 343–349. [CrossRef]
73. Goeman, J.J.; Solari, A. Multiple hypothesis testing in genomics. *Stat. Med.* **2014**, *33*, 1946–1978. [CrossRef]
74. Rubin, M. Do p Values Lose Their Meaning in Exploratory Analyses? It Depends How You Define the Familywise Error Rate. *Rev. Gen. Psychol.* **2017**, *21*, 269–275. [CrossRef]
75. Glažar, P.; Papavasileiou, P.; Rajewsky, N. circBase: A database for circular RNAs. *RNA* **2014**, *20*, 1666–1670. [CrossRef] [PubMed]
76. Bustin, S.A.; Benes, V.; Garson, J.; Hellemans, J.; Huggett, J.F.; Kubista, M.; Mueller, R.; Nolan, T.; Pfaffl, M.W.; Shipley, G.L.; et al. The MIQE Guidelines: Minimum Information for Publication of Quantitative Real-Time PCR Experiments. *Clin. Chem.* **2009**, *55*, 611–622. [CrossRef] [PubMed]
77. Jeck, W.R.; Sharpless, N.E. Detecting and characterizing circular RNAs. *Nat. Biotechnol.* **2014**, *32*, 453–461. [CrossRef]
78. Szabo, L.; Salzman, J. Detecting circular RNAs: Bioinformatic and experimental challenges. *Nat. Rev. Genet.* **2016**, *17*, 679–692. [CrossRef]
79. Bossuyt, P.M.; Reitsma, J.B.; Bruns, D.E.; Gatsonis, C.A.; Glasziou, P.P.; Irwig, L.; Lijmer, J.G.; Moher, D.; Rennie, D.; de Vet, H.C.; et al. STARD 2015: An updated list of essential items for reporting diagnostic accuracy studies. *Clin. Chem.* **2015**, *61*, 1446–1452. [CrossRef]
80. Lee, J.W.; Devanarayan, V.; Barrett, Y.C.; Weiner, R.; Allinson, J.; Fountain, S.; Keller, S.; Weinryb, I.; Green, M.; Duan, L.; et al. Fit-for-Purpose Method Development and Validation for Successful Biomarker Measurement. *Pharm. Res.* **2006**, *23*, 312–328. [CrossRef]
81. Ohl, F.; Jung, M.; Xu, C.; Stephan, C.; Rabien, A.; Burkhardt, M.; Nitsche, A.; Kristiansen, G.; Loening, S.A.; Radonic, A.; et al. Gene expression studies in prostate cancer tissue: Which reference gene should be selected for normalization? *J. Mol. Med.* **2005**, *83*, 1014–1024. [CrossRef] [PubMed]
82. Sauerbrei, W.; Taube, S.E.; McShane, L.M.; Cavenagh, M.M.; Altman, D.G. Reporting Recommendations for Tumor Marker Prognostic Studies (REMARK): An Abridged Explanation and Elaboration. *J. Natl. Cancer Inst.* **2018**, *110*, 803–811. [CrossRef]
83. Li, S.; Teng, S.; Xu, J.; Su, G.; Zhang, Y.; Zhao, J.; Zhang, S.; Wang, H.; Qin, W.; Lu, Z.J.; et al. Microarray is an efficient tool for circRNA profiling. *Brief. Bioinform.* **2018**, *20*, 1420–1433. [CrossRef]
84. Pandey, P.R.; Munk, R.; Kundu, G.; De, S.; Abdelmohsen, K.; Gorospe, M. Methods for analysis of circular RNAs. *Wiley Interdiscip. Rev. RNA* **2019**, *11*, e1566. [CrossRef]
85. Shan, G.; Shao, B.; Liu, Q.; Zeng, Y.; Fu, C.; Chen, A.; Chen, Q. circFMN2 Sponges miR-1238 to Promote the Expression of LIM-Homeobox Gene 2 in Prostate Cancer Cells. *Mol. Ther. Nucleic Acids* **2020**, *21*, 133–146. [CrossRef] [PubMed]
86. Yan, Z.; Xiao, Y.; Chen, Y.; Luo, G. Screening and identification of epithelial-to-mesenchymal transition-related circRNA and miRNA in prostate cancer. *Pathol. Res. Pract.* **2019**, *216*, 152784. [CrossRef]

87. Qiu, L.; Huang, Y.; Li, Z.; Dong, X.; Chen, G.; Xu, H.; Zeng, Y.; Cai, Z.; Liu, X.; Liu, J. Circular RNA profiling identifies circ ADAMTS 13 as a miR-484 sponge which suppresses cell proliferation in hepatocellular carcinoma. *Mol. Oncol.* **2019**, *13*, 441–455. [CrossRef]
88. Rochow, H.; Franz, A.; Jung, M.; Weickmann, S.; Ralla, B.; Kilic, E.; Stephan, C.; Fendler, A.; Jung, K. Instability of circular RNAs in clinical tissue samples impairs their reliable expression analysis using RT-qPCR: From the myth of their advantage as biomarkers to reality. *Theranostics* **2020**, *10*, 9268–9279. [CrossRef]
89. Westholm, J.O.; Miura, P.; Olson, S.; Shenker, S.; Joseph, B.; Sanfilippo, P.; Celniker, S.E.; Graveley, B.R.; Lai, E.C. Genome-wide Analysis of Drosophila Circular RNAs Reveals Their Structural and Sequence Properties and Age-Dependent Neural Accumulation. *Cell Rep.* **2014**, *9*, 1966–1980. [CrossRef] [PubMed]
90. Zhong, S.; Zhou, S.; Yang, S.; Yu, X.; Xu, H.; Wang, J.; Zhang, Q.; Lv, M.; Feng, J. Identification of internal control genes for circular RNAs. *Biotechnol. Lett.* **2019**, *41*, 1111–1119. [CrossRef]
91. Lu, T.; Cui, L.; Zhou, Y.; Zhu, C.; Fan, D.; Gong, H.; Zhao, Q.; Zhou, C.; Zhao, Y.; Lu, D.; et al. Transcriptome-wide investigation of circular RNAs in rice. *RNA* **2015**, *21*, 2076–2087. [CrossRef] [PubMed]
92. Kong, Z.; Wan, X.; Lu, Y.; Zhang, Y.; Huang, Y.; Xu, Y.; Liu, Y.; Zhao, P.; Xiang, X.; Li, L.; et al. Circular RNA circFOXO3 promotes prostate cancer progression through sponging miR-29a-3p. *J. Cell. Mol. Med.* **2020**, *24*, 799–813. [CrossRef] [PubMed]
93. Gao, Y.; Wang, J.; Zheng, Y.; Zhang, J.; Chen, S.; Zhao, F. Comprehensive identification of internal structure and alternative splicing events in circular RNAs. *Nat. Commun.* **2016**, *7*, 12060. [CrossRef] [PubMed]
94. Chakravarty, D.; Sboner, A.; Nair, S.S.; Giannopoulou, E.; Li, R.; Hennig, S.; Mosquera, J.M.; Pauwels, J.; Park, K.; Kossai, M.; et al. The oestrogen receptor alpha-regulated lncRNA NEAT1 is a critical modulator of prostate cancer. *Nat. Commun.* **2014**, *5*, 5383. [CrossRef]
95. Bai, J.; Huang, G. Role of long non-coding RNA NEAT1 in the prognosis of prostate cancer patients. *Medicine* **2020**, *99*, e20204. [CrossRef]
96. Gerszten, R.E.; Wang, T.J. The search for new cardiovascular biomarkers. *Nat. Cell Biol.* **2008**, *451*, 949–952. [CrossRef]
97. Ralla, B.; Busch, J.; Flörcken, A.; Westermann, J.; Zhao, Z.; Kilic, E.; Weickmann, S.; Jung, M.; Fendler, A.; Jung, K. miR-9-5p in Nephrectomy Specimens is a Potential Predictor of Primary Resistance to First-Line Treatment with Tyrosine Kinase Inhibitors in Patients with Metastatic Renal Cell Carcinoma. *Cancers* **2018**, *10*, 321. [CrossRef]
98. Tan, W.L.; Lim, B.T.; Anene-Nzelu, C.G.; Ackers-Johnson, M.; Dashi, A.; See, K.; Tiang, Z.; Lee, D.P.; Chua, W.W.; Luu, T.D.; et al. A landscape of circular RNA expression in the human heart. *Cardiovasc. Res.* **2017**, *113*, 298–309. [CrossRef]
99. Cieslik, M.; Chugh, R.; Wu, Y.-M.; Wu, M.; Brennan, C.; Lonigro, R.; Su, F.; Wang, R.; Siddiqui, J.; Mehra, R.; et al. The use of exome capture RNA-seq for highly degraded RNA with application to clinical cancer sequencing. *Genome Res.* **2015**, *25*, 1372–1381. [CrossRef]
100. Steyerberg, E.W.; Pencina, M.J.; Lingsma, H.F.; Kattan, M.W.; Vickers, A.J.; Van Calster, B. Assessing the incremental value of diagnostic and prognostic markers: A review and illustration. *Eur. J. Clin. Investig.* **2011**, *42*, 216–228. [CrossRef]
101. Mohler, J.L.; Antonarakis, E.S.; Armstrong, A.J.; D'Amico, A.V.; Davis, B.J.; Dorff, T.; Eastham, J.A.; Enke, C.A.; Farrington, T.A.; Higano, C.S.; et al. Prostate Cancer, Version 2.2019, NCCN Clinical Practice Guidelines in Oncology. *J. Natl. Compr. Cancer Netw.* **2019**, *17*, 479–505. [CrossRef] [PubMed]
102. Burke, H.B. Predicting Clinical Outcomes Using Molecular Biomarkers. *Biomark. Cancer* **2016**, *8*, BIC.S33380–99. [CrossRef] [PubMed]
103. Wang, J.; Zhang, Y.; Dou, Z.; Jiang, H.; Wang, Y.; Gao, X.; Xin, X. Knockdown of STIL suppresses the progression of gastric cancer by down-regulating the IGF-1/PI3K/AKT pathway. *J. Cell. Mol. Med.* **2019**, *23*, 5566–5575. [CrossRef] [PubMed]
104. Jiang, X.; Guo, S.; Zhang, Y.; Zhao, Y.; Li, X.; Jia, Y.; Xu, Y.; Ma, B. LncRNA NEAT1 promotes docetaxel resistance in prostate cancer by regulating ACSL4 via sponging miR-34a-5p and miR-204-5p. *Cell. Signal.* **2020**, *65*, 109422. [CrossRef] [PubMed]
105. Xiong, W.; Huang, C.; Deng, H.; Jian, C.; Zen, C.; Ye, K.; Zhong, Z.; Zhao, X.; Zhu, L. Oncogenic non-coding RNA NEAT1 promotes the prostate cancer cell growth through the SRC3/IGF1R/AKT pathway. *Int. J. Biochem. Cell Biol.* **2018**, *94*, 125–132. [CrossRef]
106. Steyerberg, E.W.; Harrell, F.E.; Borsboom, G.J.; Eijkemans, M.; Vergouwe, Y.; Habbema, J.F. Internal validation of predictive models. *J. Clin. Epidemiol.* **2001**, *54*, 774–781. [CrossRef]

107. Jung, M.; Mollenkopf, H.J.; Grimm, C.H.; Wagner, I.; Albrecht, M.; Waller, T.; Pilarsky, C.; Johannsen, M.; Stephan, C.; Lehrach, H.; et al. MicroRNA profiling of clear cell renal cell cancer identifies a robust signature to define renal malignancy. *J. Cell. Mol. Med.* **2009**, *13*, 3918–3928. [CrossRef]
108. Schaefer, A.; Jung, M.; Mollenkopf, H.-J.; Wagner, I.; Stephan, C.; Jentzmik, F.; Miller, K.; Lein, M.; Kristiansen, G.; Jung, K. Diagnostic and prognostic implications of microRNA profiling in prostate carcinoma. *Int. J. Cancer* **2009**, *126*, 1166–1176. [CrossRef]
109. O'Sullivan, B.; Brierley, J.; Byrd, D.; Bosman, F.; Kehoe, S.; Kossary, C.; Piñeros, M.; Van Eycken, E.; Weir, H.K.; Gospodarowicz, M. The TNM classification of malignant tumours—Towards common understanding and reasonable expectations. *Lancet Oncol.* **2017**, *18*, 849–851. [CrossRef]
110. Humphrey, P.A.; Amin, M.B.; Berney, D.M.; Billis, A.; Cao, D.; Cheng, L.; Delahunt, B.; Egevad, L.; Epstein, J.I.; Fine, S.W.; et al. Acinar Adenocarcinoma. In *WHO Classification of Tumours of the Urinary System and Male Genital Organs*, 4th ed.; Moch, H., Humphrey, P.A., Ulbright, T.M., Reuter, V.E., Eds.; International Agency for Research on Cancer: Lyon, France, 2016; pp. 152–154.
111. Jentzmik, F.; Stephan, C.; Lein, M.; Miller, K.; Kamlage, B.; Bethan, B.; Kristiansen, G.; Jung, K. Sarcosine in Prostate Cancer Tissue is not a Differential Metabolite for Prostate Cancer Aggressiveness and Biochemical Progression. *J. Urol.* **2011**, *185*, 706–711. [CrossRef]
112. Jung, K.; Reszka, R.; Kamlage, B.; Bethan, B.; Stephan, C.; Lein, M.; Kristiansen, G. Tissue metabolite profiling identifies differentiating and prognostic biomarkers for prostate carcinoma. *Int. J. Cancer* **2013**, *133*, 2914–2924. [CrossRef] [PubMed]
113. Untergasser, A.; Cutcutache, I.; Koressaar, T.; Ye, J.; Faircloth, B.C.; Remm, M.; Rozen, S.G. Primer3—New capabilities and interfaces. *Nucleic Acids Res.* **2012**, *40*, e115. [CrossRef]
114. D'Haene, B.; Mestdagh, P.; Hellemans, J.; Vandesompele, J. miRNA Expression Profiling: From Reference Genes to Global Mean Normalization. In *Next-Generation MicroRNA Expression Profiling Technology*; Humana Press: Totowa, NJ, USA, 2012; pp. 261–272. [CrossRef]
115. Hellemans, J.; Mortier, G.; De Paepe, A.; Speleman, F.; Vandesompele, J. qBase relative quantification framework and software for management and automated analysis of real-time quantitative PCR data. *Genome Biol.* **2007**, *8*, R19. [CrossRef] [PubMed]
116. Vickers, A.J.; Elkin, E.B. Decision Curve Analysis: A Novel Method for Evaluating Prediction Models. *Med. Decis. Mak.* **2006**, *26*, 565–574. [CrossRef] [PubMed]
117. Stephan, C.; Jung, K.; Semjonow, A.; Schulze-Forster, K.; Cammann, H.; Hu, X.; Meyer, H.-A.; Bögemann, M.; Miller, K.; Friedersdorff, F. Comparative Assessment of Urinary Prostate Cancer Antigen 3 and TMPRSS2: ERG Gene Fusion with the Serum [−2]Proprostate-Specific Antigen–Based Prostate Health Index for Detection of Prostate Cancer. *Clin. Chem.* **2013**, *59*, 280–288. [CrossRef] [PubMed]
118. Pencina, M.J.; D'Agostino, R.B. OverallC as a measure of discrimination in survival analysis: Model specific population value and confidence interval estimation. *Stat. Med.* **2004**, *23*, 2109–2123. [CrossRef] [PubMed]
119. Harrell, F.E., Jr.; Lee, K.L.; Mark, D.B. Multivariable prognostic models: Issues in developing models, evaluating assumptions and adequacy, and measuring and reducing errorrs. *Stat. Med.* **1996**, *15*, 361–387. [CrossRef]
120. Faul, F.; Erdfelder, E.; Lang, A.-G.; Buchner, A. G*Power 3: A flexible statistical power analysis program for the social, behavioral, and biomedical sciences. *Behav. Res. Methods* **2007**, *39*, 175–191. [CrossRef]

2

The Prognostic Role of Baseline Metabolic Tumor Burden and Systemic Inflammation Biomarkers in Metastatic Castration-Resistant Prostate Cancer Patients Treated with Radium-223: A Proof of Concept Study

Matteo Bauckneht [1,*,†], Sara Elena Rebuzzi [2,†], Alessio Signori [3], Maria Isabella Donegani [3], Veronica Murianni [2], Alberto Miceli [3], Roberto Borea [2], Stefano Raffa [3], Alessandra Damassi [2], Marta Ponzano [3], Fabio Catalano [2], Valentino Martelli [2], Cecilia Marini [1,4], Francesco Boccardo [5,6], Silvia Morbelli [1,3], Gianmario Sambuceti [1,3] and Giuseppe Fornarini [2]

1 Nuclear Medicine, IRCCS Ospedale Policlinico San Martino, 16132 Genova, Italy; cecilia.marini@unige.it (C.M.); silviadaniela.morbelli@hsanmartino.it (S.M.); sambuceti@unige.it (G.S.)
2 Medical Oncology Unit 1, IRCCS Ospedale Policlinico San Martino, 16132 Genova, Italy; saraelena89@hotmail.it (S.E.R.); murianni.veronica@gmail.com (V.M.); roby.borea@gmail.com (R.B.); alessandra.damassi@gmail.com (A.D.); catalan.fab@gmail.com (F.C.); martellivalentino91@gmail.com (V.M.); giuseppe.fornarini@hsanmartino.it (G.F.)
3 Department of Health Sciences (DISSAL), University of Genova, Largo R. Benzi 10, 16132 Genova, Italy; alessio.signori.unige@gmail.com (A.S.); isabella.donegani@gmail.com (M.I.D.); albertomiceli23@gmail.com (A.M.); Stefanoraffa@live.com (S.R.); m.ponzano@campus.unimib.it (M.P.)
4 CNR Institute of Molecular Bioimaging and Physiology (IBFM), 20090 Segrate (MI), Italy
5 Academic Unit of Medical Oncology, IRCCS Ospedale Policlinico San Martino, 16132 Genova, Italy; fboccardo@unige.it
6 Department of Internal Medicine and Medical Specialties (DiMI), School of Medicine, University of Genova, 16132 Genova, Italy
* Correspondence: matteo.bauckneht@hsanmartino.it
† These authors equally contributed as first co-authors.

Simple Summary: Radium-223 is an alpha-emitting radioisotope that selectively binds to increased bone turnover areas, such as metastatic sites, acting as a bone-seeking calcium mimetic drug. Its therapeutic function in metastatic castration-resistant prostate cancer patients relies on its capability to prolong overall survival, improve quality of life, and delay the first skeletal-related event. However, in the last few years, many studies showed that the survival benefit in the real-life patients might be lower than that initially reported, probably due to a suboptimal selection of patients with poorer prognostic clinical characteristics. In this scenario, it has emerged the urgent need for the identification of reliable biomarkers able to potentially identify patients most likely to benefit from Radium-223 since baseline. With this aim, this preliminary study is the first to combine the prognostic power of baseline FDG-PET/CT and systemic inflammation indexes in a cohort of metastatic castration-resistant prostate cancer patients undergoing Radium-223 administration.

Abstract: Over the last years has emerged the urgent need for the identification of reliable prognostic biomarkers able to potentially identify metastatic castration-resistant prostate cancer (mCRPC) patients most likely to benefit from Radium-223 (Ra-223) since baseline. In the present monocentric retrospective study, we analyzed the prognostic power of systemic inflammation biomarkers and 18F-Fluorodeoxyglucose Positron Emission Tomography/Computed Tomography (FDG-PET)-derived parameters and their potential interplay in this clinical setting. The following baseline laboratory parameters were collected in 59 mCRPC patients treated with Ra-223: neutrophil-to-lymphocyte ratio (NLR), derived NLR (dNLR), lymphocyte-to-monocyte ratio (LMR), platelets-to-lymphocyte ratio (PLR), and systemic inflammation index (SII), while maximum Standardized Uptake Value, Metabolic Tumor Volume (MTV), and Total Lesion Glycolysis (TLG) were calculated in the 48 of them submitted to baseline FDG-PET. At the univariate analysis, NLR, dNLR, MTV, and TLG were able to predict the overall survival (OS). However, only NLR and MTV were independent predictors of OS at the multivariate analysis. Additionally, the occurrence of both increased NLR and MTV at baseline identified mCRPC patients at higher risk for lower long-term survival after treatment with Ra-223. In conclusion, the degree of systemic inflammation, the quantification of the metabolically active tumor burden and their combination might represent potentially valuable tools for identifying mCRPC patients who are most likely to benefit from Ra-223. However, further studies are needed to reproduce these findings in larger settings.

Keywords: metastatic castration resistant prostate cancer; radium-223; neutrophil-to-lymphocyte ratio; lymphocyte-to-monocyte ratio; platelet-to-lymphocyte ratio; systemic inflammation index; 18F-fluorodeoxyglucose; metabolic tumor volume; total lesion glycolysis; positron emission tomography

---

1. Introduction

Bone metastases affect more than 90% of patients with metastatic castration-resistant prostate cancer (mCRPC) patients and 20–50% of them develop skeletal-related events (SREs), which represent the main cause of impaired quality of life and death [1].

Radium-223 (Ra-223) is an alpha-emitting radionuclide which selectively binds to areas of increased bone turnover, such as metastatic sites, acting as a bone-seeking calcium mimetic drug [2]. Its short-range high-energy emission induces breaks in double-strand DNA filaments and targets tumor cell death [3]. The phase III Alpharadin in Symptomatic Prostate Cancer Patients (ALSYMPCA) trial investigated Ra-223 compared to a placebo in mCRPC patients with symptomatic bone metastases, limited lymph node metastases (<3 cm), and no visceral metastases [4]. In the ALSYMPCA trial, Ra-223 was demonstrated to prolong overall survival (OS), improve quality of life, and delay the first SRE [4]. According to these results, Ra-223 was subsequently approved by the Food and Drug Administration (FDA) for mCRPC patients.

However, in the last few years, many retrospective studies showed that the survival benefit in real-life patients might be lower than that reported in the ALSYMPCA trial, probably due to a suboptimal selection of patients with poorer prognostic clinical characteristics [5–7]. Furthermore, in 2018 the European Medicine Agency (EMA) restricted the use of Ra-223 to patients with more than six osteoblastic lesions in progression after at least two prior lines of systemic therapies for mCRPC or ineligible for any available systemic mCRPC treatment [8]. However, the later timing of Ra-223 administration in the patients' clinical history might further negatively affect OS [9]. In this scenario, there is an urgent need to identify reliable biomarkers potentially able to improve the selection of patients most likely to benefit from Ra-223 treatment.

Several exploratory analyses from the ALSYMPCA trial and retrospective studies identified clinical, biochemical, and imaging parameters to predict treatment completion or survival outcomes since baseline, thus potentially improving patient selection [5,6,10–13].

Peripheral blood inflammatory parameters, such as neutrophils-to-lymphocytes (NLR), have been shown to significantly correlate with survival outcomes and therapeutic response in various cancers, including mCRPC, as potential cancer inflammation-associated markers [14–17]. These biomarkers are currently of great interest for their ready and easy accessibility in the clinical practice and their transversal role in many types of tumors and cancer treatments [15]. However, few studies have investigated their prognostic role in patients treated with Ra-223 [5,18,19]. On the other hand, we recently showed that baseline ^{18}F-Fluorodeoxyglucose Positron Emission Tomography/Computed Tomography (FDG-PET) could stratify OS in a cohort of mCRPC patients who are candidates for Ra-223 [20]. However, the comparison and the potential interplay between peripheral blood inflammatory biomarkers and metabolic FDG-PET-derived parameters still need to be investigated in this clinical setting.

Therefore, in the present proof of concept study, we analyzed the prognostic power of baseline inflammatory and functional imaging biomarkers and their potential interplay to identify mCRPC patients most likely to benefit from Ra-223.

2. Materials and Methods

2.1. Study Population

We performed a retrospective monocentric analysis of all consecutive mCRPC patients treated with Ra-223 from September 2016 to February 2020 at the IRCCS Ospedale Policlinico San Martino of Genova, Italy. The retrospective analysis was conducted under the Declaration of Helsinki, Good Clinical Practice, and local ethical and legal regulations. According to our standard procedure, all patients signed a written informed consent form, encompassing the use of anonymized data for retrospective research purposes before each imaging procedure and each Ra-223 administration.

CRPC was defined as a serum testosterone level of <50 ng/dL following surgical or pharmaceutical castration. All patients fulfilled the inclusion criteria for Ra-223 therapy and were treated according to the standard Ra-223 regimen encompassing six intravenous administrations every four weeks (55 KBq/kg) [21]. According to the established guidelines for patient selection, a bone marrow reserve fulfilling the hematologic criteria necessary to administer Ra-223 was verified [21]. During the four weeks preceding the first Ra-223 administration, each patient underwent a contrast-enhanced CT and bone scan to select mCRPC patients with symptomatic bone metastases in the absence of visceral involvement (with the exception for lymph nodes with maximum diameter < 3 cm). In the same time interval, recruited patients were submitted to FDG-PET for prognostic purposes in agreement with the emerging prognostic role of this tool in patients with mCRPC, and in accordance with the national guidelines by the Italian Association of Medical Oncology (AIOM) [22,23]. According to our standard procedure, complete blood cell count, serum chemistry, prostate-specific antigen (PSA), alkaline phosphatase (ALP), and lactate dehydrogenase (LDH) were assessed at baseline and on the same day of each Ra-223 administration.

During Ra-223 administration, patients continued androgen deprivation therapy and received the best standard of care, including antiresorptive agents (bisphosphonates/denosumab) and antalgic therapy [21]. The concomitant treatment with Abiraterone and Enzalutamide was not allowed [21].

2.2. Systemic Inflammation Indexes

We retrospectively collected white blood cells (WBC), platelets (PLT), and the absolute neutrophil (ANC), lymphocyte (ALC), and monocyte (AMC) count to obtain their ratio: NLR, derived NLR (dNLR), lymphocyte-to-monocyte ratio (LMR), platelets-to-lymphocyte ratio (PLR), and systemic inflammation index (SII). dNLR was calculated as ANC/(WBC-ANC) and SII as NLRxPLT.

2.3. Imaging Procedures and Images Analyses

FDG-PET was performed according to the European Association of Nuclear Medicine (EANM) Guidelines [24]. PET/CT scans were performed using a 16-slices PET/CT hybrid system (Hirez-Biograph 16, Siemens Medical Solutions, USA).

FDG-PET images were interpreted in consensus by three expert nuclear medicine physicians (M.B.; M.I.D.; A.M.) blinded to contrast-enhanced CT and bone scan results. From the attenuation corrected FDG-PET images, the maximum standardized uptake value (SUVmax) of the hottest bone lesion was obtained in the transaxial view. Further, a volume of interest was drawn using an SUV-based automated contouring program (Syngo Siemens workstation, Siemens Medical Solutions, USA) with an isocounter threshold based on 40% of the SUVmax, as previously recommended [25]. Total Metabolic Tumor Volume (MTV) was obtained by the sum of all skeletal and extra-skeletal lesions. Total Lesion Glycolysis (TLG) was calculated as the sum of the product of MTV of each lesion, and the SUVmean value, which, in turn, was automatically calculated within each single MTV.

Aiming to analyze the interobserver variation, a second expert PET reader (S.M.) measured MTV and TLG independently from the first group of observers.

2.4. *Survival Assessment*

Baseline inflammatory biomarkers (NLR, dNLR, LMR, PLR, SII), as well as FDG-PET-derived parameters (SUVmax, MTV, TLG), were assessed for their correlation with OS.

2.5. *Statistical Analysis*

Descriptive analyses were conducted using percentages for binary variables and means/medians for continuous variables, reporting their dispersion values.

Non-parametric Bland–Altman plots were used to evaluate median bias ad limits of agreement (2.5% and 97.5% percentiles) for MTV and TLG values measured by the two groups of PET readers [26]. A linear regression was applied to verify the eventual occurrence of proportional biases.

To assess the association of parameters, biomarkers, and clinical characteristics (independent variables) with OS, univariable and multivariable Cox regression model were used.

All parameters, biomarkers, and clinical characteristics, with a p-value < 0.10 at univariable analysis were selected for the multivariable analysis. Only those with a p-value < 0.10 were maintained in the final multivariable model.

OS was calculated from the start of treatment to death from any cause, censored at last follow-up for patients who were alive, and was estimated by mean of the Kaplan–Meier (KM) approach.

The multivariable model was performed both on the cohort with complete cases for inflammatory and FDG-PET parameters and for the whole cohort of patients after multiple imputations of missing values for FDG-PET parameters (MTV, TLG). Multiple imputation was performed using an iterative multivariate method based on chained equations. Eleven imputations were performed.

To report KM curves of OS, continuous parameters were binarized. To find the best cut-off value, the Youden index from the ROC curve for survival data at 24 months was used.

Hazard-ratios (HR) for Cox regression models were reported together with a 95% confidence interval (CI) and p-value. Due to a highly skewed distribution, for MTV and TLG, the log-transformed values were used in the analyses for a better interpretation. Gleason Score at diagnosis was categorized into three classes for clinical interpretation, as previously described [27]. Similarly, bone scan lesions were categorized in <6, 6–20, and >20, as performed in a sub-analysis of the ALSYMPCA study [4].

To assess the ability of each continuous parameter to discriminate between dead and censored patients, the Harrell's c-index for censored data was calculated for all inflammatory and FDG-PET parameters.

Further, a calibration plot to assess the accuracy of the prediction for an individual patient according to single parameters and multivariate model was realized. A joint test was performed to investigate the overall evidence for linear miscalibration.

All statistical analyses were performed using Stata (v.16; StataCorp; 4905 Lakeway Drive College Station, Texas, TX, USA).

3. Results

3.1. Patients' and Treatment Characteristics

Fifty-nine mCRPC patients treated with Ra-223 were included in the analysis. Of these, 48 (81.4%) had all complete data on both inflammatory biomarkers and FDG-PET parameters. The patient, tumor, and treatment characteristics are summarized in Table 1.

Table 1. Patients' characteristics.

Patients' Characteristics	All Sample (n = 59)	Complete Cases (n = 48)
Clinical characteristics	*n* (%)	*n* (%)
Median age, years (range)	74 (51–88)	75 (51–88)
ECOG performance status		
0	22 (37)	17 (35)
1	23 (39)	18 (38)
2	14 (24)	13 (27)
Gleason score at diagnosis		
≤7	21 (36)	16 (33)
≥8	30 (51)	24 (50)
Missing data	8 (13)	8 (17)
Gleason group at diagnosis		
≤2	10 (17)	8 (17)
≥3	42 (71)	33 (69)
Missing data	7 (12)	7 (14)
Prostatectomy		
Yes	21 (36)	17 (35)
No	35 (59)	28 (58)
Missing data	3 (5)	3 (7)
Radical radiotherapy		
Yes	4 (7)	3 (6)
No	48 (81)	40 (83)
Missing data	7 (12)	5 (11)
Metastatic disease at diagnosis		
Yes	28 (47)	22 (46)
No	27 (46)	23 (48)
Missing data	4 (7)	3 (6)
Metastases		
Bone metastases	43 (73)	35 (73)
Bone and lymph node metastases	16 (27)	13 (27)
N bone metastases		
<6	9 (16)	8 (16)
6–20	24 (40)	20 (42)
>20	26 (44)	20 (42)
Baseline median PSA, g/L (range)	55 (0–6089)	68 (0–6089)
Baseline median ALP, U/L (range)	138 (10–1296)	154 (29–1296)
Baseline ALP, U/L		
<220	40 (68)	32 (67)
≥220	19 (32)	16 (33)
Ra-223 treatment		

Table 1. *Cont.*

Patients' Characteristics	**All Sample** (*n* = 59)	**Complete Cases** (*n* = 48)
Ra-223 treatment line		
Median (range)	3 (1–6)	3 (1–6)
First-line	3 (5)	2 (4)
Second-line	21 (36)	17 (35)
Third-line	21 (36)	17 (35)
>3rd line	14 (23)	12 (26)
EMA restriction of use compliant		
Not compliant	33 (56)	22 (54)
Compliant	26 (44)	26 (46)
Median cycles received, number (range)	5 (1–6)	4 (1–6)
Completion of 3 cycles		
Yes	46 (78)	35 (73)
No	13 (22)	13 (27)
Completion of 6 cycles		
Yes	23 (39)	18 (38)
No	36 (61)	30 (62)
Prior chemotherapy		
Yes	35 (59)	28 (58)
Docetaxel	19 (32)	15 (31)
Docetaxel and Cabazitaxel	16 (27)	13 (27)
No	24 (41)	20 (42)

ECOG: Eastern Cooperative Oncology Group, PSA: prostate-specific antigen, ALP: alkaline phosphatase, Ra-223: Radium 223, EMA: European Medicines Agency.

All patients had a histological diagnosis of prostate cancer with a median Gleason score (GS) of 8 (range 5–10) with a GS ≥ 8 in 51% of patients; 47% of patients had metastatic disease at diagnosis.

Before Ra-223 therapy initiation, the median age was 74 years (range 51–88 years) and median ECOG PS was 1 (range 0–2), with ECOG PS 0–1 in 76% of patients.

All patients underwent CT and bone scans at baseline, while 81% of the enrolled patient underwent FDG-PET at the same timepoint. CT scan revealed the occurrence of lymph node metastases in 27% of patients, while bone scan showed the presence of <6, 6–20, and >20 bone lesions in 16%, 40%, and 44% of patients, respectively. Baseline peripheral blood results were available in 100% of patients.

Ra-223 therapy was administered as first and second line therapy for CRPC in 24 patients (41%), as third line in 21 (36%) patients, and as subsequent lines in 14 patients (23%). In 26 patients (44%), Ra-223 was administered after the 2018 EMA restriction of use [8].

The median number of Ra-223 cycles was 5 (range 1–6), 78% and 39% of patients completed three and all six cycles, respectively. Eight patients (13%) are currently still in treatment with Ra-223 at the time of data analysis. Thirty-five patients (59%) received chemotherapy before Ra-223, of which 19 patients (32%) received docetaxel only and 16 patients (27%) both docetaxel and cabazitaxel.

Characteristics of patients with complete cases were similar to those of the whole cohort.

3.2. *Interobserver Agreement between PET Readers*

There was good agreement between the two groups of observers for measuring MTV and TLG. Bland–Altman plots showed a median difference of 0.26 (limits of agreements: −159.67–160.19) and −15.35 (limits of agreements: −397.07–366.37), respectively (see also Figure S1). No proportional biases were observed (p = ns for both).

3.3. Systemic Inflammation Indexes and FDG-Derived Parameters in the Prediction of OS.

All patients included in the study were assessable for survival analysis and were followed-up for a median of 10 months. The median OS (mOS) was 11.6 months (95% CI: 9.1–14.7) in the whole cohort and 10.2 (95% CI: 7.1–14.7) in 48 patients with complete data. OS was 78.8% (CI: 65.6–87.3) in the whole cohort and 73.4% (58.4–84.2) in the reduced sample at 6 months, while it was 46.5% (CI: 32.4–59.4) in the whole cohort and 46.2% (CI: 30.6–60.5) in the reduced sample, respectively. Figure 1 shows the Kaplan–Meier survival function of the study cohort with all complete data (n = 48). Results from Kaplan–Meier analyses and univariable Cox regression analyses are reported in Figures 2 and 3 and in Table 2, respectively. Univariate and multivariate analyses were conducted on the complete cases set (n = 48). A further multivariate analysis was performed considering all sample (n = 59) after multiple imputation of missing data for FDG-PET parameters.

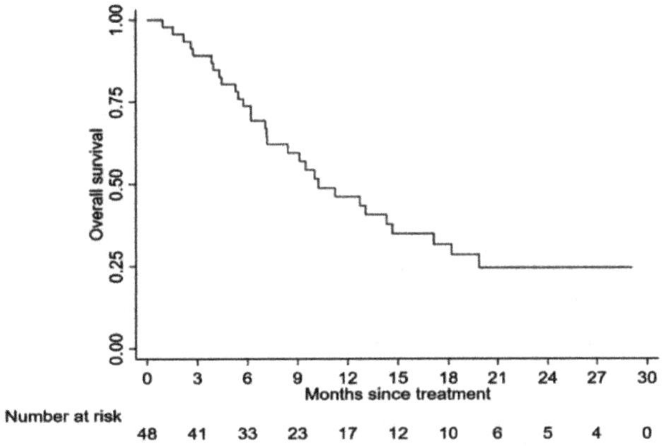

Figure 1. Survival function of the entire study cohort.

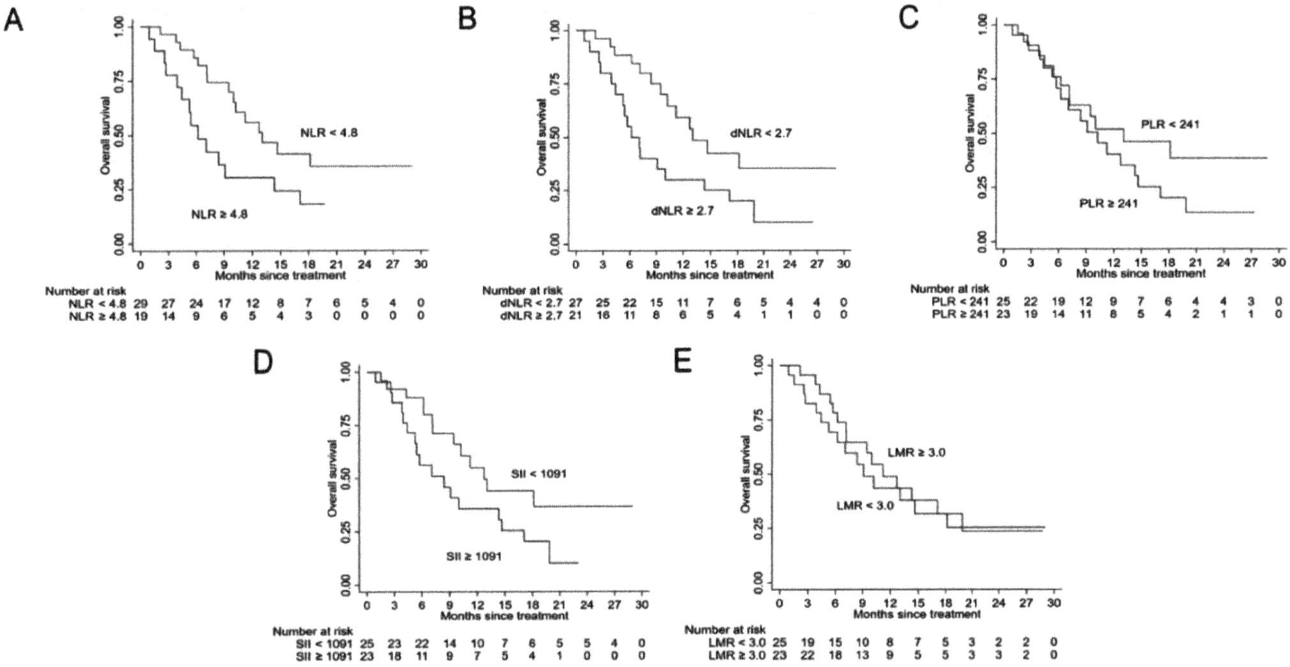

Figure 2. Kaplan–Meier curves for overall survival (OS) according to baseline systemic inflammatory indexes. Panels (**A–E**) show OS prediction according to neutrophil-to-lymphocyte ratio (NLR), derived-NLR (d-NLR), platelets-to-lymphocyte ratio (PLR), systemic inflammation index (SII), and lymphocyte-to-monocyte ration (LMR), respectively.

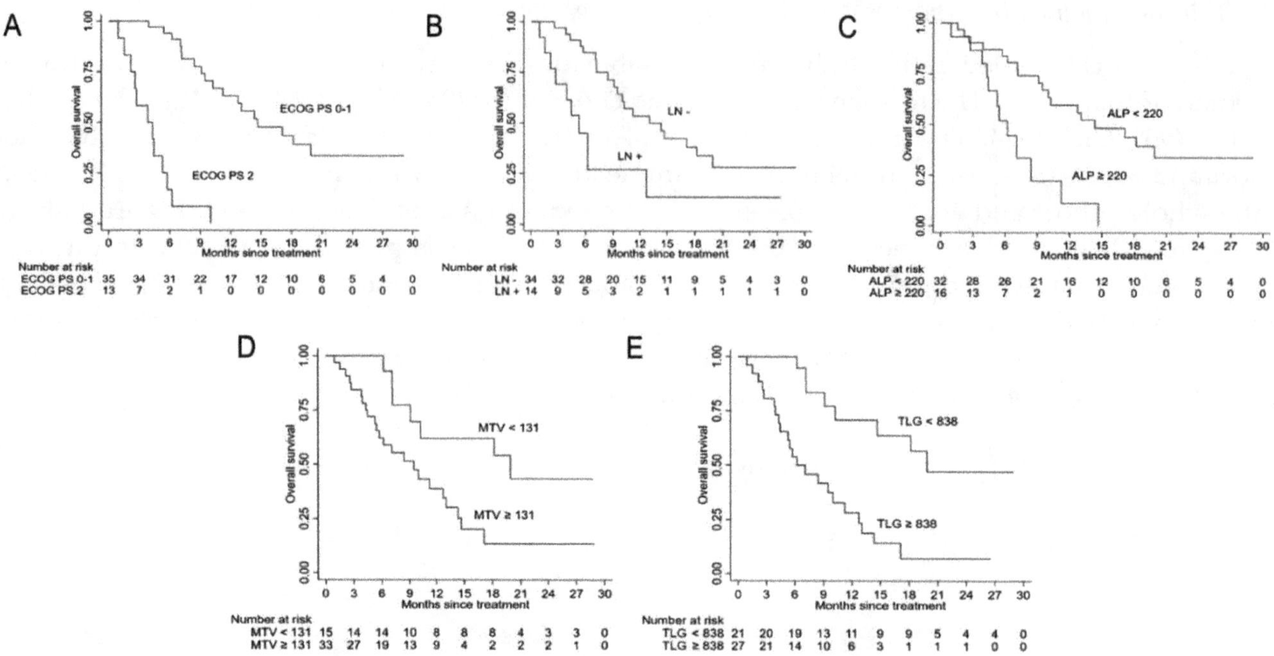

Figure 3. Kaplan–Meier curves for OS according to baseline clinical and FDG-PET parameters. Panels (**A**–**E**) show the prediction of OS according to ECOG PS, the presence of pathological lymph nodes (LN+), baseline ALP, MTV, and TLG, respectively.

Lower ECOG PS and ALP, as well as the absence of pathological lymph nodes, were associated with higher OS. Among systemic inflammation indexes, only NLR and dNLR reached the statistical significance at the univariate analysis (Table 2, Figure 2). In both cases, higher OS was observed for lower values of these systemic inflammation parameters. Similarly, lower MTV and TLG correlated with an increased OS (Table 2, Figure 3).

Low to moderate *c*-index, testing the discriminative ability, was observed for almost all inflammation parameters while MTV and TLG showed a higher *c*-index of 0.75. Both these parameters also seemed to have good accuracy in prediction (Figure 4) as also confirmed by a not significant result of the test for miscalibration (*p*-value = 0.49 for MTV and 0.64 for TLG).

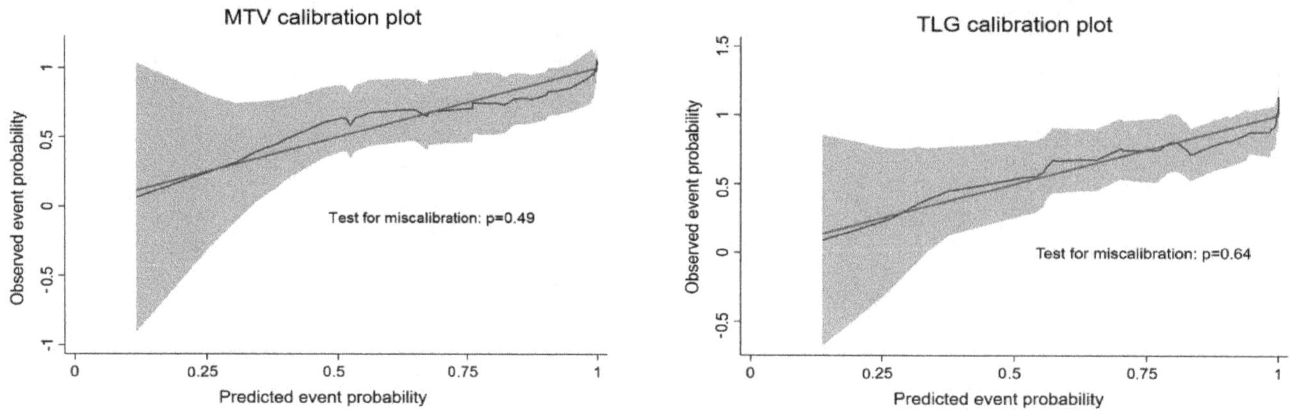

Figure 4. Calibration plot showing the relationship between the predicted and observed probability of death at 24 months for the two Fluorodeoxyglucose (FDG)-derived parameters. A well-calibrated parameter shows a 1:1 relationship between predicted and observed probability represented by a 45° line (green line). The predicted probability (red line) is based, respectively, on MTV (**left panel**) and TLG (**right panel**) and is remarkably close to the green line representing a good calibration. This is also confirmed by a not significant test for miscalibration.

The same parameters with prognostic value at the univariate analysis (apart from ALP, dNLR, and TLG) remained independently associated at the multivariate analysis for OS. The Harrell's C-index for this multivariable model was 0.81 in the reduced cohort (without imputation of missing value) and 0.79 in the whole cohort where FDG-PET parameters were imputed for the missing 11 patients.

Table 2. Systemic inflammation indexes, FDG-derived parameters, and clinical characteristics in the prediction of OS.

Biomarkers	Univariate Analyses on Complete Cases ($n = 48$)			Multivariate Analyses on Complete Cases ($n = 48$)		Multivariate Analyses on All Aample ($n = 59$)	
	HR (95% CI)	*p* Value	*c*-Index	HR (95% CI)	*p* Value	HR (95% CI)	*p* Value
Inflammatory biomarkers							
NLR (1-unit)	1.08 (1.01–1.17)	0.042	0.63	1.09 (1.00–1.20)	0.049	1.09 (1.01–1.19)	0.025
d-NLR (1-unit)	1.27 (1.02–1.58)	0.036	0.65				
LMR (1-unit)	0.95 (0.74–1.21)	0.67	0.57				
PLR (100-unit)	1.03 (0.90–1.18)	0.63	0.56				
SII (100-unit)	1.02 (0.99–1.05)	0.25	0.58				
FDG-PET parameters							
SUV max (1-unit)	1.04 (0.96–1.14)	0.33	0.53				
MTV (1-unit on log scale)	2.23 (1.52–3.25)	<0.001	0.75	1.60 (1.09–2.34)	0.016	1.74 (1.22–2.50)	0.002
TLG (1-unit on log-scale)	2.06 (1.46–2.90)	<0.001	0.75				
Patients' characteristics							
ECOG PS							
0–1	1.00 (ref)	<0.001	-	1.00 (ref)	<0.001	1.00 (ref)	<0.001
2	13.4 (5.29–33.74)			7.92 (2.74–22.90)		7.37 (2.94–18.47)	
Gleason group							
<3	1.00 (ref)	0.26	-				
≥3	1.63 (0.70–3.82)						
Lymph node metastases							
No	1.00 (ref)	0.007	-	1.00 (ref)	0.039	1.00 (ref)	0.002
Yes	2.89 (1.33–6.29)			2.66 (1.05–6.75)		3.76 (1.65–8.56)	
N° bone metastases							
<6	1.00 (ref)		-				
6–20	1.63 (0.46–5.76)	0.45					
>20	2.66 (0.74–9.53)	0.13					
ALP							
<220	1.00 (ref)	0.001	-				
≥220	3.79 (1.70–8.49)						
Treatment characteristics							
	Radium therapy line						
1–2	1.00 (ref)	0.92	-				
≥3	1.04 (0.50–2.14)						
Previous chemotherapy							
No	1.00 (ref)	0.44	-				
Yes	1.33 (0.64–2.76)						

NLR: neutrophil to lymphocyte ratio, d–NLR: derived NLR, LMR: lymphocyte to monocyte ratio, PLR: platelet to lymphocyte ratio, SII: systemic inflammation index, FDG–PET: fluorodeoxyglucose positron emission tomography, SUV: standardized uptake value, MTV: metabolic tumor volume, TLG: total lesion glycolysis, ECOG: Eastern Cooperative Oncology Group, PS: performance status, N°: number, ALP: alkaline phosphatase, Ra–233: radium–223.

3.4. The Combination of Systemic Inflammation Indexes and FDG–Derived Parameters in the Prediction of OS

Baseline NLR and MTV, both independently associated with OS in the Cox proportional hazard analyses, were thus combined. This allowed us to define an immune-metabolic-prognostic index (IMPI), as previously described by Castello et al. [28]. The combination of the above-mentioned parameters allowed us to identify three groups with different risk as it follows: low risk (neither NLR ≥ 4.8 nor MTV ≥ 131, IMPI = 0), intermediate risk (NLR ≥ 4.8 or MTV ≥ 131, IMPI = 1), and high risk (NLR ≥ 4.8 and MTV ≥ 131, IMPI = 2).

Among the 48 patients evaluable for IMPI, 10 (20.8%) had low risk, 24 (50%) had intermediate risk, and 14 (29.2%) had high risk. Median OS was 18.2 months (95% CI 7.1–30 months), 12.7 months (95% CI 9.1–25.3 months), 5.3 months (95% CI 2.6–8.4 months) for the low, intermediate, and high IMPI groups, respectively. While no significant differences were observed between low and intermediate groups ($p = 0.27$), the high IMPI group was significantly different with respect to the remaining classes ($p = 0.001$ vs. low, and $p = 0.001$ vs. intermediate). Results from the Kaplan–Meier analysis of IMPI are reported in Figure 5. The prognostic power of IMPI was confirmed including this score in a multivariable model incorporating ECOG-PS, and lymph node metastases ($p = 0.001$).

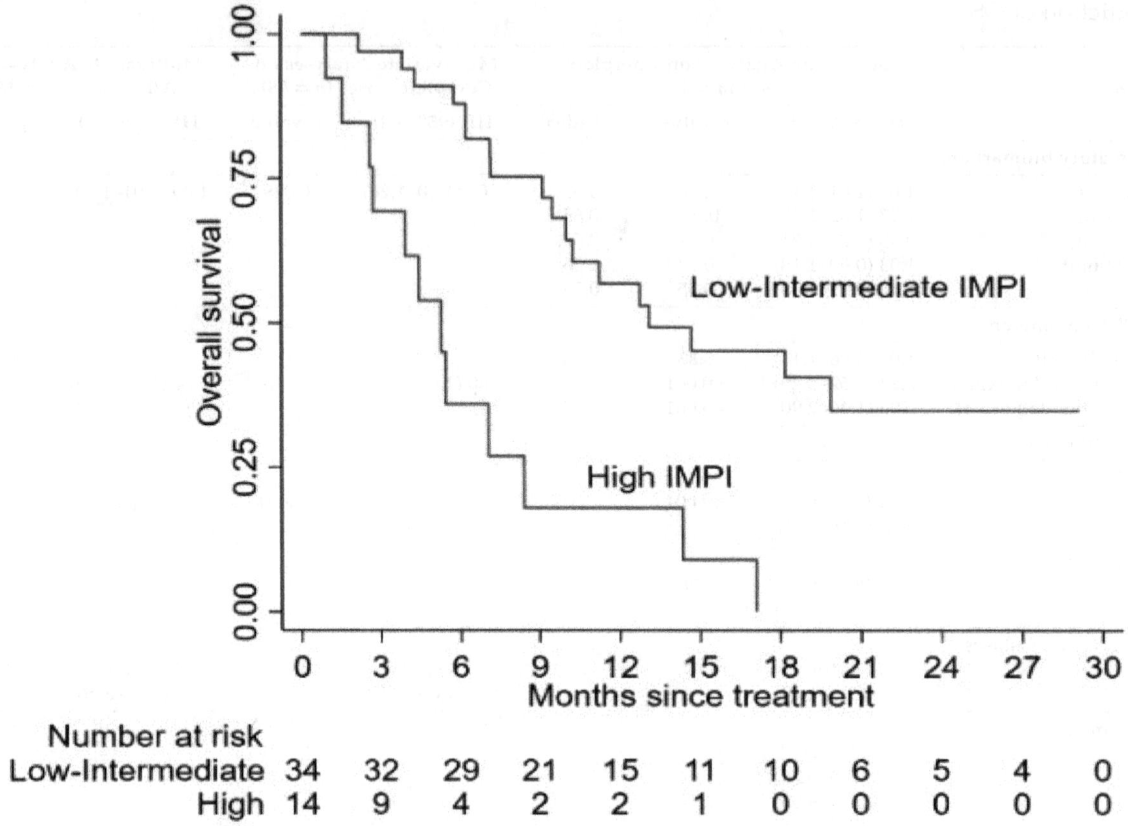

Figure 5. Kaplan–Meier curves for OS according to the immune-metabolic-prognostic index (IMPI). The figure shows the prediction of OS according to the IMPI, based on baseline NLR and MTV, categorizing patients in two groups: high risk (2 factors), and low-intermediate risk (0–1 factor).

4. Discussion

Ra–223 is one of the therapeutic options for mCRPC patients and was approved after the survival benefit observed in the phase III ALSYMPCA trial (mOS 15 versus 11 months) [4]. Nonetheless, in real-life experience, lower survival outcomes (mOS ranging from 8 to 13 months) compared to the results of the registration trial were observed [5]. This weaker survival benefit might be at least partially related to the suboptimal patients' selection process, which was further complicated by the restriction of the use of Ra-223 started in 2018 [29]. In fact, mCRPC candidates to Ra-223 therapy have weaker clinical characteristics compared to those included in clinical trials. Moreover, among the treatment options for mCRPC patients, the right collocation of Ra-223 treatment is not well-established as no comparative and sequential clinical trials are currently available [19]. There is, therefore, an unmet need to identify baseline clinical, biochemical, or imaging biomarkers able to improve the prognostic stratification of patients undergoing Ra-223.

In recent years, many studies tried to identify biomarkers to better select patients most likely to benefit from Ra-223 and, therefore, to optimize treatment strategies. These are important to gain as much as possible in efficacy with few side effects, to improve survival outcomes of mCRPC and healthcare costs. Widely studied clinical variables with prognostic value in Ra-223 patients included ECOG PS, previous lines of therapy and prior chemotherapy [6,7,12,30]. Furthermore, the number of Ra-223 administered cycles was associated with OS [30,31]. Among laboratory variables, baseline

PSA, LDH, and, especially, ALP (as an indirect index of disease burden) and hemoglobin (as an index of bone marrow reserve) have been shown to provide relevant prognostic insights in these patients [6,7,11,12,30,32].

Similar to previous studies, in our patient's cohort we observed a lower mOS compared to that reported in the ALSYMPCA trial [4]. Moreover, the independent prognostic value of baseline clinical variables such as the ECOG PS, the presence of lymph node metastases and ALP levels was confirmed. Unlike previous studies, we extended our analysis to systemic inflammatory biomarkers as well as to FDG-PET-derived parameters.

Tumor microenvironment and systemic inflammation are known to influence therapeutic response and clinical outcomes [33,34]. Hence, many inflammatory biomarkers are currently under investigation as tools to predict the therapeutic effect or prognosis in different types of advanced cancer [35]. NLR is the most studied, and it is widely established that higher levels of NLR predict poor OS regardless of the tumor type, stage and treatment [14,36]. Other types of inflammatory biomarkers were also assessed for their prognostic role in cancer [37–40]. Among them, NLR, PLR and SII have been shown to be prognostic in mCRCP patients treated with both chemotherapy or new-generation hormonal agents [16,17,41–45]. However, few data on peripheral blood biomarkers are available in mCRPC patients treated with Ra-223. In the last years, few real-world studies showed a reliable, independent disease-related prognostic power of NLR in this setting, mainly related to the prediction of OS and, to a lesser extent, of PFS [5,19,46]. To the best of our knowledge, the present study represents the first analysis of different types of inflammatory biomarkers as prognostic factors in mCRPC patients undergoing Ra-223. However, while both NLR and dNRL were characterized by a prognostic power at the univariate analysis, only a lower baseline NLR was independently associated with longer OS.

On the other hand, FDG-PET-derived parameters displaying the extent (MTV) and the intensity (TLG) of the metabolically active disease burden were predictors of OS. This result reproduces our previous study, which, however, was conducted on a smaller patient sample [20]. Furthermore, in the present study, the multivariate Cox regression analysis showed that the prognostic power of MTV was independent of the one provided by the degree of systemic inflammation.

On the pathophysiological ground, obtained results might improve the comprehension of the still poorly defined molecular mechanisms underlying FDG accumulation in advanced CRPC patients. Indeed, while FDG-PET is not useful in naïve prostate cancer as it shows low FDG-avidity, CRPC patients are characterized by higher levels of FDG uptake, particularly in chemotherapy-refractory patients [47]. The progressive increased FDG avidity in the later stages of CRPC might be explained (at least theoretically) by two different mechanisms. On one side, the overexpression of GLUT-1 in cell membranes and the enhanced Warburg effect characterizing PC cells in advanced stages might justify this phenomenon [48,49]. On the other hand, emerging data support the role of local inflammation and, in particular, of FDG-avid macrophage and lymphocyte recruitment in the tumor microenvironment, as tumor-promoting factors driving PC from the hormone-sensitive stage to refractivity [50,51]. The observed independence between the prognostic power of FDG-PET imaging and systemic inflammation indexes (which roughly measure the degree of tumor inflammation) might imply the prevalence of the former rather than the latter pathway as the underlying mechanism of FDG uptake in mCRPC. In this scenario, the detection of FDG-avid de-differentiated (eventually low osteoblastic) metastatic disease might mirror greater tumor aggressiveness, possibly predicting the lower Ra-223 accumulation and the consequent low-response rate, regardless of the systemic inflammation state (Figure 6) [20,52]. The same considerations also allow us to interpret the observed capability of the composite of pretreatment NLR and MTV (termed IMPI) to stratify the OS. Indeed, patients at the higher IMPI risk class might be characterized by the occurrence of both tumor microenvironment inflammation and de-differentiation, leading to a worst long-term survival and Ra-223 treatment outcome.

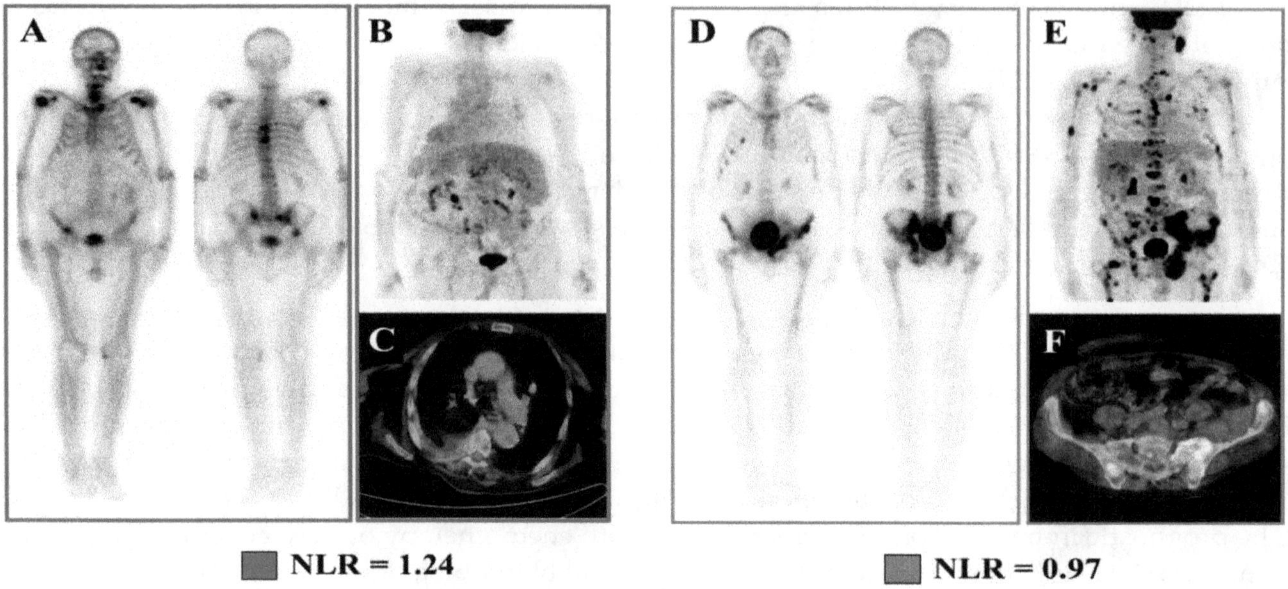

Figure 6. An emblematic example of a mismatch between the metabolic burden of metastatic disease and the systemic inflammation state. At baseline, these two patients showed similar degrees of metastatic burden at bone scan (Panels (**A–D**)) and similar NLR values, while FDG–PET showed a relevant mismatch in the extent of the metabolically active metastatic burden (Panels (**B–E**) show the Maximum intensity projection PET images, while Panels (**C–F**) show the axial section of the hottest bone lesion; MTV = 79.1 cm^3 and 985.4 cm^3, respectively).

Our study has several limitations. First, a major limitation is represented by its retrospective and monocentric nature and the consequent low number of patients analyzed. Indeed, the observed prognostic inadequacy of the systemic inflammatory indexes other than NLR (and its derived counterpart) might be related to the present study's low statistical power. On the other hand, in a subgroup of 11 patients, baseline FDG-PET was not performed. We tried to overcome this limitation through the imputation of missing values. However, the current data should be considered preliminary, while a better-defined comparison between these biomarkers needs to be assessed in a larger multicentric setting. According to this, we are currently planning a retrospective multicenter study to evaluate further the prognostic and predictive value of peripheral blood biomarkers and FDG-PET in Ra-223-treated patients. In this setting, also the immune-metabolic-prognostic index will require further validation. However, despite the sample of our patients was small, it was highly representative of the population enrolled in the ALSYMCA trial [4] as it can be observed comparing the clinical characteristics of the two studies. Similarly, the prognostic role of well-known prognostic factors (ECOG, ALP, lymph node metastases) was confirmed anyway, as further proof of its representativeness. Lastly, the monocentric nature of the analyses may also represent one of the strengths of this study. In fact, all the enrolled patients were submitted to FDG imaging using the same PET/CT scanner, avoiding the possible influence of the inter-scanner variability on PET results, possibly hampering SUVmax, MTV, and TLG reproducibility [53]. Besides the dimension of the patient's cohort, the few clinical collected variables might also represent a potential limitation of the present study. According to this, due to the intrinsic limitations of retrospective data collection, the steroid use by each patient before Ra-223 administration was not recorded and considered as a possible confounding factor. Indeed, corticosteroids might have increased baseline NLR in some patients, introducing potential bias in the data interpretation. However, Lorente et al. previously reported an independent association between baseline NLR and OS in a cohort of mCRPC patients undergoing second-line chemotherapy, regardless of the corticosteroid use at baseline [54]. Moreover, the use of corticosteroids for palliation of symptoms in advanced mCRPC with bone-involvement is well established in clinical practice, and this characteristic of the study cohort highly reflects the setting of the real-world. Larger multicentric studies are required to disclose the robustness of NLR concerning steroid administration in mCRPC patients undergoing Ra-223.

5. Conclusions

The degree of systemic inflammation and the quantification of the metabolically active tumor burden through FDG-PET imaging provide independent prognostic insights in mCRPC patients undergoing Ra-223. The combination of these biomarkers might represent a potentially valuable tool for identifying mCRPC patients who are most likely to benefit from Ra-223 since baseline. Larger studies are needed to further evaluate this hypothesis and, eventually, to confirm these preliminary results.

Author Contributions: Conceptualization, S.E.R., G.F., M.B.; data collection, M.B., M.I.D., A.M., S.R., S.M., S.E.R., F.C., R.B., A.D., V.M. (Veronica Murianni), V.M. (Valentino Martelli), F.B.; Statistical analysis, A.S., M.P.; writing—original draft preparation, S.E.R., M.B., A.S., G.F., F.C., R.B., A.D., V.M. (Veronica Murianni), V.M. (Valentino Martelli); writing—review and editing, M.B., A.S., G.F.; funding acquisition, M.B., C.M., G.S. All authors have read and agreed to the published version of the manuscript.

References

1. Yong, C.; Onukwugha, E.; Mullins, C.D. Clinical and economic burden of bone metastasis and skeletal-related events in prostate cancer. *Curr. Opin. Oncol.* **2014**, *26*, 274–283. [CrossRef] [PubMed]
2. Harrison, M.R.; Wong, T.Z.; Armstrong, A.J.; George, D.J. Radium-223 chloride: A potential new treatment for castration–resistant prostate cancer patients with metastatic bone disease. *Cancer Manag. Res.* **2013**, *5*, 1. [CrossRef] [PubMed]
3. Ritter, M.A.; Cleaver, J.E.; Tobias, C.A. High-LET radiations induce a large proportion of non-rejoining DNA breaks. *Nature* **1977**, *266*, 653–655. [CrossRef] [PubMed]
4. Parker, C.; Nilsson, S.; Heinrich, D.; Helle, S.I.; O'Sullivan, J.M.; Fosså, S.D.; Chodacki, A.; Wiechno, P.; Logue, J.; Seke, M.; et al. Alpha emitter radium-223 and survival in metastatic prostate cancer. *N. Engl. J. Med.* **2013**, *369*, 213–223. [CrossRef] [PubMed]
5. Parikh, S.; Murray, L.; Kenning, L.; Bottomley, D.; Din, O.; Dixit, S.; Ferguson, C.; Handforth, C.; Joseph, L.; Mokhtar, D.; et al. Real-world Outcomes and Factors Predicting Survival and Completion of Radium 223 in Metastatic Castrate-resistant Prostate Cancer. *Clin. Oncol.* **2018**, *30*, 548–555. [CrossRef] [PubMed]
6. Wong, W.W.; Anderson, E.M.; Mohammadi, H.; Daniels, T.B.; Schild, S.E.; Keole, S.R.; Choo, C.R.; Tzou, K.S.; Bryce, A.H.; Ho, T.H.; et al. Factors Associated with Survival Following Radium-223 Treatment for Metastatic Castration-resistant Prostate Cancer. *Clin. Genitourin. Cancer* **2017**, *15*, e969–e975. [CrossRef] [PubMed]
7. Frantellizzi, V.; Farcomeni, A.; Follacchio, G.A.; Pacilio, M.; Pellegrini, R.; Pani, R.; De Vincentis, G. A 3-variable prognostic score (3-PS) for overall survival prediction in metastatic castration-resistant prostate cancer treated with 223Radium-dichloride. *Ann. Nucl. Med.* **2018**, *32*, 142–148. [CrossRef]
8. EMA. EMA Restricts Use of Prostate Cancer Medicine XOFIGO. Available online: https://www.ema.europa.eu/en/news/ema--restricts--use--prostate--cancer--medicine--xofigo#:~{}:text=The%20European%20Medicines%20Agency%20(EMA,who%20cannot%20receive%20other%20treatments (accessed on 20 October 2020).
9. Kuppen, M.C.; Westgeest, H.M.; van der Doelen, M.J.; van den Eertwegh, A.J.; Coenen, J.L.; Aben, K.K.; van den Bergh, A.C.; Bergman, A.M.; den Bosch, J.V.; Celik, F.; et al. Real-world outcomes of radium-223 dichloride for metastatic castration resistant prostate cancer. *Future Oncol.* **2020**, *16*, 1371–1384. [CrossRef]
10. Stolten, M.D.; Steinberger, A.E.; Cotogno, P.M.; Ledet, E.M.; Lewis, B.E.; Sartor, O. Parameters Associated with 6 Cycles of Radium-223 Dichloride Therapy in Metastatic Castrate-Resistant Prostate Cancer. *Int. J. Radiat. Oncol.* **2015**, *93*, E196. [CrossRef]
11. Etchebehere, E.C.; Milton, D.R.; Araujo, J.C.; Swanston, N.M.; Macapinlac, H.A.; Rohren, E.M. Factors affecting 223Ra therapy: Clinical experience after 532 cycles from a single institution. *Eur. J. Nucl. Med. Mol. Imaging* **2016**, *43*, 8–20. [CrossRef]

12. Sartor, O.; Coleman, R.E.; Nilsson, S.; Heinrich, D.; Helle, S.I.; O'Sullivan, J.M.; Vogelzang, N.J.; Bruland, Ø.; Kobina, S.; Wilhelm, S.; et al. An exploratory analysis of alkaline phosphatase, lactate dehydrogenase, and prostate-specific antigen dynamics in the phase 3 ALSYMPCA trial with radium-223. *Ann. Oncol.* **2017**, *28*, 1090–1097. [CrossRef]
13. Prelaj, A.; Rebuzzi, S.E.; Buzzacchino, F.; Pozzi, C.; Ferrara, C.; Frantellizzi, V.; Follacchio, G.A.; Civitelli, L.; De Vincentis, G.; Tomao, S.; et al. Radium-223 in patients with metastatic castration-resistant prostate cancer: Efficacy and safety in clinical practice. *Oncol. Lett.* **2019**, *17*, 1467–1476. [CrossRef] [PubMed]
14. Templeton, A.J.; McNamara, M.G.; Šeruga, B.; Vera-Badillo, F.E.; Aneja, P.; Ocaña, A.; Leibowitz-Amit, R.; Sonpavde, G.; Knox, J.J.; Tran, B.; et al. Prognostic Role of Neutrophil-to-Lymphocyte Ratio in Solid Tumors: A Systematic Review and Meta-Analysis. *JNCI J. Natl. Cancer Inst.* **2014**, *106*. [CrossRef] [PubMed]
15. Prelaj, A.; Rebuzzi, S.E.; Pizzutilo, P.; Bilancia, M.; Montrone, M.; Pesola, F.; Longo, V.; Del Bene, G.; Lapadula, V.; Cassano, F.; et al. EPSILoN: A Prognostic Score Using Clinical and Blood Biomarkers in Advanced Non-Small-Cell Lung Cancer Treated with Immunotherapy. *Clin. Lung Cancer* **2020**, *21*, 365–377.e5. [CrossRef]
16. Guan, Y.; Xiong, H.; Feng, Y.; Liao, G.; Tong, T.; Pang, J. Revealing the prognostic landscape of neutrophil-to-lymphocyte ratio and platelet-to-lymphocyte ratio in metastatic castration-resistant prostate cancer patients treated with abiraterone or enzalutamide: A meta-analysis. *Prostate Cancer Prostatic Dis.* **2020**, *23*, 220–231. [CrossRef] [PubMed]
17. Man, Y.; Chen, Y. Systemic immune-inflammation index, serum albumin, and fibrinogen impact prognosis in castration–resistant prostate cancer patients treated with first-line docetaxel. *Int. Urol. Nephrol.* **2019**, *51*, 2189–2199. [CrossRef]
18. McKay, R.R.; Jacobus, S.; Fiorillo, M.; Ledet, E.M.; Cotogna, P.M.; Steinberger, A.E.; Jacene, H.A.; Sartor, O.; Taplin, M.-E. Radium-223 Use in Clinical Practice and Variables Associated with Completion of Therapy. *Clin. Genitourin. Cancer* **2017**, *15*, e289–e298. [CrossRef] [PubMed]
19. Maruzzo, M.; Basso, U.; Borsatti, E.; Evangelista, L.; Alongi, F.; Caffo, O.; Maines, F.; Galuppo, S.; De Vivo, R.; Zustovich, F.; et al. Results from a Large, Multicenter, Retrospective Analysis on Radium223 Use in Metastatic Castration-Resistant Prostate Cancer (mCRPC) in the Triveneto Italian Region. *Clin. Genitourin. Cancer* **2019**, *17*, e187–e194. [CrossRef]
20. Bauckneht, M.; Capitanio, S.; Donegani, M.I.; Zanardi, E.; Miceli, A.; Murialdo, R.; Raffa, S.; Tomasello, L.; Vitti, M.; Cavo, A.; et al. Role of Baseline and Post-Therapy 18F-FDG PET in the Prognostic Stratification of Metastatic Castration-Resistant Prostate Cancer (mCRPC) Patients Treated with Radium-223. *Cancers* **2019**, *12*, 31. [CrossRef]
21. Poeppel, T.D.; Handkiewicz-Junak, D.; Andreeff, M.; Becherer, A.; Bockisch, A.; Fricke, E.; Geworski, L.; Heinzel, A.; Krause, B.J.; Krause, T.; et al. EANM guideline for radionuclide therapy with radium-223 of metastatic castration-resistant prostate cancer. *Eur. J. Nucl. Med. Mol. Imaging* **2018**, *45*, 824–845. [CrossRef]
22. Jadvar, H. Imaging evaluation of prostate cancer with 18F-fluorodeoxyglucose PET/CT: Utility and limitations. *Eur. J. Nucl. Med. Mol. Imaging* **2013**, *40*, 5–10. [CrossRef] [PubMed]
23. AIOM Guidelines on Prostate Cancer. 2019. Available online: https://www.aiom.it/linee--guida--aiom--carcinoma--della--prostata--2019/ (accessed on 20 October 2020).
24. Boellaard, R.; Delgado–Bolton, R.; Oyen, W.J.G.; Giammarile, F.; Tatsch, K.; Eschner, W.; Verzijlbergen, F.J.; Barrington, S.F.; Pike, L.C.; Weber, W.A.; et al. FDG PET/CT: EANM procedure guidelines for tumour imaging: Version 2.0. *Eur. J. Nucl. Med. Mol. Imaging* **2015**, *42*, 328–354. [CrossRef] [PubMed]
25. Kruse, V.I.B.E.K.E.; Mees, G.; Maes, A.; D'Asseler, Y.V.E.S.; Borms, M.; Cocquyt, V.; Van De Wiele, C. Reproducibility of FDG PET based metabolic tumor volume measurements and of their FDG distribution within. *Q. J. Nucl. Med. Mol. Imaging* **2015**, *59*, 462–468. [PubMed]
26. Bland, J.M.; Altman, D.G. Measuring agreement in method comparison studies. *Stat. Methods Med. Res.* **1999**, *8*, 135–160. [CrossRef]
27. Epstein, J.I.; Egevad, L.; Srigley, J.R.; Humphrey, P.A. The 2014 International Society of Urological Pathology (ISUP) Consensus Conference on Gleason Grading of Prostatic Carcinoma. *Am. J. Surg. Pathol.* **2016**, *40*, 9. [CrossRef]
28. Castello, A.; Toschi, L.; Rossi, S.; Mazziotti, E.; Lopci, E. The immune-metabolic-prognostic index and clinical outcomes in patients with non-small cell lung carcinoma under checkpoint inhibitors. *J. Cancer Res. Clin. Oncol.* **2020**, *146*, 1235–1243. [CrossRef]

29. Van den Wyngaert, T.; Tombal, B. The changing role of radium-223 in metastatic castrate-resistant prostate cancer: Has the EMA missed the mark with revising the label? *Q. J. Nucl. Med. Mol. Imaging* **2019**, *63*, 170–182. [CrossRef]
30. van der Doelen, M.J.; Mehra, N.; Hermsen, R.; Janssen, M.J.R.; Gerritsen, W.R.; van Oort, I.M. Patient Selection for Radium-223 Therapy in Patients with Bone Metastatic Castration-Resistant Prostate Cancer: New Recommendations and Future Perspectives. *Clin. Genitourin. Cancer* **2019**, *17*, 79–87. [CrossRef]
31. Saad, F.; Carles, J.; Gillessen, S.; Heidenreich, A.; Heinrich, D.; Gratt, J.; Lévy, J.; Miller, K.; Nilsson, S.; Petrenciuc, O.; et al. Radium-223 and concomitant therapies in patients with metastatic castration-resistant prostate cancer: An international, early access, open-label, single-arm phase 3b trial. *Lancet Oncol.* **2016**, *17*, 1306–1316. [CrossRef]
32. Vogelzang, N.J.; Coleman, R.E.; Michalski, J.M.; Nilsson, S.; O'Sullivan, J.M.; Parker, C.; Widmark, A.; Thuresson, M.; Xu, L.; Germino, J.; et al. Hematologic Safety of Radium-223 Dichloride: Baseline Prognostic Factors Associated with Myelosuppression in the ALSYMPCA Trial. *Clin. Genitourin. Cancer* **2017**, *15*, 42–52.e8. [CrossRef]
33. Hanahan, D.; Weinberg, R.A. Hallmarks of Cancer: The Next Generation. *Cell* **2011**, *144*, 646–674. [CrossRef] [PubMed]
34. Wu, T.; Dai, Y. Tumor microenvironment and therapeutic response. *Cancer Lett.* **2017**, *387*, 61–68. [CrossRef] [PubMed]
35. Chen, L.; Kong, X.; Yan, C.; Fang, Y.; Wang, J. The Research Progress on the Prognostic Value of the Common Hematological Parameters in Peripheral Venous Blood in Breast Cancer. *Onco Targets Ther.* **2020**, *13*, 1397–1412. [CrossRef] [PubMed]
36. Tang, L.; Li, X.; Wang, B.; Luo, G.; Gu, L.; Chen, L.; Liu, K.; Gao, Y.; Zhang, X. Prognostic Value of Neutrophil-to-Lymphocyte Ratio in Localized and Advanced Prostate Cancer: A Systematic Review and Meta-Analysis. *PLoS ONE* **2016**, *11*, e0153981. [CrossRef]
37. Dolan, R.D.; McSorley, S.T.; Horgan, P.G.; Laird, B.; McMillan, D.C. The role of the systemic inflammatory response in predicting outcomes in patients with advanced inoperable cancer: Systematic review and meta -analysis. *Crit. Rev. Oncol. Hematol.* **2017**, *116*, 134–146. [CrossRef]
38. Templeton, A.J.; Ace, O.; McNamara, M.G.; Al-Mubarak, M.; Vera-Badillo, F.E.; Hermanns, T.; Šeruga, B.; Ocana, A.; Tannock, I.F.; Amir, E. Prognostic Role of Platelet to Lymphocyte Ratio in Solid Tumors: A Systematic Review and Meta-Analysis. *Cancer Epidemiol. Biomark. Prev.* **2014**, *23*, 1204–1212. [CrossRef]
39. Zhong, J.H.; Huang, D.H.; Chen, Z.Y. Prognostic role of systemic immune-inflammation index in solid tumors: A systematic review and meta-analysis. *Oncotarget* **2017**, *8*, 75381–75388. [CrossRef]
40. Mao, Y.; Chen, D.; Duan, S.; Zhao, Y.; Wu, C.; Zhu, F.; Chen, C.; Chen, Y. Prognostic impact of pretreatment lymphocyte-to-monocyte ratio in advanced epithelial cancers: A meta-analysis. *Cancer Cell Int.* **2018**, *18*, 201. [CrossRef]
41. Nuhn, P.; Vaghasia, A.M.; Goyal, J.; Zhou, X.C.; Carducci, M.A.; Eisenberger, M.A.; Antonarakis, E.S. Association of pretreatment neutrophil-to-lymphocyte ratio (NLR) and overall survival (OS) in patients with metastatic castration-resistant prostate cancer (mCRPC) treated with first-line docetaxel: NLR predicts OS in men with mCRPC receiving docetaxel. *BJU Int.* **2014**, *114*, E11–E17. [CrossRef]
42. Sonpavde, G.; Pond, G.R.; Armstrong, A.J.; Clarke, S.J.; Vardy, J.L.; Templeton, A.J.; Wang, S.-L.; Paolini, J.; Chen, I.; Chow-Maneval, E.; et al. Prognostic Impact of the Neutrophil-to-Lymphocyte Ratio in Men with Metastatic Castration-Resistant Prostate Cancer. *Clin. Genitourin. Cancer* **2014**, *12*, 317–324. [CrossRef]
43. Lozano Martínez, A.J.; Moreno Cano, R.; Escobar Páramo, S.; Salguero Aguilar, R.; Gonzalez Billalabeitia, E.; García Fernández, R.; De La Fuente Muñoz, I.; Romero Borque, A.; Porras Martínez, M.; Lopez Soler, F.; et al. Platelet-lymphocyte and neutrophil-lymphocyte ratios are prognostic but not predictive of response to abiraterone acetate in metastatic castration-resistant prostate cancer. *Clin. Transl. Oncol.* **2017**, *19*, 1531–1536. [CrossRef] [PubMed]
44. Loubersac, T.; Nguile-Makao, M.; Pouliot, F.; Fradet, V.; Toren, P. Neutrophil-to-lymphocyte Ratio as a Predictive Marker of Response to Abiraterone Acetate: A Retrospective Analysis of the COU302 Study. *Eur. Urol. Oncol.* **2020**, *3*, 298–305. [CrossRef] [PubMed]

45. Lolli, C.; Caffo, O.; Scarpi, E.; Aieta, M.; Conteduca, V.; Maines, F.; Bianchi, E.; Massari, F.; Veccia, A.; Chiuri, V.E.; et al. Systemic Immune-Inflammation Index Predicts the Clinical Outcome in Patients with mCRPC Treated with Abiraterone. *Front. Pharmacol.* **2016**, *7*. [CrossRef] [PubMed]
46. Jiang, X.Y.; Atkinson, S.; Pearson, R.; Leaning, D.; Cumming, S.; Burns, A.; Azzabi, A.; Frew, J.; McMenemin, R.; Pedley, I.D. Optimising Radium 223 Therapy for Metastatic Castration-Resistant Prostate Cancer-5-year Real-World Outcome: Focusing on Treatment Sequence and Quality of Life. *Clin. Oncol.* **2020**, S0936655520301965. [CrossRef]
47. Jadvar, H.; Desai, B.; Ji, L.; Conti, P.S.; Dorff, T.B.; Groshen, S.G.; Pinski, J.K.; Quinn, D.I. Baseline 18F-FDG PET/CT Parameters as Imaging Biomarkers of Overall Survival in Castrate-Resistant Metastatic Prostate Cancer. *J. Nucl. Med.* **2013**, *54*, 1195–1201. [CrossRef]
48. Eidelman, E.; Twum-Ampofo, J.; Ansari, J.; Siddiqui, M.M. The Metabolic Phenotype of Prostate Cancer. *Front. Oncol.* **2017**, *7*, 131. [CrossRef] [PubMed]
49. Meziou, S.; Ringuette Goulet, C.; Hovington, H.; Lefebvre, V.; Lavallée, É.; Bergeron, M.; Brisson, H.; Champagne, A.; Neveu, B.; Lacombe, D.; et al. GLUT1 expression in high-risk prostate cancer: Correlation with 18F-FDG-PET/CT and clinical outcome. *Prostate Cancer Prostatic Dis.* **2020**. [CrossRef]
50. Jin, R.J.; Lho, Y.; Connelly, L.; Wang, Y.; Yu, X.; Saint Jean, L.; Case, T.C.; Ellwood-Yen, K.; Sawyers, C.L.; Bhowmick, N.A.; et al. The Nuclear Factor-B Pathway Controls the Progression of Prostate Cancer to Androgen-Independent Growth. *Cancer Res.* **2008**, *68*, 6762–6769. [CrossRef]
51. Ammirante, M.; Luo, J.-L.; Grivennikov, S.; Nedospasov, S.; Karin, M. B-cell-derived lymphotoxin promotes castration-resistant prostate cancer. *Nature* **2010**, *464*, 302–305. [CrossRef]
52. Fox, J.J.; Gavane, S.C.; Blanc-Autran, E.; Nehmeh, S.; Gönen, M.; Beattie, B.; Vargas, H.A.; Schöder, H.; Humm, J.L.; Fine, S.W.; et al. Positron Emission Tomography/Computed Tomography-Based Assessments of Androgen Receptor Expression and Glycolytic Activity as a Prognostic Biomarker for Metastatic Castration-Resistant Prostate Cancer. *JAMA Oncol.* **2018**, *4*, 217. [CrossRef]
53. Keyes, J.W. SUV: Standard Uptake or Silly Useless Value? *J. Nucl. Med.* **1995**, *36*, 1836–1839. [PubMed]
54. Lorente, D.; Mateo, J.; Templeton, A.J.; Zafeiriou, Z.; Bianchini, D.; Ferraldeschi, R.; Bahl, A.; Shen, L.; Su, Z.; Sartor, O.; et al. Baseline neutrophil-lymphocyte ratio (NLR) is associated with survival and response to treatment with second-line chemotherapy for advanced prostate cancer independent of baseline steroid use. *Ann. Oncol.* **2015**, *26*, 750–755. [CrossRef] [PubMed]

3

Nanoparticles as Theranostic Vehicles in Experimental and Clinical Applications—Focus on Prostate and Breast Cancer

Jörgen Elgqvist [1,2]

[1] Department of Medical Physics and Biomedical Engineering, Sahlgrenska University Hospital, 413 45 Gothenburg, Sweden; jorgen.elgqvist@vgregion.se or jorgen.elgqvist@gu.se
[2] Department of Physics, University of Gothenburg, 412 96 Gothenburg, Sweden

Academic Editor: Carsten Stephan

Abstract: Prostate and breast cancer are the second most and most commonly diagnosed cancer in men and women worldwide, respectively. The American Cancer Society estimates that during 2016 in the USA around 430,000 individuals were diagnosed with one of these two types of cancers, and approximately 15% of them will die from the disease. In Europe, the rate of incidences and deaths are similar to those in the USA. Several different more or less successful diagnostic and therapeutic approaches have been developed and evaluated in order to tackle this issue and thereby decrease the death rates. By using nanoparticles as vehicles carrying both diagnostic and therapeutic molecular entities, individualized targeted theranostic nanomedicine has emerged as a promising option to increase the sensitivity and the specificity during diagnosis, as well as the likelihood of survival or prolonged survival after therapy. This article presents and discusses important and promising different kinds of nanoparticles, as well as imaging and therapy options, suitable for theranostic applications. The presentation of different nanoparticles and theranostic applications is quite general, but there is a special focus on prostate cancer. Some references and aspects regarding breast cancer are however also presented and discussed. Finally, the prostate cancer case is presented in more detail regarding diagnosis, staging, recurrence, metastases, and treatment options available today, followed by possible ways to move forward applying theranostics for both prostate and breast cancer based on promising experiments performed until today.

Keywords: nanoparticles; theranostics; nanomedicine; prostate cancer; breast cancer

1. Introduction

In order to be able to combine both a therapeutic and a diagnostic function into a single molecular entity, the research on and development of theranostic nanoparticles (TNPs) have increased continuously during the last couple of years (the MeSH (Medical Subject Headings) term "theranostics" gave 0 hits for 2004 but 801 for 2016 on Pubmed) [1–8]. These type of nanosized drug vehicles have been developed and tested in different settings such as, for example, iron oxide, gadolinium, gold, manganese, or polymeric nanoparticles (NPs), quantum dots, and liposomes for the diagnosis and treatment of various diseases [1–18]. The dimensions of these different molecular nanostructures is generally less than 100 nm, and two of the common goals for all different settings is to maximize the drug loading capacity, and increase the specificity of the TNPs towards cancer cells [1]. The key benefit of TNPs is that they have the possibility to increase the therapeutic efficacy, partly due to ameliorated drug circulation times increasing the tumor uptake, but also to lessen the risk of unwanted toxic effects on healthy tissue [16–20]. Another important feature of the TNPs is that the diagnostic and therapeutic functionality could be localized to the exact same position due to the attachment of both these agents on the same molecular drug vehicle. Compared to other larger molecular vehicles these small NPs has a larger surface-area-to-volume ratio. This feature allows the TNPs to reach the capillary bed while at the same time carry a large variety of therapeutic and diagnostic agents themselves.

When considering the use of NPs for cancer treatment or diagnosis, the enhanced permeability and retention (EPR) effect plays a central role, although this effect seems to vary among individuals in the human population [2,19,21]. The EPR effect is also believed not to be present or even similar for all types of tumors, as well as not being the only parameter responsible for the efficacy of a certain NP application [22]. Parameters such as the level of unwanted drug release into the systemic circulation and the intra-tumoral allocation as well as the amount and kinetics of the intra-tumoral drug release will also determine the final efficacy [22].

However, the EPR effect can make TNPs accumulate, and be retained, to a higher degree in tumor tissue as compared to normal tissue, due to leakiness of the increased vasculature in the tumor tissue [19,20,23]. Magnetic resonance imaging (MRI) is a valuable tool for image and evaluate the degree of accumulation due to its high spatial resolution in both tumors and healthy tissue [24]. During MRI, Gd(III) (Gd^{3+}) based contrast agents are very effective and highly paramagnetic substances, enhancing the contrast by increasing the T1 relaxation rate R1 (=1/T1), due to its rare electronic configuration of seven unpaired electron spins. By combining Gd(III) with different kind of NPs it would be possible to increase the accumulation and retention time in tumors, and therefore even more increase the MRI contrast [25–34]. TNPs could then be developed with the Gd(III)-based MRI contrast agent combined with, for example, a therapeutic drug for cancer such as gemcitabine [35,36].

Another strong argument for developing a NP based anti-cancer technology is that it could enable earlier detection of the disease. Early detection is most often absolutely crucial and decides whether a cancer patient will have the possibility to be cured, or just receive a treatment extending survival before finally succumbing to the disease. It is a well-known fact that the major cause of mortality in cancer is due to tumor metastasis [37–39]. In most cases, the dissemination of the cancerous disease is caused by tumor cells that have shed from the primary tumor and enters into the systemic circulation, i.e., circulating tumor cells CTCs. The idea of CTCs was first noticed by Dr. Tomas Ashworth already in 1869 [40]. However, while CTCs can only be confirmed and monitored in patients having a more or less advanced cancerous disease [39,41–54], the goal for a nanomedical approach would be to detect the CTCs at a much earlier time point compared to what is possible today [55,56].

The significance of the TNP technology regarding cancer in general is that it potentially could diagnose better, using multimodal imaging, and at the same time more effectively treat these diseases, especially in the disseminated cases. To achieve this, different types of isotopes could be attached to the TNPs. By attaching, for example, specific monoclonal antibodies (mAbs), fraction of mAbs, or peptides to these multifunctional TNPs highly specific and therefore targeted imaging and radiation therapies could be achieved. Personalized medicine might be possible using TNPs, since the imaging of drug accumulation in individual patients would be possible. Such imaging would refer to both tumor as well as healthy tissue and would then make it possible to estimate and predict, to a better degree than what is possible today, the therapeutic efficacy, and also make possible adjustments of ongoing regimens [2,19–21,23].

This article presents different type of NPs, imaging, and therapy options, as well as promising theranostic applications utilizing those techniques, with a focus on prostate cancer (PCa) and breast cancer (BC). Relevant PCa and BC references are presented and discussed in every section, but towards the end of the article the PCa case is given extra focus regarding diagnosis, staging, recurrence, metastases, and treatment options available today. Finally, possible ways to move forward applying theranostics for both PCa and BC are suggested and discussed based on promising experiments performed until today.

2. Nanoparticles for Prostate and Breast Cancer

The development of different and innovative NPs for various medical applications has increased tremendously during the past couple of years. Despite some problems with relatively low tumor uptake in some cancer applications, there is today a number of promising alternatives that have been tested or are under the development [57–90]. Below follows a presentation of important and interesting NP alternatives suitable for PCa and BC, some of which already have been tested for these type of diseases while some are still to be explored more thoroughly. For example, since the Nobel Prize in 2010 to Dr. Geim and Dr. Novoselov for their pioneering work on the two-dimensional material graphene, several promising NPs have since been suggested, developed, and tested based on that material. A prerequisite although, before any translation into clinical use of any NPs, is a meticulous survey of their pharmacological and toxicological properties. The presentation below summarizes the most important general characteristics of the NP options, and to what extent they have been used in the PCa and BC context so far. When possible, theranostic applications are referenced to and discussed shortly for each type of NP. In addition to theranostic applications, some studies in which only an imaging or therapeutic approach has been used are also referenced to for each type of NP.

2.1. *Iron Oxide Nanoparticles*

Due to their magnetic properties, with a diameter ranging from a few nanometers up to approximately 100 nm, iron oxide particles have been evaluated and used in several magnetic resonance technology-based biomedical applications such as multifunctional theranostic complexes combining tumor targeting, imaging as well as cancer nanotherapy in personalized cancer treatment [91–100]. The superparamagnetic iron oxide NPs (SPIONs) are most often used, and the subpopulation of ultrasmall SPIONs denoted as USPIOs defined as having a diameter of less than ~20 nm. A schematic representation of an iron oxide NP is shown in Figure 1. Three main variants of this NP are magnetite (Fe_3O_4), hematite (α-Fe_2O_3), and maghemite (γ-Fe_2O_3). The two latter being differently structured (rhombohedral and cubic, respectively) allotropic oxidized forms of magnetite. γ-Fe_2O_3 and Fe_3O_4 are preferred in medical applications due to their lack of toxicity and good biocompatibility in humans. Since SPIONSs tend to aggregate due to magnetic, van der Waals, and/or hydrophilic/hydrophobic forces it is important to minimize this effect in biomedical applications by different kind of surface modifications, for example, by PEGylation. PEGylation of a NP means attaching polyethylene glycol (PEG) molecules to its surface, thereby not only hindering aggregation but also masking the NP from the immune system. Other type of coatings can also be necessary for certain applications. For example, if SPIONs is used as a contrast agent during photoacoustic imaging, using near-infrared (IR) light, the NPs could be coated with silica (SiO_2), enhancing the light absorption compared to the bare iron oxide NP [101–103]. Regarding diagnosis iron oxide NPs have been used for atherosclerotic evaluation, gene expression analysis, inflammation, angiogenesis, stem-cell tracking and also for cancer diagnosis.

Specifically, for PCa and BC there is ongoing research on different applications using these kind of NPs [93,104–115]. For example, regarding PCa, Zhu et al. have performed synthesis, characterization, an in vitro binding assay, and an in vivo magnetic resonance imaging (MRI) evaluation of prostate specific membrane antigen (PSMA) targeting SPIONs. They showed specific uptake of their polypeptide-based SPIONs by the PSMA expressing cells, and that the MRI signal could be specifically enhanced. They concluded that PSMA-targeting SPIONs might provide a new strategy for imaging PCa [107]. As an example regarding BC, Pasha Shaik et al. recently performed experiments on blocking the IL4-α receptor (IL4Rα) using PEGylated SPIONs to inhibit BC cell proliferation [111]. They found that for 4T1 cells, blocking of this receptor caused a significant decrease in cell viability and induced apoptosis. They also concluded that a combined treatment using SPION-IL4Rα-doxorubicin caused significant increases in cell death, apoptosis, and oxidative stress, compared to either SPION-IL4Rα or doxorubicin alone.

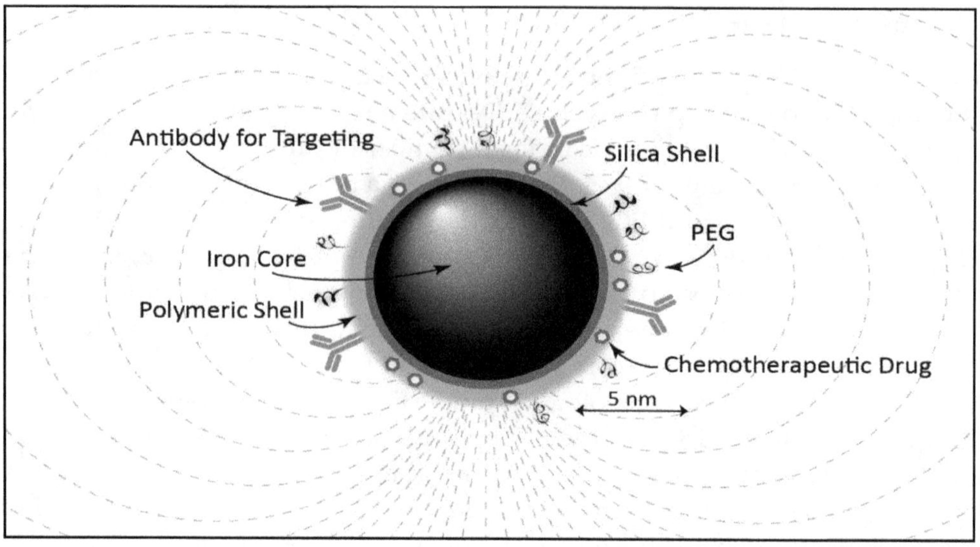

Figure 1. Functionalized iron-oxide nanoparticle. Functional biocompatible polymers are grafted onto an inorganic core of magnetite (Fe_3O_4) or maghemite (Fe_2O_3) through an anchoring group, such as an amine, carboxylic acid or phosphonic acid group. The polymeric shell improves the stability of the iron oxide nanoparticles (NPs) in solution, and also allows the encapsulation of, for example, therapeutic agents. An alternative coating in the form of a fluorescent silica (SiO_2) produces a type of iron oxide NPs often referred to as SCIONs, i.e., silica coated iron oxide NPs. It should be noted that the polymeric shell has to be very opaque in order not to block the fluorescent silica-based core, if used simultaneous. Most commonly, experiments with only a polymeric or a silica core have been evaluated. The custom size of an iron oxide NP is in the range of 10–20 nm, as exemplified by a 10 nm in diameter iron core in the figure. Indicated in the figure are also the magnetic field lines created by this type of NP.

2.2. Gadolinium, Manganese, Gold, Silver, and Platinum Nanoparticles

For many years, gadolinium (Gd^{3+}, Gd(III)) has been used in different contrast media for magnetic resonance imaging (MRI) during, for example, angiography or brain tumor imaging due to its paramagnetic characteristics, ability to shorten the T1 relaxation time, and to cross a degraded blood-brain barrier [116]. The research on contrast media based on the paramagnetic element manganese (Mn^{2+}, Mn(II)) intended for MRI and NPs has just started to accelerate in recent years. For example, carbon and Mn^{2+} based NPs have been evaluated as contrast agents for MRI, or as manganese enhance MRI (MEMRI) during in vivo studies or for functional brain imaging [117–122]. Different applications such as Mn(II)–Au NPs as MRI contrast agents in stem cell labeling or Mn(II) based prussian blue($Fe_7(CN)_{18}$)-based NPs as a theranostic agent having ultrahigh pH-responsive longitudinal relaxivity have also been investigated [123,124].

Gold NPs (AuNPs) in the form of nano-cages, -spheres, -beacons, -stars, -shells, -seeds, -sheets, or nanorods is being evaluated in many different settings, for example, for both PCa and BC (Figure 2) [8,125–141]. By changing the AuNPs' shape, size, or surface characteristics it is possible to fine-tune their properties in order to maximize their applicability as a tool for cancer diagnosis, photo-dynamic/thermal therapy, therapy-drug carrier, radiotherapy drug enhancer, targeted gene therapy, or as a combined theranostic nanovehicle [142–155]. Regarding the gene therapy approach, in which for example, small-interference RNA (siRNA) could be utilized in order to knock out specific gene expressions in cancer cells, it has received increased attention recent years. For example, Guo et al. have recently shown interesting results on the PCa cells PC-3 and LNCaP indicating that two of their investigated formulations with transferrin and folate-receptor targeting ligands respectively (AuNPs-PEG-Tf and AuNPs-PEI-FA) show potential as non-viral gene delivery vectors in the treatment of PCa [141]. The photo-dynamic/thermal technique has also shown some progress recent years for both PCa and BC [156–165]. For example, Oh et al. have shown promising PCa cell killing efficacy by using a 55 nm small icosahedral phage that was engineered to display a gold-binding peptide as well as a PCa cell-binding peptide and applying a 60 mW/cm^2 light irradiation [156]. Mkandawire et al. have recently investigated an alternative way to treat BC cells inducing apoptosis by targeting their mitochondria using AuNPs during photothermal treatment [164]. Regarding tumor detection, surface enhanced Raman spectroscopy (SERS) can be used for in vivo applications, and some studies have been performed recent years investigating its applicability for PCa and BC [129,161,166–170]. Ramaya et al. investigated the overexpression of prostate specific antigen (PSA) in LNCaP cells by using tetraphenylethylene (TPE) appended organic fluorogens adsorbed on AuNPs. Indoline-based TPE-AuNPs were efficient recognizing PSA overexpressing LNCaP cells using SERS mapping. For BC for example, Butler et al. investigated MCF-7 (Michigan Cancer Foundation-7) cells incubated with 150 nm AuNPs and concluded that they were a good starting point for near-infrared (NIR) or infrared (IR) SERS analysis [168].

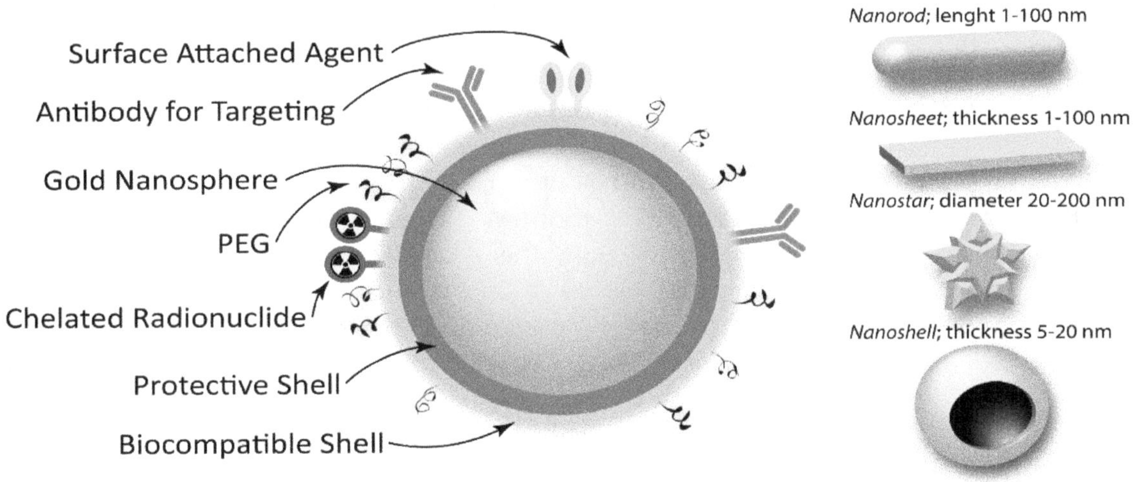

Figure 2. Image showing an example of a nanosphere of gold (Au). Gold nanoparticles (NPs) can also be based on, for example, nano-rods, -sheets, -stars, -or nanoshells, as indicated to the right with typical dimensions. The Au-nanospheres are most often produced in the size interval of 5 to 400 nm in diameter, approximately. The characteristics of AuNPs, and therefore their application possibilities, strongly depend on size, shape, and surface functionalities. Indicated in the image are also a protective and a biocompatible shell encapsulating the Au nanosphere, enabling the attachment of different kind of targeting vectors, imaging agents, therapeutic drugs, as well as polyethylene glycol (PEG) molecules. The latter an important parameter in order to protect the NPs from the immune system, to avoid reticuloendothelial system (RES) uptake, and to minimize nonspecific binding.

The use of silver NPs (AgNPs) for medical applications has not been as intense as that of AuNPs. Regarding PCa and BC, however, there have been some studies published for different applications during recent years [171–182]. For example, Wang et al. developed a Ag-hybridized-silica-NP-based electrochemical immunosensor for the sensing of PSA in human serum with promising results [172], and Swanner et al. investigated the radiosensitizing and cytotoxic effect on triple-negative BC using AgNPs with good results at doses that have little effect on nontumorigenic BC cells [178].

Platinum-based NPs (PtNPs) is also a technique with a relatively low number of publications for PCa and BC applications, and then most often in the context of AuNPs, FeONPs, or for immunosensor applications [183–192]. Cui et al. developed an immunoassay based on mesoporous PtNPs, evaluated its efficacy against the BC tumor markers CA125, CA153, and CEA, and concluded its high potential clinic value [185]. Spain et al. recently proposed an electrochemical immunosensor based on PtNPs conjugated to a recombinant scFv antibody for the detection of PSA during PCa diagnosis, and showed that picomolar PSA concentrations could be detected without the need for further PCR or nucleic-acid-sequence-based amplification (NASBA) techniques [188].

2.3. Quantum and Cornell Dots

The semi-conductor metal based NPs called quantum dots (QDs) have, due to their adjustable properties, been used and tested in many electronic applications such as LCD displays and solar cells [193,194]. However, lately they are also evaluated in cancer research and medical-imaging applications and are usually fabricated in sizes of approximately 2–7 nm in diameter [195–197]. Examples of such, from blood rapidly excreted NPs based on combinations of different semi-conductor and heavy metals, are CdSe, CdS, PbS ZnS, InP, and CdTe, having fluorescence emission spectra in the region of 450–950 nm depending mainly on size and which type of coating the QDs have for a certain application [198,199]. A common coating is polyethylene glycol (PEG), which has the effect of increasing the blood circulation time by decreasing the kidney clearance.

Due to concerns regarding the heavy metal involvement in the QDs alternatives have been developed. One such option is the silica based Cornell dots (C dots) [200], first invented by Uli Wiesner (Wiesner Group, Cornell University, USA). The spherically shaped C dots are constructed with a silica based core, in which fluorescent molecules (fluorophores) are embedded, surrounded by a PEGylated silica shell [201]. In order to turn these C dots into targeted cancer probes one possibility is then to label chains in the PEG molecule with peptides or (fraction of) monoclonal antibodies (mAbs) that are site specific for certain cancer cell receptors. If the cancer cell bound C dots are illuminated using a near-infrared light source they fluoresce and can then serve as, for example, optical guidance for surgeons. Besides this diagnostic and surgical tool the C dots can of course also be labeled with suitable anticancer drugs or radioactive isotopes, and therefore also serve as a nanovehicle for targeted cancer therapy. It should be noted that PEGylation of C dots causes them to be rapidly excreted via the kidneys, as opposed to the QDs, decreasing blood circulation times [202–205]. A first clinical trial performed at the Memorial Sloan Kettering Cancer Center (MSKCC) in New York, USA, investigated radioactive iodine-labeled 7 nm C dots on five metastatic melanoma patients regarding positron emission tomography (PET) traceability and toxicity. The results showed that, under the U.S. Food and Drug Administration's (FDA's) Investigational New Drug (IND) guidelines, these type of NPs were safe for the use in humans [204].

Regarding applications for PCa and BC there are some publications using QDs or C dots [86,206–209]. For example, Zhao et al. recently evaluated QDs in a Cerenkov-imaging PCa model. [210]. They developed three different near-infrared QDs and ^{89}Zr dual-labeled NPs and demonstrated the applicability of such self-illuminating NPs for imaging of lymph nodes and PCa tumors. For BC, applications of QDs is exemplified with a paper by Bwatanglang et al., in which they present results after investigating folic-acid functionalized chitosan-encapsulated QDs [208]. They found both enhanced binding affinity and internalization of their NP platform for folate receptor-overexpressing MCF-7 and MDA-MB-231 cells, and therefore concluded it to be a promising candidate for theranostic applications.

2.4. Carbon Based Nanoparticles

The research on NPs based on carbon and allotropes of carbon such as fullerenes and graphene (e.g., nanohorns or nanotubes) have increased in recent years (Figure 3) [57,58,211–215]. These kind of NPs have received increased attention due to their chemical stability, favorable surface chemistry, high drug loading capacity, as well as high degree of variability. When it comes to medical applications attention has been particularly directed towards applications such as drug delivery, photothermal therapy, and imaging. Examples of this kind of NPs are fullerenes (spherical (i.e., buckyballs), ellipsoidal, or tube-shaped), carbon nanotubes (CNTs) such as single-walled CNTs (SWCNTs), double-walled CNTs (DWCNTs), or multi-walled CNTs (MWCNTs), carbon quantum dots (CQDs), graphene quantum dots (GQDs), and graphene oxide (GO). Regarding fullerenes they have been evaluated and utilized as for both X-ray and MRI imaging contrast agents, but also in applications for bringing a therapeutic substance to its target, such as gene delivery [216]. Different forms of CNTs can all be produced and chemically modified enabling labeling with, for example, radioactive isotopes [217,218]. Although promising applications of CNTs have been shown the question regarding toxicity of this nanovehicle is still under debate [219]. For example, it has been demonstrated that under certain circumstances the CNTs are able to cross the cell membranes of healthy tissue and induce harmful inflammatory and fibrotic responses, as well as cell death [220–224]. It should be noted though, that elevated risks are especially connected to chronic exposure to CNTs, which is not the case for medical applications for which the administration is performed under a limited period of time.

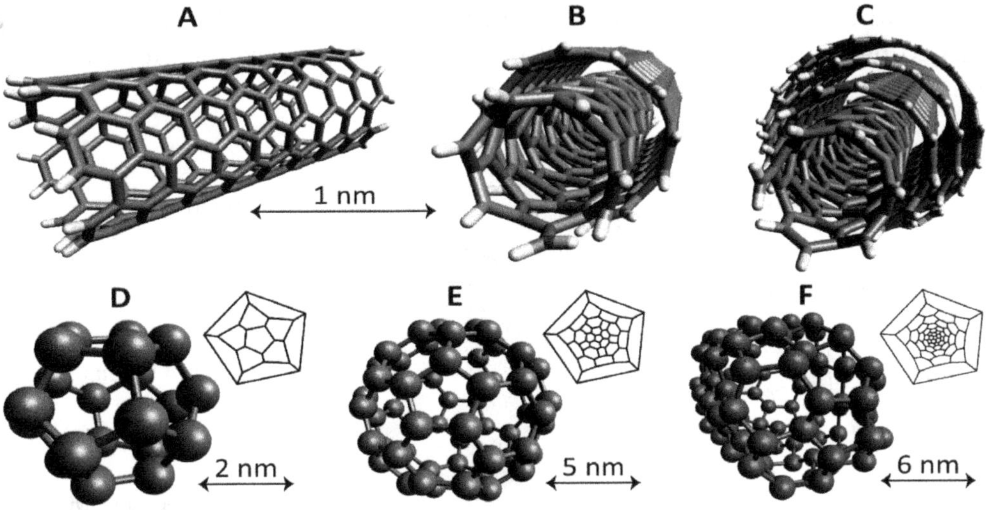

Figure 3. Examples of carbon-based nanotubes and fullerenes. (**A**) Single-walled carbon nanotube (SWCNT); (**B**) Double-walled carbon nanotube (DWCNT); (**C**) Multi-walled carbon nanotube (MWCNT); (**D**) Fullerene based on 20 carbon atoms (20-fullerene); (**E**) Fullerene based on 60 carbon atoms (60-fullerene); and (**F**) Fullerene based on 100 carbon atoms (100-fullerene). The top size indicator applies for panels **A**–**C**. The 3D-structures were created using Avogadro molecule editor. For panels **A**–**C** a rod-based representation, and for panels **D**–**F** a ball-based representation, was chosen for best clarity of the 3D-distribution of carbon atoms and the covalent bindings between them. For panels **D**–**F** is also shown 2D-representations of the fullerene structures, as well as individual size indicators. Note, the 100-fullerene has an obloid-like structure for its global energy minima, compared to the spherical 20- and 60-fullerenes, as discussed, for example, by Yoshida et al. [225].

Regarding PCa and BC applications utilizing carbon-based NPs there is an increasing number of publications during the last couple of years, both for imaging and therapy but also for different kind of electrochemical biosensor systems [226–234]. For instance, regarding PCa, Heydari-Bafrooei et al. and Pan et al. have both developed different kind of CNT-based biosensor systems able to detect prostate specific antigen (PSA) in serum and vascular endothelial growth factor (VEGF) and PSA in serum, respectively, for early diagnosis of PCa [227,229]. For example, regarding BC, Misra et al. developed a carbon NP-DNA complex (CNPLex) used to transfect green fluorescent protein (GFP) reporter gene containing plasmid DNA (pDNA) pEGFP-N1 targeting BC cells MCF-7 and MDA-MB231 with promising results [234].

2.5. *Liposomes*

The phospholipid, principally phosphatidylcholine, based bilayer structure, constituting the body of the spherical vesicle called liposome, can be arranged in such a way as to produce a small unilamellar liposome vesicle (SUV) (Ø < 100 nm), large unilamellar vesicle (LUV) (Ø = 100–1000 nm), giant unilamellar vesicle (GUV) (Ø > 1000 nm), multilamellar vesicle (MLV), or a cylindrically shaped nanocochleate vesicle (NCV). An example of a hypothetical spherical unilamellar liposome is shown in Figure 4. The MLV's are constructed by one or more unilamellar liposomes being encapsulated within a larger one. By disrupting the bilayer structure by ultra-sonication the liposomes can be prepared and loaded with, for example, different pharmaceutical drugs, either hydrophobic or hydrophilic. In such a way, the liposomes can act as vehicles for drugs directed against different diseases. The persistent and important work over several decades by the biophysicist Alec D Bengham on liposomes paved the way for its application as NPs in current biomedical research [235]. Depending on which type of liposome under consideration, the size ranges from around 20–100 nm (SUV), 100–1000 nm (LUV), to over 1000 nm for the MLV, and up to 200 µm for the GUV. The negative charges of the hydrophilic phospholipid heads on the surface of the liposome could be utilized for binding positively charged molecules and/or radioisotopes by electrostatic interaction [236]. Also, by specifically blocking these negatively charged heads using PEGylation, it is possible to increase the blood circulation time by minimizing the kidney clearance rate [237].

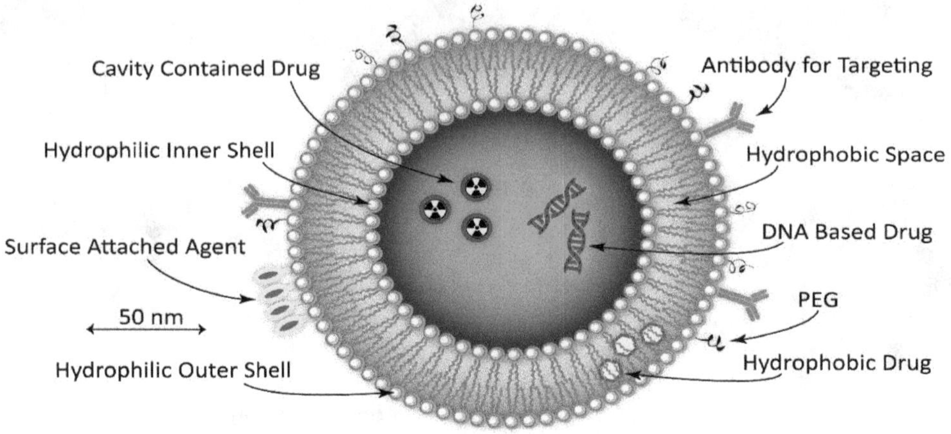

Figure 4. Schematic presentation of a spherical PEGylated liposome. Indicated are the different available spaces and surfaces that could carry different kind of targeting molecules as well as therapeutic drugs and imaging agents. In this hypothetical example, an antibody chelated to the outer surface is used for targeting. On that surface is also attached an imaging agent. Some kind of therapeutic drug is carried by the hydrophobic space between outer and inner shell. And in the core cavity, two hydrophilic drugs are situated, here exemplified by a radionuclide and a DNA-based drug such as strings of DNA, RNA, or small-interference RNA (siRNA). Unilamellar liposomes lies mostly in the size range of >150 nm, exemplified by a 200 nm liposome in the figure.

Studies utilizing liposomal-based NPs for PCa and BC theranostic techniques are few [238–247], although applications for therapy or imaging alone are significantly more frequently published [248–261]. For example, Yeh et al. recently published results from experiments investigating peptide-conjugated liposomal NPs in a theranostic approach for PCa. They found that the administration of liposomal doxorubicin and vinorelbine conjugated with targeting peptides increased the inhibition human PCa growth, and concluded that the targeting peptide SP204 has significant potential for both targeted imaging and therapy of PCa [238]. A liposomal-based theranostic approach against BC could be exemplified by the work by Rizzitelli et al. in which they evaluated the release of doxorubicin from liposomes monitored by MRI and triggered by ultrasound stimuli. The treatment led to a complete tumor regression in their BC mouse model [241].

2.6. *Polymer Based Nanoparticles*

These type of biodegradable block-copolymer based NPs can encapsulate and carry relatively large pharmaceutical molecules such as proteins, individual genes, or pieces of DNA [262]. Examples of polymers used for these types of NPs are polycyanoacrylate (PCA), poly D,L-glycolide (PLG), polylactic acid (PLA), polylactide-*co*-glycolide (PLGA), poly(isohexyl cyanoacrylate) (PIHCA), or polybutyl cyanoacrylate (PBCA) [262]. Among these polymers, PBCA and PIHCA have shown to be the fastest regarding biodegradability. For example, 24 h post an intravenous injection of PBCA it showed a level of reduction in the order of 80% [263]. PIHCA is currently undergoing clinical trials in phase III for hepatocellular carcinomas using the drug doxorubicin (Livatag® (Doxorubicin Transdrug™), Paris, France). Three main NP structures, or micelles, can be achieved using polymers, namely nanocapsules, nanospheres, and nanoparticles. In the first case the pharmaceutical is encapsulated and completely surrounded by a spherical or rod-shaped shell of block-copolymers. In the second case, the pharmaceutical is embedded in a polymeric spherically shaped matrix. In the last case, the pharmaceutical is attached on the surface of the polymer based nanostructure [262]. The encapsulated, embedded, or attached pharmaceutical can of course be a radioactive agent of some sort [264]. Covalent pegylation of polymeric NPs can increase blood circulation times as well as facilitate uptake of the drug at targets aimed for [265]. Dendrons and symmetrical dendrimers (Figure 5) are a type of branched polymer based macromolecule that could be used as NPs [266,267]. Dendrimers have attracted much attention regarding theranostic applications, and the subject could easily fill a review on its own [268–270]. For example, hyperbranched PAMAM (polyamidoamine) dendrimer, based on hydrophilic ethylene diamine and investigated for medical purposes, can be labelled with monoclonal antibodies due to suitable amino groups in its structure [271]. The PAMAMs can be produced with multifunctional terminal surfaces and a narrow molecular weight distribution [272]. Finally, polymersomes is a type of polymeric NP for which amphiphilic synthetic block-copolymers are utilized to construct the membrane of the vesicle. Polymersomes have many similarities with liposomes, built by natural lipids (see above), but exhibit decreased permeability and increased stability compared to liposomes. The polymersomes have a size span of approximately 50–5000 nm.

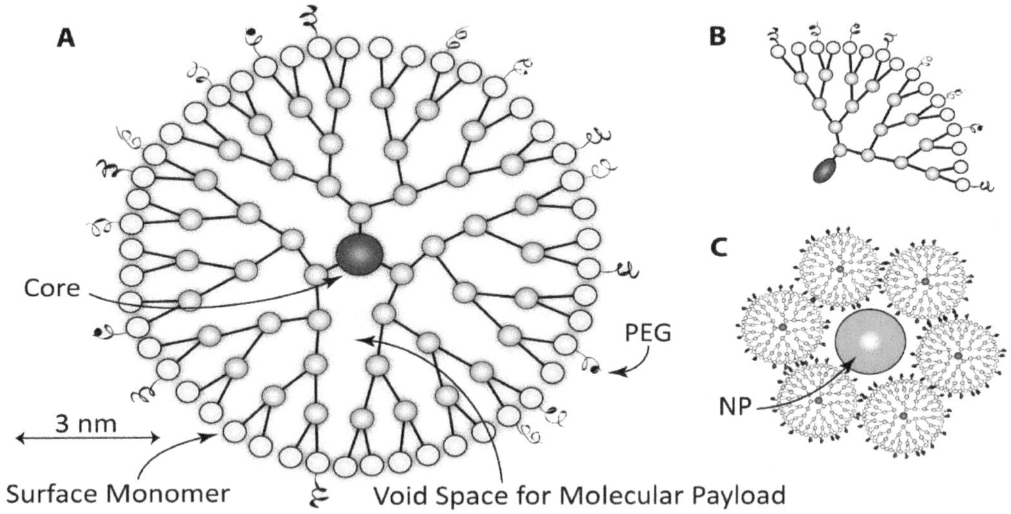

Figure 5. Schematic presentation of one type of spherical PEGylated dendrimer based on a central core (**A**), which in itself can be a dendrimer or some other type of NP (i.e., if so, a NP-cored dendrimer (NPCD)). A standard size of a dendrimer shown in A is 5–10 nm, exemplified by a 10 nm dendrimer in the figure. The surface monomers enable attachment of imaging and/or drug payloads, also able to be entrapped in the void space. The network of covalently bound interior monomers connects the surface monomers to the core. The number of radially emerging branch points defines the generation of the dendrimer; in this case four, denoted G-4. If instead, NPs are situated inside the network of monomers the term used is dendrimer-encapsulated nanoparticles (DENPs). Hyper-branched polymers are a variant similar to dendrimers, except that the branches emanating from the core differ from each other with regard to number of branch points. To the right is shown an example of a dendron (**B**), i.e., a small fragment of a dendrimer that also could be used as a NP. An example of a dendrimer-stabilized nanoparticle (DSNP) is shown in the lower right corner (**C**). Depending on if the functionalization is located on the surface, in the void space, or at the core of the dendrimer it is usually denoted as surface, interior, or core functionalized, or as a combination of all three possibilities.

There are very few theranostic polymer-based NP studies reported for both PCa and BC. In one such study Ling et al. evaluated multifunctional dual docetaxel/superparamagnetic iron oxide (SPIONs) loaded polymer vesicles (147 nm in diameter) for both imaging and therapy of PCa [273]. Enhanced cellular uptake and anti-proliferative effect for the PC3 cell line was observed which, in conjunction with the SPION-based MRI possibility, made the authors conclude that these polymer-based NP vesicles were promising for simultaneous imaging, drug delivery, and real-time monitoring of the therapeutic effect. For BC, a theranostic polymer based technique has been published by Abbasi et al. in which they experimented with Mn-oxide and docetaxel co-loaded fluorescent polymer-based NPs for dual-modal imaging and therapy of BC [274]. The authors concluded this type of polymer-based NP as a good candidate for cancer theranostic applications. Other interesting, however not yet fully theranostic, applications of polymer-based NP for PCa and BC have been published [275–279].

2.7. *Solid Lipid Nanoparticles*

The methodology of solid lipid NPs (SLNPs, or SLNs) is a promising emerging research field of lipid nanotechnology [280–285], which offers good possibilities to incorporate drugs into nanosized targeted vehicles having great biotolerability and low biotoxicity due to their constitution of physiological lipids [286]. Examples of such lipids are mono-, di-, and tri-glycerides, steroids, and fatty acids. Among the advantages of SLNPs could be mentioned the possibility of incorporating both hydro- and lipophilic drugs, good drug stability, and the lack of organic solvents in its composition [286]. The size of the SLNPs vary between 10 and 1000 nm, and the most common geometrical shape is spherical (Figure 6). The core is composed of solid lipids which is stabilized by emulsifiers, which also has the effect of decreasing the risk of NP agglomeration [286,287].

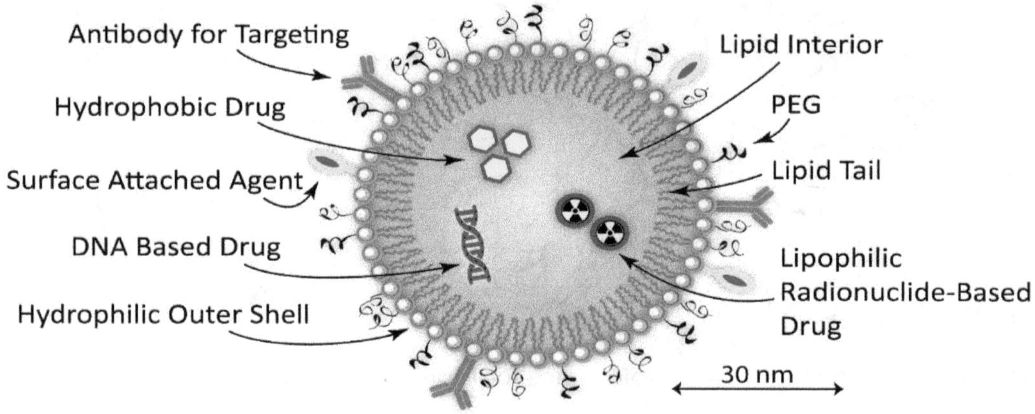

Figure 6. Solid lipid NP (SLNP). Although liquid lipid NPs are possible to produce, the most common form of lipid-based NPs investigated for medical purposes are SLNPs. The lipids most often used are fatty acids or different forms of glycerides. The smallest forms of SLNPs are in the shape of micelles, in which the fully dehydrated tails of the phosphatidylcholine molecules meet in the center, producing SLNPs in the size of 10 nm in diameter. Typical sizes for SLNPs are, however, most commonly in the interval of 5 to 500 nm in radii, exemplified by a hypothetical SLNP with a radius of approximately 30 nm in the figure.

Until today, no fully theranostic application has been reported for neither PCa nor BC utilizing SLNPs. However, some studies have been published investigating the possibility using this NP system for either imaging or therapy alone [288–298]. For example, Radaic et al. investigated the possibility of gene therapy using SLNPs and tested the capacity of their NPs to accommodate DNA (and withstand DNase degradation), their colloidal stability and in vitro cytotoxicity, as well as the transfection efficiency in PCa cells [288]. For BC, Jain et al. recently published results investigating the anticancer efficacy of lycopene loaded SLNPs [294]. They found that the concentration and time dependent cell survival of MCF-7 BC cells was significantly reduced by LYC-SLNPs, as compared to their free lycopene counterparts.

3. Multimodal Imaging Options for Prostate and Breast Cancer

The use of various biomedical imaging techniques in preclinical and clinical applications, during both diagnosis and treatment has increased tremendously during the past decades, and is now considered a central part in many of such applications. Computed tomography, positron emission tomography, single photon emission computed tomography, magnetic resonance imaging, ultrasound imaging, Cherenkov luminescence imaging, photoacoustic imaging, and optical imaging are examples of images techniques used, and still under development. The images these different technologies produce enable early detection, screening, image-guided treatment, as well as the possibility of estimating the level of progression or retrogression of the disease investigated [299]. By using a NP-based targeted vehicle it is possible to use combinations of these imaging techniques simultaneously in order to increase the level of accuracy, possibly also at a cellular or even a molecular level. This NP-based multifunctionality in biomedical imaging could be referred to as multimodal imaging (MMI). Most often, only two imaging techniques is utilized simultaneously, which then is referred to as bimodal imaging (BMI). Below follows a condensed presentation of each of these different biomedical imaging techniques and their basic characteristics. When applicable, examples on how they have been used in NP-settings for PCa and BC applications so far, e.g., in MMI or BMI contexts, are shortly mentioned and referenced to.

3.1. Computed Tomography and Tomosynthesis

Regarding computed tomography (CT), contrast enhancers such as barium or iodine compounds (e.g., Gastrografin) could be used to increase the absorption of X-rays and thereby enhancing the contrast of tissues in an image, taking up these contrast agents. A targeted NP platform carrying such contrast enhancers could thus improve the anatomical visualization of organs and other structures, compared to non-targeted regions. But also some NPs themselves can improve the contrast, exemplified by AuNPs increasing the contrast approximately three times as compared to the same amount of iodine [300]. Differently sized AuNPs have been evaluated for micro CT for example, and some are under the consideration for approval for use in the clinic [301–303]. A low-density lipoprotein (LDL)-based iodinated nanoparticle targeting the LDL receptor (LDLR), expressed in PCa, for example, has also been evaluated for CT imaging [304–306], as well as polyvinyl pyrrolidone coated bismuth sulfide (Bi_2S_3) based nanocrystals [307]. For tomosynthesis, the same general principle applies as described above for CT, namely that the contrast in an image could be increased approximately three times using AuNPs as compared to using the same amount of iodine-based contrast agent. For contrast-enhanced breast tomosynthesis (CE DBT), temporal or dual-energy subtraction techniques are of course still possible to use regardless of which type of contrast agent is utilized [308].

Most applications of CT in NP contexts are based on positron emission and single photon emission computed tomography (see below). However, one example in which CT has been used is described by Kim et al., in which they investigated a multifunctional gold-based NP system for both contrast-enhanced imaging and therapy of PCa [309]. RNA-aptamer functionalized gold NPs targeting PSMA enabled specific imaging of PCa. When also loaded with doxorubicin their theranostic NPs showed good therapeutic efficacy against LNCaP cells. For BC, a study performed by Naha et al. evaluated gold silver alloy NPs as an imaging probe for BC screening using conventional CT as well as dual-energy mammography (DEM) [310]. In vivo experiments in mice exhibited good tumor accumulation of the NPs and produced high contrast DEM and CT images, enabling the authors to conclude that their NP system has potential for both blood pool imaging and BC screening.

3.2. Positron Emission and Single Photon Emission Computed Tomography

Radio imaging using positron emission tomography (PET) and/or single photon emission computed tomography (SPECT) they have been evaluated for several NP applications using both organic and inorganic NPs, for example, in PET/CT or SPECT/CT settings [311–314]. Using a NP platform makes it possible to increase the contrast in an image due to the possibility to label each NP with a large number of radionuclides. For PET, examples of radionuclides used in such applications are ^{18}F, ^{124}I and ^{64}Cu, and for SPECT examples are ^{125}I and ^{125}Cd.

Regarding PCa, PET (or PET/CT) and SPECT (or SPECT/CT) has been used in several NP applications [131,315–321]. For example, Pressley et al. evaluated an amphiphilic NP for natriuretic peptide clearance receptor (NPRC) targeting and DOTA (1,4,7,10-tetraazacyclododecane-1,4,7,10-tetraacetic acid) chelator for high specific activity ^{64}Cu PET-radiolabeling. PET/CT images revealed high blood pool retention, low renal clearance, enhanced tumor uptake, and decreased hepatic burden relative to a nontargeted NP version [317], indicating the possibility of a new nanoagent for PCa PET imaging, according to the authors. In NP-based BC applications, PET and SPECT have been utilized in several studies [322–326]. For example, Lee et al. recently published a study in which they assessed the EPR effect in nineteen patients with HER2-positive metastatic BC using a ^{64}Cu-labeled NP (^{64}Cu-labeled HER2-targeted PEGylated liposomal doxorubicin) using PET/CT [322]. The authors concluded that the results provide evidence and quantification of the EPR effect in human metastatic BC tumors, as well as support NP-deposition imaging as a potential technique for identifying patients well-suited for NP-based therapeutics.

3.3. Magnetic Resonance Imaging

The magnetic resonance imaging (MRI), or magnetic resonance tomography (MRT), technology is today widely used for imaging physiological processes as well as the anatomy during both preclinical research and in the clinic [327]. Varieties of this technique includes functional MRI (fMRI), measuring levels of cerebral blood flow, as well as techniques to increase the contrast in MRI images such as dynamic contrast-enhanced MRI (DCE-MRI), utilizing a contrast agent such as gadolinium, and diffusion-weighted MRI (DW-MRI), utilizing the Brownian motion of water molecules. The MRI tool plays an important role in the staging of PCa (see below in section Prostate Cancer) and will most likely be applicable and show an increased importance also for other types of cancers, such as BC, for both diagnosis and staging, especially if used in a NP setting, discussed in this paper.

The ^{19}F-based MRI [328–332] offers many advantages, despite the difficulty of providing suitable non-toxic ^{19}F-based compounds in sufficient amounts for in vivo imaging, compared to common proton-based ^{1}H-MRI such as decreased background levels, quantitative determination of pharmacokinetics, and estimation of tissue oxygenation [300,333,334]. The use of ^{19}F-MRI in NP applications is a developing research field investigating, for example, the applicability compared to SPIONs, the efficacy of fluorinated dendrimers and multifunctional micelle-based core–shell NPs, and the detection of folate-receptor positive tumors in a ^{19}F/florescence-based bimodal imaging setting [331,335–337]. Just recently, a ^{19}F based nanoemulsion has been FDA approved for noninvasive clinical cell-tracking imaging [338].

Regarding MRI/MRT used in PCa related NP settings the number of publications is constantly increasing [104,339–344]. Jin et al., for example, evaluated MRI-guided focal NP-based (porphysomes) photothermal therapy (see below) in an orthotropic PCa mouse model, and concluded that it might be an effective and safe technique to treat PCa, with a low risk of progression of disease [343]. For BC, there is also a large number of publications [91,345–349]. In a study by Turino et al. L-ferritine-coated paclitaxel- and Gd-loaded NPs were evaluated for simultaneous delivery of a therapeutic drug and a MRI-contrast agent in a MCF7 BC model [345]. According to the authors, the theranostic potential of this NP system was demonstrated by, for example, evaluating signal-intensity enhancements in T1-weighted MRI images.

As for CT, by combining the MR-imaging mode with PET enables localization and biodistribution at the same time. Very few studies are however reported until today using this technique in NP settings for PCa and BC [350–352].

3.4. Ultrasound Imaging

During ultrasound imaging (USI), utilizing contrast agents to improve the contrast, particle sizes used often exceed 250 nm. Although the most commonly used size definition for NPs is 1–100 nm, the USI contrast agents is still appropriate to mention here since USI can play an important role in MMI. Two examples of commercially available USI contrast agents are Definity and Optison based on microbubbles. Both type of bubbles contain octafluoropropane gas, while Definity uses a phospholipid spherical shell and Optison an albumin based shell to enclose the gas. Experimentally, SPIONs, liposomes, AuNPs, and nanodroplets have also been evaluated as contrast agents and drug carriers during NP-based US applications [353–358]. All types of microbubbles can serve as platforms for not only imaging, but also for the distribution of drugs for therapy by encapsulating the drug into the bubbles [359,360]. Targeted microbubbles for use during both imaging and therapy, or at the same time as targeted theranostic vehicles, can be achieved by attaching ligands on the surface of the bubbles which specifically bind to receptors on, for example, tumor cells.

In the study by Tong et al. mentioned above for PCa, a protamine cationic microbubble (Ø $\approx$ 500 nm) was constructed for simultaneous gene therapy (androgen-receptor siRNA) and ultrasound imaging [360]. The authors concluded that the gene-transfection efficiency was better than that of a liposomes-based comparable system, and that their microbubble system could be used as a gene-loading and ultrasound-imaging technique of tumors. For BC, Zhao et al. recently investigated a near-infrared (808 nm) photothermal responsive dual aptamers-targeted docetaxel-containing NPs for both cancer therapy and USI [353]. The dual-ligand functionalization increased uptake in MCF-7 cells and made USI possible at tumor site. The authors therefore concluded their system to be a promising theranostic option involving light-thermal response, dual ligand targeted triplex therapy (chemotherapy, photothermal therapy, and biological therapy), and USI.

3.5. Cherenkov Luminescence Imaging

The Cherenkov luminescence imaging (CLI) technology, named after Pavel Alekseyevich Cherenkov who shared the Nobel Prize in physics in 1958 for the discovery of the now called Cherenkov effect, has during recent years emerged as an alternative imaging technique for several different applications [361–367]. The electromagnetic Cherenkov radiation, emitted when charged particles passes through a medium at a speed greater than light propagates through the same medium, could be used to image, for example, the uptake of a charged-particle emitter in tumors during radioimmunotherapy. There are very few publications on PCa and BC using CLI [368–371], among which very few have a NP approach. Lohrman et al. found a positive correlation between the radioactivity uptake and CLI signal from the ^{90}Y labeled gastrin-releasing peptide-receptor (GRPR) antagonist DOTA-AR in xenografted PCa tumors [370]. Regarding using CLI in NP applications besides PCa and BC there are some publications [372–375]. For example, Madru et al. investigated the usability ^{68}Ga-labeled SPIONs for multi-modality PET/MR/CLI imaging of sentinel lymph nodes (SLNs). Based on promising biodistribution experiments, the authors concluded that ^{68}Ga-SPIONs can enhance the identification of SLNs by combining PET and MR imaging, and potential also enable Cherenkov luminescent-guided resection of SLNs [372].

3.6. Photoacoustic Imaging

A relatively new emerging imaging modality is photoacoustic imaging (PAI), although already with some PCa and BC orientated studies published the past decade [376–383]. PAI could be achieved by irradiating a biological site with a pulsed laser-beam in the megahertz range, which energy is then absorbed by, for example, targeted NPs. The absorbed energy creates acoustic pressure waves, caused by thermoelastic expansion, in the irradiated site. These waves could then be detected by using an ultrasonic transducer, enabling an image to be constructed. If instead of using a laser, pulses in radio-frequency range are used, the technique is called thermoacoustic imaging (TAI). Su et al. investigated recently mesoporous-silica coated and PEG modified multifunctional doxorubicin-loaded prussian-blue nanocubes (PB@mSiO_2-PEG/DOX). Good both MRI and PAI ability, as well as a synergistic photothermal and chemical therapeutic efficacy, for BC was found [377]. For PCa, Levi et al. evaluated a PAI agent (AA3G-740) targeting the gastrin-releasing peptide receptor (GRPR), highly overexpressed in PCa [380]. The study showed that, even for poorly vascularized tumors, AA3G-740 was able to bind to GRPR and led to a significantly higher photoacoustic signal relative to a control agent.

Regarding NP applications using PAI there are some studies published for both PCa and BC [230,382,384–391]. By using PCa cells, Tian et al., for example, constructed PEGylated and RGD (Arginine-Glycine-Aspartic)-peptide functionalized AuNPs and evaluated them as a contrast agent for PAI of single PCa cells. The authors concluded that these NPs provide a platform for detection and imaging of individual cancer cells, with a potential impact on clinical diagnostic [384]. Pham et al. used mouse models based on orthotopic primary triple-negative BC xenografts (including patient-derived xenografts) to evaluate the efficacy of bevacizumab (a VEGF pathway-targeting antiangiogenic drug) in combination with CRLX101, an NP-drug conjugate containing camptothecin (a cytotoxic quinoline alkaloid inhibiting DNA topoisomerase). PAI was used in the study to show that the use of CRLX101 led to an improved tumor perfusion as well as reduced hypoxia. The authors concluded that pairing antiangiogenic therapy with a cytotoxic NP construct may be a promising way to treat metastatic BC [391].

3.7. Optical Imaging

The Optical imaging (OI) technology (sometimes referred to as biophotonics), the inclusive term often used for different types of infrared, ultraviolet, and visible light, as well as sometimes also photoacoustic (see above) applications in biomedical imaging, have a number of interesting publications regarding NP applications for both PCa and BC [319,392–400]. Generally, a NP-based OI approach could enable or optimize an optical excitation energy in, for example, tumor tissue, enable multispectral imaging by combining spectroscopy and OI, or make possible multiplex imaging by using different color emitters for different targets simultaneously [300]. For cancer applications, Ahir et al. recently developed a copper oxide-nanowire NP decorated with folic acid and studied its effect on triple negative BC (TNBC). They found that their NPs induced apoptosis and retarded migration of the TNBC cells, and used optical fluorescence imaging to monitor its distribution in tumors and different organs [392]. Regarding PCa, Behnam et al. constructed and investigated a PSMA-targeted bionized nanoferrite (BNF) NP in an experimental PCa model [319]. The study used near-infrared fluorescence microscopy, SPECT, Prussian blue staining, immunohistochemistry, and biodistribution to show an enhanced NP uptake in PSMA-positive tumors, with a maximum uptake 48 h post injection.

3.8. Electron Microscopy

Regarding electron microscopy (EM) in general, but especially transmission electron microscopy (TEM), it has an important role to play for the in vitro and ex vivo analyses due to its often sub-nanometer spatial resolution. Nanoparticles based on heavy elements such as gold could therefore be used for TEM applications in order to retrieve information on, for example, NP distribution on the organelle level. So far though, this technique has only been used occasionally in PCa and BC NP applications. Since EM is not considered to be an imaging technique possible to use in theranostic contexts, its value lies instead in in vitro and ex vivo analyses, as mentioned above, or during the production process of the NPs in order to be able to characterize them properly [401–408].

4. Multimodal Therapy Options for Prostate and Breast Cancer

Due to differences in metabolic and chemical stability, level of solubility in blood serum and interstitial fluid, degree of toxicity, and most important level of specificity for a certain tumor type as well as potency once properly targeted, several different drugs have been evaluated and some approved for targeted therapies against cancer [409,410]. For a detailed compilation of the NP-based technology and therapy of cancer in general the reader is referred to Professor P.N. Prasad's fine textbook on the subject [300]. A NP-based therapeutic, in some cases also potentially synergistic, multifunctionality can be referred to as multimodal therapy (MMT), or if only two therapies are used simultaneously, as bimodal therapy (BMT). Below follows a presentation of different therapy options that all could be implemented in various NP settings. The basic characteristics and principles of each modality are presented briefly. References are also listed and some specific examples on how some of the available therapy modalities have been utilized in NP-settings for PCa and BC are discussed shortly, e.g., in MMT or BMT contexts.

4.1. Chemotherapy

Treatments using chemotherapy (CTH), since many years successfully applied and still under development for a wide category of cancers including PCa and BC, has limitations due its relatively high degree of non-specificity, inducing toxicity [411–415]. A targeted NP-based approach has shown to be beneficial and has been evaluated by many research teams. Some such NP-based CTH drugs have been FDA approved; the albumin-paclitaxel-based Abraxane® and the PEG-doxorubicin-based Doxil® for metastasized BC, the latter being the first FDA approved nanodrug [416,417]. But also other formulations are being evaluated in the clinic, or have already been approved or are being marketed in, for example, Europe. Such examples for BC is the non-pegylated liposomal-doxorubicin-based Myocet® or the polymeric micelle-paclitaxel-based Genexol-PM® [418,419]. An update from 2014 of FDA approved NP-based cancer drugs, and also others at various stages of development, has been published [420]. Regarding targeting of NP-based CTH drugs research are ongoing in order to, instead of relying on the passive targeting caused by the EPR effect, develop strategies for active targeting using, for example, mAbs (or fraction of mAbs) directed against the PSA receptor in the PCa case [421].

However, a large number of studies, using different techniques, have been published with a NP and CTH-based approach for both PCa and BC, of which only a tiny fraction are listed here [105,253,315,353,422–431]. For example, Belz et al. recently designed ultra-small silica NPs containing the radiosensitizing drug docetaxel for combined chemoradiation therapy, with potential benefit for patients with PCa [425]. For BC, Li et al. found synergistic inhibition of both migration and invasion of 4T1 BC cells by doubly loaded NPs (docetaxel + the Akt inhibitor quercetin), via the Akt/matrix metallopeptidase 9 (MMP-9) pathway [431].

4.2. Gene Therapy

The gene therapy (GTH) alternative has during the last two decades evolved as a promising tool for the treatment of cancer, either as a stand-alone therapy or in conjunction with chemotherapy, surgery, and/or radiation therapy [432,433]. The development of GTH towards treatment based on an individual's specific genome, immune status, and tumor characteristics, together with new vectors for transferring the genetic material such as synthetic viruses as well as non-viral methods will further refine this still experimental, treatment option [434]. By adopting an NP-based GTH approach, the treatment is believed to be improved even further, especially when implemented as TNPs enabling imaging simultaneous with therapy. For the two main groups of genes associated with cancer, i.e., tumor-suppressor genes and oncogenes, examples of nucleic-acid based therapeutic molecules that are being evaluated for GTH are cytotoxic or corrective genes, small interfering RNA (siRNA) or short hairpin RNA (shRNA) [435].

Regarding NP-based GTH techniques for BC there are very few, however an increasing number, publications the last decade [234,436–444]. Su et al., for example, investigated recently the efficacy of a combinational technique including photothermal therapy (see below), CTH, and GTH for triple negative BC [442]. Indocyanine green, paclitaxel, and survivin siRNA was integrated into a NP and was found to exhibit very good tumor efficacy with low toxicity. The protein survivin, encoded by the *BIRC5* oncogene in the human genome, and which inhibits the caspase activation and therefore downregulates the apoptotic pathway, has received much attention lately. Several attempts, also including NPs, have been made to distribute anti-survivin siRNA in order to silence the BIRC5 gene [445–447]. For NP-based GTH applications for PCa, there are also quite few publications the last decade [141,448–452]. Guo et al. investigated, for example, gene silencing using siRNA-based AuNPs for LNCaP cells, overexpressing PSMA. With AuNPs conjugated with folate-receptor targeting ligands it was found that siRNA was specifically delivered into the LNCaP cells, and produced enhanced endogenous gene silencing [141].

4.3. Photon Activation Therapy

The photon activation therapy (PAT), sometimes also referred to as photon activated therapy, involving Auger electrons and mentioned for the first time for medical applications over three decades ago, shows a limited amount of publications but is an interesting option for TNPs and therefore discussed here [453–461]. The PAT technique is based on the principle of specific tumor localization of a high-Z compound such as platinum (Pt), incorporated in, for example, a CTH drug, after which synchrotron radiation or X-rays directed against the tumor site is used to, via the photoelectric effect, trigger a cascade release of high linear energy transfer (high-LET) Auger electrons. Except Pt, other nuclides investigated for PAT have been Au, Tl, Gd, I, and Fe. In the Pt case, the photon energy suitable for triggering this effect should be just above the binding energy of the K-shell electrons, i.e., 78.4 keV. As for α-particles, the mean LET value for Auger electrons is considerable higher than that of, for example, beta-particles; ~100, ~15, and ~0.2 keV/μm, respectively. This means that, as for α-particles, the Auger electrons will create densely ionization tracks causing damages in the cells, such as double strand breaks (DSB), which are very difficult to repair. An additional advantage with Auger electrons, compared to α-particles, is that their range in tissue is on the nanometer scale, compared to 50–100 μm for α-particles. So, provided that the Auger-electron emitting nuclide is being properly targeted in close proximity to, or incorporated into, the DNA of the tumor cells, a highly targeted high-LET irradiation will be achieved.

Regarding PCa and BC utilizing a NP-based PAT approach there is only one study published, having only a tentative BC relevance [462]. In that experiment Choi et al. investigated the therapeutic efficacy on colon cancer tumor-bearing mice injected with FeO NPs and irradiated using 7.1 keV synchrotron X-rays, an energy near the Fe K-shell binding energy. For example, one group that received FeO NPs and an absorbed tumor dose of 10 Gy showed 80% complete tumor regression after 15–35 days. As noted by the authors however, the use of 7.1 keV X-rays, having a high tissue attenuation, makes the treatment only suitable for superficial skin malignancies, and possibly also for superficial chest wall recurrence of BC.

4.4. Photodynamic Therapy

Photodynamic therapy (PDT), also referred to as photochemotherapy, utilizes a photosensitizing chemical substance called a photosensitizer (PS) that is irradiated with light at certain wavelengths to induce the production of molecular oxygen in the form of reactive oxygen species (ROS). The ROS, e.g., superoxide, peroxide, singlet oxygen, or hydroxyl radicals, have the capacity to induce cell death at the site of production and can therefore, if targeted properly, be used as a therapeutic option against several diseases [463]. Acne and psoriasis, or to some extent even herpes experimentally, are treated using PDT. But also different type of cancers, in particular different types of skin cancer, are being treated with PDT techniques [464]. Both wavelength and fluence of the light are important parameters to monitor in order to target and trigger the PS properly, using a laser-equipped endoscope as a special case for reaching, for example, intestinal cancers [465].

An interesting version of PDT is the two-photon excitation (TPE) based PDT for the treatment of cancer. This technique combine the advantages of TPE near-infrared (NIR) photosensitizers and nanotechnology and has been reviewed by Shen et al. [466]. The absorption of two relatively low-energy NIR photons will enable the emission of high-energy photons in the visible spectrum, which in its turn will sensitize oxygen producing singlet oxygen and reactive oxygen species (ROS) able to kill targeted cancer cells due to its cytotoxic effect. Compared to single-photon based PDT the possibility of reaching further into tissues, due to the relatively long wavelength of the light used in TPE PDT, has great advantages enabling to reach tumors more deep seated. There are some publications using the TPE technique, both for imaging and therapy, in different NP and theranostic settings [467–471]. The paper by Gary-Bobo et al. [471] was the first two-photon based PDT experiment in vivo using NPs.

Regarding PCa, PDT approaches have been evaluated both preclinically and for patients [472,473]. Especially, studies using PDT as a theranostic approach for PCa has lately also been published. For example, Chen et al. recently investigated a low-molecular-weight theranostic photosensitizer denoted YC-9 for PSMA-targeted optical imaging and PDT [474]. The study indicates that YC-9 is a promising therapeutic agent for targeted PDT of PSMA-expressing tissues, such as PCa. Similarly, Wang et al. synthesized two PSMA-targeting PDT conjugates (PSMA-1-Pc413 and PSMA-1-IR700), both having the potential to aid in the detection and resection of PCa [475]. Lin et al. developed a novel nano-platform for targeted delivery of heat, ROS, as well as the heat shock-protein 90 (Hsp90) inhibitor for the treatment of PCa [476]. Vaillant et al. investigated targeting a membrane lectin using a mannose-6-phosphate analogue grafted onto the surface of functionalized mesoporous silica NPOs [477].

For BC, several approaches have been evaluated. For example, Feng et al. investigated a multimodality theranostic agent based on mesoporous copper sulfide NPs encapsulating doxorubicin, enabling both PAI as well as chemo- and ROS generating phototherapy of BC [400]. Against TNBC, Choi et al. developed photosensitizer-conjugated and camptothecin-encapsulated hyaluronic acid NPs as enzyme-activatable theranostic NPs for near-infrared fluorescence imaging and photodynamic/chemo dual therapy [478]. Both in vitro and in vivo, Wang et al. performed experiments evaluating the effects of sinoporphyrin sodium-mediated PDT on tumor cell proliferation and metastasis for the highly metastatic 4T1 BC cells and a mouse xenograft model [479]. Targeting the TrkC (tropomyosin receptor kinase C) receptor, which tends to be overexpressed in metastatic BC, with a ROS photosensitizer-labeled small molecule enabled Kue et al. to investigate the therapeutic efficacy of PDT in nude mice [480]. Finally, Shemesh et al. used a liposomal-based theranostic delivery system, with indocyanine green as a photosensitizer, for investigating real-time biodistribution monitoring as well as the efficacy of PDT against TNBC [244].

4.5. Photothermal Therapy

The photothermal therapy (PTT) approach builds on the PDT principle (see above) in that it via passive (e.g., via the EPR effect) or active (e.g., via mAbs) tumor accumulation of nanoheaters/photosensitizers enables a localized temperature increase. This could cause the destruction of DNA/RNA molecules as well as proteins, leading to cell death by membrane rupture or necrosis [300,481]. The difference of PTT compared to PDT is that the former does not need oxygen present in order to induce cell killing. Especially one version of PTT has attracted increased attention, namely plasmonic PTT (PPTT) [482–484]. The PPTT technology is based on the principle that when AuNPs are irradiated using infrared or near-infrared light coherent excitation of its conduction electrons at the surface will take place, due to the surface plasmon resonance (SPR) effect. When these electrons deexcite, they will produce localized heat waves causing wanted cell destruction.

Regarding PCa and BC there are several publications investigating PTT in different NP settings [91,156,228,230,247,343,422,485,486]. For example, Hosoya et al. evaluated a theranostic hydrogel-based NP platform combining both targeting of the tumor cells, photon-to-heat conversion, as well as triggered drug delivery enabling controlled release of the anticancer drug and multimodal imaging [247]. Their results showed the possibility of simultaneous targeted delivery of an anticancer drug and noninvasive imaging for both PCa and BC in a mouse model. Also, Cantu et al. investigated polymeric NPs (<100 nm in diameter) in a photothermal ablation setting. When experimenting on MDA-MB-231 BC cells they were able to show complete cancer cell ablation in vitro using an 808-nm laser, indicating the potential benefit of their NP platform utilizing the PTT technology.

4.6. Radioimmunotherapy

The cancer treatment modality termed radioimmunotherapy (RIT) is since many years a well-established technique to specifically irradiate targeted tumor cells using monoclonal antibodies (mAbs), or fraction of mAbs, labeled with suitable radioactive isotopes such as α-, β-, or Auger-electron emitters. Review papers regarding the current RIT status for PCa and BC is referred to for further reading [487–492]. Regarding NP-based platforms for cancer utilizing RIT, sometimes referred to as radioimmunonanoparticles (RINPs), there is a small but increasing number of publications [493–496]. For PCa and BC, there have been only a few papers presenting some promising results [497–501]. Natarajan et al., for example, published a paper in 2008 presenting a potential theranostic approach in a PCa and BC experiment [501]. They developed a novel ^{111}In-radioconjugate NP based on anti-MUC-1-scFv antibody fragments and functionalized NPs.

4.7. Neutron Capture Therapy

The radiation-based technique called neutron capture therapy (NCT) is based on a neutron source in order to generate a targeted internal radiation therapy at the specific tumor site, and has been described in several publications [300,502–504]. The technique is still a highly active research area, and applications in which it is evaluated now also includes theranostic NP-based settings [505]. Most applications so far have been exploiting the nuclear reaction ^{10}B(n,α)^{7}Li, i.e., bombarding boron atoms with thermal neutrons to produce internally emitted α-particles. This technique is called boron neutron capture therapy (BNCT). The isotope ^{157}Gd has also been evaluated for NCT, although it has been questioned due to toxicity concerns regarding Gd^{3+} ions. However, chelation using DTPA has been promising and capable of producing stable Gd-DTPA complexes, and therefore nontoxic. The isotope ^{157}Gd has some advantages over ^{10}B, including, for example, a 67 times higher cross section for thermal neutrons as well as Gd^{3+} ions being paramagnetic and thereby able to function as contrast enhancers during MRI [300]. Regarding NP-based applications of NCT, it could help to increase the accumulation of ^{10}B or ^{157}Gd in the targeted tumor tissue. Liposome-based NP techniques is a possible approach and some experiments have shown promising results [504,506–508].

Regarding PCa and BC there are very few studies published using NP-based NCT techniques. Only two BC-related publications are to be found on PubMed, investigating dendrimer- and lipid-based gadolinium NPs [509,510].

4.8. Magnetic Therapy

In addition, for magnetic NPs being able to serve as contrast enhancers during MRI (see above), these type of NPs could also be used for therapy, i.e., magnetic therapy (MTH), and thus used as a theranostic platform. Both alternating-current (AC) and direct-current (DC) based magnetic fields could be utilized for this type of technique, although the most commonly used option called magnetic hyperthermia uses AC-based magnetic fields [300]. The Brownian and Neel relaxation processes are the two sources of heat generation during the AC-based magnetic hyperthermia option [511]. The smaller the NP used the more the Neel relaxation process will dominate over the Brownian in contributing to the heat generation in targeted tissue. If instead using a DC-based magnetic field is used the process of magnetocytolysis is utilized in order to induce cellular disruption.

Regarding PCa and BC related applications using a NP-based MTH technique there are only a few publications available [493,512–516]. For example, Han et al. recently evaluated a theranostic strategy based on Fe_3O_4/Au NPs used for prostate-specific antigen detection, MRI, as well as magnetic hyperthermia [512]. For BC, Yao et al. recently investigated a multifunction therapy platform based on silica NP and quantum dots for controlled and targeted drug (doxorubicin) release, NIR-based PTT, and AC-based magnetic hyperthermia in a 4T1 BC model, indicating a significant synergistic therapeutic effect [515].

5. The Prostate Cancer Case

TNPs might play an important role in the future for the detection, diagnosis, and staging, as well as for the therapy of cancerous diseases at different stages. In order to specifically up-date the reader on the current situation regarding the statistics, diagnosis options, staging, recurrence, metastases, as well as some available treatment options for PCa, a short presentation of this is given below.

5.1. Background Statistics

Worldwide, PCa is the second most frequently diagnosed cancer in men, and the fourth most common in both sexes combined. Approximately 1.1 million men were diagnosed with PCa in the world during 2012, which is approximately 15% of all cancers diagnosed in men [517]. Prostate cancer is also the fifth leading cause of death related to cancer in men, with 307,000 deaths worldwide during 2012 [517]. In the USA, PCa is the second leading cause of cancer-related deaths and the second most frequently diagnosed cancer, while in Europe it is number one. The American Cancer Society estimated that 180,890 men would be diagnosed with PCa during 2016 in USA, and about 26,120 would die from the diseases [518]. The International Agency for Research on Cancer (IARC) concluded that during 2012 in Europe close to 345,000 men were diagnosed with PCa. Although more effort has been directed towards early detection through screening, 72,000 men died of PCa in Europe in 2012 [519–526]. Notably, there is less variation in mortality worldwide than is observed for the incidence. This is explained by the PSA testing having greater effect on incidence than on the mortality [517]. The development of improved therapy modalities should therefore be prioritized and targeted therapies based on TNPs are promising candidates to increase the therapeutic efficacy and chance for survival of this category of patients. Several studies of the therapeutic efficacy and toxicity of RIT against PCa have been performed [492,527–544].

5.2. Diagnosis, Staging, Recurrence, and Metastases

A transrectal ultrasonography—guided pathologic examinational procedure is applied during tumor diagnosis of PCa. The extent of the localized PCa tumor is also estimated by digital rectal examination and PSA testing, sometimes supplemented using CT, bone scanning, or multiparametric MRI [545]. The staging procedure for malignant PCa tumors as outlined in the National Comprehensive Cancer Network (NCCN) guidelines [546], should follow the TNM (Tumor—regional lymph Nodes—Metastasis) classification developed by the Union for International Cancer Control (UICC) and published by the American Joint Committee on Cancer (AJCC), as well as the International Federation of Gynecology and Obstetrics (FIGO), staging manuals [547].

Positron emission tomography in combination with CT is used for the staging of lymph-node metastasis involvement. Depending on stage, ^{18}F-FDG, ^{18}F-choline, or ^{11}C PET could be used [548–556]. The use of PET in combination with MRI may also help detect PCa as well as improve accuracy of staging [557–560]. Regarding the estimation if the PCa under investigation is clinically insignificant/indolent (CIPC) or significant/aggressive the Epstein criteria could be used, taken into account its limitations and many variations [561–566]. Better criteria deciding CIPC or not CIPC could help minimize the amount of under- and overtreated men having PCa [521]. Regardless whether CIPC or not CIPC, monitoring the disease is usually performed using PSA testing, complemented with MRI and/or PET/CT if PSA level is rising [567].

Regarding the treatment of localized PCa radiation therapy (RT) and radical prostectomy (RP) are established protocols, although resulting in up to 50% of PSA recurrence often referred to as biochemical recurrence (BCR) [568]. The PSA doubling time, the Gleason score, and the pathologic T-stage determines the time between BCR and when metastases are confirmed [488,569]. In order to be able to determine if the recurrence is local or in the form of metastases, ^{11}C-choline based PET/CT and/or MRI are often used [488,545,551,570–573]. Regarding metastases, the skeleton and regional lymph nodes are the most common sites, with >80% of the men succumbing to PCa having metastases in the skeleton [574]. Bone scintigraphy, as SPECT in conjunction with CT (SPECT/CT), using Technetium-99 (^{99m}Tc)-methylene di-phosphonate is often used to estimate the degree of metastases in the skeleton [567,575]. The use of ^{18}F-fluoride PET/CT might also be an option to be used for detecting and classifying metastases in the skeleton [545].

6. Theranostic Nanoparticles for Prostate and Breast Cancer

For cancer applications in general there is an increasing number of publications regarding multifunctional TNPs, exemplified by a limited selection of references [1,76,576–591]. For PCa and BC there is only a limited number of publications, some of which already have been mentioned above in conjunction with the presentation of the different type of NPs as well as different imaging and therapy options available for TNPs [1,131,230,345,358,476–478,592,593]. As TNPs combine into one nanovehicle both imaging and therapy, the presentation of selected representative examples below illustrate some of these combinations evaluated so far for PCa and BC.

Lin et al. developed and evaluated a novel multifunctional NP-based platform for simultaneous imaging and therapy of PCa using LNCaP and PC3 cells in a mouse model [476]. The imaging was achieved by using NIR activatable fluorescence NPs enabling optical imaging and therefore real-time monitoring of the drug delivery. The therapy was achieved by simultaneous targeted delivery of heat, ROS, and heat-chock protein 90 (Hsp90) inhibitor. Their porphyrine-based system was able to generate enough heat and ROS simultaneous with light activation in order to achieve a dual PTT/PDT therapy. The developed formulations of Hsp90 inhibitors also enabled a decrease of the level of pro-survival and angiogenic signaling induced by the PTT and PDT treatment, which sensitizes the tumor cells to the phototherapy. The authors concluded that by using their PCa-specific and image-guided minimally invasive NP-based PTT/PDT drug delivery system, in conjunction with the Hsp90 inhibitors, could enhance the therapeutic efficacy for PCa.

In a paper by Vaillant et al. it was investigated the possibility of developing and using a targeting molecule against the cation-independent mannose 6-phosphate receptor (M6PR), over-expressed in especially the LNCaP cell line [477]. The targeting molecule was a mannose 6-phosphate analogue, synthesized in six steps, which was grafted onto functionalized silica NPs. Experiments were performed both in vitro and in vivo using PDT and showed promising results regarding both targeting, imaging, and therapy of PCa. Regarding the developed biomarker and the M6PR investigated, the authors especially emphasize that the target fulfill important characteristics, namely (i) over-expression in 84% of PCa tissues; (ii) no expression in normal tissues or non-cancerous hypertrophy of prostate; and (iii) over-expression in low-grade cancers. Therefore, M6PR is according to the authors a promising target for non-invasive personalized therapy of PCa, with the possibility of future theranostic applications.

In a paper by Agemy et al. the targeting of the tumor vasculature was investigated for both therapy and imaging of PCa [358]. By screening phage-displayed peptide libraries they identified specific targets in the vessels of PCa tumors. One such peptide, the penta-peptide Cys-Arg-Glu-Lys-Ala, recognizes a fibrin-fibronectin complex located in tumor vasculature. By using SPIONs coated with this peptide in 22Rv1-and LAPC9-PCa cells xenograft mice models an accumulation in tumor vessels was achieved after intravenous injection, which in its turn caused additional clotting and thereby additional sites for the TNPs to bind to in the tumors. No clotting was seen in other parts of the body. Imaging was performed by MRI. The addition of an anti-cancer drug, to these tumor vasculature-blocking TNPs, is hypothesized by the authors to increase the therapeutic efficacy even further.

In a study by Li et al. a BC xenograft-mice model was used to evaluate the imaging and therapeutic efficacy of self-assembled gemcitabine-Gd(III)-based pegylated 50 nm TNPs [1]. The anti-cancer drug gemcitabine combined with the MRI contrast agent Gd(III) used in this setting for the BC cell line MDA-MB-231 showed a high in vivo antitumor efficacy compared to saline control; median tumor volume equal to 188 and 695 mm^3 28 days post injection, respectively. The level of toxicity was indistinguishable compared to controls, drug loading capacity of the TNPs higher than compared to other systems [35,36], and the in vivo MRI-signaling efficacy comparable with other similar NPs [30,594].

In vitro experiments were performed by Choi et al. in which they evaluated enzyme-activatable TNPs for NIR-fluorescence imaging and a combination of PDT and CTH of TNBC [478]. The photosensitizer chlorin e6 (Ce6) conjugated to hyaluronic acid (HA) formed Ce6-HA NPs by self-assembly. Then, the anticancer topoisomerase-1 inhibitor camptothecin (CPT) was encapsulated inside these NPs forming the final TNPs. Treatment using the enzyme hyaluronidase induced activation of singlet oxygen generation and NIR fluorescence, as well as the release of CPT from the TNPs. The light irradiation of treated TNBC cells further enhanced the therapeutic efficacy significantly. An up-dated and well written review on the subject of targeted NPs for image-guided treatment of TNBC has been written by Miller-Kleinhenz et al. and discusses, for example, subtypes, biomarkers, and potential surface targets for TNBC [242].

Ansari et al. demonstrated in a study the feasibility of a TNP incorporating both tumor specificity, enzyme-activated prodrugs, and in vivo imaging possibilities by conjugating the FDA-approved magnetic iron-oxide NP ferumoxytol to a matrix metalloproteinase-activatable peptide conjugate of the colchicine analogue azademethyl-colchicine [592]. Intravenous injections of the TNPs into MMTV-PyMT (mouse mammary tumor virus-polyoma middle-T-antigen) BC tumor-bearing mice resulted in a significant anti-tumor efficacy compared to controls, with no detectable normal-tissue toxicity, explained by a significant tumor accumulation of the TNPs shown by MRI. The results are important since the MMTV-PyMT cells are considered to be a good model for BC metastasis [595]. It should be noted that by March 30, 2015, FDA changed its prescription instructions for the ferumoxytol-based anemia drug Feraheme® due to risk of serious allergic reactions [596].

In conclusion, theranostic NPs applied in an individualized targeted nanomedicine setting have a high potential to become one of the most valuable technologies for the detection, diagnosis, and therapy of PCa and BC. The tumor cell specific multifunctionality of such nanovehicles could enable earlier detection of the diseases, as well as increased sensitivity and specificity during diagnosis. The TNPs also have the potential to increase the likelihood of survival as well as decreasing systemic toxicity for treated patients, compared to the options available today. There are many combinatorial possibilities when constructing TNPs, and all of them have pros and cons as illustrated in this paper. Clinical trials need to be performed in order to give the U.S. Food and Drug Administration, its European Union equivalence European Medicines Agency, and other national medicine-regulatory authorities, the possibility to evaluate relevant TNP options further. This will hopefully add to the list of NP-based drugs under clinical evaluation or already clinically approved, and listed in Table 1 below, also theranostic applications for both PCa and BC.

Table 1. Nanoparticle-based drugs for PCa and BC, approved or under clinical evaluation. Listed are also examples of drugs for solid cancers in general, since they also might be applicable to PCa and BC in the future.

Cancer	Specific Indication	Nanoparticle	Drug	Product	Phase	Company
PCa	US enhancement imaging	Phospholipid microbubbles	-	SonoVue®	Phase III	Bracco Diagnostics Inc.
	Metastatic CRPC	Polymeric	Docetaxel	BIND-014 (Accurin™)	Phase II	Pfizer Inc/BIND Therapeutics Inc.
	Hormone refractive PCa	Albumin-based NP	Paclitaxel	Abraxane®	Phase II	Celgene Corporation
	Androgen independant PCa	Liposome	Doxorubicin	Doxil®	Phase II	Janssen Pharmaceuticals Inc.
	-	Iron NP	Iron NP	Magnablate	Phase I/0	University College London Hospitals
BC	Metastatic BC	Liposome	Doxorubicin	Myocet™	Approved	Teva UK Ltd.
	Metastatic BC	Albumin-based NP	Paclitaxel	Abraxane™	Approved	Celgene Corporation
	-	Micelle (polymeric)	Paclitaxel	Genexol-PM™	Approved	Samyang Pharmaceuticals Co.
	US enhancement imaging	Lipid microspheres	-	Definity®	Approved	Lantheus Medical Imaging Inc.
	Metastatic BC	Liposome	Paclitaxel	LIPUSU®	Phase IV	Nanjing Luye Sike Pharmaceutical Co., Ltd.
	Metastatic BC	Polymeric conjugate	Irinotecan	NKTR-102	Phase III	Nektar Therapeutics
	Refractory chest wall BC	Liposome	Doxorubicin	ThermoDox™	Phase II/I	Celsion Co.
	-	Micelle (polymeric)	Paclitaxel	NK105	Phase III	NanoCarrier Co., Ltd.
	Advanced/metastatic BC	HER2-liposome	Doxorubicin	-MM-302	Phase III/II/I	Merrimack Pharmaceuticals Inc.
	Tripple-negative metastatic BC	Liposome	Doxorubicin	Doxil®	Phase II	Janssen Pharmaceuticals Inc.
	-	Liposome	Doxorubicin	Caelyx®	Phase II	Janssen-Cilag Ltd.
	Tripple-negative metastatic BC	Liposome	Paclitaxel	EndoTAG-1	Phase II	MediGene AG
	Metastatic	Liposome	Paclitaxel	LEP-ETU	Phase II	Insys Therapeutics Inc.
	Advanced recurrent/metastatic BC	Liposome	Mitoxantrone	Mitoxantrone HCL Liposome	Phase II	CSPC ZhongQi Pharmaceutical Technology
	Metastatic BC	Micelle (polymeric)	Paclitaxel	Nanoxel™	Phase I	Samyang Pharmaceuticals Co.
	US enhancement imaging	Phospholipid microbubbles	-	SonoVue®	Pilot	Bracco Imaging Inc.
	Metastatic/locally recurrent	Micelle (polymeric)	Paclitaxel	Cynviloq	Not provided	Sorrento Therapeutics Inc.
Solid cancers	Advanced tumors	Liposome	Curcumin	Lipocurc	Phase II/I	SignPath Pharma Inc.
	Advanced tumors	Micelle	Gemcitabine/Cisplatin	NC-6004 Nanoplatin	Phase II/I	NanoCarrier Co., Ltd.
	Advanced tumors	Cyclodextrin-based NP	Docetaxel	CRLX301	Phase II/I	Cerulean Pharma Inc.
	-	Micelle (polymeric)	Docetaxel/Taxotere	Docetaxel-PM DOPNP201	Phase I	Samyang Pharmaceuticals Co.
	-	Micelle	Docetaxel	CriPec	Phase I	Cristal Therapeutics
	Advanced tumors	Micelle (polymeric)	Cisplatin/paclitaxel	NC-4016 DACH-Platin micelle	Phase I	NanoCarrier Co Ltd/MD Anderson Cancer Center
	-	Liposome	Eribulin mesylate	Halaven E7389-LF	Phase I	Eisai Co., Ltd.
	-	Liposome	Mitomycin-C	Promitil®	Phase I	LipoMedix Pharmaceuticals Inc.
	Refractory/recurrent tumors	Liposome	Topotecan, docetaxel, CP	SGT-53	Phase I	SynerGene Therapeutics Inc.
	-	Liposome	RB94 plasmid DNA	SGT-94	Phase I	SynerGene Therapeutics Inc.
	Advanced tumors	Liposome	^{188}Re-BMEDA	^{188}Re-BMEDA	Phase I	INER, Taiwan
	Advanced tumors	Albumin-based NP	Thiocolchicine	ABI-011	Phase I	NantBioScience Inc.
	-	Lipid	DsiRNA	DCR-MYC	Phase I	Dicerna Pharmaceuticals Inc.
	Advanced recurrent tumors	Liposome	siRNA	siRNA-EphA2-DOPC	Phase I	MD Anderson Cancer Center
	Advanced/refractory tumors	Liposome	Cisplatin	LiPlaCis	Phase I	Oncology Venture/LiPlasome Pharma A/S
	Advanced solid tumors	Polymeric	AZD2811, Irinotecan	AZD2811 (Accurin™)	Phase I	AztraZeneca/BIND Therapeutics Inc.

US = Ultra sound; CRPC = Castration resistant prostate cancer; PSMA = Prostate-specific membrane antigen; AZD2811—Aurora B kinase inhibitor; DsiRNA = Double stranded small interfering RNA; siRNA = small interfering RNA; CP = Cyclophosphamide; NP = Nanoparticle; EndoTag = Endothelial targeting agent; LEP-ETU = liposome entrapped paclitaxel easy-to-us; LIPUSU = Paclitaxel liposome for injection; BMEDA = (2-mercaptoethyl)-*N′*,*N′*-diethylethylenediamine.

References

1. Li, L.; Tong, R.; Li, M.; Kohane, D.S. Self-assembled gemcitabine-gadolinium nanoparticles for magnetic resonance imaging and cancer therapy. *Acta Biomater.* **2016**, *33*, 34–39. [CrossRef] [PubMed]
2. Rizzo, L.Y.; Theek, B.; Storm, G.; Kiessling, F.; Lammers, T. Recent progress in nanomedicine: Therapeutic, diagnostic and theranostic applications. *Curr. Opin. Biotechnol.* **2013**, *24*, 1159–1166. [CrossRef] [PubMed]
3. Lee, G.Y.; Qian, W.P.; Wang, L.; Wang, Y.A.; Staley, C.A.; Satpathy, M.; Nie, S.; Mao, H.; Yang, L. Theranostic nanoparticles with controlled release of gemcitabine for targeted therapy and MRI of pancreatic cancer. *ACS Nano* **2013**, *7*, 2078–2089. [CrossRef] [PubMed]
4. Tian, Q.; Hu, J.; Zhu, Y.; Zou, R.; Chen, Z.; Yang, S.; Li, R.; Su, Q.; Han, Y.; Liu, X. Sub-10 nm Fe_3O_4@$Cu_{2-x}S$ core-shell nanoparticles for dual-modal imaging and photothermal therapy. *J. Am. Chem. Soc.* **2013**, *135*, 8571–8577. [CrossRef] [PubMed]
5. Bardhan, R.; Lal, S.; Joshi, A.; Halas, N.J. Theranostic nanoshells: From probe design to imaging and treatment of cancer. *Acc. Chem. Res.* **2011**, *44*, 936–946. [CrossRef] [PubMed]
6. Huang, P.; Rong, P.; Lin, J.; Li, W.; Yan, X.; Zhang, M.G.; Nie, L.; Niu, G.; Lu, J.; Wang, W.; et al. Triphase interface synthesis of plasmonic gold bellflowers as near-infrared light mediated acoustic and thermal theranostics. *J. Am. Chem. Soc.* **2014**, *136*, 8307–8313. [CrossRef] [PubMed]
7. Kim, J.; Piao, Y.; Hyeon, T. Multifunctional nanostructured materials for multimodal imaging, and simultaneous imaging and therapy. *Chem. Soc. Rev.* **2009**, *38*, 372–390. [CrossRef] [PubMed]
8. Giljohann, D.A.; Seferos, D.S.; Daniel, W.L.; Massich, M.D.; Patel, P.C.; Mirkin, C.A. Gold nanoparticles for biology and medicine. *Angew. Chem. Int. Ed. Engl.* **2010**, *49*, 3280–3294. [CrossRef] [PubMed]
9. Liu, G.; Zhang, G.; Hu, J.; Wang, X.; Zhu, M.; Liu, S. Hyperbranched self-immolative polymers (HSIPS) for programmed payload delivery and ultrasensitive detection. *J. Am. Chem. Soc.* **2015**, *137*, 11645–11655. [CrossRef] [PubMed]
10. Sanna, V.; Pala, N.; Sechi, M. Targeted therapy using nanotechnology: Focus on cancer. *Int. J. Nanomed.* **2014**, *9*, 467–483.
11. Doane, T.L.; Burda, C. The unique role of nanoparticles in nanomedicine: Imaging, drug delivery and therapy. *Chem. Soc. Rev.* **2012**, *41*, 2885–2911. [CrossRef] [PubMed]
12. Kim, B.Y.; Rutka, J.T.; Chan, W.C. Nanomedicine. *N. Engl. J. Med.* **2010**, *363*, 2434–2443. [CrossRef] [PubMed]
13. Riehemann, K.; Schneider, S.W.; Luger, T.A.; Godin, B.; Ferrari, M.; Fuchs, H. Nanomedicine—Challenge and perspectives. *Angew. Chem. Int. Ed. Engl.* **2009**, *48*, 872–897. [CrossRef] [PubMed]
14. Zhang, L.; Gu, F.X.; Chan, J.M.; Wang, A.Z.; Langer, R.S.; Farokhzad, O.C. Nanoparticles in medicine: Therapeutic applications and developments. *Clin. Pharmacol. Ther.* **2008**, *83*, 761–769. [CrossRef] [PubMed]
15. Peer, D.; Karp, J.M.; Hong, S.; Farokhzad, O.C.; Margalit, R.; Langer, R. Nanocarriers as an emerging platform for cancer therapy. *Nat. Nanotechnol.* **2007**, *2*, 751–760. [CrossRef] [PubMed]
16. Langer, R. Polymer-controlled drug delivery systems. *Acc. Chem. Res.* **1993**, *26*, 537–542. [CrossRef]
17. Tong, R.; Chiang, H.H.; Kohane, D.S. Photoswitchable nanoparticles for in vivo cancer chemotherapy. *Proc. Natl. Acad. Sci. USA* **2013**, *110*, 19048–19053. [CrossRef] [PubMed]
18. Cheng, L.; Wang, C.; Feng, L.; Yang, K.; Liu, Z. Functional nanomaterials for phototherapies of cancer. *Chem. Rev.* **2014**, *114*, 10869–10939. [CrossRef] [PubMed]
19. Carmeliet, P.; Jain, R.K. Principles and mechanisms of vessel normalization for cancer and other angiogenic diseases. *Nat. Rev. Drug Discov.* **2011**, *10*, 417–427. [CrossRef] [PubMed]
20. Perrault, S.D.; Walkey, C.; Jennings, T.; Fischer, H.C.; Chan, W.C. Mediating tumor targeting efficiency of nanoparticles through design. *Nano Lett.* **2009**, *9*, 1909–1915. [CrossRef] [PubMed]
21. Miller, M.A.; Gadde, S.; Pfirschke, C.; Engblom, C.; Sprachman, M.M.; Kohler, R.H.; Yang, K.S.; Laughney, A.M.; Wojtkiewicz, G.; Kamaly, N.; et al. Predicting therapeutic nanomedicine efficacy using a companion magnetic resonance imaging nanoparticle. *Sci. Transl. Med.* **2015**, *7*, 314ra183. [CrossRef] [PubMed]
22. Hare, J.I.; Lammers, T.; Ashford, M.B.; Puri, S.; Storm, G.; Barry, S.T. Challenges and strategies in anti-cancer nanomedicine development: An industry perspective. *Adv. Drug Deliv. Rev.* **2017**, *108*, 25–38. [CrossRef] [PubMed]

23. Matsumura, Y.; Maeda, H. A new concept for macromolecular therapeutics in cancer chemotherapy: Mechanism of tumoritropic accumulation of proteins and the antitumor agent smancs. *Cancer Res.* **1986**, *46*, 6387–6392. [PubMed]
24. Caravan, P.; Ellison, J.J.; McMurry, T.J.; Lauffer, R.B. Gadolinium(III) chelates as MRI contrast agents: Structure, dynamics, and applications. *Chem. Rev.* **1999**, *99*, 2293–2352. [CrossRef] [PubMed]
25. Walker, E.A.; Fenton, M.E.; Salesky, J.S.; Murphey, M.D. Magnetic resonance imaging of benign soft tissue neoplasms in adults. *Radiol. Clin. N. Am.* **2011**, *49*, 1197–1217. [CrossRef] [PubMed]
26. Liu, T.; Li, X.; Qian, Y.; Hu, X.; Liu, S. Multifunctional pH-disintegrable micellar nanoparticles of asymmetrically functionalized β-cyclodextrin-based star copolymer covalently conjugated with doxorubicin and DOTA-Gd moieties. *Biomaterials* **2012**, *33*, 2521–2531. [CrossRef] [PubMed]
27. Kircher, M.F.; de la Zerda, A.; Jokerst, J.V.; Zavaleta, C.L.; Kempen, P.J.; Mittra, E.; Pitter, K.; Huang, R.; Campos, C.; Habte, F.; et al. A brain tumor molecular imaging strategy using a new triple-modality MRI-photoacoustic-raman nanoparticle. *Nat. Med.* **2012**, *18*, 829–834. [CrossRef] [PubMed]
28. Kielar, F.; Tei, L.; Terreno, E.; Botta, M. Large relaxivity enhancement of paramagnetic lipid nanoparticles by restricting the local motions of the Gd(III) chelates. *J. Am. Chem. Soc.* **2010**, *132*, 7836–7837. [CrossRef] [PubMed]
29. Mi, P.; Kokuryo, D.; Cabral, H.; Kumagai, M.; Nomoto, T.; Aoki, I.; Terada, Y.; Kishimura, A.; Nishiyama, N.; Kataoka, K. Hydrothermally synthesized pegylated calcium phosphate nanoparticles incorporating Gd-DTPA for contrast enhanced MRI diagnosis of solid tumors. *J. Control. Release* **2014**, *174*, 63–71. [CrossRef] [PubMed]
30. Mi, P.; Cabral, H.; Kokuryo, D.; Rafi, M.; Terada, Y.; Aoki, I.; Saga, T.; Takehiko, I.; Nishiyama, N.; Kataoka, K. Gd-DTPA-loaded polymer-metal complex micelles with high relaxivity for MR cancer imaging. *Biomaterials* **2013**, *34*, 492–500. [CrossRef] [PubMed]
31. Frias, J.C.; Williams, K.J.; Fisher, E.A.; Fayad, Z.A. Recombinant hdl-like nanoparticles: A specific contrast agent for MRI of atherosclerotic plaques. *J. Am. Chem. Soc.* **2004**, *126*, 16316–16317. [CrossRef] [PubMed]
32. Li, X.; Qian, Y.; Liu, T.; Hu, X.; Zhang, G.; You, Y.; Liu, S. Amphiphilic multiarm star block copolymer-based multifunctional unimolecular micelles for cancer targeted drug delivery and mr imaging. *Biomaterials* **2011**, *32*, 6595–6605. [CrossRef] [PubMed]
33. Fossheim, S.L.; Fahlvik, A.K.; Klaveness, J.; Muller, R.N. Paramagnetic liposomes as MRI contrast agents: Influence of liposomal physicochemical properties on the in vitro relaxivity. *Magn. Reson. Imaging* **1999**, *17*, 83–89. [CrossRef]
34. Perrier, M.; Gallud, A.; Ayadi, A.; Kennouche, S.; Porredon, C.; Gary-Bobo, M.; Larionova, J.; Goze-Bac, C.; Zanca, M.; Garcia, M.; et al. Investigation of cyano-bridged coordination nanoparticles Gd(3+)/[Fe(Cn)6](3-)/D-mannitol as T1-weighted MRI contrast agents. *Nanoscale* **2015**, *7*, 11899–11903. [CrossRef] [PubMed]
35. Hu, X.; Liu, G.; Li, Y.; Wang, X.; Liu, S. Cell-penetrating hyperbranched polyprodrug amphiphiles for synergistic reductive milieu-triggered drug release and enhanced magnetic resonance signals. *J. Am. Chem. Soc.* **2015**, *137*, 362–368. [CrossRef] [PubMed]
36. Lee, S.M.; Song, Y.; Hong, B.J.; MacRenaris, K.W.; Mastarone, D.J.; O'Halloran, T.V.; Meade, T.J.; Nguyen, S.T. Modular polymer-caged nanobins as a theranostic platform with enhanced magnetic resonance relaxivity and pH-responsive drug release. *Angew. Chem. Int. Ed. Engl.* **2010**, *49*, 9960–9964. [CrossRef] [PubMed]
37. Budd, G.T. Let me do more than count the ways: What circulating tumor cells can tell us about the biology of cancer. *Mol. Pharm.* **2009**, *6*, 1307–1310. [CrossRef] [PubMed]
38. Bray, F.; Moller, B. Predicting the future burden of cancer. *Nat. Rev. Cancer* **2006**, *6*, 63–74. [CrossRef] [PubMed]
39. Danila, D.C.; Fleisher, M.; Scher, H.I. Circulating tumor cells as biomarkers in prostate cancer. *Clin. Cancer Res.* **2011**, *17*, 3903–3912. [CrossRef] [PubMed]
40. Ashworth, T.R. A case of cancer in which cells similar to those in the tumours were seen in the blood after death. *Med. J. Aust.* **1869**, *14*, 146–147.
41. Pantel, K.; Alix-Panabieres, C.; Riethdorf, S. Cancer micrometastases. *Nat. Rev. Clin. Oncol.* **2009**, *6*, 339–351. [CrossRef] [PubMed]
42. Gupta, G.P.; Massague, J. Cancer metastasis: Building a framework. *Cell* **2006**, *127*, 679–695. [CrossRef] [PubMed]

43. Fehm, T.; Sagalowsky, A.; Clifford, E.; Beitsch, P.; Saboorian, H.; Euhus, D.; Meng, S.; Morrison, L.; Tucker, T.; Lane, N.; et al. Cytogenetic evidence that circulating epithelial cells in patients with carcinoma are malignant. *Clin. Cancer Res.* **2002**, *8*, 2073–2084. [PubMed]
44. Sleijfer, S.; Gratama, J.W.; Sieuwerts, A.M.; Kraan, J.; Martens, J.W.; Foekens, J.A. Circulating tumour cell detection on its way to routine diagnostic implementation? *Eur. J. Cancer* **2007**, *43*, 2645–2650. [CrossRef] [PubMed]
45. Fidler, I.J. The pathogenesis of cancer metastasis: The 'seed and soil' hypothesis revisited. *Nat. Rev. Cancer* **2003**, *3*, 453–458. [CrossRef] [PubMed]
46. Hayes, D.F.; Smerage, J. Is there a role for circulating tumor cells in the management of breast cancer? *Clin. Cancer Res.* **2008**, *14*, 3646–3650. [CrossRef] [PubMed]
47. Pantel, K.; Riethdorf, S. Pathology: Are circulating tumor cells predictive of overall survival? *Nat. Rev. Clin. Oncol.* **2009**, *6*, 190–191. [CrossRef] [PubMed]
48. Aceto, N.; Bardia, A.; Miyamoto, D.T.; Donaldson, M.C.; Wittner, B.S.; Spencer, J.A.; Yu, M.; Pely, A.; Engstrom, A.; Zhu, H.; et al. Circulating tumor cell clusters are oligoclonal precursors of breast cancer metastasis. *Cell* **2014**, *158*, 1110–1122. [CrossRef] [PubMed]
49. Miller, M.C.; Doyle, G.V.; Terstappen, L.W. Significance of circulating tumor cells detected by the cellsearch system in patients with metastatic breast colorectal and prostate cancer. *J. Oncol.* **2010**, *2010*, 617421. [CrossRef] [PubMed]
50. Swaby, R.F.; Cristofanilli, M. Circulating tumor cells in breast cancer: A tool whose time has come of age. *BMC Med.* **2011**, *9*, 43. [CrossRef] [PubMed]
51. Hekimian, K.; Meisezahl, S.; Trompelt, K.; Rabenstein, C.; Pachmann, K. Epithelial cell dissemination and readhesion: Analysis of factors contributing to metastasis formation in breast cancer. *ISRN Oncol.* **2012**, *2012*, 601810. [CrossRef] [PubMed]
52. O'Hara, S.M.; Moreno, J.G.; Zweitzig, D.R.; Gross, S.; Gomella, L.G.; Terstappen, L.W. Multigene reverse transcription-PCR profiling of circulating tumor cells in hormone-refractory prostate cancer. *Clin. Chem.* **2004**, *50*, 826–835. [CrossRef] [PubMed]
53. Attard, G.; Swennenhuis, J.F.; Olmos, D.; Reid, A.H.; Vickers, E.; A'Hern, R.; Levink, R.; Coumans, F.; Moreira, J.; Riisnaes, R.; et al. Characterization of *ERG, AR* and *PTEN* gene status in circulating tumor cells from patients with castration-resistant prostate cancer. *Cancer Res.* **2009**, *69*, 2912–2918. [CrossRef] [PubMed]
54. Coumans, F.A.; Doggen, C.J.; Attard, G.; de Bono, J.S.; Terstappen, L.W. All circulating EpCam+CK+CD45-objects predict overall survival in castration-resistant prostate cancer. *Ann. Oncol.* **2010**, *21*, 1851–1857. [CrossRef] [PubMed]
55. Chen, F.; Hong, H.; Zhang, Y.; Valdovinos, H.F.; Shi, S.; Kwon, G.S.; Theuer, C.P.; Barnhart, T.E.; Cai, W. In vivo tumor targeting and image-guided drug delivery with antibody-conjugated, radiolabeled mesoporous silica nanoparticles. *ACS Nano* **2013**, *7*, 9027–9039. [CrossRef] [PubMed]
56. Gupta, P.B.; Onder, T.T.; Jiang, G.; Tao, K.; Kuperwasser, C.; Weinberg, R.A.; Lander, E.S. Identification of selective inhibitors of cancer stem cells by high-throughput screening. *Cell* **2009**, *138*, 645–659. [CrossRef] [PubMed]
57. Zhu, S.; Xu, G. Single-walled carbon nanohorns and their applications. *Nanoscale* **2010**, *2*, 2538–2549. [CrossRef] [PubMed]
58. Kaur, R.; Badea, I. Nanodiamonds as novel nanomaterials for biomedical applications: Drug delivery and imaging systems. *Int. J. Nanomed.* **2013**, *8*, 203–220.
59. Clift, M.J.; Stone, V. Quantum dots: An insight and perspective of their biological interaction and how this relates to their relevance for clinical use. *Theranostics* **2012**, *2*, 668–680. [CrossRef] [PubMed]
60. Taylor, A.; Wilson, K.M.; Murray, P.; Fernig, D.G.; Levy, R. Long-term tracking of cells using inorganic nanoparticles as contrast agents: Are we there yet? *Chem. Soc. Rev.* **2012**, *41*, 2707–2717. [CrossRef] [PubMed]
61. Bae, K.H.; Chung, H.J.; Park, T.G. Nanomaterials for cancer therapy and imaging. *Mol. Cells* **2011**, *31*, 295–302. [CrossRef] [PubMed]
62. Wilhelm, S.; Tavares, A.J.; Dai, Q.; Ohta, S.; Audet, J.; Dvorak, H.F.; Chan, W.C.W. Analysis of nanoparticle delivery to tumours. *Nat. Rev. Mater.* **2016**, *1*, 1–12. [CrossRef]
63. Cheng, C.J.; Tietjen, G.T.; Saucier-Sawyer, J.K.; Saltzman, W.M. A holistic approach to targeting disease with polymeric nanoparticles. *Nat. Rev. Drug Discov.* **2015**, *14*, 239–247. [CrossRef] [PubMed]

64. Ding, Y.; Jiang, Z.; Saha, K.; Kim, C.S.; Kim, S.T.; Landis, R.F.; Rotello, V.M. Gold nanoparticles for nucleic acid delivery. *Mol. Ther.* **2014**, *22*, 1075–1083. [CrossRef] [PubMed]
65. Kasprzak, B.; Miskiel, S.; Markowska, J. Nanooncology in ovarian cancer treatment. *Eur. J. Gynaecol. Oncol.* **2016**, *37*, 161–163. [PubMed]
66. Hu, J.J.; Xiao, D.; Zhang, X.Z. Advances in peptide functionalization on mesoporous silica nanoparticles for controlled drug release. *Small* **2016**, *12*, 3344–3359. [CrossRef] [PubMed]
67. Mocan, L.; Matea, C.T.; Bartos, D.; Mosteanu, O.; Pop, T.; Mocan, T.; Iancu, C. Advances in cancer research using gold nanoparticles mediated photothermal ablation. *Clujul Med.* **2016**, *89*, 199–202. [CrossRef] [PubMed]
68. Lu, B.; Huang, X.; Mo, J.; Zhao, W. Drug delivery using nanoparticles for cancer stem-like cell targeting. *Front. Pharmacol.* **2016**, *7*, 84. [CrossRef] [PubMed]
69. Genchi, G.G.; Marino, A.; Rocca, A.; Mattoli, V.; Ciofani, G. Barium titanate nanoparticles: Promising multitasking vectors in nanomedicine. *Nanotechnology* **2016**, *27*, 232001. [CrossRef] [PubMed]
70. Dolati, S.; Sadreddini, S.; Rostamzadeh, D.; Ahmadi, M.; Jadidi-Niaragh, F.; Yousefi, M. Utilization of nanoparticle technology in rheumatoid arthritis treatment. *Biomed. Pharmacother.* **2016**, *80*, 30–41. [CrossRef] [PubMed]
71. Santoso, M.R.; Yang, P.C. Magnetic nanoparticles for targeting and imaging of stem cells in myocardial infarction. *Stem Cells Int.* **2016**, *2016*. [CrossRef] [PubMed]
72. Li, X.; Tsibouklis, J.; Weng, T.; Zhang, B.; Yin, G.; Feng, G.; Cui, Y.; Savina, I.N.; Mikhalovska, L.I.; Sandeman, S.R.; et al. Nano carriers for drug transport across the blood brain barrier. *J. Drug Target.* **2017**, *25*, 17–28. [CrossRef] [PubMed]
73. Beloqui, A.; des Rieux, A.; Preat, V. Mechanisms of transport of polymeric and lipidic nanoparticles across the intestinal barrier. *Adv. Drug Deliv. Rev.* **2016**, *106*, 242–255. [CrossRef] [PubMed]
74. Nishiyama, N.; Matsumura, Y.; Kataoka, K. Development of polymeric micelles for targeting intractable cancers. *Cancer Sci.* **2016**, *107*, 867–874. [CrossRef] [PubMed]
75. Ulbrich, K.; Hola, K.; Subr, V.; Bakandritsos, A.; Tucek, J.; Zboril, R. Targeted drug delivery with polymers and magnetic nanoparticles: Covalent and noncovalent approaches, release control, and clinical studies. *Chem. Rev.* **2016**, *116*, 5338–5431. [CrossRef] [PubMed]
76. Shahbazi, R.; Ozpolat, B.; Ulubayram, K. Oligonucleotide-based theranostic nanoparticles in cancer therapy. *Nanomedicine (lond.)* **2016**, *11*, 1287–1308. [CrossRef] [PubMed]
77. Yuan, Y.; Cai, T.; Xia, X.; Zhang, R.; Cai, Y.; Chiba, P. Nanoparticle delivery of anticancer drugs overcomes multidrug resistance in breast cancer. *Drug Deliv.* **2016**, *23*, 3350–3357. [CrossRef] [PubMed]
78. Zhou, M.; Tian, M.; Li, C. Copper-based nanomaterials for cancer imaging and therapy. *Bioconjug. Chem.* **2016**, *27*, 1188–1199. [CrossRef] [PubMed]
79. Rajabi, M.; Mousa, S.A. Lipid nanoparticles and their application in nanomedicine. *Curr. Pharm. Biotechnol.* **2016**, *17*, 662–672. [CrossRef] [PubMed]
80. Rao, P.V.; Nallappan, D.; Madhavi, K.; Rahman, S.; Jun Wei, L.; Gan, S.H. Phytochemicals and biogenic metallic nanoparticles as anticancer agents. *Oxid. Med. Cell. Longev.* **2016**, *2016*. [CrossRef] [PubMed]
81. Ma, D.D.; Yang, W.X. Engineered nanoparticles induce cell apoptosis: Potential for cancer therapy. *Oncotarget* **2016**, *7*, 40882–40903. [CrossRef] [PubMed]
82. Shabestari Khiabani, S.; Farshbaf, M.; Akbarzadeh, A.; Davaran, S. Magnetic nanoparticles: Preparation methods, applications in cancer diagnosis and cancer therapy. *Artif. Cells Nanomed. Biotechnol.* **2016**, *45*, 6–17. [CrossRef] [PubMed]
83. Lemaster, J.E.; Jokerst, J.V. What is new in nanoparticle-based photoacoustic imaging? *Wiley Interdiscip. Rev. Nanomed. Nanobiotechnol.* **2016**, *9*, e1404. [CrossRef] [PubMed]
84. Liu, H.; Zhang, J.; Chen, X.; Du, X.S.; Zhang, J.L.; Liu, G.; Zhang, W.G. Application of iron oxide nanoparticles in glioma imaging and therapy: From bench to bedside. *Nanoscale* **2016**, *8*, 7808–7826. [CrossRef] [PubMed]
85. Fathi Karkan, S.; Mohammadhosseini, M.; Panahi, Y.; Milani, M.; Zarghami, N.; Akbarzadeh, A.; Abasi, E.; Hosseini, A.; Davaran, S. Magnetic nanoparticles in cancer diagnosis and treatment: A review. *Artif. Cells Nanomed. Biotechnol.* **2016**, *45*, 1–5. [CrossRef] [PubMed]
86. Radenkovic, D.; Kobayashi, H.; Remsey-Semmelweis, E.; Seifalian, A.M. Quantum dot nanoparticle for optimization of breast cancer diagnostics and therapy in a clinical setting. *Nanomedicine* **2016**, *12*, 1581–1592. [CrossRef] [PubMed]

87. Pratt, E.C.; Shaffer, T.M.; Grimm, J. Nanoparticles and radiotracers: Advances toward radionanomedicine. *Wiley Interdiscip. Rev. Nanomed. Nanobiotechnol.* **2016**, *8*, 872–890. [CrossRef] [PubMed]
88. Pasqua, L.; Leggio, A.; Sisci, D.; Ando, S.; Morelli, C. Mesoporous silica nanoparticles in cancer therapy: Relevance of the targeting function. *Mini Rev. Med. Chem.* **2016**, *16*, 743–753. [CrossRef] [PubMed]
89. Rancoule, C.; Magne, N.; Vallard, A.; Guy, J.B.; Rodriguez-Lafrasse, C.; Deutsch, E.; Chargari, C. Nanoparticles in radiation oncology: From bench-side to bedside. *Cancer Lett.* **2016**, *375*, 256–262. [CrossRef] [PubMed]
90. Alam, F.; Naim, M.; Aziz, M.; Yadav, N. Unique roles of nanotechnology in medicine and cancer-II. *Indian J. Cancer* **2015**, *52*, 1–9. [CrossRef] [PubMed]
91. Yang, R.M.; Fu, C.P.; Fang, J.Z.; Xu, X.D.; Wei, X.H.; Tang, W.J.; Jiang, X.Q.; Zhang, L.M. Hyaluronan-modified superparamagnetic iron oxide nanoparticles for bimodal breast cancer imaging and photothermal therapy. *Int. J. Nanomed.* **2017**, *12*, 197–206. [CrossRef] [PubMed]
92. Oddo, L.; Cerroni, B.; Domenici, F.; Bedini, A.; Bordi, F.; Chiessi, E.; Gerbes, S.; Paradossi, G. Next generation ultrasound platforms for theranostics. *J. Colloid Interface Sci.* **2017**, *491*, 151–160. [CrossRef] [PubMed]
93. Dadras, P.; Atyabi, F.; Irani, S.; Ma'mani, L.; Foroumadi, A.; Mirzaie, Z.H.; Ebrahimi, M.; Dinarvand, R. Formulation and evaluation of targeted nanoparticles for breast cancer theranostic system. *Eur. J. Pharm. Sci.* **2017**, *97*, 47–54. [CrossRef] [PubMed]
94. Huang, Y.; Mao, K.; Zhang, B.; Zhao, Y. Superparamagnetic iron oxide nanoparticles conjugated with folic acid for dual target-specific drug delivery and MRI in cancer theranostics. *Mater. Sci. Eng. C Mater. Biol. Appl.* **2017**, *70*, 763–771. [CrossRef] [PubMed]
95. Sun, L.; Joh, D.Y.; Al-Zaki, A.; Stangl, M.; Murty, S.; Davis, J.J.; Baumann, B.C.; Alonso-Basanta, M.; Kaol, G.D.; Tsourkas, A.; et al. Theranostic application of mixed gold and superparamagnetic iron oxide nanoparticle micelles in glioblastoma multiforme. *J. Biomed. Nanotechnol.* **2016**, *12*, 347–356. [CrossRef] [PubMed]
96. Shevtsov, M.; Multhoff, G. Recent developments of magnetic nanoparticles for theranostics of brain tumor. *Curr. Drug Metab.* **2016**, *17*, 737–744. [CrossRef] [PubMed]
97. Zarrin, A.; Sadighian, S.; Rostamizadeh, K.; Firuzi, O.; Hamidi, M.; Mohammadi-Samani, S.; Miri, R. Design, preparation, and in vitro characterization of a trimodally-targeted nanomagnetic onco-theranostic system for cancer diagnosis and therapy. *Int. J. Pharm.* **2016**, *500*, 62–76. [CrossRef] [PubMed]
98. Bakhtiary, Z.; Saei, A.A.; Hajipour, M.J.; Raoufi, M.; Vermesh, O.; Mahmoudi, M. Targeted superparamagnetic iron oxide nanoparticles for early detection of cancer: Possibilities and challenges. *Nanomedicine* **2016**, *12*, 287–307. [CrossRef] [PubMed]
99. Kandasamy, G.; Maity, D. Recent advances in superparamagnetic iron oxide nanoparticles (SPIONs) for in vitro and in vivo cancer nanotheranostics. *Int. J. Pharm.* **2015**, *496*, 191–218. [CrossRef] [PubMed]
100. Bulte, J.W.; Kraitchman, D.L. Iron oxide mr contrast agents for molecular and cellular imaging. *NMR Biomed.* **2004**, *17*, 484–499. [CrossRef] [PubMed]
101. Alwi, R.; Telenkov, S.; Mandelis, A.; Leshuk, T.; Gu, F.; Oladepo, S.; Michaelian, K. Silica-coated super paramagnetic iron oxide nanoparticles (SPION) as biocompatible contrast agent in biomedical photoacoustics. *Biomed. Opt. Express* **2012**, *3*, 2500–2509. [CrossRef] [PubMed]
102. Bohmer, N.; Jordan, A. Caveolin-1 and CDC42 mediated endocytosis of silica-coated iron oxide nanoparticles in HeLa cells. *Beilstein J. Nanotechnol.* **2015**, *6*, 167–176. [CrossRef] [PubMed]
103. Nyalosaso, J.L.; Rascol, E.; Pisani, C.; Dorandeu, C.; Dumail, X.; Maynadier, M.; Gary-Bobo, M.; Kee Him, J.L.; Bron, P.; Garcia, M.; et al. Synthesis, decoration, and cellular effects of magnetic mesoporous silica nanoparticles. *RSC Adv.* **2016**, *6*, 7275–7283. [CrossRef]
104. Winter, A.; Engels, S.; Kowald, T.; Paulo, T.S.; Gerullis, H.; Chavan, A.; Wawroschek, F. Magnetic sentinel lymph node detection in prostate cancer after intraprostatic injection of superparamagnetic iron oxide nanoparticles. *Aktuelle Urol.* **2017**. [CrossRef]
105. Sabnis, S.; Sabnis, N.A.; Raut, S.; Lacko, A.G. Superparamagnetic reconstituted high-density lipoprotein nanocarriers for magnetically guided drug delivery. *Int. J. Nanomed.* **2017**, *12*, 1453–1464. [CrossRef] [PubMed]
106. Nagesh, P.K.; Johnson, N.R.; Boya, V.K.; Chowdhury, P.; Othman, S.F.; Khalilzad-Sharghi, V.; Hafeez, B.B.; Ganju, A.; Khan, S.; Behrman, S.W.; et al. PSMA targeted docetaxel-loaded superparamagnetic iron oxide nanoparticles for prostate cancer. *Colloids Surf. B Biointerfaces* **2016**, *144*, 8–20. [CrossRef] [PubMed]

107. Zhu, Y.; Sun, Y.; Chen, Y.; Liu, W.; Jiang, J.; Guan, W.; Zhang, Z.; Duan, Y. In vivo molecular MRI imaging of prostate cancer by targeting psma with polypeptide-labeled superparamagnetic iron oxide nanoparticles. *Int. J. Mol. Sci.* **2015**, *16*, 9573–9587. [CrossRef] [PubMed]
108. Yu, M.K.; Kim, D.; Lee, I.H.; So, J.S.; Jeong, Y.Y.; Jon, S. Image-guided prostate cancer therapy using aptamer-functionalized thermally cross-linked superparamagnetic iron oxide nanoparticles. *Small* **2011**, *7*, 2241–2249. [CrossRef] [PubMed]
109. Min, K.; Jo, H.; Song, K.; Cho, M.; Chun, Y.S.; Jon, S.; Kim, W.J.; Ban, C. Dual-aptamer-based delivery vehicle of doxorubicin to both PSMA (+) and PSMA (−) prostate cancers. *Biomaterials* **2011**, *32*, 2124–2132. [CrossRef] [PubMed]
110. Prabhu, S.; Ananthanarayanan, P.; Aziz, S.K.; Rai, S.; Mutalik, S.; Sadashiva, S.R. Enhanced effect of geldanamycin nanocomposite against breast cancer cells growing in vitro and as xenograft with vanquished normal cell toxicity. *Toxicol. Appl. Pharmacol.* **2017**, *320*, 60–72. [CrossRef] [PubMed]
111. Shaik, A.P.; Shaik, A.S.; Majwal, A.A.; Faraj, A.A. Blocking IL4-α receptor using polyethylene glycol functionalized superparamagnetic iron oxide nanocarriers to inhibit breast cancer cell proliferation. *Cancer Res. Treat.* **2016**, *49*, 322–329. [CrossRef] [PubMed]
112. Chiappi, M.; Conesa, J.J.; Pereiro, E.; Sorzano, C.O.; Rodriguez, M.J.; Henzler, K.; Schneider, G.; Chichon, F.J.; Carrascosa, J.L. Cryo-soft X-ray tomography as a quantitative three-dimensional tool to model nanoparticle:Cell interaction. *J. Nanobiotechnol.* **2016**, *14*, 15. [CrossRef] [PubMed]
113. Stapf, M.; Pompner, N.; Teichgraber, U.; Hilger, I. Heterogeneous response of different tumor cell lines to methotrexate-coupled nanoparticles in presence of hyperthermia. *Int. J. Nanomed.* **2016**, *11*, 485–500. [CrossRef] [PubMed]
114. Almaki, J.H.; Nasiri, R.; Idris, A.; Majid, F.A.; Salouti, M.; Wong, T.S.; Dabagh, S.; Marvibaigi, M.; Amini, N. Synthesis, characterization and in vitro evaluation of exquisite targeting SPIONs-PEG-HER in HER2+ human breast cancer cells. *Nanotechnology* **2016**, *27*, 105601. [CrossRef] [PubMed]
115. Kievit, F.M.; Stephen, Z.R.; Veiseh, O.; Arami, H.; Wang, T.; Lai, V.P.; Park, J.O.; Ellenbogen, R.G.; Disis, M.L.; Zhang, M. Targeting of primary breast cancers and metastases in a transgenic mouse model using rationally designed multifunctional spions. *ACS Nano* **2012**, *6*, 2591–2601. [CrossRef] [PubMed]
116. Lentschig, M.G.; Reimer, P.; Rausch-Lentschig, U.L.; Allkemper, T.; Oelerich, M.; Laub, G. Breath-hold gadolinium-enhanced MR angiography of the major vessels at 1.0 t: Dose-response findings and angiographic correlation. *Radiology* **1998**, *208*, 353–357. [CrossRef] [PubMed]
117. Lin, Y.J.; Koretsky, A.P. Manganese ion enhances t1-weighted MRI during brain activation: An approach to direct imaging of brain function. *Magn. Reson. Med.* **1997**, *38*, 378–388. [CrossRef] [PubMed]
118. Zhen, Z.; Xie, J. Development of manganese-based nanoparticles as contrast probes for magnetic resonance imaging. *Theranostics* **2012**, *2*, 45–54. [CrossRef] [PubMed]
119. Silva, A.C.; Lee, J.H.; Aoki, I.; Koretsky, A.P. Manganese-enhanced magnetic resonance imaging (MEMRI): Methodological and practical considerations. *NMR Biomed.* **2004**, *17*, 532–543. [CrossRef] [PubMed]
120. Koretsky, A.P.; Silva, A.C. Manganese-enhanced magnetic resonance imaging (MEMRI). *NMR Biomed.* **2004**, *17*, 527–531. [CrossRef] [PubMed]
121. Paratala, B.S.; Jacobson, B.D.; Kanakia, S.; Francis, L.D.; Sitharaman, B. Physicochemical characterization, and relaxometry studies of micro-graphite oxide, graphene nanoplatelets, and nanoribbons. *PLoS ONE* **2012**, *7*, e38185. [CrossRef] [PubMed]
122. Harisinghani, M.G.; Jhaveri, K.S.; Weissleder, R.; Schima, W.; Saini, S.; Hahn, P.F.; Mueller, P.R. MRI contrast agents for evaluating focal hepatic lesions. *Clin. Radiol.* **2001**, *56*, 714–725. [CrossRef] [PubMed]
123. Hunyadi Murph, S.; Jacobs, S.; Liu, J.; Hu, T.; Siegfired, M.; Serkiz, S.; Hudson, J. Manganese–gold nanoparticles as an MRI positive contrast agent in mesenchymal stem cell labeling. *J. Nanopart. Res.* **2012**, *14*, 658. [CrossRef]
124. Cai, X.; Gao, W.; Ma, M.; Wu, M.; Zhang, L.; Zheng, Y.; Chen, H.; Shi, J. Nanoparticles: A prussian blue-based core-shell hollow-structured mesoporous nanoparticle as a smart theranostic agent with ultrahigh pH-responsive longitudinal relaxivity (adv. Mater. 41/2015). *Adv. Mater.* **2015**, *27*, 6382–6389. [CrossRef] [PubMed]
125. Peng, G.; Tisch, U.; Adams, O.; Hakim, M.; Shehada, N.; Broza, Y.Y.; Billan, S.; Abdah-Bortnyak, R.; Kuten, A.; Haick, H. Diagnosing lung cancer in exhaled breath using gold nanoparticles. *Nat. Nanotechnol.* **2009**, *4*, 669–673. [CrossRef] [PubMed]

126. Samadian, H.; Hosseini-Nami, S.; Kamrava, S.K.; Ghaznavi, H.; Shakeri-Zadeh, A. Folate-conjugated gold nanoparticle as a new nanoplatform for targeted cancer therapy. *J. Cancer Res. Clin. Oncol.* **2016**, *142*, 2217–2229. [CrossRef] [PubMed]
127. Gossai, N.P.; Naumann, J.A.; Li, N.S.; Zamora, E.A.; Gordon, D.J.; Piccirilli, J.A.; Gordon, P.M. Drug conjugated nanoparticles activated by cancer cell specific mRNA. *Oncotarget* **2016**, *7*, 38243–38256. [CrossRef] [PubMed]
128. Gupta, A.; Moyano, D.F.; Parnsubsakul, A.; Papadopoulos, A.; Wang, L.S.; Landis, R.F.; Das, R.; Rotello, V.M. Ultra-stable biofunctionalizable gold nanoparticles. *ACS Appl. Mater. Interfaces* **2016**, *8*, 14096–14101. [CrossRef] [PubMed]
129. Ramya, A.N.; Joseph, M.M.; Nair, J.B.; Karunakaran, V.; Narayanan, N.; Maiti, K.K. New insight of tetraphenylethylene-based raman signatures for targeted SERS nanoprobe construction toward prostate cancer cell detection. *ACS Appl. Mater. Interfaces* **2016**, *8*, 10220–10225. [CrossRef] [PubMed]
130. Spaliviero, M.; Harmsen, S.; Huang, R.; Wall, M.A.; Andreou, C.; Eastham, J.A.; Touijer, K.A.; Scardino, P.T.; Kircher, M.F. Detection of lymph node metastases with SERRS nanoparticles. *Mol. Imaging Biol.* **2016**, *18*, 677–685. [CrossRef] [PubMed]
131. Moeendarbari, S.; Tekade, R.; Mulgaonkar, A.; Christensen, P.; Ramezani, S.; Hassan, G.; Jiang, R.; Oz, O.K.; Hao, Y.; Sun, X. Theranostic nanoseeds for efficacious internal radiation therapy of unresectable solid tumors. *Sci. Rep.* **2016**, *6*. [CrossRef] [PubMed]
132. Tsai, L.C.; Hsieh, H.Y.; Lu, K.Y.; Wang, S.Y.; Mi, F.L. EGCG/gelatin-doxorubicin gold nanoparticles enhance therapeutic efficacy of doxorubicin for prostate cancer treatment. *Nanomedicine (Lond.)* **2016**, *11*, 9–30. [CrossRef] [PubMed]
133. Morshed, R.A.; Muroski, M.E.; Dai, Q.; Wegscheid, M.L.; Auffinger, B.; Yu, D.; Han, Y.; Zhang, L.; Wu, M.; Cheng, Y.; et al. Cell penetrating peptide-modified gold nanoparticles for the delivery of doxorubicin to brain metastatic breast cancer. *Mol. Pharm.* **2016**, *13*, 1843–1854. [CrossRef] [PubMed]
134. Her, S.; Cui, L.; Bristow, R.G.; Allen, C. Dual action enhancement of gold nanoparticle radiosensitization by pentamidine in triple negative breast cancer. *Radiat. Res.* **2016**, *185*, 549–562. [CrossRef] [PubMed]
135. Rizk, N.; Christoforou, N.; Lee, S. Optimization of anti-cancer drugs and a targeting molecule on multifunctional gold nanoparticles. *Nanotechnology* **2016**, *27*, 185704. [CrossRef] [PubMed]
136. Zhou, F.; Feng, B.; Yu, H.; Wang, D.; Wang, T.; Liu, J.; Meng, Q.; Wang, S.; Zhang, P.; Zhang, Z.; et al. Cisplatin prodrug-conjugated gold nanocluster for fluorescence imaging and targeted therapy of the breast cancer. *Theranostics* **2016**, *6*, 679–687. [CrossRef] [PubMed]
137. Yook, S.; Lu, Y.; Jeong, J.J.; Cai, Z.; Tong, L.; Alwarda, R.; Pignol, J.P.; Winnik, M.A.; Reilly, R.M. Stability and biodistribution of thiol-functionalized and ^{177}Lu-labeled metal chelating polymers bound to gold nanoparticles. *Biomacromolecules* **2016**, *17*, 1292–1302. [CrossRef] [PubMed]
138. Huang, X.; Jain, P.K.; El-Sayed, I.H.; El-Sayed, M.A. Determination of the minimum temperature required for selective photothermal destruction of cancer cells with the use of immunotargeted gold nanoparticles. *Photochem. Photobiol.* **2006**, *82*, 412–417. [CrossRef] [PubMed]
139. Huang, X.; El-Sayed, I.H.; Qian, W.; El-Sayed, M.A. Cancer cell imaging and photothermal therapy in the near-infrared region by using gold nanorods. *J. Am. Chem. Soc.* **2006**, *128*, 2115–2120. [CrossRef] [PubMed]
140. Chen, W.; Zhang, S.; Yu, Y.; Zhang, H.; He, Q. Structural-engineering rationales of gold nanoparticles for cancer theranostics. *Adv. Mater.* **2016**, *28*, 8567–8585. [CrossRef] [PubMed]
141. Guo, J.; O'Driscoll, C.M.; Holmes, J.D.; Rahme, K. Bioconjugated gold nanoparticles enhance cellular uptake: A proof of concept study for siRNA delivery in prostate cancer cells. *Int. J. Pharm.* **2016**, *509*, 16–27. [CrossRef] [PubMed]
142. Stuchinskaya, T.; Moreno, M.; Cook, M.J.; Edwards, D.R.; Russell, D.A. Targeted photodynamic therapy of breast cancer cells using antibody-phthalocyanine-gold nanoparticle conjugates. *Photochem. Photobiol. Sci.* **2011**, *10*, 822–831. [CrossRef] [PubMed]
143. Brown, S.D.; Nativo, P.; Smith, J.A.; Stirling, D.; Edwards, P.R.; Venugopal, B.; Flint, D.J.; Plumb, J.A.; Graham, D.; Wheate, N.J. Gold nanoparticles for the improved anticancer drug delivery of the active component of oxaliplatin. *J. Am. Chem. Soc.* **2010**, *132*, 4678–4684. [CrossRef] [PubMed]
144. Chen, Y.W.; Liu, T.Y.; Chen, P.J.; Chang, P.H.; Chen, S.Y. A high-sensitivity and low-power theranostic nanosystem for cell sers imaging and selectively photothermal therapy using anti-EGFR-conjugated reduced graphene oxide/mesoporous silica/aunps nanosheets. *Small* **2016**, *12*, 1458–1468. [CrossRef] [PubMed]

145. Ashraf, S.; Pelaz, B.; del Pino, P.; Carril, M.; Escudero, A.; Parak, W.J.; Soliman, M.G.; Zhang, Q.; Carrillo-Carrion, C. Gold-based nanomaterials for applications in nanomedicine. *Top. Curr. Chem.* **2016**, *370*, 169–202. [PubMed]
146. Conde, J.; de la Fuente, J.M.; Baptista, P.V. Nanomaterials for reversion of multidrug resistance in cancer: A new hope for an old idea? *Front. Pharmacol.* **2013**, *4*, 134. [CrossRef] [PubMed]
147. Han, G.; Ghosh, P.; Rotello, V.M. Multi-functional gold nanoparticles for drug delivery. *Adv. Exp. Med. Biol.* **2007**, *620*, 48–56. [PubMed]
148. Conde, J.; Tian, F.; Hernandez, Y.; Bao, C.; Cui, D.; Janssen, K.P.; Ibarra, M.R.; Baptista, P.V.; Stoeger, T.; de la Fuente, J.M. In vivo tumor targeting via nanoparticle-mediated therapeutic siRNA coupled to inflammatory response in lung cancer mouse models. *Biomaterials* **2013**, *34*, 7744–7753. [CrossRef] [PubMed]
149. McMahon, S.J.; Hyland, W.B.; Muir, M.F.; Coulter, J.A.; Jain, S.; Butterworth, K.T.; Schettino, G.; Dickson, G.R.; Hounsell, A.R.; O'Sullivan, J.M.; et al. Biological consequences of nanoscale energy deposition near irradiated heavy atom nanoparticles. *Sci. Rep.* **2011**, *1*. [CrossRef] [PubMed]
150. Conde, J.; Larguinho, M.; Cordeiro, A.; Raposo, L.R.; Costa, P.M.; Santos, S.; Diniz, M.S.; Fernandes, A.R.; Baptista, P.V. Gold-nanobeacons for gene therapy: Evaluation of genotoxicity, cell toxicity and proteome profiling analysis. *Nanotoxicology* **2014**, *8*, 521–532. [CrossRef] [PubMed]
151. Conde, J.; Rosa, J.; de la Fuente, J.M.; Baptista, P.V. Gold-nanobeacons for simultaneous gene specific silencing and intracellular tracking of the silencing events. *Biomaterials* **2013**, *34*, 2516–2523. [CrossRef] [PubMed]
152. Cabral, R.M.; Baptista, P.V. Anti-cancer precision theranostics: A focus on multifunctional gold nanoparticles. *Expert Rev. Mol. Diagn.* **2014**, *14*, 1041–1052. [CrossRef] [PubMed]
153. Song, J.; Wang, F.; Yang, X.; Ning, B.; Harp, M.G.; Culp, S.H.; Hu, S.; Huang, P.; Nie, L.; Chen, J.; et al. Gold nanoparticle coated carbon nanotube ring with enhanced raman scattering and photothermal conversion property for theranostic applications. *J. Am. Chem. Soc.* **2016**, *138*, 7005–7015. [CrossRef] [PubMed]
154. Croissant, J.G.; Qi, C.; Maynadier, M.; Cattoen, X.; Wong Chi Man, M.; Raehm, L.; Mongin, O.; Blanchard-Desce, M.; Garcia, M.; Gary-Bobo, M.; et al. Multifunctional gold-mesoporous silica nanocomposites for enhanced two-photon imaging and therapy of cancer cells. *Front. Mol. Biosci.* **2016**, *3*, 1. [CrossRef] [PubMed]
155. Croissant, J.; Maynadier, M.; Mongin, O.; Hugues, V.; Blanchard-Desce, M.; Chaix, A.; Cattoen, X.; Wong Chi Man, M.; Gallud, A.; Gary-Bobo, M.; et al. Enhanced two-photon fluorescence imaging and therapy of cancer cells via gold@bridged silsesquioxane nanoparticles. *Small* **2015**, *11*, 295–299. [CrossRef] [PubMed]
156. Oh, M.H.; Yu, J.H.; Kim, I.; Nam, Y.S. Genetically programmed clusters of gold nanoparticles for cancer cell-targeted photothermal therapy. *ACS Appl. Mater. Interfaces* **2015**, *7*, 22578–22586. [CrossRef] [PubMed]
157. Jimenez-Mancilla, N.; Ferro-Flores, G.; Santos-Cuevas, C.; Ocampo-Garcia, B.; Luna-Gutierrez, M.; Azorin-Vega, E.; Isaac-Olive, K.; Camacho-Lopez, M.; Torres-Garcia, E. Multifunctional targeted therapy system based on (99M)TC/(177) Lu-labeled gold nanoparticles-TAT(49–57)-lys(3)-bombesin internalized in nuclei of prostate cancer cells. *J. Labelled Comp. Radiopharm.* **2013**, *56*, 663–671. [CrossRef] [PubMed]
158. Szlachcic, A.; Pala, K.; Zakrzewska, M.; Jakimowicz, P.; Wiedlocha, A.; Otlewski, J. FGF1-gold nanoparticle conjugates targeting FGFR efficiently decrease cell viability upon NIR irradiation. *Int. J. Nanomed.* **2012**, *7*, 5915–5927.
159. Van de Broek, B.; Devoogdt, N.; D'Hollander, A.; Gijs, H.L.; Jans, K.; Lagae, L.; Muyldermans, S.; Maes, G.; Borghs, G. Specific cell targeting with nanobody conjugated branched gold nanoparticles for photothermal therapy. *ACS Nano* **2011**, *5*, 4319–4328. [CrossRef] [PubMed]
160. Lukianova-Hleb, E.Y.; Oginsky, A.O.; Samaniego, A.P.; Shenefelt, D.L.; Wagner, D.S.; Hafner, J.H.; Farach-Carson, M.C.; Lapotko, D.O. Tunable plasmonic nanoprobes for theranostics of prostate cancer. *Theranostics* **2011**, *1*, 3–17. [CrossRef] [PubMed]
161. Lu, W.; Singh, A.K.; Khan, S.A.; Senapati, D.; Yu, H.; Ray, P.C. Gold nano-popcorn-based targeted diagnosis, nanotherapy treatment, and in situ monitoring of photothermal therapy response of prostate cancer cells using surface-enhanced raman spectroscopy. *J. Am. Chem. Soc.* **2010**, *132*, 18103–18114. [CrossRef] [PubMed]
162. Kang, J.H.; Ko, Y.T. Lipid-coated gold nanocomposites for enhanced cancer therapy. *Int. J. Nanomed.* **2015**, *10*, 33–45.
163. Banu, H.; Sethi, D.K.; Edgar, A.; Sheriff, A.; Rayees, N.; Renuka, N.; Faheem, S.M.; Premkumar, K.; Vasanthakumar, G. Doxorubicin loaded polymeric gold nanoparticles targeted to human folate receptor upon laser photothermal therapy potentiates chemotherapy in breast cancer cell lines. *J. Photochem. Photobiol. B* **2015**, *149*, 116–128. [CrossRef] [PubMed]

164. Mkandawire, M.M.; Lakatos, M.; Springer, A.; Clemens, A.; Appelhans, D.; Krause-Buchholz, U.; Pompe, W.; Rodel, G.; Mkandawire, M. Induction of apoptosis in human cancer cells by targeting mitochondria with gold nanoparticles. *Nanoscale* **2015**, *7*, 10634–10640. [CrossRef] [PubMed]
165. Yang, L.; Tseng, Y.T.; Suo, G.; Chen, L.; Yu, J.; Chiu, W.J.; Huang, C.C.; Lin, C.H. Photothermal therapeutic response of cancer cells to aptamer-gold nanoparticle-hybridized graphene oxide under nir illumination. *ACS Appl. Mater. Interfaces* **2015**, *7*, 5097–5106. [CrossRef] [PubMed]
166. Lechtman, E.; Mashouf, S.; Chattopadhyay, N.; Keller, B.M.; Lai, P.; Cai, Z.; Reilly, R.M.; Pignol, J.P. A Monte Carlo-based model of gold nanoparticle radiosensitization accounting for increased radiobiological effectiveness. *Phys. Med. Biol.* **2013**, *58*, 3075–3087. [CrossRef] [PubMed]
167. Jain, S.; Coulter, J.A.; Hounsell, A.R.; Butterworth, K.T.; McMahon, S.J.; Hyland, W.B.; Muir, M.F.; Dickson, G.R.; Prise, K.M.; Currell, F.J.; et al. Cell-specific radiosensitization by gold nanoparticles at megavoltage radiation energies. *Int. J. Radiat. Oncol. Biol. Phys.* **2011**, *79*, 531–539. [CrossRef] [PubMed]
168. Butler, H.J.; Fogarty, S.W.; Kerns, J.G.; Martin-Hirsch, P.L.; Fullwood, N.J.; Martin, F.L. Gold nanoparticles as a substrate in bio-analytical near-infrared surface-enhanced Raman spectroscopy. *Analyst* **2015**, *140*, 3090–3097. [CrossRef] [PubMed]
169. Kalmodia, S.; Harjwani, J.; Rajeswari, R.; Yang, W.; Barrow, C.J.; Ramaprabhu, S.; Krishnakumar, S.; Elchuri, S.V. Synthesis and characterization of surface-enhanced Raman-scattered gold nanoparticles. *Int. J. Nanomed.* **2013**, *8*, 4327–4338. [CrossRef] [PubMed]
170. Zhu, J.; Zhou, J.; Guo, J.; Cai, W.; Liu, B.; Wang, Z.; Sun, Z. Surface-enhanced Raman spectroscopy investigation on human breast cancer cells. *Chem. Cent. J.* **2013**, *7*, 37. [CrossRef] [PubMed]
171. Firdhouse, M.J.; Lalitha, P. Biosynthesis of silver nanoparticles using the extract of -antiproliferative effect against prostate cancer cells. *Cancer Nanotechnol.* **2013**, *4*, 137–143. [CrossRef] [PubMed]
172. Wang, H.; Zhang, Y.; Yu, H.; Wu, D.; Ma, H.; Li, H.; Du, B.; Wei, Q. Label-free electrochemical immunosensor for prostate-specific antigen based on silver hybridized mesoporous silica nanoparticles. *Anal. Biochem.* **2013**, *434*, 123–127. [CrossRef] [PubMed]
173. Nayak, D.; Minz, A.P.; Ashe, S.; Rauta, P.R.; Kumari, M.; Chopra, P.; Nayak, B. Synergistic combination of antioxidants, silver nanoparticles and chitosan in a nanoparticle based formulation: Characterization and cytotoxic effect on MCF-7 breast cancer cell lines. *J. Colloid Interface Sci.* **2016**, *470*, 142–152. [CrossRef] [PubMed]
174. Karunamuni, R.; Naha, P.C.; Lau, K.C.; Al-Zaki, A.; Popov, A.V.; Delikatny, E.J.; Tsourkas, A.; Cormode, D.P.; Maidment, A.D. Development of silica-encapsulated silver nanoparticles as contrast agents intended for dual-energy mammography. *Eur. Radiol.* **2016**, *26*, 3301–3309. [CrossRef] [PubMed]
175. Farah, M.A.; Ali, M.A.; Chen, S.M.; Li, Y.; Al-Hemaid, F.M.; Abou-Tarboush, F.M.; Al-Anazi, K.M.; Lee, J. Silver nanoparticles synthesized from adenium obesum leaf extract induced DNA damage, apoptosis and autophagy via generation of reactive oxygen species. *Colloids Surf. B Biointerfaces* **2016**, *141*, 158–169. [CrossRef] [PubMed]
176. Jannathul Firdhouse, M.; Lalitha, P. Apoptotic efficacy of biogenic silver nanoparticles on human breast cancer MCF-7 cell lines. *Prog. Biomater.* **2015**, *4*, 113–121.
177. Casanas Pimentel, R.G.; Robles Botero, V.; San Martin Martinez, E.; Gomez Garcia, C.; Hinestroza, J.P. Soybean agglutinin-conjugated silver nanoparticles nanocarriers in the treatment of breast cancer cells. *J. Biomater. Sci. Polym. Ed.* **2016**, *27*, 218–234. [CrossRef] [PubMed]
178. Swanner, J.; Mims, J.; Carroll, D.L.; Akman, S.A.; Furdui, C.M.; Torti, S.V.; Singh, R.N. Differential cytotoxic and radiosensitizing effects of silver nanoparticles on triple-negative breast cancer and non-triple-negative breast cells. *Int. J. Nanomed.* **2015**, *10*, 3937–3953.
179. Gurunathan, S.; Park, J.H.; Han, J.W.; Kim, J.H. Comparative assessment of the apoptotic potential of silver nanoparticles synthesized by bacillus tequilensis and calocybe indica in MDA-MB-231 human breast cancer cells: Targeting p53 for anticancer therapy. *Int. J. Nanomed.* **2015**, *10*, 4203–4222. [CrossRef] [PubMed]
180. Wei, L.; Lu, J.; Xu, H.; Patel, A.; Chen, Z.S.; Chen, G. Silver nanoparticles: Synthesis, properties, and therapeutic applications. *Drug Discov. Today* **2015**, *20*, 595–601. [CrossRef] [PubMed]
181. Thompson, E.A.; Graham, E.; MacNeill, C.M.; Young, M.; Donati, G.; Wailes, E.M.; Jones, B.T.; Levi-Polyachenko, N.H. Differential response of MCF-7, MDA-MB-231, and MCF-10a cells to hyperthermia, silver nanoparticles and silver nanoparticle-induced photothermal therapy. *Int. J. Hyperth.* **2014**, *30*, 312–323. [CrossRef] [PubMed]

182. Chung, I.M.; Park, I.; Seung-Hyun, K.; Thiruvengadam, M.; Rajakumar, G. Plant-mediated synthesis of silver nanoparticles: Their characteristic properties and therapeutic applications. *Nanoscale Res. Lett.* **2016**, *11*, 40. [CrossRef] [PubMed]
183. Ghoneum, A.; Zhu, H.; Woo, J.; Zabinyakov, N.; Sharma, S.; Gimzewski, J.K. Biophysical and morphological effects of nanodiamond/nanoplatinum solution (DPV576) on metastatic murine breast cancer cells in vitro. *Nanotechnology* **2014**, *25*, 465101. [CrossRef] [PubMed]
184. Xiao, C.; Liu, Y.L.; Xu, J.Q.; Lv, S.W.; Guo, S.; Huang, W.H. Real-time monitoring of H_2O_2 release from single cells using nanoporous gold microelectrodes decorated with platinum nanoparticles. *Analyst* **2015**, *140*, 3753–3758. [CrossRef] [PubMed]
185. Cui, Z.; Wu, D.; Zhang, Y.; Ma, H.; Li, H.; Du, B.; Wei, Q.; Ju, H. Ultrasensitive electrochemical immunosensors for multiplexed determination using mesoporous platinum nanoparticles as nonenzymatic labels. *Anal. Chim. Acta* **2014**, *807*, 44–50. [CrossRef] [PubMed]
186. Sengupta, P.; Basu, S.; Soni, S.; Pandey, A.; Roy, B.; Oh, M.S.; Chin, K.T.; Paraskar, A.S.; Sarangi, S.; Connor, Y.; et al. Cholesterol-tethered platinum II-based supramolecular nanoparticle increases antitumor efficacy and reduces nephrotoxicity. *Proc. Natl. Acad. Sci. USA* **2012**, *109*, 11294–11299. [CrossRef] [PubMed]
187. Teow, Y.; Valiyaveettil, S. Active targeting of cancer cells using folic acid-conjugated platinum nanoparticles. *Nanoscale* **2010**, *2*, 2607–2613. [CrossRef] [PubMed]
188. Spain, E.; Gilgunn, S.; Sharma, S.; Adamson, K.; Carthy, E.; O'Kennedy, R.; Forster, R.J. Detection of prostate specific antigen based on electrocatalytic platinum nanoparticles conjugated to a recombinant SCFV antibody. *Biosens. Bioelectron.* **2016**, *77*, 759–766. [CrossRef] [PubMed]
189. Zhang, B.; Liu, B.; Chen, G.; Tang, D. Redox and catalysis 'all-in-one' infinite coordination polymer for electrochemical immunosensor of tumor markers. *Biosens. Bioelectron.* **2015**, *64*, 6–12. [CrossRef] [PubMed]
190. Kumar, A.; Huo, S.; Zhang, X.; Liu, J.; Tan, A.; Li, S.; Jin, S.; Xue, X.; Zhao, Y.; Ji, T.; et al. Neuropilin-1-targeted gold nanoparticles enhance therapeutic efficacy of platinum(IV) drug for prostate cancer treatment. *ACS Nano* **2014**, *8*, 4205–4220. [CrossRef] [PubMed]
191. Taylor, R.M.; Sillerud, L.O. Paclitaxel-loaded iron platinum stealth immunomicelles are potent MRI imaging agents that prevent prostate cancer growth in a psma-dependent manner. *Int. J. Nanomed.* **2012**, *7*, 4341–4352. [CrossRef] [PubMed]
192. Taylor, R.M.; Huber, D.L.; Monson, T.C.; Ali, A.M.; Bisoffi, M.; Sillerud, L.O. Multifunctional iron platinum stealth immunomicelles: Targeted detection of human prostate cancer cells using both fluorescence and magnetic resonance imaging. *J. Nanopart. Res.* **2011**, *13*, 4717–4729. [CrossRef] [PubMed]
193. Chuang, C.H.; Brown, P.R.; Bulovic, V.; Bawendi, M.G. Improved performance and stability in quantum dot solar cells through band alignment engineering. *Nat. Mater.* **2014**, *13*, 796–801. [CrossRef] [PubMed]
194. Sun, Q.; Wang, A.; Li, L.; Wang, D.; Zhu, T.; Xu, J.; Yang, C.; Li, Y. Bright, multicoloured light-emitting diodes based on quantum dots. *Nat. Photonics* **2007**, *1*, 717–722. [CrossRef]
195. Fang, M.; Peng, C.W.; Pang, D.W.; Li, Y. Quantum dots for cancer research: Current status, remaining issues, and future perspectives. *Cancer Biol. Med.* **2012**, *9*, 151–163. [PubMed]
196. Jamieson, T.; Bakhshi, R.; Petrova, D.; Pocock, R.; Imani, M.; Seifalian, A.M. Biological applications of quantum dots. *Biomaterials* **2007**, *28*, 4717–4732. [CrossRef] [PubMed]
197. Hotz, C.Z. Applications of quantum dots in biology: An overview. *Methods Mol. Biol.* **2005**, *303*, 1–17. [PubMed]
198. Barar, J.; Omidi, Y. Surface modified multifunctional nanomedicines for simultaneous imaging and therapy of cancer. *Bioimpacts* **2014**, *4*, 3–14. [PubMed]
199. Choi, H.S.; Frangioni, J.V. Nanoparticles for biomedical imaging: Fundamentals of clinical translation. *Mol. Imaging* **2010**, *9*, 291–310. [PubMed]
200. Ow, H.; Larson, D.R.; Srivastava, M.; Baird, B.A.; Webb, W.W.; Wiesner, U. Bright and stable core-shell fluorescent silica nanoparticles. *Nano Lett.* **2005**, *5*, 113–117. [CrossRef] [PubMed]
201. Larson, D.; Ow, H.; Vishwasrao, H.; Heikal, A.; Wiesner, U.; Webb, W. Silica nanoparticle architecture determines radiative properties of encapsulated fluorophores. *Chem. Mater.* **2008**, *20*, 2677–2684. [CrossRef]
202. Burns, A.A.; Vider, J.; Ow, H.; Herz, E.; Penate-Medina, O.; Baumgart, M.; Larson, S.M.; Wiesner, U.; Bradbury, M. Fluorescent silica nanoparticles with efficient urinary excretion for nanomedicine. *Nano Lett.* **2009**, *9*, 442–448. [CrossRef] [PubMed]

203. Schipper, M.L.; Cheng, Z.; Lee, S.W.; Bentolila, L.A.; Iyer, G.; Rao, J.; Chen, X.; Wu, A.M.; Weiss, S.; Gambhir, S.S. Micropet-based biodistribution of quantum dots in living mice. *J. Nucl. Med.* **2007**, *48*, 1511–1518. [CrossRef] [PubMed]
204. Phillips, E.; Penate-Medina, O.; Zanzonico, P.B.; Carvajal, R.D.; Mohan, P.; Ye, Y.; Humm, J.; Gonen, M.; Kalaigian, H.; Schoder, H.; et al. Clinical translation of an ultrasmall inorganic optical-PET imaging nanoparticle probe. *Sci. Transl. Med.* **2014**, *6*, 260ra149. [CrossRef] [PubMed]
205. Choi, H.S.; Liu, W.; Misra, P.; Tanaka, E.; Zimmer, J.P.; Itty Ipe, B.; Bawendi, M.G.; Frangioni, J.V. Renal clearance of quantum dots. *Nat. Biotechnol.* **2007**, *25*, 1165–1170. [CrossRef] [PubMed]
206. Thakur, M.; Mewada, A.; Pandey, S.; Bhori, M.; Singh, K.; Sharon, M.; Sharon, M. Milk-derived multi-fluorescent graphene quantum dot-based cancer theranostic system. *Mater. Sci. Eng. C Mater. Biol. Appl.* **2016**, *67*, 468–477. [CrossRef] [PubMed]
207. Wang, J.; Wang, F.; Li, F.; Zhang, W.; Shen, Y.; Zhou, D.; Guo, S. A multifunctional poly(curcumin) nanomedicine for dual-modal targeted delivery, intracellular responsive release, dual-drug treatment and imaging of multidrug resistant cancer cells. *J. Mater. Chem. B Mater. Biol. Med.* **2016**, *4*, 2954–2962. [CrossRef] [PubMed]
208. Bwatanglang, I.B.; Mohammad, F.; Yusof, N.A.; Abdullah, J.; Hussein, M.Z.; Alitheen, N.B.; Abu, N. Folic acid targeted MN:Zns quantum dots for theranostic applications of cancer cell imaging and therapy. *Int. J. Nanomed.* **2016**, *11*, 413–428.
209. Lin, Z.; Ma, Q.; Fei, X.; Zhang, H.; Su, X. A novel aptamer functionalized cuins2 quantum dots probe for daunorubicin sensing and near infrared imaging of prostate cancer cells. *Anal. Chim. Acta* **2014**, *818*, 54–60. [CrossRef] [PubMed]
210. Zhao, Y.; Shaffer, T.M.; Das, S.; Perez-Medina, C.; Mulder, W.J.; Grimm, J. Near-infrared quantum dot and ^{89}Zr dual-labeled nanoparticles for in vivo Cerenkov imaging. *Bioconjug. Chem.* **2017**, *28*, 600–608. [CrossRef] [PubMed]
211. Klumpp, C.; Kostarelos, K.; Prato, M.; Bianco, A. Functionalized carbon nanotubes as emerging nanovectors for the delivery of therapeutics. *Biochim. Biophys. Acta* **2006**, *1758*, 404–412. [CrossRef] [PubMed]
212. Partha, R.; Conyers, J.L. Biomedical applications of functionalized fullerene-based nanomaterials. *Int. J. Nanomed.* **2009**, *4*, 261–275.
213. Karousis, N.; Suarez-Martinez, I.; Ewels, C.P.; Tagmatarchis, N. Structure, properties, functionalization, and applications of carbon nanohorns. *Chem. Rev.* **2016**, *116*, 4850–4883. [CrossRef] [PubMed]
214. Serpell, C.J.; Kostarelos, K.; Davis, B.G. Can carbon nanotubes deliver on their promise in biology? Harnessing unique properties for unparalleled applications. *ACS Cent. Sci.* **2016**, *2*, 190–200. [CrossRef] [PubMed]
215. Bhattacharya, K.; Mukherjee, S.P.; Gallud, A.; Burkert, S.C.; Bistarelli, S.; Bellucci, S.; Bottini, M.; Star, A.; Fadeel, B. Biological interactions of carbon-based nanomaterials: From coronation to degradation. *Nanomedicine* **2016**, *12*, 333–351. [CrossRef] [PubMed]
216. Lalwani, G.; Sitharaman, B. Multifunctional fullerene- and metallofullerene-based nanobiomaterials. *Nano Life* **2013**, *3*, 1342003. [CrossRef]
217. Ruggiero, A.; Villa, C.H.; Bander, E.; Rey, D.A.; Bergkvist, M.; Batt, C.A.; Manova-Todorova, K.; Deen, W.M.; Scheinberg, D.A.; McDevitt, M.R. Paradoxical glomerular filtration of carbon nanotubes. *Proc. Natl. Acad. Sci. USA* **2010**, *107*, 12369–12374. [CrossRef] [PubMed]
218. Kostarelos, K.; Bianco, A.; Prato, M. Promises, facts and challenges for carbon nanotubes in imaging and therapeutics. *Nat. Nanotechnol.* **2009**, *4*, 627–633. [CrossRef] [PubMed]
219. Zhang, Y.; Petibone, D.; Xu, Y.; Mahmood, M.; Karmakar, A.; Casciano, D.; Ali, S.; Biris, A.S. Toxicity and efficacy of carbon nanotubes and graphene: The utility of carbon-based nanoparticles in nanomedicine. *Drug Metab. Rev.* **2014**, *46*, 232–246. [CrossRef] [PubMed]
220. Porter, A.E.; Gass, M.; Muller, K.; Skepper, J.N.; Midgley, P.A.; Welland, M. Direct imaging of single-walled carbon nanotubes in cells. *Nat. Nanotechnol.* **2007**, *2*, 713–717. [CrossRef] [PubMed]
221. Kolosnjaj, J.; Szwarc, H.; Moussa, F. Toxicity studies of carbon nanotubes. *Adv. Exp. Med. Biol.* **2007**, *620*, 181–204. [PubMed]
222. Poland, C.A.; Duffin, R.; Kinloch, I.; Maynard, A.; Wallace, W.A.; Seaton, A.; Stone, V.; Brown, S.; Macnee, W.; Donaldson, K. Carbon nanotubes introduced into the abdominal cavity of mice show asbestos-like

pathogenicity in a pilot study. *Nat. Nanotechnol.* **2008**, *3*, 423–428. [CrossRef] [PubMed]
223. Lam, C.W.; James, J.T.; McCluskey, R.; Arepalli, S.; Hunter, R.L. A review of carbon nanotube toxicity and assessment of potential occupational and environmental health risks. *Crit. Rev. Toxicol.* **2006**, *36*, 189–217. [CrossRef] [PubMed]
224. Corredor, C.; Hou, W.; Klein, S.; Moghadam, B.; Goryll, M.; Doudrick, K.; Westerhoff, P.; Posner, J. Disruption of model cell membranes by carbon nanotubes. *Carbon* **2013**, *60*, 67–75. [CrossRef]
225. Yoshida, M.; Goto, H.; Hirose, Y.; Zhao, X.; Osawa, E. Prediction of favorable isomeric structures for the c100 to c120 giant fullerenes. An application of the phason line criteria. *Electron. J. Theor. Chem.* **1996**, *1*, 163–171. [CrossRef]
226. Castro Nava, A.; Cojoc, M.; Peitzsch, C.; Cirillo, G.; Kurth, I.; Fuessel, S.; Erdmann, K.; Kunhardt, D.; Vittorio, O.; Hampel, S.; et al. Development of novel radiochemotherapy approaches targeting prostate tumor progenitor cells using nanohybrids. *Int. J. Cancer* **2015**, *137*, 2492–2503. [CrossRef] [PubMed]
227. Heydari-Bafrooei, E.; Shamszadeh, N.S. Electrochemical bioassay development for ultrasensitive aptasensing of prostate specific antigen. *Biosens. Bioelectron.* **2017**, *91*, 284–292. [CrossRef] [PubMed]
228. Thapa, R.K.; Youn, Y.S.; Jeong, J.H.; Choi, H.G.; Yong, C.S.; Kim, J.O. Graphene oxide-wrapped pegylated liquid crystalline nanoparticles for effective chemo-photothermal therapy of metastatic prostate cancer cells. *Colloids Surf. B Biointerfaces* **2016**, *143*, 271–277. [CrossRef] [PubMed]
229. Pan, L.H.; Kuo, S.H.; Lin, T.Y.; Lin, C.W.; Fang, P.Y.; Yang, H.W. An electrochemical biosensor to simultaneously detect vegf and psa for early prostate cancer diagnosis based on graphene oxide/ssdna/plla nanoparticles. *Biosens. Bioelectron.* **2017**, *89*, 598–605. [CrossRef] [PubMed]
230. Yang, L.; Cheng, J.; Chen, Y.; Yu, S.; Liu, F.; Sun, Y.; Chen, Y.; Ran, H. Phase-transition nanodroplets for real-time photoacoustic/ultrasound dual-modality imaging and photothermal therapy of sentinel lymph node in breast cancer. *Sci. Rep.* **2017**, *7*, 45213. [CrossRef] [PubMed]
231. Misra, S.K.; Srivastava, I.; Tripathi, I.; Daza, E.; Ostadhossein, F.; Pan, D. Macromolecularly "caged" carbon nanoparticles for intracellular trafficking via switchable photoluminescence. *J. Am. Chem. Soc.* **2017**, *139*, 1746–1749. [CrossRef] [PubMed]
232. Du, J.; Zhang, Y.; Ming, J.; Liu, J.; Zhong, L.; Liang, Q.; Fan, L.; Jiang, J. Evaluation of the tracing effect of carbon nanoparticle and carbon nanoparticle-epirubicin suspension in axillary lymph node dissection for breast cancer treatment. *World J. Surg. Oncol.* **2016**, *14*, 164. [CrossRef] [PubMed]
233. Wu, X.; Lin, Q.; Chen, G.; Lu, J.; Zeng, Y.; Chen, X.; Yan, J. Sentinel lymph node detection using carbon nanoparticles in patients with early breast cancer. *PLoS ONE* **2015**, *10*, e0135714. [CrossRef] [PubMed]
234. Misra, S.K.; Ohoka, A.; Kolmodin, N.J.; Pan, D. Next generation carbon nanoparticles for efficient gene therapy. *Mol. Pharm.* **2015**, *12*, 375–385. [CrossRef] [PubMed]
235. Bangham, A.D. Lipid bilayers and biomembranes. *Annu. Rev. Biochem.* **1972**, *41*, 753–776. [CrossRef] [PubMed]
236. Abou, D.S.; Thorek, D.L.; Ramos, N.N.; Pinkse, M.W.; Wolterbeek, H.T.; Carlin, S.D.; Beattie, B.J.; Lewis, J.S. ^{89}Zr-labeled paramagnetic octreotide-liposomes for PET-MR imaging of cancer. *Pharm. Res.* **2013**, *30*, 878–888. [CrossRef] [PubMed]
237. Laverman, P.; Brouwers, A.H.; Dams, E.T.; Oyen, W.J.; Storm, G.; van Rooijen, N.; Corstens, F.H.; Boerman, O.C. Preclinical and clinical evidence for disappearance of long-circulating characteristics of polyethylene glycol liposomes at low lipid dose. *J. Pharmacol. Exp. Ther.* **2000**, *293*, 996–1001. [PubMed]
238. Yeh, C.Y.; Hsiao, J.K.; Wang, Y.P.; Lan, C.H.; Wu, H.C. Peptide-conjugated nanoparticles for targeted imaging and therapy of prostate cancer. *Biomaterials* **2016**, *99*, 1–15. [CrossRef] [PubMed]
239. Lin, Q.; Jin, C.S.; Huang, H.; Ding, L.; Zhang, Z.; Chen, J.; Zheng, G. Nanoparticle-enabled, image-guided treatment planning of target specific rnai therapeutics in an orthotopic prostate cancer model. *Small* **2014**, *10*, 3072–3082. [CrossRef] [PubMed]
240. Yaari, Z.; da Silva, D.; Zinger, A.; Goldman, E.; Kajal, A.; Tshuva, R.; Barak, E.; Dahan, N.; Hershkovitz, D.; Goldfeder, M.; et al. Theranostic barcoded nanoparticles for personalized cancer medicine. *Nat. Commun.* **2016**, *7*, 13325. [CrossRef] [PubMed]
241. Rizzitelli, S.; Giustetto, P.; Faletto, D.; Delli Castelli, D.; Aime, S.; Terreno, E. The release of doxorubicin from liposomes monitored by MRI and triggered by a combination of us stimuli led to a complete tumor regression in a breast cancer mouse model. *J. Control. Release* **2016**, *230*, 57–63. [CrossRef] [PubMed]

242. Miller-Kleinhenz, J.M.; Bozeman, E.N.; Yang, L. Targeted nanoparticles for image-guided treatment of triple-negative breast cancer: Clinical significance and technological advances. *Wiley Interdiscip. Rev. Nanomed. Nanobiotechnol.* **2015**, *7*, 797–816. [CrossRef] [PubMed]
243. Rizzitelli, S.; Giustetto, P.; Cutrin, J.C.; Delli Castelli, D.; Boffa, C.; Ruzza, M.; Menchise, V.; Molinari, F.; Aime, S.; Terreno, E. Sonosensitive theranostic liposomes for preclinical in vivo MRI-guided visualization of doxorubicin release stimulated by pulsed low intensity non-focused ultrasound. *J. Control. Release* **2015**, *202*, 21–30. [CrossRef] [PubMed]
244. Shemesh, C.S.; Moshkelani, D.; Zhang, H. Thermosensitive liposome formulated indocyanine green for near-infrared triggered photodynamic therapy: In vivo evaluation for triple-negative breast cancer. *Pharm. Res.* **2015**, *32*, 1604–1614. [CrossRef] [PubMed]
245. He, Y.; Zhang, L.; Zhu, D.; Song, C. Design of multifunctional magnetic iron oxide nanoparticles/mitoxantrone-loaded liposomes for both magnetic resonance imaging and targeted cancer therapy. *Int. J. Nanomed.* **2014**, *9*, 4055–4066. [CrossRef] [PubMed]
246. Muthu, M.S.; Kulkarni, S.A.; Raju, A.; Feng, S.S. Theranostic liposomes of TPGS coating for targeted co-delivery of docetaxel and quantum dots. *Biomaterials* **2012**, *33*, 3494–3501. [CrossRef] [PubMed]
247. Hosoya, H.; Dobroff, A.S.; Driessen, W.H.; Cristini, V.; Brinker, L.M.; Staquicini, F.I.; Cardo-Vila, M.; D'Angelo, S.; Ferrara, F.; Proneth, B.; et al. Integrated nanotechnology platform for tumor-targeted multimodal imaging and therapeutic cargo release. *Proc. Natl. Acad. Sci. USA* **2016**, *113*, 1877–1882. [CrossRef] [PubMed]
248. Lee, J.B.; Zhang, K.; Tam, Y.Y.; Quick, J.; Tam, Y.K.; Lin, P.J.; Chen, S.; Liu, Y.; Nair, J.K.; Zlatev, I.; et al. A glu-urea-lys ligand-conjugated lipid nanoparticle/siRNA system inhibits androgen receptor expression in vivo. *Mol. Ther. Nucleic Acids* **2016**, *5*, e348. [CrossRef] [PubMed]
249. Sharkey, C.C.; Li, J.; Roy, S.; Wu, Q.; King, M.R. Two-stage nanoparticle delivery of piperlongumine and tumor necrosis factor-related apoptosis-inducing ligand (Trail) anti-cancer therapy. *Technology* **2016**, *4*, 60–69. [CrossRef] [PubMed]
250. Bhosale, R.R.; Gangadharappa, H.V.; Hani, U.; Osmani, R.A.; Vaghela, R.; Kulkarni, P.K.; Venkata, K.S. Current perspectives on novel drug delivery systems and therapies for management of prostate cancer: An inclusive review. *Curr. Drug Targets* **2016**. [CrossRef]
251. Majzoub, R.N.; Wonder, E.; Ewert, K.K.; Kotamraju, V.R.; Teesalu, T.; Safinya, C.R. Rab11 and lysotracker markers reveal correlation between endosomal pathways and transfection efficiency of surface-functionalized cationic liposome-DNA nanoparticles. *J. Phys. Chem. B* **2016**, *120*, 6439–6453. [CrossRef] [PubMed]
252. Wang, F.; Chen, L.; Zhang, R.; Chen, Z.; Zhu, L. RGD peptide conjugated liposomal drug delivery system for enhance therapeutic efficacy in treating bone metastasis from prostate cancer. *J. Control. Release* **2014**, *196*, 222–233. [CrossRef] [PubMed]
253. Nguyen, V.D.; Zheng, S.; Han, J.; Le, V.H.; Park, J.O.; Park, S. Nanohybrid magnetic liposome functionalized with hyaluronic acid for enhanced cellular uptake and near-infrared-triggered drug release. *Colloids Surf. B Biointerfaces* **2017**, *154*, 104–114. [CrossRef] [PubMed]
254. Sneider, A.; Jadia, R.; Piel, B.; VanDyke, D.; Tsiros, C.; Rai, P. Engineering remotely triggered liposomes to target triple negative breast cancer. *Oncomedicine* **2017**, *2*, 1–13. [CrossRef] [PubMed]
255. Bayraktar, R.; Pichler, M.; Kanlikilicer, P.; Ivan, C.; Bayraktar, E.; Kahraman, N.; Aslan, B.; Oguztuzun, S.; Ulasli, M.; Arslan, A.; et al. Microrna 603 acts as a tumor suppressor and inhibits triple-negative breast cancer tumorigenesis by targeting elongation factor 2 kinase. *Oncotarget* **2016**, *8*, 11641–11658. [CrossRef] [PubMed]
256. Fernandes, R.S.; Silva, J.O.; Monteiro, L.O.; Leite, E.A.; Cassali, G.D.; Rubello, D.; Cardoso, V.N.; Ferreira, L.A.; Oliveira, M.C.; de Barros, A.L. Doxorubicin-loaded nanocarriers: A comparative study of liposome and nanostructured lipid carrier as alternatives for cancer therapy. *Biomed. Pharmacother.* **2016**, *84*, 252–257. [CrossRef] [PubMed]
257. Alaarg, A.; Jordan, N.Y.; Verhoef, J.J.; Metselaar, J.M.; Storm, G.; Kok, R.J. Docosahexaenoic acid liposomes for targeting chronic inflammatory diseases and cancer: An in vitro assessment. *Int. J. Nanomed.* **2016**, *11*, 5027–5040. [CrossRef] [PubMed]
258. Amiri, B.; Ebrahimi-Far, M.; Saffari, Z.; Akbarzadeh, A.; Soleimani, E.; Chiani, M. Preparation, characterization and cytotoxicity of silibinin-containing nanoniosomes in T47D human breast carcinoma cells. *Asian Pac. J. Cancer Prev.* **2016**, *17*, 3835–3838. [PubMed]

259. Qian, R.C.; Cao, Y.; Long, Y.T. Binary system for microrna-targeted imaging in single cells and photothermal cancer therapy. *Anal. Chem.* **2016**, *88*, 8640–8647. [CrossRef] [PubMed]
260. Cao, H.; Dan, Z.; He, X.; Zhang, Z.; Yu, H.; Yin, Q.; Li, Y. Liposomes coated with isolated macrophage membrane can target lung metastasis of breast cancer. *ACS Nano* **2016**, *10*, 7738–7748. [CrossRef] [PubMed]
261. Jiang, L.; He, B.; Pan, D.; Luo, K.; Yi, Q.; Gu, Z. Anti-cancer efficacy of paclitaxel loaded in PH triggered liposomes. *J. Biomed. Nanotechnol.* **2016**, *12*, 79–90. [CrossRef] [PubMed]
262. Soppimath, K.S.; Aminabhavi, T.M.; Kulkarni, A.R.; Rudzinski, W.E. Biodegradable polymeric nanoparticles as drug delivery devices. *J. Control. Release* **2001**, *70*, 1–20. [CrossRef]
263. Kreuter, J. Drug delivery to the central nervous system by polymeric nanoparticles: What do we know? *Adv. Drug Deliv. Rev.* **2014**, *71*, 2–14. [CrossRef] [PubMed]
264. Rossin, R.; Pan, D.; Qi, K.; Turner, J.L.; Sun, X.; Wooley, K.L.; Welch, M.J. ^{64}Cu-labeled folate-conjugated shell cross-linked nanoparticles for tumor imaging and radiotherapy: Synthesis, radiolabeling, and biologic evaluation. *J. Nucl. Med.* **2005**, *46*, 1210–1218. [PubMed]
265. Salmaso, S.; Caliceti, P. Stealth properties to improve therapeutic efficacy of drug nanocarriers. *J. Drug Deliv.* **2013**, *2013*. [CrossRef] [PubMed]
266. Roberts, J.C.; Adams, Y.E.; Tomalia, D.; Mercer-Smith, J.A.; Lavallee, D.K. Using starburst dendrimers as linker molecules to radiolabel antibodies. *Bioconjug. Chem.* **1990**, *1*, 305–308. [CrossRef] [PubMed]
267. Tomalia, D.; Naylor, A.; Goddard, W. Starburst dendrimers: Molecular-level control of size, shape, surface-chemistry, topology, and flexibility from atoms to macroscopic matter. *Angew. Chem. Int. Ed. Engl.* **1990**, *29*, 138–175. [CrossRef]
268. Sk, U.H.; Kojima, C. Dendrimers for theranostic applications. *Biomol. Concepts* **2015**, *6*, 205–217. [CrossRef] [PubMed]
269. Sharma, A.; Mejia, D.; Maysinger, D.; Kakkar, A. Design and synthesis of multifunctional traceable dendrimers for visualizing drug delivery. *RSC Adv.* **2014**, *4*, 19242–19245. [CrossRef]
270. Sharma, A.; Khatchadourian, A.; Khanna, K.; Sharma, R.; Kakkar, A.; Maysinger, D. Multivalent niacin nanoconjugates for delivery to cytoplasmic lipid droplets. *Biomaterials* **2011**, *32*, 1419–1429. [CrossRef] [PubMed]
271. Wu, C.; Brechbiel, M.; Kozak, R.; Gansow, O. Metal-chelate-dendrimer-antibody constructs for use in radioimmunotherapy and imaging. *Bioorg. Med. Chem. Lett.* **1994**, *4*, 449–454. [CrossRef]
272. Wangler, C.; Moldenhauer, G.; Saffrich, R.; Knapp, E.M.; Beijer, B.; Schnolzer, M.; Wangler, B.; Eisenhut, M.; Haberkorn, U.; Mier, W. Pamam structure-based multifunctional fluorescent conjugates for improved fluorescent labelling of biomacromolecules. *Chemistry* **2008**, *14*, 8116–8130. [CrossRef]
273. Ling, Y.; Wei, K.; Luo, Y.; Gao, X.; Zhong, S. Dual docetaxel/superparamagnetic iron oxide loaded nanoparticles for both targeting magnetic resonance imaging and cancer therapy. *Biomaterials* **2011**, *32*, 7139–7150. [CrossRef]
274. Abbasi, A.Z.; Prasad, P.; Cai, P.; He, C.; Foltz, W.D.; Amini, M.A.; Gordijo, C.R.; Rauth, A.M.; Wu, X.Y. Manganese oxide and docetaxel co-loaded fluorescent polymer nanoparticles for dual modal imaging and chemotherapy of breast cancer. *J. Control. Release* **2015**, *209*, 186–196. [CrossRef] [PubMed]
275. Farokhzad, O.C.; Jon, S.; Khademhosseini, A.; Tran, T.N.; Lavan, D.A.; Langer, R. Nanoparticle-aptamer bioconjugates: A new approach for targeting prostate cancer cells. *Cancer Res.* **2004**, *64*, 7668–7672. [CrossRef] [PubMed]
276. He, C.; Cai, P.; Li, J.; Zhang, T.; Lin, L.; Abbasi, A.Z.; Henderson, J.T.; Rauth, A.M.; Wu, X.Y. Blood-brain barrier-penetrating amphiphilic polymer nanoparticles deliver docetaxel for the treatment of brain metastases of triple negative breast cancer. *J. Control. Release* **2017**, *246*, 98–109. [CrossRef]
277. Pramanik, A.; Laha, D.; Dash, S.K.; Chattopadhyay, S.; Roy, S.; Das, D.K.; Pramanik, P.; Karmakar, P. An in vivo study for targeted delivery of copper-organic complex to breast cancer using chitosan polymer nanoparticles. *Mater. Sci. Eng. C Mater. Biol. Appl.* **2016**, *68*, 327–337. [CrossRef]
278. Zhou, Z.; Munyaradzi, O.; Xia, X.; Green, D.; Bong, D. High-capacity drug carriers from common polymer amphiphiles. *Biomacromolecules* **2016**, *17*, 3060–3066. [CrossRef] [PubMed]
279. Danafar, H.; Sharafi, A.; Kheiri Manjili, H.; Andalib, S. Sulforaphane delivery using MPEG-PCL co-polymer nanoparticles to breast cancer cells. *Pharm. Dev. Technol.* **2016**, 1–10. [CrossRef] [PubMed]

280. Rostami, E.; Kashanian, S.; Azandaryani, A.H.; Faramarzi, H.; Dolatabadi, J.E.; Omidfar, K. Drug targeting using solid lipid nanoparticles. *Chem. Phys. Lipids* **2014**, *181*, 56–61. [CrossRef] [PubMed]
281. Rostami, E.; Kashanian, S.; Azandaryani, A.H. Preparation of solid lipid nanoparticles as drug carriers for levothyroxine sodium with in vitro drug delivery kinetic characterization. *Mol. Biol. Rep.* **2014**, *41*, 3521–3527. [CrossRef] [PubMed]
282. Mashaghi, S.; Jadidi, T.; Koenderink, G.; Mashaghi, A. Lipid nanotechnology. *Int. J. Mol. Sci.* **2013**, *14*, 4242–4282. [CrossRef] [PubMed]
283. Uner, M.; Yener, G. Importance of solid lipid nanoparticles (SLN) in various administration routes and future perspectives. *Int. J. Nanomed.* **2007**, *2*, 289–300.
284. Muller, R.H.; Mader, K.; Gohla, S. Solid lipid nanoparticles (SLN) for controlled drug delivery—A review of the state of the art. *Eur. J. Pharm. Biopharm.* **2000**, *50*, 161–177. [CrossRef]
285. Zur Muhlen, A.; Schwarz, C.; Mehnert, W. Solid lipid nanoparticles (SLN) for controlled drug delivery—Drug release and release mechanism. *Eur. J. Pharm. Biopharm.* **1998**, *45*, 149–155. [CrossRef]
286. Mehnert, W.; Mader, K. Solid lipid nanoparticles: Production, characterization and applications. *Adv. Drug Deliv. Rev.* **2001**, *47*, 165–196. [CrossRef]
287. Jenning, V.; Thunemann, A.F.; Gohla, S.H. Characterisation of a novel solid lipid nanoparticle carrier system based on binary mixtures of liquid and solid lipids. *Int. J. Pharm.* **2000**, *199*, 167–177. [CrossRef]
288. Radaic, A.; de Paula, E.; de Jesus, M.B. Factorial design and development of solid lipid nanoparticles (SLN) for gene delivery. *J. Nanosci. Nanotechnol.* **2015**, *15*, 1793–1800. [CrossRef] [PubMed]
289. Akanda, M.H.; Rai, R.; Slipper, I.J.; Chowdhry, B.Z.; Lamprou, D.; Getti, G.; Douroumis, D. Delivery of retinoic acid to LNCaP human prostate cancer cells using solid lipid nanoparticles. *Int. J. Pharm.* **2015**, *493*, 161–171. [CrossRef] [PubMed]
290. Swami, R.; Singh, I.; Jeengar, M.K.; Naidu, V.G.; Khan, W.; Sistla, R. Adenosine conjugated lipidic nanoparticles for enhanced tumor targeting. *Int. J. Pharm.* **2015**, *486*, 287–296. [CrossRef] [PubMed]
291. de Jesus, M.B.; Radaic, A.; Hinrichs, W.L.; Ferreira, C.V.; de Paula, E.; Hoekstra, D.; Zuhorn, I.S. Inclusion of the helper lipid dioleoyl-phosphatidylethanolamine in solid lipid nanoparticles inhibits their transfection efficiency. *J. Biomed. Nanotechnol.* **2014**, *10*, 355–365. [CrossRef] [PubMed]
292. Carbone, C.; Tomasello, B.; Ruozi, B.; Renis, M.; Puglisi, G. Preparation and optimization of PIT solid lipid nanoparticles via statistical factorial design. *Eur. J. Med. Chem.* **2012**, *49*, 110–117. [CrossRef] [PubMed]
293. De Jesus, M.B.; Ferreira, C.V.; de Paula, E.; Hoekstra, D.; Zuhorn, I.S. Design of solid lipid nanoparticles for gene delivery into prostate cancer. *J. Control. Release* **2010**, *148*, e89–e90. [CrossRef] [PubMed]
294. Jain, A.; Sharma, G.; Kushwah, V.; Thakur, K.; Ghoshal, G.; Singh, B.; Jain, S.; Shivhare, U.S.; Katare, O.P. Fabrication and functional attributes of lipidic nanoconstructs of lycopene: An innovative endeavour for enhanced cytotoxicity in MCF-7 breast cancer cells. *Colloids Surf. B Biointerfaces* **2017**, *152*, 482–491. [CrossRef] [PubMed]
295. Campos, J.; Varas-Godoy, M.; Haidar, Z.S. Physicochemical characterization of chitosan-hyaluronan-coated solid lipid nanoparticles for the targeted delivery of paclitaxel: A proof-of-concept study in breast cancer cells. *Nanomedicine (Lond.)* **2017**, *12*, 473–490. [CrossRef] [PubMed]
296. Wang, F.; Li, L.; Liu, B.; Chen, Z.; Li, C. Hyaluronic acid decorated pluronic p85 solid lipid nanoparticles as a potential carrier to overcome multidrug resistance in cervical and breast cancer. *Biomed. Pharmacother.* **2017**, *86*, 595–604. [CrossRef] [PubMed]
297. Liu, J.; Meng, T.; Yuan, M.; Wen, L.; Cheng, B.; Liu, N.; Huang, X.; Hong, Y.; Yuan, H.; Hu, F. MicroRNA-200c delivered by solid lipid nanoparticles enhances the effect of paclitaxel on breast cancer stem cell. *Int. J. Nanomed.* **2016**, *11*, 6713–6725. [CrossRef] [PubMed]
298. Cavaco, M.C.; Pereira, C.; Kreutzer, B.; Gouveia, L.F.; Silva-Lima, B.; Brito, A.M.; Videira, M. Evading p-glycoprotein mediated-efflux chemoresistance using solid lipid nanoparticles. *Eur. J. Pharm. Biopharm.* **2017**, *110*, 76–84. [CrossRef] [PubMed]
299. Hou, A.H.; Swanson, D.; Barqawi, A.B. Modalities for imaging of prostate cancer. *Adv. Urol.* **2009**. [CrossRef] [PubMed]
300. Prasad, P. *Introduction to Nanomedicine and Nanobioengineering*; John Wiley & Sons, Inc.: Hoboken, NJ, USA, 2012; p. 590.
301. Hainfeld, J.F.; Slatkin, D.N.; Focella, T.M.; Smilowitz, H.M. Gold nanoparticles: A new X-ray contrast agent. *Br. J. Radiol.* **2006**, *79*, 248–253. [CrossRef] [PubMed]

302. Nebuloni, L.; Kuhn, G.A.; Muller, R. A comparative analysis of water-soluble and blood-pool contrast agents for in vivo vascular imaging with micro-ct. *Acad. Radiol* **2013**, *20*, 1247–1255. [CrossRef] [PubMed]
303. Clark, D.P.; Ghaghada, K.; Moding, E.J.; Kirsch, D.G.; Badea, C.T. In vivo characterization of tumor vasculature using iodine and gold nanoparticles and dual energy micro-CT. *Phys. Med. Biol.* **2013**, *58*, 1683–1704. [CrossRef] [PubMed]
304. Wan, F.; Qin, X.; Zhang, G.; Lu, X.; Zhu, Y.; Zhang, H.; Dai, B.; Shi, G.; Ye, D. Oxidized low-density lipoprotein is associated with advanced-stage prostate cancer. *Tumour Biol.* **2015**, *36*, 3573–3582. [CrossRef] [PubMed]
305. Hill, M.L.; Corbin, I.R.; Levitin, R.B.; Cao, W.; Mainprize, J.G.; Yaffe, M.J.; Zheng, G. In vitro assessment of poly-iodinated triglyceride reconstituted low-density lipoprotein: Initial steps toward ct molecular imaging. *Acad. Radiol.* **2010**, *17*, 1359–1365. [CrossRef] [PubMed]
306. Furuya, Y.; Sekine, Y.; Kato, H.; Miyazawa, Y.; Koike, H.; Suzuki, K. Low-density lipoprotein receptors play an important role in the inhibition of prostate cancer cell proliferation by statins. *Prostate Int.* **2016**, *4*, 56–60. [CrossRef] [PubMed]
307. Ai, K.; Liu, Y.; Liu, J.; Yuan, Q.; He, Y.; Lu, L. Large-scale synthesis of Bi_2S_3 nanodots as a contrast agent for in vivo X-ray computed tomography imaging. *Adv. Mater.* **2011**, *23*, 4886–4891. [CrossRef] [PubMed]
308. Carton, A.K.; Gavenonis, S.C.; Currivan, J.A.; Conant, E.F.; Schnall, M.D.; Maidment, A.D. Dual-energy contrast-enhanced digital breast tomosynthesis—A feasibility study. *Br. J. Radiol.* **2010**, *83*, 344–350. [CrossRef] [PubMed]
309. Kim, D.; Jeong, Y.Y.; Jon, S. A drug-loaded aptamer-gold nanoparticle bioconjugate for combined ct imaging and therapy of prostate cancer. *ACS Nano* **2010**, *4*, 3689–3696. [CrossRef] [PubMed]
310. Naha, P.C.; Lau, K.C.; Hsu, J.C.; Hajfathalian, M.; Mian, S.; Chhour, P.; Uppuluri, L.; McDonald, E.S.; Maidment, A.D.; Cormode, D.P. Gold silver alloy nanoparticles (GSAN): An imaging probe for breast cancer screening with dual-energy mammography or computed tomography. *Nanoscale* **2016**, *8*, 13740–13754. [CrossRef] [PubMed]
311. Devaraj, N.K.; Keliher, E.J.; Thurber, G.M.; Nahrendorf, M.; Weissleder, R. ^{18}F labeled nanoparticles for in vivo PET-CT imaging. *Bioconjug. Chem.* **2009**, *20*, 397–401. [CrossRef] [PubMed]
312. Welch, M.J.; Hawker, C.J.; Wooley, K.L. The advantages of nanoparticles for pet. *J. Nucl. Med.* **2009**, *50*, 1743–1746. [CrossRef] [PubMed]
313. Chrastina, A.; Schnitzer, J.E. Iodine-125 radiolabeling of silver nanoparticles for in vivo SPECT imaging. *Int. J. Nanomed.* **2010**, *5*, 653–659.
314. Woodward, J.; Kennel, S.; Mirzadeh, S.; Dai, S.; Wall, J.; Richey, T.; Avanell, J.; Rondinone, A. In vivo SPECT/CT imaging and biodistribution using radioactive 125-CDTE/ZnS nanoparticles. *Nanotechnology* **2007**, *18*, 175103. [CrossRef]
315. Wong, P.; Li, L.; Chea, J.; Delgado, M.K.; Crow, D.; Poku, E.; Szpikowska, B.; Bowles, N.; Channappa, D.; Colcher, D.; et al. Pet imaging of ^{64}Cu-DOTA-SCFV-anti-psma lipid nanoparticles (LNPS): Enhanced tumor targeting over anti-PSMA SCFV or untargeted LNPS. *Nucl. Med. Biol.* **2017**, *47*, 62–68. [CrossRef] [PubMed]
316. Zhao, Y.; Sultan, D.; Detering, L.; Luehmann, H.; Liu, Y. Facile synthesis, pharmacokinetic and systemic clearance evaluation, and positron emission tomography cancer imaging of (6)(4)Cu-Au alloy nanoclusters. *Nanoscale* **2014**, *6*, 13501–13509. [CrossRef] [PubMed]
317. Pressly, E.D.; Pierce, R.A.; Connal, L.A.; Hawker, C.J.; Liu, Y. Nanoparticle PET/CT imaging of natriuretic peptide clearance receptor in prostate cancer. *Bioconjug. Chem.* **2013**, *24*, 196–204. [CrossRef] [PubMed]
318. Shen, Y.; Ma, Z.; Chen, F.; Dong, Q.; Hu, Q.; Bai, L.; Chen, J. Effective photothermal chemotherapy with docetaxel-loaded gold nanospheres in advanced prostate cancer. *J. Drug Target.* **2015**, *23*, 568–576. [CrossRef] [PubMed]
319. Behnam Azad, B.; Banerjee, S.R.; Pullambhatla, M.; Lacerda, S.; Foss, C.A.; Wang, Y.; Ivkov, R.; Pomper, M.G. Evaluation of a PSMA-targeted BNF nanoparticle construct. *Nanoscale* **2015**, *7*, 4432–4442. [CrossRef] [PubMed]
320. Lee, C.; Lo, S.T.; Lim, J.; da Costa, V.C.; Ramezani, S.; Oz, O.K.; Pavan, G.M.; Annunziata, O.; Sun, X.; Simanek, E.E. Design, synthesis and biological assessment of a triazine dendrimer with approximately 16 paclitaxel groups and 8 PEG groups. *Mol. Pharm.* **2013**, *10*, 4452–4461. [CrossRef] [PubMed]
321. Mendoza-Sanchez, A.N.; Ferro-Flores, G.; Ocampo-Garcia, B.E.; Morales-Avila, E.; de, M.R.F.; De Leon-Rodriguez, L.M.; Santos-Cuevas, C.L.; Medina, L.A.; Rojas-Calderon, E.L.; Camacho-Lopez, M.A.

Lys3-bombesin conjugated to 99mTc-labelled gold nanoparticles for in vivo gastrin releasing peptide-receptor imaging. *J. Biomed. Nanotechnol.* **2010**, *6*, 375–384. [CrossRef] [PubMed]
322. Lee, H.; Shields, A.F.; Siegel, B.A.; Miller, K.D.; Krop, I.; Ma, C.X.; LoRusso, P.M.; Munster, P.N.; Campbell, K.; Gaddy, D.F.; et al. ^{64}Cu-MM-302 positron emission tomography quantifies variability of enhanced permeability and retention of nanoparticles in relation to treatment response in patients with metastatic breast cancer. *Clin. Cancer Res.* **2017**. [CrossRef] [PubMed]
323. Aanei, I.L.; ElSohly, A.M.; Farkas, M.E.; Netirojjanakul, C.; Regan, M.; Taylor Murphy, S.; O'Neil, J.P.; Seo, Y.; Francis, M.B. Biodistribution of antibody-MS2 viral capsid conjugates in breast cancer models. *Mol. Pharm.* **2016**, *13*, 3764–3772. [CrossRef] [PubMed]
324. Perez-Medina, C.; Abdel-Atti, D.; Zhang, Y.; Longo, V.A.; Irwin, C.P.; Binderup, T.; Ruiz-Cabello, J.; Fayad, Z.A.; Lewis, J.S.; Mulder, W.J.; et al. A modular labeling strategy for in vivo pet and near-infrared fluorescence imaging of nanoparticle tumor targeting. *J. Nucl. Med.* **2014**, *55*, 1706–1711. [CrossRef] [PubMed]
325. Wang, Y.; Black, K.C.; Luehmann, H.; Li, W.; Zhang, Y.; Cai, X.; Wan, D.; Liu, S.Y.; Li, M.; Kim, P.; et al. Comparison study of gold nanohexapods, nanorods, and nanocages for photothermal cancer treatment. *ACS Nano* **2013**, *7*, 2068–2077. [CrossRef] [PubMed]
326. Tseng, Y.C.; Xu, Z.; Guley, K.; Yuan, H.; Huang, L. Lipid-calcium phosphate nanoparticles for delivery to the lymphatic system and SPECT/CT imaging of lymph node metastases. *Biomaterials* **2014**, *35*, 4688–4698. [CrossRef] [PubMed]
327. Kilcoyne, A.; Price, M.C.; McDermott, S.; Harisinghani, M.G. Imaging on nodal staging of prostate cancer. *Future Oncol.* **2017**, *13*, 551–565. [CrossRef] [PubMed]
328. Ruiz-Cabello, J.; Barnett, B.P.; Bottomley, P.A.; Bulte, J.W. Fluorine (^{19}F) MRS and MRI in biomedicine. *NMR Biomed.* **2011**, *24*, 114–129. [CrossRef] [PubMed]
329. Schmieder, A.H.; Caruthers, S.D.; Keupp, J.; Wickline, S.A.; Lanza, G.M. Recent advances in fluorine magnetic resonance imaging with perfluorocarbon emulsions. *Engineering (Beijing)* **2015**, *1*, 475–489. [PubMed]
330. Chen, H.; Song, M.; Tang, J.; Hu, G.; Xu, S.; Guo, Z.; Li, N.; Cui, J.; Zhang, X.; Chen, X.; et al. Ultrahigh (19)f loaded cu1.75s nanoprobes for simultaneous ^{19}F magnetic resonance imaging and photothermal therapy. *ACS Nano* **2016**, *10*, 1355–1362. [CrossRef] [PubMed]
331. Muhammad, G.; Jablonska, A.; Rose, L.; Walczak, P.; Janowski, M. Effect of MRI tags: Spio nanoparticles and ^{19}F nanoemulsion on various populations of mouse mesenchymal stem cells. *Acta Neurobiol. Exp. (Wars)* **2015**, *75*, 144–159. [PubMed]
332. Amiri, H.; Srinivas, M.; Veltien, A.; van Uden, M.J.; de Vries, I.J.; Heerschap, A. Cell tracking using ^{19}F magnetic resonance imaging: Technical aspects and challenges towards clinical applications. *Eur. Radiol.* **2015**, *25*, 726–735. [CrossRef] [PubMed]
333. Maxwell, R.J.; Frenkiel, T.A.; Newell, D.R.; Bauer, C.; Griffiths, J.R. ^{19}F nuclear magnetic resonance imaging of drug distribution in vivo: The disposition of an antifolate anticancer drug in mice. *Magn. Reson. Med.* **1991**, *17*, 189–196. [CrossRef] [PubMed]
334. Kim, J.G.; Zhao, D.; Song, Y.; Constantinescu, A.; Mason, R.P.; Liu, H. Interplay of tumor vascular oxygenation and tumor PO2 observed using near-infrared spectroscopy, an oxygen needle electrode, and 19f mr po2 mapping. *J. Biomed. Opt.* **2003**, *8*, 53–62. [CrossRef] [PubMed]
335. Yu, W.; Yang, Y.; Bo, S.; Li, Y.; Chen, S.; Yang, Z.; Zheng, X.; Jiang, Z.X.; Zhou, X. Design and synthesis of fluorinated dendrimers for sensitive ^{19}F MRI. *J. Org. Chem.* **2015**, *80*, 4443–4449. [CrossRef] [PubMed]
336. Matsushita, H.; Mizukami, S.; Sugihara, F.; Nakanishi, Y.; Yoshioka, Y.; Kikuchi, K. Multifunctional core-shell silica nanoparticles for highly sensitive ^{19}F magnetic resonance imaging. *Angew. Chem. Int. Ed. Engl.* **2014**, *53*, 1008–1011. [CrossRef] [PubMed]
337. Bae, P.K.; Jung, J.; Lim, S.J.; Kim, D.; Kim, S.K.; Chung, B.H. Bimodal perfluorocarbon nanoemulsions for nasopharyngeal carcinoma targeting. *Mol. Imaging Biol.* **2013**, *15*, 401–410. [CrossRef] [PubMed]
338. Ahrens, E.T.; Helfer, B.M.; O'Hanlon, C.F.; Schirda, C. Clinical cell therapy imaging using a perfluorocarbon tracer and fluorine-19 MRI. *Magn. Reson. Med.* **2014**, *72*, 1696–1701. [CrossRef] [PubMed]
339. Cho, S.; Park, W.; Kim, D.H. Silica-coated metal chelating-melanin nanoparticles as a dual-modal contrast enhancement imaging and therapeutic agent. *ACS Appl. Mater. Interfaces* **2017**, *9*, 101–111. [CrossRef] [PubMed]

340. Moghanaki, D.; Turkbey, B.; Vapiwala, N.; Ehdaie, B.; Frank, S.J.; McLaughlin, P.W.; Harisinghani, M. Advances in prostate cancer magnetic resonance imaging and positron emission tomography-computed tomography for staging and radiotherapy treatment planning. *Semin. Radiat. Oncol.* **2017**, *27*, 21–33. [CrossRef] [PubMed]
341. Jayapaul, J.; Arns, S.; Bunker, M.; Weiler, M.; Rutherford, S.; Comba, P.; Kiessling, F. In vivo evaluation of riboflavin receptor targeted fluorescent USPIO in mice with prostate cancer xenografts. *Nano Res.* **2016**, *9*, 1319–1333. [CrossRef] [PubMed]
342. Kilcoyne, A.; Harisinghani, M.G.; Mahmood, U. Prostate cancer imaging and therapy: Potential role of nanoparticles. *J. Nucl. Med.* **2016**, *57*, 105S–110S. [CrossRef] [PubMed]
343. Jin, C.S.; Overchuk, M.; Cui, L.; Wilson, B.C.; Bristow, R.G.; Chen, J.; Zheng, G. Nanoparticle-enabled selective destruction of prostate tumor using MRI-guided focal photothermal therapy. *Prostate* **2016**, *76*, 1169–1181. [CrossRef] [PubMed]
344. Hurley, K.R.; Ring, H.L.; Etheridge, M.; Zhang, J.; Gao, Z.; Shao, Q.; Klein, N.D.; Szlag, V.M.; Chung, C.; Reineke, T.M.; et al. Predictable heating and positive MRI contrast from a mesoporous silica-coated iron oxide nanoparticle. *Mol. Pharm.* **2016**, *13*, 2172–2183. [CrossRef] [PubMed]
345. Turino, L.N.; Ruggiero, M.R.; Stefania, R.; Cutrin, J.C.; Aime, S.; Geninatti Crich, S. Ferritin decorated PLGA/paclitaxel loaded nanoparticles endowed with an enhanced toxicity toward MCF-7 breast tumor cells. *Bioconjug. Chem.* **2017**, *28*, 1283–1290. [CrossRef] [PubMed]
346. Shamsi, M.; Pirayesh Islamian, J. Breast cancer: Early diagnosis and effective treatment by drug delivery tracing. *Nucl. Med. Rev. Cent. East. Eur.* **2017**, *20*, 45–48. [CrossRef] [PubMed]
347. Shan, X.H.; Wang, P.; Xiong, F.; Lu, H.Y.; Hu, H. Detection of human breast cancer cells using a 2-deoxy-D-glucose-functionalized superparamagnetic iron oxide nanoparticles. *Cancer Biomark.* **2017**. [CrossRef] [PubMed]
348. Keshtkar, M.; Shahbazi-Gahrouei, D.; Khoshfetrat, S.M.; Mehrgardi, M.A.; Aghaei, M. Aptamer-conjugated magnetic nanoparticles as targeted magnetic resonance imaging contrast agent for breast cancer. *J. Med. Signals Sens.* **2016**, *6*, 243–247. [PubMed]
349. Zhang, L.; Varma, N.R.; Gang, Z.Z.; Ewing, J.R.; Arbab, A.S.; Ali, M.M. Targeting triple negative breast cancer with a small-sized paramagnetic nanoparticle. *J. Nanomed. Nanotechnol.* **2016**, *7*, 404. [CrossRef] [PubMed]
350. Moon, S.H.; Yang, B.Y.; Kim, Y.J.; Hong, M.K.; Lee, Y.S.; Lee, D.S.; Chung, J.K.; Jeong, J.M. Development of a complementary PET/MR dual-modal imaging probe for targeting prostate-specific membrane antigen (PSMA). *Nanomedicine* **2016**, *12*, 871–879. [CrossRef] [PubMed]
351. Hu, H.; Li, D.; Liu, S.; Wang, M.; Moats, R.; Conti, P.S.; Li, Z. Integrin α2β1 targeted GdVO4:Eu ultrathin nanosheet for multimodal PET/MR imaging. *Biomaterials* **2014**, *35*, 8649–8658. [CrossRef] [PubMed]
352. Aryal, S.; Key, J.; Stigliano, C.; Landis, M.D.; Lee, D.Y.; Decuzzi, P. Positron emitting magnetic nanoconstructs for PET/MR imaging. *Small* **2014**, *10*, 2688–2696. [CrossRef] [PubMed]
353. Zhao, F.; Zhou, J.; Su, X.; Wang, Y.; Yan, X.; Jia, S.; Du, B. A smart responsive dual aptamers-targeted bubble-generating nanosystem for cancer triplex therapy and ultrasound imaging. *Small* **2017**. [CrossRef] [PubMed]
354. Xu, L.; Wan, C.; Du, J.; Li, H.; Liu, X.; Yang, H.; Li, F. Synthesis, characterization, and in vitro evaluation of targeted gold nanoshelled poly(D,L-lactide-*co*-glycolide) nanoparticles carrying anti p53 antibody as a theranostic agent for ultrasound contrast imaging and photothermal therapy. *J. Biomater. Sci. Polym. Ed.* **2017**, *28*, 415–430. [CrossRef] [PubMed]
355. Baghbani, F.; Moztarzadeh, F.; Mohandesi, J.A.; Yazdian, F.; Mokhtari-Dizaji, M. Novel alginate-stabilized doxorubicin-loaded nanodroplets for ultrasounic theranosis of breast cancer. *Int. J. Biol. Macromol.* **2016**, *93*, 512–519. [CrossRef] [PubMed]
356. Lee, J.Y.; Carugo, D.; Crake, C.; Owen, J.; de Saint Victor, M.; Seth, A.; Coussios, C.; Stride, E. Nanoparticle-loaded protein-polymer nanodroplets for improved stability and conversion efficiency in ultrasound imaging and drug delivery. *Adv. Mater.* **2015**, *27*, 5484–5492. [CrossRef] [PubMed]
357. Wang, S.; Dai, Z.; Ke, H.; Qu, E.; Qi, X.; Zhang, K.; Wang, J. Contrast ultrasound-guided photothermal therapy using gold nanoshelled microcapsules in breast cancer. *Eur. J. Radiol.* **2014**, *83*, 117–122. [CrossRef] [PubMed]

358. Agemy, L.; Sugahara, K.N.; Kotamraju, V.R.; Gujraty, K.; Girard, O.M.; Kono, Y.; Mattrey, R.F.; Park, J.H.; Sailor, M.J.; Jimenez, A.I.; et al. Nanoparticle-induced vascular blockade in human prostate cancer. *Blood* **2010**, *116*, 2847–2856. [CrossRef] [PubMed]
359. Yang, H.; Deng, L.; Li, T.; Shen, X.; Yan, J.; Zuo, L.; Wu, C.; Liu, Y. Multifunctional PLGA nanobubbles as theranostic agents: Combining doxorubicin and P-GP siRNA co-delivery into human breast cancer cells and ultrasound cellular imaging. *J. Biomed. Nanotechnol.* **2015**, *11*, 2124–2136. [CrossRef] [PubMed]
360. Tong, H.P.; Wang, L.F.; Guo, Y.L.; Li, L.; Fan, X.Z.; Ding, J.; Huang, H.Y. Preparation of protamine cationic nanobubbles and experimental study of their physical properties and in vivo contrast enhancement. *Ultrasound Med. Biol.* **2013**, *39*, 2147–2157. [CrossRef] [PubMed]
361. Thorek, D.; Robertson, R.; Bacchus, W.A.; Hahn, J.; Rothberg, J.; Beattie, B.J.; Grimm, J. Cerenkov imaging —A new modality for molecular imaging. *Am. J. Nucl. Med. Mol. Imaging* **2012**, *2*, 163–173. [PubMed]
362. Black, K.C.; Ibricevic, A.; Gunsten, S.P.; Flores, J.A.; Gustafson, T.P.; Raymond, J.E.; Samarajeewa, S.; Shrestha, R.; Felder, S.E.; Cai, T.; et al. In vivo fate tracking of degradable nanoparticles for lung gene transfer using pet and cerenkov imaging. *Biomaterials* **2016**, *98*, 53–63. [CrossRef] [PubMed]
363. Spinelli, A.E.; Schiariti, M.P.; Grana, C.M.; Ferrari, M.; Cremonesi, M.; Boschi, F. Cerenkov and radioluminescence imaging of brain tumor specimens during neurosurgery. *J. Biomed. Opt.* **2016**, *21*, 50502. [CrossRef] [PubMed]
364. Schwenck, J.; Fuchs, K.; Eilenberger, S.H.; Rolle, A.M.; Castaneda Vega, S.; Thaiss, W.M.; Maier, F.C. Fluorescence and Cerenkov luminescence imaging. Applications in small animal research. *Nuklearmedizin* **2016**, *55*, 63–70. [PubMed]
365. Pandya, D.N.; Hantgan, R.; Budzevich, M.M.; Kock, N.D.; Morse, D.L.; Batista, I.; Mintz, A.; Li, K.C.; Wadas, T.J. Preliminary therapy evaluation of ^{225}Ac-DOTA-c(RGDyK) demonstrates that cerenkov radiation derived from ^{225}Ac daughter decay can be detected by optical imaging for in vivo tumor visualization. *Theranostics* **2016**, *6*, 698–709. [CrossRef] [PubMed]
366. Shimamoto, M.; Gotoh, K.; Hasegawa, K.; Kojima, A. Hybrid light imaging using cerenkov luminescence and liquid scintillation for preclinical optical imaging in vivo. *Mol. Imaging Biol.* **2016**, *18*, 500–509. [CrossRef] [PubMed]
367. Andreozzi, J.M.; Zhang, R.; Gladstone, D.J.; Williams, B.B.; Glaser, A.K.; Pogue, B.W.; Jarvis, L.A. Cherenkov imaging method for rapid optimization of clinical treatment geometry in total skin electron beam therapy. *Med. Phys.* **2016**, *43*, 993–1003. [CrossRef] [PubMed]
368. Wibmer, A.G.; Burger, I.A.; Sala, E.; Hricak, H.; Weber, W.A.; Vargas, H.A. Molecular imaging of prostate cancer. *Radiographics* **2016**, *36*, 142–159. [CrossRef] [PubMed]
369. Vargas, H.A.; Grimm, J.; O, F.D.; Sala, E.; Hricak, H. Molecular imaging of prostate cancer: Translating molecular biology approaches into the clinical realm. *Eur. Radiol.* **2015**, *25*, 1294–1302. [CrossRef] [PubMed]
370. Lohrmann, C.; Zhang, H.; Thorek, D.L.; Desai, P.; Zanzonico, P.B.; O'Donoghue, J.; Irwin, C.P.; Reiner, T.; Grimm, J.; Weber, W.A. Cerenkov luminescence imaging for radiation dose calculation of a (9)(0)Y-labeled gastrin-releasing peptide receptor antagonist. *J. Nucl. Med.* **2015**, *56*, 805–811. [CrossRef] [PubMed]
371. Hu, Z.; Chi, C.; Liu, M.; Guo, H.; Zhang, Z.; Zeng, C.; Ye, J.; Wang, J.; Tian, J.; Yang, W.; et al. Nanoparticle-mediated radiopharmaceutical-excited fluorescence molecular imaging allows precise image-guided tumor-removal surgery. *Nanomedicine* **2017**, *13*, 1323–1331. [CrossRef] [PubMed]
372. Madru, R.; Tran, T.A.; Axelsson, J.; Ingvar, C.; Bibic, A.; Stahlberg, F.; Knutsson, L.; Strand, S.E. ^{68}Ga-labeled superparamagnetic iron oxide nanoparticles (SPIONs) for multi-modality PET/MR/Cherenkov luminescence imaging of sentinel lymph nodes. *Am. J. Nucl. Med. Mol. Imaging* **2013**, *4*, 60–69. [PubMed]
373. Hu, Z.; Zhao, M.; Qu, Y.; Zhang, X.; Zhang, M.; Liu, M.; Guo, H.; Zhang, Z.; Wang, J.; Yang, W.; et al. In vivo 3-dimensional radiopharmaceutical-excited fluorescence tomography. *J. Nucl. Med.* **2017**, *58*, 169–174. [CrossRef] [PubMed]
374. Lee, S.B.; Yoon, G.; Lee, S.W.; Jeong, S.Y.; Ahn, B.C.; Lim, D.K.; Lee, J.; Jeon, Y.H. Combined positron emission tomography and Cerenkov luminescence imaging of sentinel lymph nodes using pegylated radionuclide-embedded gold nanoparticles. *Small* **2016**, *12*, 4894–4901. [CrossRef] [PubMed]
375. Tanha, K.; Pashazadeh, A.M.; Pogue, B.W. Review of biomedical Cerenkov luminescence imaging applications. *Biomed. Opt. Express* **2015**, *6*, 3053–3065. [CrossRef] [PubMed]
376. Zhang, M.; Kim, H.S.; Jin, T.; Yi, A.; Moon, W.K. Ultrasound-guided photoacoustic imaging for the selective

detection of EGFR-expressing breast cancer and lymph node metastases. *Biomed. Opt. Express* **2016**, *7*, 1920–1931. [CrossRef] [PubMed]
377. Su, Y.; Teng, Z.; Yao, H.; Wang, S.; Tian, Y.; Zhang, Y.; Liu, W.; Tian, W.; Zheng, L.; Lu, N.; et al. A multifunctional PB@mSiO$_2$-PEG/DOX nanoplatform for combined photothermal-chemotherapy of tumor. *ACS Appl. Mater. Interfaces* **2016**, *8*, 17038–17046. [CrossRef] [PubMed]
378. Feng, H.; Xia, X.; Li, C.; Song, Y.; Qin, C.; Zhang, Y.; Lan, X. Tyr as a multifunctional reporter gene regulated by the tet-on system for multimodality imaging: An in vitro study. *Sci. Rep.* **2015**, *5*, 15502. [CrossRef] [PubMed]
379. Zhang, T.; Cui, H.; Fang, C.Y.; Cheng, K.; Yang, X.; Chang, H.C.; Forrest, M.L. Targeted nanodiamonds as phenotype-specific photoacoustic contrast agents for breast cancer. *Nanomedicine (Lond.)* **2015**, *10*, 573–587. [CrossRef] [PubMed]
380. Levi, J.; Sathirachinda, A.; Gambhir, S.S. A high-affinity, high-stability photoacoustic agent for imaging gastrin-releasing peptide receptor in prostate cancer. *Clin. Cancer Res.* **2014**, *20*, 3721–3729. [CrossRef] [PubMed]
381. Dogra, V.S.; Chinni, B.K.; Valluru, K.S.; Joseph, J.V.; Ghazi, A.; Yao, J.L.; Evans, K.; Messing, E.M.; Rao, N.A. Multispectral photoacoustic imaging of prostate cancer: Preliminary ex vivo results. *J. Clin. Imaging Sci.* **2013**, *3*, 41. [CrossRef] [PubMed]
382. Kim, G.; Huang, S.W.; Day, K.C.; O'Donnell, M.; Agayan, R.R.; Day, M.A.; Kopelman, R.; Ashkenazi, S. Indocyanine-green-embedded pebbles as a contrast agent for photoacoustic imaging. *J. Biomed. Opt.* **2007**, *12*, 044020. [CrossRef] [PubMed]
383. Kim, C.; Favazza, C.; Wang, L.V. In vivo photoacoustic tomography of chemicals: High-resolution functional and molecular optical imaging at new depths. *Chem. Rev.* **2010**, *110*, 2756–2782. [CrossRef] [PubMed]
384. Tian, C.; Qian, W.; Shao, X.; Xie, Z.; Cheng, X.; Liu, S.; Cheng, Q.; Liu, B.; Wang, X. Plasmonic nanoparticles with quantitatively controlled bioconjugation for photoacoustic imaging of live cancer cells. *Adv. Sci. (Weinh)* **2016**, *3*, 1600237. [CrossRef] [PubMed]
385. Olafsson, R.; Bauer, D.R.; Montilla, L.G.; Witte, R.S. Real-time, contrast enhanced photoacoustic imaging of cancer in a mouse window chamber. *Opt. Express* **2010**, *18*, 18625–18632. [CrossRef] [PubMed]
386. Zhang, H. Cyclic arg-gly-asp-polyethyleneglycol-single-walled carbon nanotubes. In *Molecular Imaging and Contrast Agent Database (Micad)*; Bethesda: Washington DC MD, USA, 2004.
387. Xia, J.; Feng, G.; Xia, X.; Hao, L.; Wang, Z. Nh4hco3 gas-generating liposomal nanoparticle for photoacoustic imaging in breast cancer. *Int. J. Nanomed.* **2017**, *12*, 1803–1813. [CrossRef] [PubMed]
388. Biffi, S.; Petrizza, L.; Garrovo, C.; Rampazzo, E.; Andolfi, L.; Giustetto, P.; Nikolov, I.; Kurdi, G.; Danailov, M.B.; Zauli, G.; et al. Multimodal near-infrared-emitting plus silica nanoparticles with fluorescent, photoacoustic, and photothermal capabilities. *Int. J. Nanomed.* **2016**, *11*, 4865–4874.
389. Hu, D.; Liu, C.; Song, L.; Cui, H.; Gao, G.; Liu, P.; Sheng, Z.; Cai, L. Indocyanine green-loaded polydopamine-iron ions coordination nanoparticles for photoacoustic/magnetic resonance dual-modal imaging-guided cancer photothermal therapy. *Nanoscale* **2016**, *8*, 17150–17158. [CrossRef] [PubMed]
390. Cai, X.; Liu, X.; Liao, L.D.; Bandla, A.; Ling, J.M.; Liu, Y.H.; Thakor, N.; Bazan, G.C.; Liu, B. Encapsulated conjugated oligomer nanoparticles for real-time photoacoustic sentinel lymph node imaging and targeted photothermal therapy. *Small* **2016**, *12*, 4873–4880. [CrossRef] [PubMed]
391. Pham, E.; Yin, M.; Peters, C.G.; Lee, C.R.; Brown, D.; Xu, P.; Man, S.; Jayaraman, L.; Rohde, E.; Chow, A.; et al. Preclinical efficacy of bevacizumab with crlx101, an investigational nanoparticle-drug conjugate, in treatment of metastatic triple-negative breast cancer. *Cancer Res.* **2016**, *76*, 4493–4503. [CrossRef] [PubMed]
392. Feng, Q.; Zhang, Y.; Zhang, W.; Shan, X.; Yuan, Y.; Zhang, H.; Hou, L.; Zhang, Z. Tumor-targeted and multi-stimuli responsive drug delivery system for near-infrared light induced chemo-phototherapy and photoacoustic tomography. *Acta Biomater.* **2016**, *38*, 129–142. [CrossRef] [PubMed]
393. Ahir, M.; Bhattacharya, S.; Karmakar, S.; Mukhopadhyay, A.; Mukherjee, S.; Ghosh, S.; Chattopadhyay, S.; Patra, P.; Adhikary, A. Tailored-CuO-nanowire decorated with folic acid mediated coupling of the mitochondrial-ROS generation and MIR425-PTEN axis in furnishing potent anti-cancer activity in human triple negative breast carcinoma cells. *Biomaterials* **2016**, *76*, 115–132. [CrossRef] [PubMed]
394. Zevon, M.; Ganapathy, V.; Kantamneni, H.; Mingozzi, M.; Kim, P.; Adler, D.; Sheng, Y.; Tan, M.C.; Pierce, M.; Riman, R.E.; et al. CXCR-4 targeted, short wave infrared (SWIR) emitting nanoprobes for enhanced deep tissue imaging and micrometastatic cancer lesion detection. *Small* **2015**, *11*, 6347–6357. [CrossRef] [PubMed]

395. Ozel, T.; White, S.; Nguyen, E.; Moy, A.; Brenes, N.; Choi, B.; Betancourt, T. Enzymatically activated near infrared nanoprobes based on amphiphilic block copolymers for optical detection of cancer. *Lasers Surg. Med.* **2015**. [CrossRef]
396. Yuan, J.P.; Wang, L.W.; Qu, A.P.; Chen, J.M.; Xiang, Q.M.; Chen, C.; Sun, S.R.; Pang, D.W.; Liu, J.; Li, Y. Quantum dots-based quantitative and in situ multiple imaging on ki67 and cytokeratin to improve ki67 assessment in breast cancer. *PLoS ONE* **2015**, *10*, e0122734. [CrossRef] [PubMed]
397. D'Angelis do, E.S.B.C.; Correa, J.R.; Medeiros, G.A.; Barreto, G.; Magalhaes, K.G.; de Oliveira, A.L.; Spencer, J.; Rodrigues, M.O.; Neto, B.A. Carbon dots (C-dots) from cow manure with impressive subcellular selectivity tuned by simple chemical modification. *Chemistry* **2015**, *21*, 5055–5060. [CrossRef] [PubMed]
398. Li, J.; Jiang, X.; Guo, Y.; An, S.; Kuang, Y.; Ma, H.; He, X.; Jiang, C. Linear-dendritic copolymer composed of polyethylene glycol and all-trans-retinoic acid as drug delivery platform for paclitaxel against breast cancer. *Bioconjug. Chem.* **2015**, *26*, 418–426. [CrossRef] [PubMed]
399. Montecinos, V.P.; Morales, C.H.; Fischer, T.H.; Burns, S.; San Francisco, I.F.; Godoy, A.S.; Smith, G.J. Selective targeting of bioengineered platelets to prostate cancer vasculature: New paradigm for therapeutic modalities. *J. Cell Mol. Med.* **2015**, *19*, 1530–1537. [CrossRef] [PubMed]
400. Yu, Y.; Huang, T.; Wu, Y.; Ma, X.; Yu, G.; Qi, J. In Vitro and in vivo imaging of prostate tumor using NAYF4: Yb, Er up-converting nanoparticles. *Pathol. Oncol. Res.* **2014**, *20*, 335–341. [CrossRef] [PubMed]
401. Laprise-Pelletier, M.; Lagueux, J.; Cote, M.F.; LaGrange, T.; Fortin, M.A. Low-dose prostate cancer brachytherapy with radioactive palladium-gold nanoparticles. *Adv. Healthc. Mater.* **2017**, *6*. [CrossRef] [PubMed]
402. Li, W.; Yalcin, M.; Lin, Q.; Ardawi, M.M.; Mousa, S.A. Self-assembly of green tea catechin derivatives in nanoparticles for oral lycopene delivery. *J. Control. Release* **2017**, *248*, 117–124. [CrossRef] [PubMed]
403. Netala, V.R.; Bethu, M.S.; Pushpalatha, B.; Baki, V.B.; Aishwarya, S.; Rao, J.V.; Tartte, V. Biogenesis of silver nanoparticles using endophytic fungus pestalotiopsis microspora and evaluation of their antioxidant and anticancer activities. *Int. J. Nanomed.* **2016**, *11*, 5683–5696. [CrossRef] [PubMed]
404. Jazayeri, M.H.; Amani, H.; Pourfatollah, A.A.; Avan, A.; Ferns, G.A.; Pazoki-Toroudi, H. Enhanced detection sensitivity of prostate-specific antigen via PSA-conjugated gold nanoparticles based on localized surface plasmon resonance: GNP-coated anti-PSA/LSPR as a novel approach for the identification of prostate anomalies. *Cancer Gene. Ther.* **2016**, *23*, 365–369. [CrossRef] [PubMed]
405. Ray, S.; Ghosh Ray, S.; Mandal, S. Development of bicalutamide-loaded PLGA nanoparticles: Preparation, characterization and in vitro evaluation for the treatment of prostate cancer. *Artif. Cells Nanomed. Biotechnol.* **2016**, 1–11. [CrossRef] [PubMed]
406. Huo, Y.; Singh, P.; Kim, Y.J.; Soshnikova, V.; Kang, J.; Markus, J.; Ahn, S.; Castro-Aceituno, V.; Mathiyalagan, R.; Chokkalingam, M.; et al. Biological synthesis of gold and silver chloride nanoparticles by glycyrrhiza uralensis and in vitro applications. *Artif. Cells Nanomed. Biotechnol.* **2017**, 1–13. [CrossRef] [PubMed]
407. Mokhtari, M.J.; Koohpeima, F.; Mohammadi, H. A comparison inhibitory effects of cisplatin and MNPS-PEG-cisplatin on the adhesion capacity of bone metastatic breast cancer. *Chem. Biol. Drug Des.* **2017**. [CrossRef] [PubMed]
408. Bhuvaneswari, R.; Xavier, R.J.; Arumugam, M. Facile synthesis of multifunctional silver nanoparticles using mangrove plant *Excoecaria agallocha* L. For its antibacterial, antioxidant and cytotoxic effects. *J. Parasit. Dis.* **2017**, *41*, 180–187. [CrossRef] [PubMed]
409. Lacroix, M. *Targeted Therapies in Cancer*; Nova Sciences Publishers: Hauppauge, NY, USA, 2014.
410. Abramson, R. Overview of Targeted Therapies for Cancer. Available online: https://www.mycancergenome.org/content/molecular-medicine/overview-of-targeted-therapies-for-cancer/ (accessed on 13 June 2016).
411. Collignon, J.; Lousberg, L.; Schroeder, H.; Jerusalem, G. Triple-negative breast cancer: Treatment challenges and solutions. *Breast Cancer (Dove Med Press)* **2016**, *8*, 93–107. [PubMed]
412. Kontani, K.; Hashimoto, S.I.; Murazawa, C.; Norimura, S.; Tanaka, H.; Ohtani, M.; Fujiwara-Honjo, N.; Date, M.; Teramoto, K.; Houchi, H.; et al. Indication of metronomic chemotherapy for metastatic breast cancer: Clinical outcomes and responsive subtypes. *Mol. Clin. Oncol.* **2016**, *4*, 947–953. [CrossRef] [PubMed]
413. Bateman, J.C.; Carlton, H.N. The role of chemotherapy in the treatment of breast cancer. *Surgery* **1960**, *47*, 895–907. [PubMed]

414. Nakano, M.; Shoji, S.; Higure, T.; Kawakami, M.; Tomonaga, T.; Terachi, T.; Uchida, T. Low-dose docetaxel, estramustine and prednisolone combination chemotherapy for castration-resistant prostate cancer. *Mol. Clin. Oncol.* **2016**, *4*, 942–946. [CrossRef] [PubMed]
415. Herbst, W.P. The present picture in chemotherapy in prostatic carcinoma. *J. Urol.* **1947**, *57*, 296–299. [PubMed]
416. Albumin-bound paclitaxel (abraxane) for advanced breast cancer. *Med. Lett. Drugs Ther.* **2005**, *47*, 39–40.
417. Barenholz, Y. Doxil—The first FDA-approved nano-drug: Lessons learned. *J. Control. Release* **2012**, *160*, 117–134. [CrossRef] [PubMed]
418. Chan, S.; Davidson, N.; Juozaityte, E.; Erdkamp, F.; Pluzanska, A.; Azarnia, N.; Lee, L.W. Phase III trial of liposomal doxorubicin and cyclophosphamide compared with epirubicin and cyclophosphamide as first-line therapy for metastatic breast cancer. *Ann. Oncol.* **2004**, *15*, 1527–1534. [CrossRef] [PubMed]
419. Lee, K.S.; Chung, H.C.; Im, S.A.; Park, Y.H.; Kim, C.S.; Kim, S.B.; Rha, S.Y.; Lee, M.Y.; Ro, J. Multicenter phase II trial of genexol-pm, a cremophor-free, polymeric micelle formulation of paclitaxel, in patients with metastatic breast cancer. *Breast Cancer Res. Treat.* **2008**, *108*, 241–250. [CrossRef] [PubMed]
420. Pillai, G. Nanomedicines for cancer therapy: An update of FDA approved and those under various stages of development. *SOJ Pharm. Pharm. Sci.* **2014**, *1*, 13.
421. Wang, M.; Thanou, M. Targeting nanoparticles to cancer. *Pharmacol. Res.* **2010**, *62*, 90–99. [CrossRef] [PubMed]
422. Zhang, C.; Zhao, X.; Guo, S.; Lin, T.; Guo, H. Highly effective photothermal chemotherapy with pH-responsive polymer-coated drug-loaded melanin-like nanoparticles. *Int. J. Nanomed.* **2017**, *12*, 1827–1840. [CrossRef] [PubMed]
423. Bakht, M.K.; Oh, S.W.; Hwang, D.W.; Lee, Y.S.; Youn, H.; Porter, L.A.; Cheon, G.J.; Kwak, C.; Lee, D.S.; Kang, K.W. The potential roles of radionanomedicine and radioexosomic in prostate cancer research and treatment. *Curr. Pharm. Des.* **2017**. [CrossRef] [PubMed]
424. Lopes, A.M.; Chen, K.Y.; Kamei, D.T. A transferrin variant as the targeting ligand for polymeric nanoparticles incorporated in 3-D PLGA porous scaffolds. *Mater. Sci. Eng. C Mater. Biol. Appl.* **2017**, *73*, 373–380. [CrossRef] [PubMed]
425. Belz, J.; Castilla-Ojo, N.; Sridhar, S.; Kumar, R. Radiosensitizing silica nanoparticles encapsulating docetaxel for treatment of prostate cancer. *Methods Mol. Biol.* **2017**, *1530*, 403–409. [PubMed]
426. Yan, J.; Wang, Y.; Jia, Y.; Liu, S.; Tian, C.; Pan, W.; Liu, X.; Wang, H. Co-delivery of docetaxel and curcumin prodrug via dual-targeted nanoparticles with synergistic antitumor activity against prostate cancer. *Biomed. Pharmacother.* **2017**, *88*, 374–383. [CrossRef] [PubMed]
427. Huang, W.Y.; Lin, J.N.; Hsieh, J.T.; Chou, S.C.; Lai, C.H.; Yun, E.J.; Lo, U.G.; Pong, R.C.; Lin, J.H.; Lin, Y.H. Nanoparticle targeting CD44-positive cancer cells for site-specific drug delivery in prostate cancer therapy. *ACS Appl. Mater. Interfaces* **2016**, *8*, 30722–30734. [CrossRef] [PubMed]
428. Bharali, D.J.; Sudha, T.; Cui, H.; Mian, B.M.; Mousa, S.A. Anti-CD24 nano-targeted delivery of docetaxel for the treatment of prostate cancer. *Nanomedicine* **2017**, *13*, 263–273. [CrossRef] [PubMed]
429. Qu, N.; Lee, R.J.; Sun, Y.; Cai, G.; Wang, J.; Wang, M.; Lu, J.; Meng, Q.; Teng, L.; Wang, D.; et al. Cabazitaxel-loaded human serum albumin nanoparticles as a therapeutic agent against prostate cancer. *Int. J. Nanomed.* **2016**, *11*, 3451–3459.
430. Pirayesh Islamian, J.; Hatamian, M.; Aval, N.A.; Rashidi, M.R.; Mesbahi, A.; Mohammadzadeh, M.; Asghari Jafarabadi, M. Targeted superparamagnetic nanoparticles coated with 2-deoxy-d-gloucose and doxorubicin more sensitize breast cancer cells to ionizing radiation. *Breast* **2017**, *33*, 97–103. [CrossRef] [PubMed]
431. Li, J.; Zhang, J.; Wang, Y.; Liang, X.; Wusiman, Z.; Yin, Y.; Shen, Q. Synergistic inhibition of migration and invasion of breast cancer cells by dual docetaxel/quercetin-loaded nanoparticles via Akt/MMP-9 pathway. *Int. J. Pharm.* **2017**, *523*, 300–309. [CrossRef] [PubMed]
432. Stratton, M.R. Exploring the genomes of cancer cells: Progress and promise. *Science* **2011**, *331*, 1553–1558. [CrossRef] [PubMed]
433. Merz, B. Gene therapy may have future role in cancer treatment. *JAMA* **1987**, *257*, 150–151. [CrossRef] [PubMed]
434. Kozielski, K.L.; Rui, Y.; Green, J.J. Non-viral nucleic acid containing nanoparticles as cancer therapeutics. *Expert. Opin. Drug Deliv.* **2016**, *13*, 1475–1487. [CrossRef] [PubMed]

435. Gogtay, N.J.; Sridharan, K. Therapeutic nucleic acids: Current clinical status. *Br. J. Clin. Pharmacol.* **2016**, *82*, 659–672.
436. Yu, Y.; Yao, Y.; Yan, H.; Wang, R.; Zhang, Z.; Sun, X.; Zhao, L.; Ao, X.; Xie, Z.; Wu, Q. A tumor-specific microRNA recognition system facilitates the accurate targeting to tumor cells by magnetic nanoparticles. *Mol. Ther. Nucleic Acids* **2016**, *5*, e318. [CrossRef] [PubMed]
437. Rejeeth, C.; Vivek, R. Comparison of two silica based nonviral gene therapy vectors for breast carcinoma: Evaluation of the p53 delivery system in balb/C mice. *Artif. Cells Nanomed. Biotechnol.* **2017**, *45*, 489–494. [CrossRef] [PubMed]
438. Rejeeth, C.; Salem, A. Novel luminescent silica nanoparticles (LSN): p53 Gene delivery system in breast cancer in vitro and in vivo. *J. Pharm. Pharmacol.* **2016**, *68*, 305–315. [CrossRef] [PubMed]
439. Li, T.; Shen, X.; Chen, Y.; Zhang, C.; Yan, J.; Yang, H.; Wu, C.; Zeng, H.; Liu, Y. Polyetherimide-grafted Fe_3O_4@SiO_2 nanoparticles as theranostic agents for simultaneous VEGF siRNA delivery and magnetic resonance cell imaging. *Int. J. Nanomed.* **2015**, *10*, 4279–4291. [CrossRef] [PubMed]
440. Zhou, H.; Wei, J.; Dai, Q.; Wang, L.; Luo, J.; Cheang, T.; Wang, S. $CaCo_3$/CaIP6 composite nanoparticles effectively deliver AKT1 small interfering rna to inhibit human breast cancer growth. *Int. J. Nanomed.* **2015**, *10*, 4255–4266.
441. Nourbakhsh, M.; Jaafari, M.R.; Lage, H.; Abnous, K.; Mosaffa, F.; Badiee, A.; Behravan, J. Nanolipoparticles-mediated MDR1 siRNA delivery reduces doxorubicin resistance in breast cancer cells and silences MDR1 expression in xenograft model of human breast cancer. *Iran J. Basic Med. Sci.* **2015**, *18*, 385–392. [PubMed]
442. Su, S.; Tian, Y.; Li, Y.; Ding, Y.; Ji, T.; Wu, M.; Wu, Y.; Nie, G. "Triple-punch" strategy for triple negative breast cancer therapy with minimized drug dosage and improved antitumor efficacy. *ACS Nano* **2015**, *9*, 1367–1378. [CrossRef] [PubMed]
443. Dong, D.; Gao, W.; Liu, Y.; Qi, X.R. Therapeutic potential of targeted multifunctional nanocomplex co-delivery of siRNA and low-dose doxorubicin in breast cancer. *Cancer Lett.* **2015**, *359*, 178–186. [CrossRef] [PubMed]
444. Huang, Y.P.; Hung, C.M.; Hsu, Y.C.; Zhong, C.Y.; Wang, W.R.; Chang, C.C.; Lee, M.J. Suppression of breast cancer cell migration by small interfering RNA delivered by polyethylenimine-functionalized graphene oxide. *Nanoscale Res. Lett.* **2016**, *11*, 247. [CrossRef] [PubMed]
445. Arami, S.; Rashidi, M.R.; Mahdavi, M.; Fathi, M.; Entezami, A.A. Synthesis and characterization of Fe_3O_4-PEG-LAC-chitosan-PEI nanoparticle as a survivin siRNA delivery system. *Hum. Exp. Toxicol.* **2017**, *36*, 227–237. [CrossRef] [PubMed]
446. Unsoy, G.; Gunduz, U. Targeted silencing of survivin in cancer cells by siRNA loaded chitosan magnetic nanoparticles. *Expert Rev. Anticancer Ther.* **2016**, *16*, 789–797. [CrossRef] [PubMed]
447. Park, D.H.; Cho, J.; Kwon, O.J.; Yun, C.O.; Choy, J.H. Biodegradable inorganic nanovector: Passive versus active tumor targeting in siRNA transportation. *Angew. Chem. Int. Ed. Engl.* **2016**, *55*, 4582–4586. [CrossRef] [PubMed]
448. McBride, J.W.; Massey, A.S.; McCaffrey, J.; McCrudden, C.M.; Coulter, J.A.; Dunne, N.J.; Robson, T.; McCarthy, H.O. Development of TMTP-1 targeted designer biopolymers for gene delivery to prostate cancer. *Int. J. Pharm.* **2016**, *500*, 144–153. [CrossRef] [PubMed]
449. Xing, Z.; Gao, S.; Duan, Y.; Han, H.; Li, L.; Yang, Y.; Li, Q. Delivery of dnazyme targeting aurora kinase a to inhibit the proliferation and migration of human prostate cancer. *Int. J. Nanomed.* **2015**, *10*, 5715–5727.
450. Fitzgerald, K.A.; Guo, J.; Tierney, E.G.; Curtin, C.M.; Malhotra, M.; Darcy, R.; O'Brien, F.J.; O'Driscoll, C.M. The use of collagen-based scaffolds to simulate prostate cancer bone metastases with potential for evaluating delivery of nanoparticulate gene therapeutics. *Biomaterials* **2015**, *66*, 53–66. [CrossRef] [PubMed]
451. Zhang, T.; Xue, X.; He, D.; Hsieh, J.T. A prostate cancer-targeted polyarginine-disulfide linked pei nanocarrier for delivery of microrna. *Cancer Lett.* **2015**, *365*, 156–165. [CrossRef] [PubMed]
452. Huang, R.Y.; Chiang, P.H.; Hsiao, W.C.; Chuang, C.C.; Chang, C.W. Redox-sensitive polymer/SPIO nanocomplexes for efficient magnetofection and mr imaging of human cancer cells. *Langmuir* **2015**, *31*, 6523–6531. [CrossRef] [PubMed]
453. Ceresa, C.; Nicolini, G.; Semperboni, S.; Requardt, H.; Le Duc, G.; Santini, C.; Pellei, M.; Bentivegna, A.; Dalpra, L.; Cavaletti, G.; et al. Synchrotron-based photon activation therapy effect on cisplatin pre-treated human glioma stem cells. *Anticancer Res.* **2014**, *34*, 5351–5355. [PubMed]

454. Bakhshabadi, M.; Ghorbani, M.; Meigooni, A.S. Photon activation therapy: A Monte Carlo study on dose enhancement by various sources and activation media. *Australas. Phys. Eng. Sci. Med.* **2013**, *36*, 301–311. [CrossRef] [PubMed]
455. Ceresa, C.; Nicolini, G.; Requardt, H.; Le Duc, G.; Cavaletti, G.; Bravin, A. The effect of photon activation therapy on cisplatin pre-treated human tumour cell lines: Comparison with conventional X-ray irradiation. *J. Biol. Regul. Homeost. Agents* **2013**, *27*, 477–485. [PubMed]
456. Ceberg, C.; Jonsson, B.A.; Prezado, Y.; Pommer, T.; Nittby, H.; Englund, E.; Grafstrom, G.; Edvardsson, A.; Stenvall, A.; Stromblad, S.; et al. Photon activation therapy of RG2 glioma carrying fischer rats using stable thallium and monochromatic synchrotron radiation. *Phys. Med. Biol.* **2012**, *57*, 8377–8391. [CrossRef] [PubMed]
457. Laster, B.H.; Dixon, D.W.; Novick, S.; Feldman, J.P.; Seror, V.; Goldbart, Z.I.; Kalef-Ezra, J.A. Photon activation therapy and brachytherapy. *Brachytherapy* **2009**, *8*, 324–330. [CrossRef] [PubMed]
458. Suortti, P.; Thomlinson, W. Medical applications of synchrotron radiation. *Phys Med Biol* **2003**, *48*, R1–R35. [CrossRef] [PubMed]
459. Laster, B.H.; Thomlinson, W.C.; Fairchild, R.G. Photon activation of iododeoxyuridine: Biological efficacy of auger electrons. *Radiat. Res.* **1993**, *133*, 219–224. [CrossRef] [PubMed]
460. Miller, R.W.; DeGraff, W.; Kinsella, T.J.; Mitchell, J.B. Evaluation of incorporated iododeoxyuridine cellular radiosensitization by photon activation therapy. *Int. J. Radiat. Oncol. Biol. Phys.* **1987**, *13*, 1193–1197. [CrossRef]
461. Fairchild, R.G.; Bond, V.P. Photon activation therapy. *Strahlentherapie* **1984**, *160*, 758–763. [PubMed]
462. Choi, G.H.; Seo, S.J.; Kim, K.H.; Kim, H.T.; Park, S.H.; Lim, J.H.; Kim, J.K. Photon activated therapy (PAT) using monochromatic synchrotron X-rays and iron oxide nanoparticles in a mouse tumor model: Feasibility study of PAT for the treatment of superficial malignancy. *Radiat. Oncol.* **2012**, *7*, 184. [CrossRef] [PubMed]
463. Dolmans, D.E.; Fukumura, D.; Jain, R.K. Photodynamic therapy for cancer. *Nat. Rev. Cancer* **2003**, *3*, 380–387. [CrossRef] [PubMed]
464. Chen, J.; Keltner, L.; Christophersen, J.; Zheng, F.; Krouse, M.; Singhal, A.; Wang, S.S. New technology for deep light distribution in tissue for phototherapy. *Cancer J.* **2002**, *8*, 154–163. [CrossRef] [PubMed]
465. Sneider, A.; VanDyke, D.; Paliwal, S.; Rai, P. Remotely triggered nano-theranostics for cancer applications. *Nanotheranostics (Syd.)* **2017**, *1*, 1–22. [CrossRef] [PubMed]
466. Shen, Y.; Shuhendler, A.J.; Ye, D.; Xu, J.J.; Chen, H.Y. Two-photon excitation nanoparticles for photodynamic therapy. *Chem. Soc. Rev.* **2016**, *45*, 6725–6741. [CrossRef] [PubMed]
467. Chen, R.; Zhang, J.; Chelora, J.; Xiong, Y.; Kershaw, S.V.; Li, K.F.; Lo, P.K.; Cheah, K.W.; Rogach, A.L.; Zapien, J.A.; et al. Ruthenium(ii) complex incorporated uio-67 metal-organic framework nanoparticles for enhanced two-photon fluorescence imaging and photodynamic cancer therapy. *ACS Appl. Mater. Interfaces* **2017**, *9*, 5699–5708. [CrossRef] [PubMed]
468. Shen, X.; Li, S.; Li, L.; Yao, S.Q.; Xu, Q.H. Highly efficient, conjugated-polymer-based nano-photosensitizers for selectively targeted two-photon photodynamic therapy and imaging of cancer cells. *Chemistry* **2015**, *21*, 2214–2221. [CrossRef] [PubMed]
469. Secret, E.; Maynadier, M.; Gallud, A.; Chaix, A.; Bouffard, E.; Gary-Bobo, M.; Marcotte, N.; Mongin, O.; El Cheikh, K.; Hugues, V.; et al. Two-photon excitation of porphyrin-functionalized porous silicon nanoparticles for photodynamic therapy. *Adv. Mater.* **2014**, *26*, 7643–7648. [CrossRef] [PubMed]
470. Zhao, T.; Yu, K.; Li, L.; Zhang, T.; Guan, Z.; Gao, N.; Yuan, P.; Li, S.; Yao, S.Q.; Xu, Q.H.; et al. Gold nanorod enhanced two-photon excitation fluorescence of photosensitizers for two-photon imaging and photodynamic therapy. *ACS Appl. Mater. Interfaces* **2014**, *6*, 2700–2708. [CrossRef] [PubMed]
471. Gary-Bobo, M.; Mir, Y.; Rouxel, C.; Brevet, D.; Basile, I.; Maynadier, M.; Vaillant, O.; Mongin, O.; Blanchard-Desce, M.; Morere, A.; et al. Mannose-functionalized mesoporous silica nanoparticles for efficient two-photon photodynamic therapy of solid tumors. *Angew. Chem. Int. Ed. Engl.* **2011**, *50*, 11425–11429. [CrossRef] [PubMed]
472. Swartling, J.; Axelsson, J.; Ahlgren, G.; Kalkner, K.M.; Nilsson, S.; Svanberg, S.; Svanberg, K.; Andersson-Engels, S. System for interstitial photodynamic therapy with online dosimetry: First clinical experiences of prostate cancer. *J. Biomed. Opt.* **2010**, *15*, 058003. [CrossRef] [PubMed]

473. Swartling, J.; Hoglund, O.V.; Hansson, K.; Sodersten, F.; Axelsson, J.; Lagerstedt, A.S. Online dosimetry for temoporfin-mediated interstitial photodynamic therapy using the canine prostate as model. *J. Biomed. Opt.* **2016**, *21*, 28002. [CrossRef] [PubMed]
474. Chen, Y.; Chatterjee, S.; Lisok, A.; Minn, I.; Pullambhatla, M.; Wharram, B.; Wang, Y.; Jin, J.; Bhujwalla, Z.M.; Nimmagadda, S.; et al. A psma-targeted theranostic agent for photodynamic therapy. *J. Photochem. Photobiol. B* **2017**, *167*, 111–116. [CrossRef] [PubMed]
475. Wang, X.; Tsui, B.; Ramamurthy, G.; Zhang, P.; Meyers, J.; Kenney, M.E.; Kiechle, J.; Ponsky, L.; Basilion, J.P. Theranostic agents for photodynamic therapy of prostate cancer by targeting prostate-specific membrane antigen. *Mol. Cancer Ther.* **2016**, *15*, 1834–1844. [CrossRef] [PubMed]
476. Lin, T.Y.; Guo, W.; Long, Q.; Ma, A.; Liu, Q.; Zhang, H.; Huang, Y.; Chandrasekaran, S.; Pan, C.; Lam, K.S.; et al. Hsp90 inhibitor encapsulated photo-theranostic nanoparticles for synergistic combination cancer therapy. *Theranostics* **2016**, *6*, 1324–1335. [CrossRef] [PubMed]
477. Vaillant, O.; El Cheikh, K.; Warther, D.; Brevet, D.; Maynadier, M.; Bouffard, E.; Salgues, F.; Jeanjean, A.; Puche, P.; Mazerolles, C.; et al. Mannose-6-phosphate receptor: A target for theranostics of prostate cancer. *Angew. Chem. Int. Ed. Engl.* **2015**, *54*, 5952–5956. [CrossRef] [PubMed]
478. Choi, J.; Kim, H.; Choi, Y. Theranostic nanoparticles for enzyme-activatable fluorescence imaging and photodynamic/chemo dual therapy of triple-negative breast cancer. *Quant. Imaging Med. Surg.* **2015**, *5*, 656–664. [PubMed]
479. Wang, X.; Hu, J.; Wang, P.; Zhang, S.; Liu, Y.; Xiong, W.; Liu, Q. Analysis of the in vivo and in vitro effects of photodynamic therapy on breast cancer by using a sensitizer, sinoporphyrin sodium. *Theranostics* **2015**, *5*, 772–786. [CrossRef] [PubMed]
480. Kue, C.S.; Kamkaew, A.; Lee, H.B.; Chung, L.Y.; Kiew, L.V.; Burgess, K. Targeted PDT agent eradicates trkc expressing tumors via photodynamic therapy (PDT). *Mol. Pharm.* **2015**, *12*, 212–222. [CrossRef] [PubMed]
481. El-Sayed, I.H. Nanotechnology in head and neck cancer: The race is on. *Curr Oncol Rep* **2010**, *12*, 121–128. [CrossRef] [PubMed]
482. Huang, X.; El-Sayed, M.A. Plasmonic photo-thermal therapy (PPTT). *Alex. J. Med.* **2011**, *47*, 1–9. [CrossRef]
483. Huang, X.; Jain, P.K.; El-Sayed, I.H.; El-Sayed, M.A. Plasmonic photothermal therapy (PPTT) using gold nanoparticles. *Lasers Med. Sci.* **2008**, *23*, 217–228. [CrossRef] [PubMed]
484. Turcheniuk, K.; Dumych, T.; Bilyy, R.; Turcheniuk, V.; Bouckaert, J.; Vovk, V.; Chopyak, V.; Zaitsev, V.; Mariot, P.; Prevarskaya, N.; et al. Plasmonic photothermal cancer therapy with gold nanorods/reduced graphene oxide core/shell nanocomposites. *RSC Adv.* **2016**, *6*, 1600–1610. [CrossRef]
485. Peng, J.; Dong, M.; Ran, B.; Li, W.; Hao, Y.; Yang, Q.; Tan, L.; Shi, K.; Qian, Z. "One-for-all" type, biodegradable prussian blue/manganese dioxide hybrid nanocrystal for tri-modal imaging guided photothermal therapy and oxygen regulation of breast cancer. *ACS Appl. Mater. Interfaces* **2017**, *9*, 13875–13886. [CrossRef] [PubMed]
486. Cantu, T.; Walsh, K.; Pattani, V.P.; Moy, A.J.; Tunnell, J.W.; Irvin, J.A.; Betancourt, T. Conductive polymer-based nanoparticles for laser-mediated photothermal ablation of cancer: Synthesis, characterization, and in vitro evaluation. *Int. J. Nanomed.* **2017**, *12*, 615–632. [CrossRef] [PubMed]
487. Haberkorn, U.; Eder, M.; Kopka, K.; Babich, J.W.; Eisenhut, M. New strategies in prostate cancer: Prostate-specific membrane antigen (PSMA) ligands for diagnosis and therapy. *Clin. Cancer Res.* **2016**, *22*, 9–15. [CrossRef] [PubMed]
488. Bouchelouche, K.; Tagawa, S.T.; Goldsmith, S.J.; Turkbey, B.; Capala, J.; Choyke, P. PET/CT imaging and radioimmunotherapy of prostate cancer. *Semin. Nucl. Med.* **2011**, *41*, 29–44. [CrossRef] [PubMed]
489. Awada, G.; Gombos, A.; Aftimos, P.; Awada, A. Emerging drugs targeting human epidermal growth factor receptor 2 (Her2) in the treatment of breast cancer. *Expert Opin. Emerg. Drugs* **2016**, *21*, 91–101. [CrossRef] [PubMed]
490. Lluch, A.; Eroles, P.; Perez-Fidalgo, J.A. Emerging EGFR antagonists for breast cancer. *Expert Opin. Emerg. Drugs* **2014**, *19*, 165–181. [CrossRef] [PubMed]
491. Doddamane, I.; Butler, R.; Jhaveri, A.; Chung, G.G.; Cheng, D. Where does radioimmunotherapy fit in the management of breast cancer? *Immunotherapy* **2013**, *5*, 895–904. [CrossRef] [PubMed]
492. Evans-Axelsson, S.; Timmermand, O.V.; Bjartell, A.; Strand, S.E.; Elgqvist, J. Radioimmunotherapy for prostate cancer—Current status and future possibilities. *Semin. Nucl. Med.* **2016**, *46*, 165–179. [CrossRef] [PubMed]

493. Zolata, H.; Afarideh, H.; Davani, F.A. Triple therapy of HER2+ cancer using radiolabeled multifunctional iron oxide nanoparticles and alternating magnetic field. *Cancer Biother. Radiopharm.* **2016**, *31*, 324–329. [CrossRef] [PubMed]
494. Wang, X.; Sun, Q.; Shen, S.; Xu, Y.; Huang, L. Nanotrastuzumab in combination with radioimmunotherapy: Can it be a viable treatment option for patients with HER2-positive breast cancer with brain metastasis? *Med. Hypotheses* **2016**, *88*, 79–81. [CrossRef] [PubMed]
495. Parakh, S.; Parslow, A.C.; Gan, H.K.; Scott, A.M. Antibody-mediated delivery of therapeutics for cancer therapy. *Expert Opin. Drug Deliv.* **2016**, *13*, 401–419. [CrossRef] [PubMed]
496. Yang, Q.; Parker, C.L.; McCallen, J.D.; Lai, S.K. Addressing challenges of heterogeneous tumor treatment through bispecific protein-mediated pretargeted drug delivery. *J. Control. Release* **2015**, *220*, 715–726. [CrossRef] [PubMed]
497. Yook, S.; Cai, Z.; Lu, Y.; Winnik, M.A.; Pignol, J.P.; Reilly, R.M. Radiation nanomedicine for egfr-positive breast cancer: Panitumumab-modified gold nanoparticles complexed to the beta-particle-emitter, ^{177}Lu. *Mol. Pharm.* **2015**, *12*, 3963–3972. [CrossRef] [PubMed]
498. Rasaneh, S.; Rajabi, H.; Johari Daha, F. Activity estimation in radioimmunotherapy using magnetic nanoparticles. *Chin. J. Cancer Res.* **2015**, *27*, 203–208. [PubMed]
499. Bushman, J.; Vaughan, A.; Sheihet, L.; Zhang, Z.; Costache, M.; Kohn, J. Functionalized nanospheres for targeted delivery of paclitaxel. *J. Control. Release* **2013**, *171*, 315–321. [CrossRef] [PubMed]
500. D'Huyvetter, M.; Aerts, A.; Xavier, C.; Vaneycken, I.; Devoogdt, N.; Gijs, M.; Impens, N.; Baatout, S.; Ponsard, B.; Muyldermans, S.; et al. Development of ^{177}Lu-nanobodies for radioimmunotherapy of her2-positive breast cancer: Evaluation of different bifunctional chelators. *Contrast Media Mol. Imaging* **2012**, *7*, 254–264. [CrossRef] [PubMed]
501. Natarajan, A.; Xiong, C.Y.; Gruettner, C.; DeNardo, G.L.; DeNardo, S.J. Development of multivalent radioimmunonanoparticles for cancer imaging and therapy. *Cancer Biother. Radiopharm.* **2008**, *23*, 82–91. [CrossRef] [PubMed]
502. Nedunchezhian, K.; Aswath, N.; Thiruppathy, M.; Thirugnanamurthy, S. Boron neutron capture therapy—A literature review. *J. Clin. Diagn. Res.* **2016**, *10*, ZE01–ZE04. [CrossRef] [PubMed]
503. Mirzaei, H.R.; Sahebkar, A.; Salehi, R.; Nahand, J.S.; Karimi, E.; Jaafari, M.R.; Mirzaei, H. Boron neutron capture therapy: Moving toward targeted cancer therapy. *J. Cancer Res. Ther.* **2016**, *12*, 520–525. [CrossRef] [PubMed]
504. Luderer, M.J.; de la Puente, P.; Azab, A.K. Advancements in tumor targeting strategies for boron neutron capture therapy. *Pharm. Res.* **2015**, *32*, 2824–2836. [CrossRef] [PubMed]
505. Alberti, D.; Protti, N.; Franck, M.; Stefania, R.; Bortolussi, S.; Altieri, S.; Deagostino, A.; Aime, S.; Geninatti Crich, S. Theranostic nanoparticles loaded with imaging probes and rubrocurcumin for combined cancer therapy by folate receptor targeting. *Chem. Med. Chem.* **2017**, *12*, 502–509. [CrossRef] [PubMed]
506. Peters, T.; Grunewald, C.; Blaickner, M.; Ziegner, M.; Schutz, C.; Iffland, D.; Hampel, G.; Nawroth, T.; Langguth, P. Cellular uptake and in vitro antitumor efficacy of composite liposomes for neutron capture therapy. *Radiat. Oncol.* **2015**, *10*, 52. [CrossRef] [PubMed]
507. Heber, E.M.; Hawthorne, M.F.; Kueffer, P.J.; Garabalino, M.A.; Thorp, S.I.; Pozzi, E.C.; Monti Hughes, A.; Maitz, C.A.; Jalisatgi, S.S.; Nigg, D.W.; et al. Therapeutic efficacy of boron neutron capture therapy mediated by boron-rich liposomes for oral cancer in the hamster cheek pouch model. *Proc. Natl. Acad. Sci. USA* **2014**, *111*, 16077–16081. [CrossRef] [PubMed]
508. Tachikawa, S.; Miyoshi, T.; Koganei, H.; El-Zaria, M.E.; Vinas, C.; Suzuki, M.; Ono, K.; Nakamura, H. Spermidinium closo-dodecaborate-encapsulating liposomes as efficient boron delivery vehicles for neutron capture therapy. *Chem. Commun. (Camb.)* **2014**, *50*, 12325–12328. [CrossRef] [PubMed]
509. Kobayashi, H.; Kawamoto, S.; Bernardo, M.; Brechbiel, M.W.; Knopp, M.V.; Choyke, P.L. Delivery of gadolinium-labeled nanoparticles to the sentinel lymph node: Comparison of the sentinel node visualization and estimations of intra-nodal gadolinium concentration by the magnetic resonance imaging. *J. Control. Release* **2006**, *111*, 343–351. [CrossRef] [PubMed]
510. Oyewumi, M.O.; Liu, S.; Moscow, J.A.; Mumper, R.J. Specific association of thiamine-coated gadolinium nanoparticles with human breast cancer cells expressing thiamine transporters. *Bioconjug. Chem.* **2003**, *14*, 404–411. [CrossRef] [PubMed]

511. Fortin, J.P.; Gazeau, F.; Wilhelm, C. Intracellular heating of living cells through neel relaxation of magnetic nanoparticles. *Eur. Biophys. J.* **2008**, *37*, 223–228. [CrossRef] [PubMed]
512. Han, Y.; Lei, S.L.; Lu, J.H.; He, Y.; Chen, Z.W.; Ren, L.; Zhou, X. Potential use of sers-assisted theranostic strategy based on Fe_3O_4/Au cluster/shell nanocomposites for bio-detection, MRI, and magnetic hyperthermia. *Mater. Sci. Eng. C Mater. Biol. Appl.* **2016**, *64*, 199–207. [CrossRef] [PubMed]
513. Stocke, N.A.; Sethi, P.; Jyoti, A.; Chan, R.; Arnold, S.M.; Hilt, J.Z.; Upreti, M. Toxicity evaluation of magnetic hyperthermia induced by remote actuation of magnetic nanoparticles in 3d micrometastasic tumor tissue analogs for triple negative breast cancer. *Biomaterials* **2017**, *120*, 115–125. [CrossRef] [PubMed]
514. Oh, Y.; Moorthy, M.S.; Manivasagan, P.; Bharathiraja, S.; Oh, J. Magnetic hyperthermia and pH-responsive effective drug delivery to the sub-cellular level of human breast cancer cells by modified $coFe_2O_4$ nanoparticles. *Biochimie* **2017**, *133*, 7–19. [CrossRef] [PubMed]
515. Yao, X.; Niu, X.; Ma, K.; Huang, P.; Grothe, J.; Kaskel, S.; Zhu, Y. Graphene quantum dots-capped magnetic mesoporous silica nanoparticles as a multifunctional platform for controlled drug delivery, magnetic hyperthermia, and photothermal therapy. *Small* **2017**, *13*, 1602225. [CrossRef] [PubMed]
516. Kossatz, S.; Grandke, J.; Couleaud, P.; Latorre, A.; Aires, A.; Crosbie-Staunton, K.; Ludwig, R.; Dahring, H.; Ettelt, V.; Lazaro-Carrillo, A.; et al. Efficient treatment of breast cancer xenografts with multifunctionalized iron oxide nanoparticles combining magnetic hyperthermia and anti-cancer drug delivery. *Breast Cancer Res.* **2015**, *17*, 66. [CrossRef] [PubMed]
517. Ferlay, J.; Soerjomataram, I.; Ervik, M.; Dikshit, R.; Eser, S.; Mathers, C.; Rebelo, M.; Parkin, D.; Forman, D.; Bray, F. *Globocan 2012 v1.0, Cancer Incidence and Mortality Worldwide: Iarc Cancerbase No. 11 [Internet]*; International Agency for Research on Cancer: Lyon, France, 2013.
518. Siegel, R.L.; Miller, K.D.; Jemal, A. Cancer statistics, 2016. *CA Cancer J. Clin.* **2016**, *66*, 7–30. [CrossRef] [PubMed]
519. Hoffman, R.M.; Couper, M.P.; Zikmund-Fisher, B.J.; Levin, C.A.; McNaughton-Collins, M.; Helitzer, D.L.; VanHoewyk, J.; Barry, M.J. Prostate cancer screening decisions: Results from the national survey of medical decisions (decisions study). *Arch. Intern. Med.* **2009**, *169*, 1611–1618. [CrossRef] [PubMed]
520. Bill-Axelson, A.; Bratt, O. Words of wisdom. Re: Screening and prostate cancer mortality: Results of the european randomised study of screening for prostate cancer (ERSPC) at 13 years of follow-up. *Eur. Urol.* **2015**, *67*, 175. [CrossRef] [PubMed]
521. Heidenreich, A.; Bastian, P.J.; Bellmunt, J.; Bolla, M.; Joniau, S.; van der Kwast, T.; Mason, M.; Matveev, V.; Wiegel, T.; Zattoni, F.; et al. Eau guidelines on prostate cancer. Part 1: Screening, diagnosis, and local treatment with curative intent-update 2013. *Eur. Urol.* **2014**, *65*, 124–137. [CrossRef] [PubMed]
522. Kim, S.P.; Karnes, R.J.; Nguyen, P.L.; Ziegenfuss, J.Y.; Thompson, R.H.; Han, L.C.; Shah, N.D.; Smaldone, M.C.; Gross, C.P.; Frank, I.; et al. A national survey of radiation oncologists and urologists on recommendations of prostate-specific antigen screening for prostate cancer. *BJU Int.* **2014**, *113*, E106–E111. [CrossRef] [PubMed]
523. Loeb, S. Prostate cancer screening: Highlights from the 29th european association of urology congress Stockholm, Sweden, april 11–15, 2014. *Rev. Urol.* **2014**, *16*, 90–91. [PubMed]
524. Schroder, F.H. Screening for prostate cancer: Current status of ERSPC and screening-related issues. *Recent Results Cancer Res.* **2014**, *202*, 47–51. [PubMed]
525. Schroder, F.H.; Hugosson, J.; Roobol, M.J.; Tammela, T.L.; Zappa, M.; Nelen, V.; Kwiatkowski, M.; Lujan, M.; Maattanen, L.; Lilja, H.; et al. Screening and prostate cancer mortality: Results of the european randomised study of screening for prostate cancer (ERSPC) at 13 years of follow-up. *Lancet* **2014**, *384*, 2027–2035. [CrossRef]
526. Schroder, F.H. Erspc, plco studies and critique of cochrane review 2013. *Recent Results Cancer Res.* **2014**, *202*, 59–63. [PubMed]
527. Vallabhajosula, S.; Nikolopoulou, A.; Jhanwar, Y.S.; Kaur, G.; Tagawa, S.T.; Nanus, D.M.; Bander, N.H.; Goldsmith, S.J. Radioimmunotherapy of metastatic prostate cancer with ^{177}Lu-DOTA-HUJ591 anti prostate specific membrane antigen specific monoclonal antibody. *Curr. Radiopharm.* **2016**, *9*, 44–53. [CrossRef] [PubMed]
528. Van Rij, C.M.; Frielink, C.; Goldenberg, D.M.; Sharkey, R.M.; Lutje, S.; McBride, W.J.; Oyen, W.J.; Boerman, O.C. Pretargeted radioimmunotherapy of prostate cancer with an anti-TROP-2×-anti-HSG bispecific antibody and a ^{177}Lu-labeled peptide. *Cancer Biother. Radiopharm.* **2014**, *29*, 323–329. [CrossRef] [PubMed]

529. Wang, H.Y.; Lin, W.Y.; Chen, M.C.; Lin, T.; Chao, C.H.; Hsu, F.N.; Lin, E.; Huang, C.Y.; Luo, T.Y.; Lin, H. Inhibitory effects of rhenium-188-labeled herceptin on prostate cancer cell growth: A possible radioimmunotherapy to prostate carcinoma. *Int. J. Radiat. Biol.* **2013**, *89*, 346–355. [CrossRef] [PubMed]
530. Van Rij, C.M.; Lutje, S.; Frielink, C.; Sharkey, R.M.; Goldenberg, D.M.; Franssen, G.M.; McBride, W.J.; Rossi, E.A.; Oyen, W.J.; Boerman, O.C. Pretargeted immuno-pet and radioimmunotherapy of prostate cancer with an anti-TROP-2× anti-HSG bispecific antibody. *Eur. J. Nucl. Med. Mol. Imaging* **2013**, *40*, 1377–1383. [CrossRef] [PubMed]
531. Pan, M.H.; Gao, D.W.; Feng, J.; He, J.; Seo, Y.; Tedesco, J.; Wolodzko, J.G.; Hasegawa, B.H.; Franc, B.L. Biodistributions of ^{177}Lu- and ^{111}In-labeled 7e11 antibodies to prostate-specific membrane antigen in xenograft model of prostate cancer and potential use of ^{111}In-7e11 as a pre-therapeutic agent for ^{177}Lu-7e11 radioimmunotherapy. *Mol. Imaging Biol.* **2009**, *11*, 159–166. [CrossRef] [PubMed]
532. Kelly, M.P.; Lee, S.T.; Lee, F.T.; Smyth, F.E.; Davis, I.D.; Brechbiel, M.W.; Scott, A.M. Therapeutic efficacy of ^{177}Lu-CHX-A″-DTPA-hu3S193 radioimmunotherapy in prostate cancer is enhanced by EGFR inhibition or docetaxel chemotherapy. *Prostate* **2009**, *69*, 92–104. [CrossRef] [PubMed]
533. Pandit-Taskar, N.; O'Donoghue, J.A.; Morris, M.J.; Wills, E.A.; Schwartz, L.H.; Gonen, M.; Scher, H.I.; Larson, S.M.; Divgi, C.R. Antibody mass escalation study in patients with castration-resistant prostate cancer using ^{111}In-j591: Lesion detectability and dosimetric projections for 90y radioimmunotherapy. *J. Nucl. Med.* **2008**, *49*, 1066–1074. [CrossRef] [PubMed]
534. Kimura, Y.; Inoue, K.; Abe, M.; Nearman, J.; Baranowska-Kortylewicz, J. Pdgfrbeta and HIF-1α inhibition with imatinib and radioimmunotherapy of experimental prostate cancer. *Cancer Biol. Ther.* **2007**, *6*, 1763–1772. [CrossRef] [PubMed]
535. Zhao, X.Y.; Schneider, D.; Biroc, S.L.; Parry, R.; Alicke, B.; Toy, P.; Xuan, J.A.; Sakamoto, C.; Wada, K.; Schulze, M.; et al. Targeting tomoregulin for radioimmunotherapy of prostate cancer. *Cancer Res.* **2005**, *65*, 2846–2853. [CrossRef] [PubMed]
536. Vallabhajosula, S.; Goldsmith, S.J.; Kostakoglu, L.; Milowsky, M.I.; Nanus, D.M.; Bander, N.H. Radioimmunotherapy of prostate cancer using 90y- and ^{177}Lu-labeled j591 monoclonal antibodies: Effect of multiple treatments on myelotoxicity. *Clin. Cancer Res.* **2005**, *11*, 7195s–7200s. [CrossRef] [PubMed]
537. Richman, C.M.; Denardo, S.J.; O'Donnell, R.T.; Yuan, A.; Shen, S.; Goldstein, D.S.; Tuscano, J.M.; Wun, T.; Chew, H.K.; Lara, P.N.; et al. High-dose radioimmunotherapy combined with fixed, low-dose paclitaxel in metastatic prostate and breast cancer by using a muc-1 monoclonal antibody, m170, linked to indium-111/yttrium-90 via a cathepsin cleavable linker with cyclosporine to prevent human anti-mouse antibody. *Clin. Cancer Res.* **2005**, *11*, 5920–5927. [PubMed]
538. DeNardo, S.J.; Richman, C.M.; Albrecht, H.; Burke, P.A.; Natarajan, A.; Yuan, A.; Gregg, J.P.; O'Donnell, R.T.; DeNardo, G.L. Enhancement of the therapeutic index: From nonmyeloablative and myeloablative toward pretargeted radioimmunotherapy for metastatic prostate cancer. *Clin. Cancer Res.* **2005**, *11*, 7187s–7194s. [CrossRef] [PubMed]
539. Vallabhajosula, S.; Smith-Jones, P.M.; Navarro, V.; Goldsmith, S.J.; Bander, N.H. Radioimmunotherapy of prostate cancer in human xenografts using monoclonal antibodies specific to prostate specific membrane antigen (PSMA): Studies in nude mice. *Prostate* **2004**, *58*, 145–155. [CrossRef] [PubMed]
540. DeNardo, S.J.; DeNardo, G.L.; Yuan, A.; Richman, C.M.; O'Donnell, R.T.; Lara, P.N.; Kukis, D.L.; Natarajan, A.; Lamborn, K.R.; Jacobs, F.; et al. Enhanced therapeutic index of radioimmunotherapy (RIT) in prostate cancer patients: Comparison of radiation dosimetry for 1,4,7,10-tetraazacyclododecane-*n*,*n*′,*n*″,*n*‴-tetraacetic acid (DOTA)-peptide versus 2IT-DOTA monoclonal antibody linkage for rit. *Clin. Cancer Res.* **2003**, *9*, 3938S–3944S. [PubMed]
541. O'Donnell, R.T.; DeNardo, S.J.; Miers, L.A.; Lamborn, K.R.; Kukis, D.L.; DeNardo, G.L.; Meyers, F.J. Combined modality radioimmunotherapy for human prostate cancer xenografts with taxanes and 90yttrium-DOTA-peptide-CHL6. *Prostate* **2002**, *50*, 27–37. [CrossRef] [PubMed]
542. O'Donnell, R.T.; DeNardo, S.J.; Yuan, A.; Shen, S.; Richman, C.M.; Lara, P.N.; Griffith, I.J.; Goldstein, D.S.; Kukis, D.L.; Martinez, G.S.; et al. Radioimmunotherapy with ^{111}In/^{90}Y-2IT-BAD-m170 for metastatic prostate cancer. *Clin. Cancer Res.* **2001**, *7*, 1561–1568. [PubMed]
543. McDevitt, M.R.; Barendswaard, E.; Ma, D.; Lai, L.; Curcio, M.J.; Sgouros, G.; Ballangrud, A.M.; Yang, W.H.; Finn, R.D.; Pellegrini, V.; et al. An alpha-particle emitting antibody ([213bi]j591) for radioimmunotherapy of prostate cancer. *Cancer Res.* **2000**, *60*, 6095–6100. [PubMed]

544. Rydh, A.; Riklund-Ahlstrom, K.; Widmark, A.; Bergh, A.; Johansson, L.; Tavelin, B.; Nilsson, S.; Stigbrand, T.; Damber, J.E.; Hietala, S.O. Radioimmunotherapy of du-145 tumours in nude mice—A pilot study with e4, a novel monoclonal antibody against prostate cancer. *Acta Oncol.* **1999**, *38*, 1075–1079. [CrossRef] [PubMed]
545. Mottet, N.; Bellmunt, J.; Briers, E.; van den Bergh, R.; Bolla, M.; van Casteren, N.; Cornford, P.; Culine, S.; Joniau, S.; Lam, T.; et al. *Guidelines on Prostate Cancer*; European Association of Urology: Arnhem, the Netherlands, 2015; pp. 1–137.
546. NCCN. NCCN guidelines on Prostate Cancer (version 1.2015). Available online: http://www.nccn.org (accessed on 9 March 2016).
547. Edge, S.; Byrd, D.; Compton, C. *AJCC Cancer Staging*; Springer: New York, NY, USA, 2010.
548. Powles, T.; Murray, I.; Brock, C.; Oliver, T.; Avril, N. Molecular positron emission tomography and PET/CT imaging in urological malignancies. *Eur. Urol.* **2007**, *51*, 1511–1520, discussion 1520–1511. [CrossRef] [PubMed]
549. Turkbey, B.; Pinto, P.A.; Choyke, P.L. Imaging techniques for prostate cancer: Implications for focal therapy. *Nat. Rev. Urol.* **2009**, *6*, 191–203. [CrossRef] [PubMed]
550. Jana, S.; Blaufox, M.D. Nuclear medicine studies of the prostate, testes, and bladder. *Semin. Nucl. Med.* **2006**, *36*, 51–72. [CrossRef] [PubMed]
551. DeGrado, T.R.; Coleman, R.E.; Wang, S.; Baldwin, S.W.; Orr, M.D.; Robertson, C.N.; Polascik, T.J.; Price, D.T. Synthesis and evaluation of ^{18}F-labeled choline as an oncologic tracer for positron emission tomography: Initial findings in prostate cancer. *Cancer Res.* **2001**, *61*, 110–117. [PubMed]
552. Watanabe, H.; Kanematsu, M.; Kondo, H.; Kako, N.; Yamamoto, N.; Yamada, T.; Goshima, S.; Hoshi, H.; Bae, K.T. Preoperative detection of prostate cancer: A comparison with ^{11}C-choline pet, ^{18}F-fluorodeoxyglucose pet and MR imaging. *J. Magn. Reson. Imaging* **2010**, *31*, 1151–1156. [CrossRef] [PubMed]
553. Morris, M.J.; Akhurst, T.; Osman, I.; Nunez, R.; Macapinlac, H.; Siedlecki, K.; Verbel, D.; Schwartz, L.; Larson, S.M.; Scher, H.I. Fluorinated deoxyglucose positron emission tomography imaging in progressive metastatic prostate cancer. *Urology* **2002**, *59*, 913–918. [CrossRef]
554. Schoder, H.; Herrmann, K.; Gonen, M.; Hricak, H.; Eberhard, S.; Scardino, P.; Scher, H.I.; Larson, S.M. 2-^{18}Ffluoro-2-deoxyglucose positron emission tomography for the detection of disease in patients with prostate-specific antigen relapse after radical prostatectomy. *Clin. Cancer Res.* **2005**, *11*, 4761–4769. [CrossRef] [PubMed]
555. Poulsen, M.H.; Bouchelouche, K.; Hoilund-Carlsen, P.F.; Petersen, H.; Gerke, O.; Steffansen, S.I.; Marcussen, N.; Svolgaard, N.; Vach, W.; Geertsen, U.; et al. ^{18}F fluoromethylcholine (FCH) positron emission tomography/computed tomography (PET/CT) for lymph node staging of prostate cancer: A prospective study of 210 patients. *BJU Int.* **2012**, *110*, 1666–1671. [CrossRef] [PubMed]
556. Brogsitter, C.; Zophel, K.; Kotzerke, J. ^{18}F-choline, ^{11}C-choline and ^{11}C-acetate PET/CT: Comparative analysis for imaging prostate cancer patients. *Eur. J. Nucl. Med. Mol. Imaging* **2013**, *40*, S18–S27. [CrossRef] [PubMed]
557. Murphy, G.; Haider, M.; Ghai, S.; Sreeharsha, B. The expanding role of MRI in prostate cancer. *AJR Am. J. Roentgenol.* **2013**, *201*, 1229–1238. [CrossRef] [PubMed]
558. Souvatzoglou, M.; Eiber, M.; Takei, T.; Furst, S.; Maurer, T.; Gaertner, F.; Geinitz, H.; Drzezga, A.; Ziegler, S.; Nekolla, S.G.; et al. Comparison of integrated whole-body^{11}C-choline pet/mr with PET/CT in patients with prostate cancer. *Eur. J. Nucl. Med. Mol. Imaging* **2013**, *40*, 1486–1499. [CrossRef] [PubMed]
559. Wetter, A.; Lipponer, C.; Nensa, F.; Heusch, P.; Rubben, H.; Altenbernd, J.C.; Schlosser, T.; Bockisch, A.; Poppel, T.; Lauenstein, T.; et al. Evaluation of the pet component of simultaneous ^{18}F-choline PET/MRI in prostate cancer: Comparison with^{18}F-choline PET/CT. *Eur. J. Nucl. Med. Mol. Imaging* **2014**, *41*, 79–88. [CrossRef] [PubMed]
560. Eiber, M.; Takei, T.; Souvatzoglou, M.; Mayerhoefer, M.E.; Furst, S.; Gaertner, F.C.; Loeffelbein, D.J.; Rummeny, E.J.; Ziegler, S.I.; Schwaiger, M.; et al. Performance of whole-body integrated ^{18}F -FDG PET/MR in comparison to PET/CT for evaluation of malignant bone lesions. *J. Nucl. Med.* **2014**, *55*, 191–197. [CrossRef] [PubMed]
561. Van der Kwast, T.H.; Roobol, M.J. Defining the threshold for significant versus insignificant prostate cancer. *Nat. Rev. Urol.* **2013**, *10*, 473–482. [CrossRef] [PubMed]

562. Steyerberg, E.W.; Roobol, M.J.; Kattan, M.W.; van der Kwast, T.H.; de Koning, H.J.; Schroder, F.H. Prediction of indolent prostate cancer: Validation and updating of a prognostic nomogram. *J. Urol.* **2007**, *177*, 107–112, discussion 112. [CrossRef] [PubMed]
563. Epstein, J.I.; Walsh, P.C.; Carmichael, M.; Brendler, C.B. Pathologic and clinical findings to predict tumor extent of nonpalpable (stage T1C) prostate cancer. *JAMA* **1994**, *271*, 368–374. [CrossRef] [PubMed]
564. Epstein, J.I.; Chan, D.W.; Sokoll, L.J.; Walsh, P.C.; Cox, J.L.; Rittenhouse, H.; Wolfert, R.; Carter, H.B. Nonpalpable stageT1C prostate cancer: Prediction of insignificant disease using free/total prostate specific antigen levels and needle biopsy findings. *J. Urol.* **1998**, *160*, 2407–2411. [CrossRef]
565. Bastian, P.J.; Carter, B.H.; Bjartell, A.; Seitz, M.; Stanislaus, P.; Montorsi, F.; Stief, C.G.; Schroder, F. Insignificant prostate cancer and active surveillance: From definition to clinical implications. *Eur. Urol.* **2009**, *55*, 1321–1330. [CrossRef] [PubMed]
566. Oon, S.F.; Watson, R.W.; O'Leary, J.J.; Fitzpatrick, J.M. Epstein criteria for insignificant prostate cancer. *BJU Int.* **2011**, *108*, 518–525. [CrossRef] [PubMed]
567. Heidenreich, A.; Bastian, P.J.; Bellmunt, J.; Bolla, M.; Joniau, S.; van der Kwast, T.; Mason, M.; Matveev, V.; Wiegel, T.; Zattoni, F.; et al. Eau guidelines on prostate cancer. Part II: Treatment of advanced, relapsing, and castration-resistant prostate cancer. *Eur. Urol.* **2014**, *65*, 467–479. [CrossRef] [PubMed]
568. Mottet, N.; Briers, J.; van den Berg, D. Guidelines on prostate cancer. *Eur. Urol.* **2015**.
569. Pepe, P.; Fraggetta, F.; Galia, A.; Panella, P.; Pennisi, M.; Colecchia, M.; Aragona, F. Preoperative findings, pathological stage PSA recurrence in men with prostate cancer incidentally detected at radical cystectomy: Our experience in 242 cases. *Int. Urol. Nephrol.* **2014**, *46*, 1325–1328. [CrossRef] [PubMed]
570. Picchio, M.; Messa, C.; Landoni, C.; Gianolli, L.; Sironi, S.; Brioschi, M.; Matarrese, M.; Matei, D.V.; De Cobelli, F.; Del Maschio, A.; et al. Value of ^{11}C-choline-positron emission tomography for re-staging prostate cancer: A comparison with ^{18}F-fluorodeoxyglucose-positron emission tomography. *J. Urol.* **2003**, *169*, 1337–1340. [CrossRef] [PubMed]
571. Winter, A.; Uphoff, J.; Henke, R.P.; Wawroschek, F. First results of ^{11}C-choline PET/CT-guided secondary lymph node surgery in patients with psa failure and single lymph node recurrence after radical retropubic prostatectomy. *Urol. Int.* **2010**, *84*, 418–423. [CrossRef] [PubMed]
572. Fuccio, C.; Castellucci, P.; Schiavina, R.; Santi, I.; Allegri, V.; Pettinato, V.; Boschi, S.; Martorana, G.; Al-Nahhas, A.; Rubello, D.; et al. Role of ^{11}C-choline PET/CT in the restaging of prostate cancer patients showing a single lesion on bone scintigraphy. *Ann. Nucl. Med.* **2010**, *24*, 485–492. [CrossRef] [PubMed]
573. Cimitan, M.; Bortolus, R.; Morassut, S.; Canzonieri, V.; Garbeglio, A.; Baresic, T.; Borsatti, E.; Drigo, A.; Trovo, M.G. ^{18}F-fluorocholine PET/CT imaging for the detection of recurrent prostate cancer at psa relapse: Experience in 100 consecutive patients. *Eur. J. Nucl. Med. Mol. Imaging* **2006**, *33*, 1387–1398. [CrossRef] [PubMed]
574. Ibrahim, T.; Flamini, E.; Mercatali, L.; Sacanna, E.; Serra, P.; Amadori, D. Pathogenesis of osteoblastic bone metastases from prostate cancer. *Cancer* **2010**, *116*, 1406–1418. [CrossRef] [PubMed]
575. Helyar, V.; Mohan, H.K.; Barwick, T.; Livieratos, L.; Gnanasegaran, G.; Clarke, S.E.; Fogelman, I. The added value of multislice SPECT/CT in patients with equivocal bony metastasis from carcinoma of the prostate. *Eur. J. Nucl. Med. Mol. Imaging* **2010**, *37*, 706–713. [CrossRef] [PubMed]
576. Herranz-Blanco, B.; Shahbazi, M.A.; Correia, A.R.; Balasubramanian, V.; Kohout, T.; Hirvonen, J.; Santos, H.A. PH-switch nanoprecipitation of polymeric nanoparticles for multimodal cancer targeting and intracellular triggered delivery of doxorubicin. *Adv. Healthc. Mater.* **2016**, *5*, 1904–1916. [CrossRef] [PubMed]
577. Vu-Quang, H.; Vinding, M.S.; Nielsen, T.; Ullisch, M.G.; Nielsen, N.C.; Kjems, J. Theranostic tumor targeted nanoparticles combining drug delivery with dual near infrared and f magnetic resonance imaging modalities. *Nanomedicine* **2016**, *12*, 1873–1884. [CrossRef] [PubMed]
578. Hu, W.; Ma, H.; Hou, B.; Zhao, H.; Ji, Y.; Jiang, R.; Hu, X.; Lu, X.; Zhang, L.; Tang, Y.; et al. Engineering lysosome-targeting bodipy nanoparticles for photoacoustic imaging and photodynamic therapy under near-infrared light. *ACS Appl. Mater. Interfaces* **2016**, *8*, 12039–12047. [CrossRef] [PubMed]
579. Detappe, A.; Lux, F.; Tillement, O. Pushing radiation therapy limitations with theranostic nanoparticles. *Nanomedicine (Lond.)* **2016**, *11*, 997–999. [CrossRef] [PubMed]
580. Hung, C.C.; Huang, W.C.; Lin, Y.W.; Yu, T.W.; Chen, H.H.; Lin, S.C.; Chiang, W.H.; Chiu, H.C. Active tumor permeation and uptake of surface charge-switchable theranostic nanoparticles for imaging-guided photothermal/chemo combinatorial therapy. *Theranostics* **2016**, *6*, 302–317. [CrossRef] [PubMed]

581. Wang, G.; Zhang, F.; Tian, R.; Zhang, L.; Fu, G.; Yang, L.; Zhu, L. Nanotubes-embedded indocyanine green-hyaluronic acid nanoparticles for photoacoustic-imaging-guided phototherapy. *ACS Appl. Mater. Interfaces* **2016**, *8*, 5608–5617. [CrossRef] [PubMed]
582. Ghaemi, B.; Mashinchian, O.; Mousavi, T.; Karimi, R.; Kharrazi, S.; Amani, A. Harnessing the cancer radiation therapy by lanthanide-doped zinc oxide based theranostic nanoparticles. *ACS Appl. Mater. Interfaces* **2016**, *8*, 3123–3134. [CrossRef] [PubMed]
583. Gurka, M.K.; Pender, D.; Chuong, P.; Fouts, B.L.; Sobelov, A.; McNally, M.W.; Mezera, M.; Woo, S.Y.; McNally, L.R. Identification of pancreatic tumors in vivo with ligand-targeted, pH responsive mesoporous silica nanoparticles by multispectral optoacoustic tomography. *J. Control. Release* **2016**, *231*, 60–67. [CrossRef] [PubMed]
584. Andreou, C.; Pal, S.; Rotter, L.; Yang, J.; Kircher, M.F. Molecular imaging in nanotechnology and theranostics. *Mol. Imaging Biol.* **2017**, *19*, 363–372. [CrossRef] [PubMed]
585. Li, J.; Wang, S.; Shi, X.; Shen, M. Aqueous-phase synthesis of iron oxide nanoparticles and composites for cancer diagnosis and therapy. *Adv. Colloid Interface Sci.* **2017**. [CrossRef] [PubMed]
586. Lin, L.S.; Yang, X.; Zhou, Z.; Yang, Z.; Jacobson, O.; Liu, Y.; Yang, A.; Niu, G.; Song, J.; Yang, H.H.; et al. Yolk-shell nanostructure: An ideal architecture to achieve harmonious integration of magnetic-plasmonic hybrid theranostic platform. *Adv. Mater.* **2017**. [CrossRef] [PubMed]
587. Tang, L.; Zhang, F.; Yu, F.; Sun, W.; Song, M.; Chen, X.; Zhang, X.; Sun, X. Croconaine nanoparticles with enhanced tumor accumulation for multimodality cancer theranostics. *Biomaterials* **2017**, *129*, 28–36. [CrossRef] [PubMed]
588. Kuang, Y.; Zhang, K.; Cao, Y.; Chen, X.; Wang, K.; Liu, M.; Pei, R. Hydrophobic IR-780 dye encapsulated in CRGD-conjugated solid lipid nanoparticles for NIR imaging-guided photothermal therapy. *ACS Appl. Mater. Interfaces* **2017**, *9*, 12217–12226. [CrossRef] [PubMed]
589. Owen, J.; Crake, C.; Lee, J.Y.; Carugo, D.; Beguin, E.; Khrapitchev, A.A.; Browning, R.J.; Sibson, N.; Stride, E. A versatile method for the preparation of particle-loaded microbubbles for multimodality imaging and targeted drug delivery. *Drug Deliv. Transl. Res.* **2017**. [CrossRef] [PubMed]
590. Rajasekharreddy, P.; Huang, C.; Busi, S.; Rajkumari, J.; Tai, M.H.; Liu, G. Green synthesized nanomaterials as theranostic platforms for cancer treatment: Principles, challenges and the road ahead. *Curr. Med. Chem.* **2017**. [CrossRef] [PubMed]
591. Wang, Z.; Qiao, R.; Tang, N.; Lu, Z.; Wang, H.; Zhang, Z.; Xue, X.; Huang, Z.; Zhang, S.; Zhang, G.; et al. Active targeting theranostic iron oxide nanoparticles for MRI and magnetic resonance-guided focused ultrasound ablation of lung cancer. *Biomaterials* **2017**, *127*, 25–35. [CrossRef] [PubMed]
592. Ansari, C.; Tikhomirov, G.A.; Hong, S.H.; Falconer, R.A.; Loadman, P.M.; Gill, J.H.; Castaneda, R.; Hazard, F.K.; Tong, L.; Lenkov, O.D.; et al. Development of novel tumor-targeted theranostic nanoparticles activated by membrane-type matrix metalloproteinases for combined cancer magnetic resonance imaging and therapy. *Small* **2014**, *10*, 417, 566–575. [CrossRef]
593. Kiess, A.P.; Banerjee, S.R.; Mease, R.C.; Rowe, S.P.; Rao, A.; Foss, C.A.; Chen, Y.; Yang, X.; Cho, S.Y.; Nimmagadda, S.; et al. Prostate-specific membrane antigen as a target for cancer imaging and therapy. *Q. J. Nucl. Med. Mol. Imaging* **2015**, *59*, 241–268. [PubMed]
594. Hou, Y.; Qiao, R.; Fang, F.; Wang, X.; Dong, C.; Liu, K.; Liu, C.; Liu, Z.; Lei, H.; Wang, F.; et al. Nagdf4 nanoparticle-based molecular probes for magnetic resonance imaging of intraperitoneal tumor xenografts in vivo. *ACS Nano* **2013**, *7*, 330–338. [CrossRef] [PubMed]
595. Franci, C.; Zhou, J.; Jiang, Z.; Modrusan, Z.; Good, Z.; Jackson, E.; Kouros-Mehr, H. Biomarkers of residual disease, disseminated tumor cells, and metastases in the MMTV-PYMT breast cancer model. *PLoS ONE* **2013**, *8*, e58183. [CrossRef] [PubMed]
596. FDA. Fda Drug Safety Communication: Fda Strengthens Warnings and Changes Prescribing Instructions to Decrease the Risk of Serious Allergic Reactions with Anemia Drug Feraheme (Ferumoxytol). Available online: http://www.fda.gov/Drugs/DrugSafety/ucm440138.htm (accessed on 17 June 2016).

4

Akt Activation Correlates with Snail Expression and Potentially Determines the Recurrence of Prostate Cancer in Patients at Stage T2 after a Radical Prostatectomy

Wei-Yu Chen [1,2,3], Kuo-Tai Hua [4], Wei-Jiunn Lee [5,6], Yung-Wei Lin [7], Yen-Nien Liu [8], Chi-Long Chen [1,2,*], Yu-Ching Wen [6,7,*] and Ming-Hsien Chien [1,5,*]

1 Graduate Institute of Clinical Medicine, College of Medicine, Taipei Medical University, Taipei 110, Taiwan; 1047@tmu.edu.tw
2 Department of Pathology, School of Medicine, College of Medicine, Taipei Medical University, Taipei 110, Taiwan
3 Department of Pathology, Wan Fang Hospital, Taipei Medical University, Taipei 116, Taiwan
4 Graduate Institute of Toxicology, College of Medicine, National Taiwan University, Taipei 100, Taiwan; d94447003@gmail.com
5 Department of Medical Education and Research, Wan Fang Hospital, Taipei Medical University, Taipei 116, Taiwan; lwj5905@gmail.com
6 Department of Urology, School of Medicine, College of Medicine, Taipei Medical University, Taipei 110, Taiwan
7 Department of Urology, Wan Fang Hospital, Taipei Medical University, Taipei 116, Taiwan; highwei168@gmail.com
8 Graduate Institute of Cancer Biology and Drug Discovery, College of Medical Science and Technology, Taipei Medical University, Taipei 110, Taiwan; liuy@tmu.edu.tw
* Correspondence: chcl0997@yahoo.com.tw (C.-L.C.); s811007@yahoo.com.tw (Y.-C.W.); mhchien1976@gmail.com (M.-H.C.)

Academic Editor: Carsten Stephan

Abstract: Our previous work demonstrated the epithelial-mesenchymal transition factor, Snail, is a potential marker for predicting the recurrence of localized prostate cancer (PCa). Akt activation is important for Snail stabilization and transcription in PCa. The purpose of this study was to retrospectively investigate the relationship between the phosphorylated level of Akt (p-Akt) in radical prostatectomy (RP) specimens and cancer biochemical recurrence (BCR). Using a tissue microarray and immunohistochemistry, the expression of p-Akt was measured in benign and neoplastic tissues from RP specimens in 53 patients whose cancer was pathologically defined as T2 without positive margins. Herein, we observed that the p-Akt level was higher in PCa than in benign tissues and was significantly associated with the Snail level. A high p-Akt image score ($\geqslant$8) was significantly correlated with a higher histological Gleason sum, Snail image score, and preoperative prostate-specific antigen (PSA) value. Moreover, the high p-Akt image score and Gleason score sum ($\geqslant$7) showed similar discriminatory abilities for BCR according to a receiver-operator characteristic curve analysis and were correlated with worse recurrence-free survival according to a log-rank test ($p < 0.05$). To further determine whether a high p-Akt image score could predict the risk of BCR, a Cox proportional hazard model showed that only a high p-Akt image score (hazard ratio (HR): 3.12, $p = 0.05$) and a high Gleason score sum ($\geqslant$7) (HR: 1.18, $p = 0.05$) but not a high preoperative PSA value (HR: 0.62, $p = 0.57$) were significantly associated with a higher risk of developing BCR. Our data indicate that, for localized PCa patients after an RP, p-Akt can serve as a potential prognostic marker that improves predictions of BCR-free survival.

Keywords: prostate cancer; radical prostatectomy; stage T2; Akt; Snail; biochemical recurrence

1. Introduction

Globally, prostate cancer (PCa) accounts for 15% of male cancers and 6.6% of total male cancer mortality [1]. A radical prostatectomy (RP) is recognized as the gold standard for treating patients with localized PCa. The most important advantage of an RP is its potential to cure without damaging adjacent tissues and provide accurate staging because of the total removal of the organ. Although most patients are cured after surgery, around 23%–35% of PCa patients progress to biochemical recurrence (BCR) due to serum prostate-specific antigen (PSA) elevation, indicating that they have an increased risk of developing advanced PCa among 10 years after an RP [2,3]. To now, the challenge of PCa patients after an RP has been to determine which patients harbor high-risk disease requiring aggressive/curative therapy and which patients harbor indolent disease that can be managed with active surveillance.

Clinical prognostic risk factors such as the Gleason score, pathological stage, a positive surgical margin, and preoperative PSA value are used to estimate patient outcomes postoperatively [4,5]. However, the sensitivity of predicting BCR of individual patients using such parameters is insufficient [4,5]. Hence, novel biomarkers are needed to predict BCR in PCa patients after an RP to help provide better patient counseling, to help with more-precise clinical decision-making, and to search for therapeutic targets. Recently, studies have identified several molecular alterations involved in prostate recurrence. For example, we previously identified that the epithelial-mesenchymal transition (EMT) factor, Snail, is upregulated in PCa and is a predictive factor for subsequent localized PCa recurrence after an RP [6]. However, the precise mechanisms underlying Snail expression in this malignancy has not been fully elucidated.

Activation of the serine threonine kinase, Akt (phosphorylated (p)-Akt), was reported to regulate the stability and transcription of Snail in several cancer types, such as colorectal [7], oral [8], and prostate [9] cancers. A previous report indicated that p-Akt was expressed in around 8% of non-neoplastic prostate and 50% of PCa cases, indicative of its overexpression in cancer [10]. Increased Akt phosphorylation was observed in high-Gleason-score PCa and was correlated with proliferation in human PCa as estimated by the expression of the cell proliferation antigen, Ki67 [11,12]. Bedolla et al. recruited 65 PCa patients including T1~T3 stages with positive margins and showed that p-Akt is an important predictor of the risk of BCR [13]. Based on these results, we hypothesized an important role for Akt in PCa recurrence.

To further investigate the role of Akt activation in localized PCa recurrence, this study recruited 53 PCa patients at the T2 stage without positive margins after an RP. We evaluated the p-Akt expression pattern in these PCa patients using immunohistochemistry (IHC), and correlated expression levels with Snail and other clinicopathological parameters. We report for the first time that expression of p-Akt was highly correlated with Snail expression in localized PCa, and the cytoplasmic p-Akt protein level has potential to serve as an independent biomarker to improve estimation of localized PCa prognoses.

2. Results

In this study, we recruited 76 PCa patients who had not received neoadjuvant therapy and had undergone a whole-mount pathological assessment of their tumor after an RP. Next, we further excluded patients with a positive surgical margin and seminal vesicle invasion, and 53 of 76 patients who had organ-confined disease were ultimately recruited. Demographic and clinical characteristics are summarized in Table 1. Among the 53 PCa patients, the age at the time of the RP ranged 48–88 (mean, 70.7 $\pm$ 15.2) years. The histologic type of all tumors was an adenocarcinoma. According to the American Joint Committee on Cancer (AJCC) TNM staging system, tumors were classified into T2a (n = 6), T2b (n = 4), and T2c (n = 43). At a mean follow-up time of 71 months, 25 of 53 patients had BCR.

Table 1. Characteristics of prostate cancer (PCa) patients at the pT2 stage who underwent a radical prostatectomy (RP).

Characteristic	Total (%)
Total number of patients	53
Median age at RP (years)	71, mean 70.7 ± 15.2 (48–88 y/o)
Mean preoperative PSA level (ng/mL)	10.31 (1–21.64 ng/mL)
Biochemical failure	25 (47.2)
Pathological stage	
T2a	6 (11.3)
T2b	4 (7.5)
T2c	43 (81.2)
Gleason score	
⩾7	34 (64.2)
⩽6	19 (35.8)
Snail image score	
⩾8	35 (66)
⩽6	18 (34)
Phosphorylated-Akt image score	
⩾8	32 (60.4)
⩽6	21 (39.1)
Median follow-up time (months)	99, mean: 71 ± 49.5 (53–184 m)

RP, radical prostatectomy; PSA, prostate specific antigen; y/o, years old; m, months.

Figure 1A–D shows that p-Akt expression was observed in PCa tissue with a wide distribution of IHC scores. Immunostaining was almost completely restricted to the cytoplasm of epithelial tumor cells, and the pattern of expression was usually homogeneous. The p-Akt score was determined by multiplying the staining intensity (1–3) by the distribution rate (1–4) to represent p-Akt expression in PCa tissues, and representative examples of tumors showing overall low (with an image score of ⩽6) and high (with an image score of ⩾8) p-Akt expressions are illustrated in Figure 1A–D. In contrast to PCa, non-tumor adjacent tissues or benign prostatic hyperplasia (BPH) expressed p-Akt very weakly or not at all (Figure 1D,E), indicating that high levels of p-Akt were almost exclusively expressed in cancer tissues.

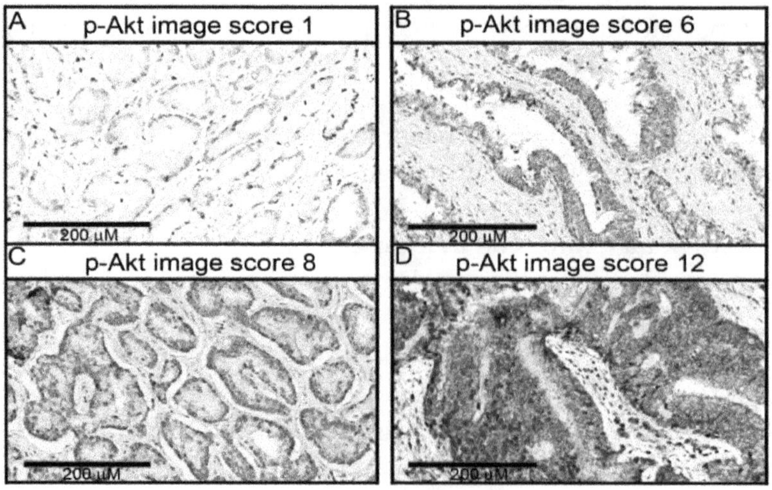

Figure 1. *Cont.*

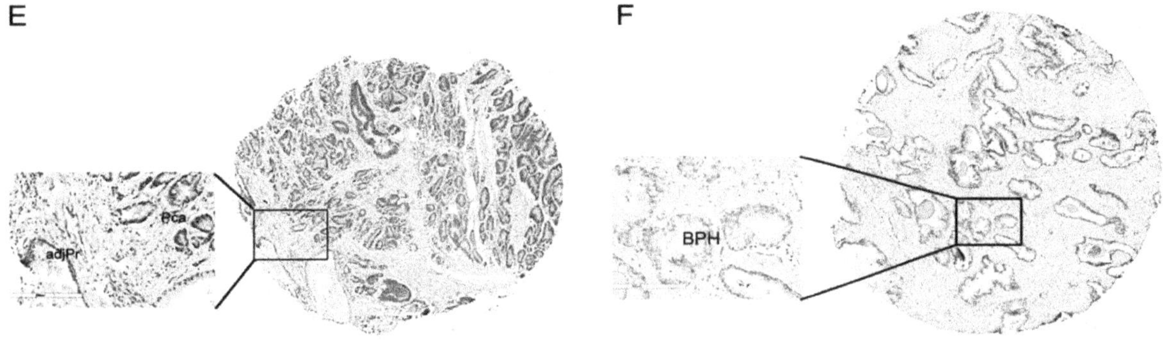

Figure 1. Phosphorylated (p)-Akt expression levels in representative primary prostate cancer (PCa) and non-neoplastic prostate tissues. Tissue microarrays (TMAs) of primary PCa and non-neoplastic prostate (benign prostatic hyperplasia; BPH) tissues were immunohistochemistry (IHC) analyzed for p-Akt. (**A**) Patient with a weak p-Akt expression level (intensity score 1 × extent score 1 = p-Akt image score 1); (**B**) Patient with T2cN0M0 cancer, a Gleason score of 3 + 4 = 7, and a moderate p-Akt expression level (intensity score 2 × extent score 3 = p-Akt image score 6); (**C**) Patient with T2cN0M0 cancer, a Gleason score of 4 + 3 = 7, and marked p-Akt immunostaining in the cytoplasm (intensity score 2 × extent score 4 = Snail image score 8); (**D**) Patient with T2cN0M0 cancer and a Gleason score of 4 + 5 = 9 and who displayed marked p-Akt immunostaining in the cytoplasm and discrete, diffuse staining in the nucleus (intensity score 3 × extent score 4 = image score 12) (200×); (**E**,**F**) No p-Akt immunostaining signal was detected in non-tumor adjacent tissues (**E**) or BPH (**F**). The high-power fields (200×) are magnified fields in the black boxed area in the right panel.

Previous studies indicated that Akt activation is important for Snail stabilization and transcription in PCa cells [9,14]. To further examine the correlation between expression levels of p-Akt and Snail in PCa, the same PCa TMA cohort was used. Representative IHC staining of p-Akt and Snail with different image scores on serial section of the same patients are shown in Figure 2A. IHC analysis of PCa specimens revealed a significant positive correlation between p-Akt and Snail expressions (Spearman correlation coefficient $r = 0.851$, $p < 0.0001$; Figure 2B).

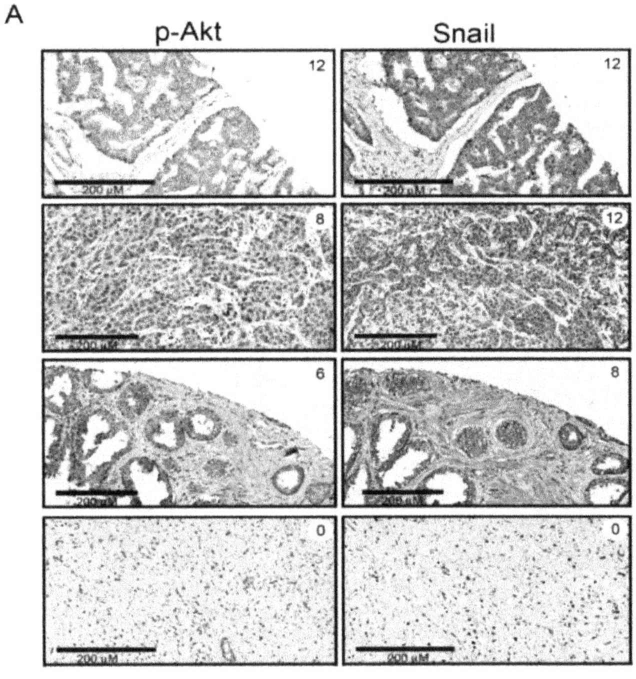

Figure 2. *Cont.*

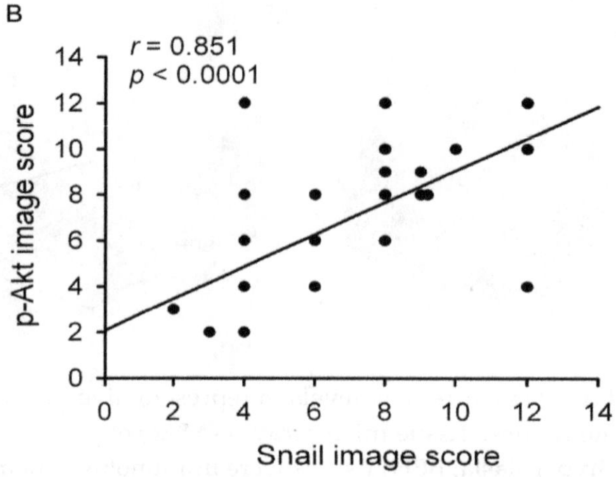

Figure 2. Phosphorylated (p)-Akt expression is positively correlated with Snail protein levels of patients with localized prostate cancer (PCa). (**A**) IHC staining analysis of p-Akt and Snail proteins in serial sections (200× magnification). Note the positive correlation of p-Akt and Snail protein expressions in tumor cells; (**B**) A significant positive correlation was observed between p-Akt expression levels and Snail expression levels (Spearman's correlation coefficients: $r = 0.851$, $p < 0.0001$).

As we showed earlier [6] , staining for Snail was significantly correlated with postoperative BCR of PCa. We further investigated relationships between p-Akt expression and selected clinicopathologic factors. Table 2 shows that among the 53 recruited patients, 32 patients (60.4%) were identified as having a high p-Akt image score (of ⩾8), and the remaining 21 patients had a low p-Akt image score (of ⩽6). High p-Akt (score of ⩾8) expression was significantly associated with a higher histological Gleason sum (score of ⩾7) ($p = 0.024$), Snail image score (score of ⩾8) ($p = 0.035$), and preoperative PSA value ($p = 0.026$). Moreover, we also observed that high p-Akt expression was significantly correlated with postoperative BCR ($p = 0.012$). Moreover, according to an ROC analysis, the areas under the ROC curve for high p-Akt image score (score of ⩾8) and Gleason score sum (score of ⩾7) were similar, indicating that the high p-Akt image score and Gleason score sum showed similar discriminatory capacities for BCR (Figure 3).

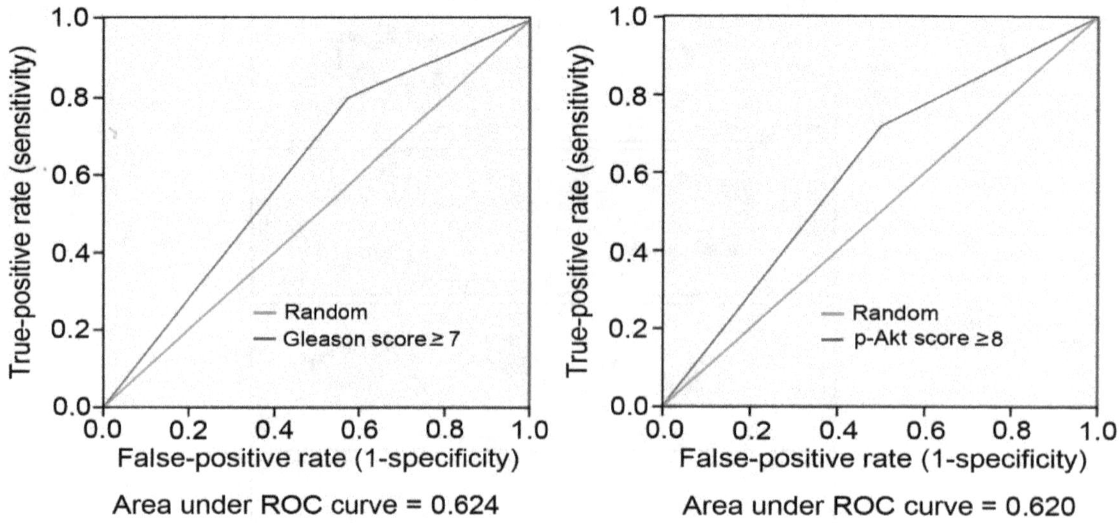

Figure 3. Sensitivity and specificity of gain of a high Gleason score or high p-Akt in specimens with respect to biochemical recurrence (BRC). Areas under the ROC (AUC) for high p-Akt image score (⩾8) and high Gleason score (⩾7) were 0.62 and 0.624, indicating similar discriminatory abilities for BRC.

Table 2. The association of phosphorylated (p)-Akt staining and clinicopathological features of prostate cancer (PCa) patients.

Characteristic	**No. of Patients (%)**		***p* Value**
	pAkt Score ⩾ 8	**pAkt Score ⩽ 6**	
Total number of patients	32 (60.4)	21 (39.6)	
Age (years)			
<50	1	0	
50–59	5	3	
60–69	11	6	
⩾70	15	12	
Pathological stage			
T2a	2 (6.25)	3 (14.3)	0.540
T2b	2 (6.25)	2 (9.5)	
T2c	28 (87.5)	16 (76.2)	
Gleason score			
⩾7	28 (87.5)	8 (38.1)	0.024
⩽6	4 (12.5)	13 (61.9)	
Snail image score			
⩾8	29 (90.6)	6 (28.6)	0.035
⩽6	3 (9.4)	15 (71.4)	
Recurrence	18 (56.3)	7 (33.3)	0.012
PSA, mean (ng/mL)	29.9	12.1	0.026

PSA: prostate specific antigen.

According to the Kaplan-Meier test, we observed that patients with higher p-Akt expression (with scores of ⩾8) had shorter recurrence-free survival times compared to those with lower expression (with scores of ⩽6) of the protein (Figure 4A). For patients who had higher p-Akt tumor expression, the median recurrence-free survival was 62 months, whereas for those who demonstrated lower p-Akt tumor expression, it was 88 months ($p = 0.03$) (Figure 4A). Moreover, results of the Kaplan-Meier test also showed that patients with a higher Gleason score sum (of ⩾7) or a higher Snail expression (with a score of ⩾8) all had significantly shorter recurrence-free survival times ($p = 0.03$ and 0.05) (Figure 4B,C). These results showed that the *p* value of the Kaplan-Meier test used to compare the higher p-Akt group was the same and smaller than the higher Gleason score group and higher Snail group, respectively.

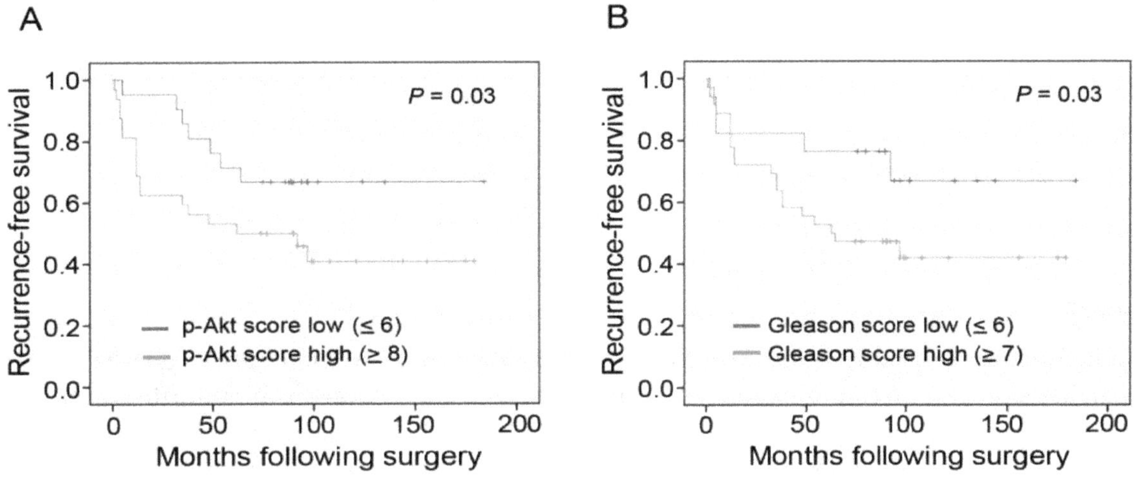

Figure 4. *Cont.*

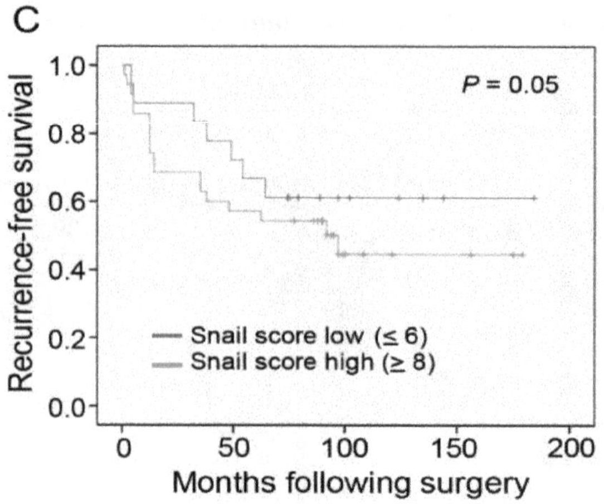

Figure 4. Kaplan-Meier survival curves showing relationships of the phosphorylated (p)-Akt image score (**A**), Gleason score sum (**B**), and Snail image score (**C**) in primary tumors with recurrence-free survival in 53 patients with clinically-localized prostate cancer. The recurrence-free survival of patients with a higher p-Akt, Snail image score (⩾8) or Gleason score sum (⩾7) was significantly lower than that of patients with a lower p-Akt, Snail image score (⩽6) or Gleason score sum (⩽6) ($p \leqslant 0.05$, log-rank test).

A Cox proportional hazard model was conducted to further explore relationships of p-Akt and Snail expressions with recurrence-free survival of the 53 patients with PCa after an RP. Table 3 summarizes the associations between the recurrence-free survival rate of the 53 patients with PCa and clinicopathologic parameters. In this analysis, we only observed that a high p-Akt image score (⩾8) (hazard ratio (HR): 3.12, $p = 0.05$) or a high Gleason score sum (⩾7) (HR: 1.18, $p = 0.05$), but not a high pre-operative PSA value (>10 ng/mL) (HR: 0.62, $p = 0.57$), was significantly correlated with worse recurrence-free survival (Table 3). In conclusion, our results suggest that a high p-Akt image score and a high histological Gleason score sum but not the preoperative PSA value can predict organ-confined PCa recurrence in our study. Moreover, we observed that patients with a high Snail image score (⩾8) also tended to correlate with BCR (HR: 1.31, $p = 0.06$). Furthermore, our data indicated that patients with a high p-Akt image score (HR: 3.12) showed a higher risk for BRC than patients with a high Gleason score sum (HR: 1.18) or a high Snail image score (HR: 1.31) (Table 3).

Table 3. Survival analyses of biochemical progression predictors in patients with prostate cancer at pT2 who underwent a radical prostatectomy (RP) according to a Cox proportional hazards regression model.

Factor	Hazard Ratio (95% CI)	*p* Value
PSA > 10 ng/mL	0.62 (0.12–3.19)	0.57
Pathological Gleason sum ⩾ 7	1.18 (0.23–1.32)	0.05
Snail image score ⩾ 8	1.31 (0.09–3.03)	0.06
P-Akt image score ⩾ 8	3.12 (0.95–10.27)	0.05

3. Discussion

PCa is the most common cancer and the second leading cause of male cancer deaths in the United States [15]. This underscores the need for a more-thorough molecular understanding of this resilient disease. Generally, patients with clinically-localized PCa will be cured after receiving radical surgery. However, a fraction of patients with localized PCa harbor microscopic localized or metastatic residual disease. The lethal consequences of PCa are related to its metastasis to other organ sites. Although the preoperative PSA value, surgical margin status, and Gleason score sum have been extensively used in assessing biochemical disease recurrence risk after RP, the sensitivities of these approaches are insufficient [16,17]. Therefore, it is of critical significance to discover a new marker for the early prediction of tumor recurrence, and earlier adjuvant therapy is very important for clinicians.

The EMT is a critical cellular mechanism during tumor progression and development of metastasis. It was suggested that the EMT is co-opted by PCa cells during their metastatic dissemination from a primary organ to secondary sites [18]. We previously showed that increased expression of the EMT promoter, Snail, in the prostatic epithelium is a good predictor of BCR following a prostatectomy [6]. The phosphatidylinositol 3′-kinase (PI3K)/Akt pathway is frequently activated in various cancers and plays an important role in promoting the EMT through regulating Snail stability in PCa [9,19]. Our current results indicated that the Akt activation status was significantly correlated with Snail expression levels in tissues from patients with clinically-localized PCa (T2 stage only). Representative IHC staining patterns of p-Akt and Snail from consecutive serial sections were nearly identical in PCa specimens, further implying their highly correlated expressions. Compared to our previous study [6], we extended the postoperative follow-up time (an average of 51 to 71 months) of localized PCa patients and further investigated the correlation between the Akt activation status in PCa specimens and BRC of patients. Our data showed that p-Akt was predominantly expressed in PCa, but not in non-neoplastic tissues. Cox proportional hazard models suggested that the p-Akt index (HR: 3.12, $p = 0.05$) is a better postoperative marker than the preoperative PSA value (HR: 0.62, $p = 0.57$) in localized PCa in our patient cohort. Although the Gleason score sum showed a similar discriminatory capacity with the p-Akt index and was also a useful predictor of BRC in our patient cohort, it was not as good as p-Akt. Compared to a high p-Akt image score, a high Gleason score sum showed a lower HR (HR: 1.18, $p = 0.05$) for BRC. Moreover, our previous study [6] indicated that the Snail index might be a useful predictor of BRC in the same patient cohort. However, after we extended the postoperative follow-up time in this study, the high Snail image score only showed a borderline significant trend ($p = 0.06$) of correlating with BRC, suggesting that p-Akt might show higher sensitivity than Snail for predicting organ-confined PCa recurrence. In addition to Snail, other transcription factors such as Slug, Zeb1, and Zeb2 are also involved in the control of EMT [20]. A previous report indicated that Akt activation can upregulate Snail and Zeb2 and promote EMT in squamous cell carcinoma [21]. However, the roles of Akt and Zeb2 in prostate cancer progression and recurrence are still unclear and worth further investigation in our future work.

High levels of p-Akt are associated with earlier recurrence, clearly indicating that p-Akt is associated with aggressiveness and disease progression in PCa. In addition to the Akt-mediated Snail expression and EMT induction in an androgen-independent PC3 cell line [14], Akt was also shown to be involved in a number of proliferative, metabolic, and antiapoptotic pathways that are dependent on PI3K signaling for activation [22]. Activated Akt was suggested to regulate a number of intracellular targets such as $p27^{Kip1}$, Bcl-2-associated death promoter (BAD), and caspase-9 which are involved in PCa progression and androgen independence [23–25]. Androgen deprivation therapy on androgen-dependent PCa cells such as LNCaP was reported to stimulate Akt activation, which finally resulted in androgen independence of the cells [26]. The pro-survival role of Akt activities was further shown in several clinical studies. For instance, increased levels of Akt or p-Akt expression were associated with a high Gleason grade and a worse prognosis in PCa [27–29]. Herein, we also showed that high levels of p-Akt were associated with more-aggressive features of the disease, as patients with high levels of p-Akt were identified as having a high PSA level and a high Gleason score.

Although the clinical application of p-Akt in predicting BCR of PCa was previously reported [10,13], the patient cohort recruited in this study was totally different from those of previous studies. Previous studies [10,13] enrolled PCa patients after an RP at different stages (pT1–pT3), and included those with lymph node metastasis, extracapsular extension, positive margins, and seminal vesicle invasion. However, in our study, we excluded PCa patients with positive margins or seminal vesicle involvement and only included true organ-confined PCa patients (pT2a–pT2c) after an RP. To our best knowledge, this is the first report to investigate the relationships of p-Akt and Snail with the prognostic role of p-Akt in patients with clinically-localized PCa. The pathological definition of

T2a–T2c stages is involvement of tumor cells in the prostate: in T2a, the tumor involves ⩽50% of one lobe; in T2b, the tumor involves >50% of one lobe, but not both lobes; and in T2c, the tumor involves both lobes [30]. A previous report indicated that tumor focality can significantly influence the BCR-free survival rate [31]. However, more-recent reports indicated that tumor focality did not predict the risk of BCR after an RP in men with clinically-localized PCa, even if the tumor involved both lobes of the prostate [32], suggesting that tumor focality might not be a suitable predictive marker for BCR in patients with organ-confined PCa. Our study observed that p-Akt expression level should be a better predictive marker of BCR in this PCa population. In addition to Akt, its downstream signaling pathways such as GSK-3β inactivation and NF-κB activation were also involved in Akt-mediated Snail expression in prostate cancer cells as well as in other cancer types [7,14,21]. Our future work will further investigate the correlation between these downstream effectors and BCR-free survival rate in patients with localized PCa.

4. Materials and Methods

4.1. Patient Selection and Specimen Collection

Pathology files of Wan Fang Hospital and Taipei Medical University Hospital were searched, and 76 radical prostatectomy specimens with a pathologic diagnosis of prostatic adenocarcinoma were found from March 1999 to December 2011. The pathologic diagnosis and Gleason scoring were microscopically reconfirmed by pathologists. Each case was pathologically staged using the 2002 American Joint Committee on Cancer TNM staging system. In our recruited patients, 13 patients with advanced stage were excluded. Another 10 patients who had positive surgical margins were also excluded from the study. Ultimately, 53 cases fulfilling the selection criteria were included for further study. Follow-up information was obtained from a cancer registration database. A PSA level of ⩾0.2 ng/mL on at least two occasions over a 2-month period was used to define biochemical failure [33].

4.2. Tissue Microarrays (TMAs)

Two independent PCa TMA sets were used in this study. PCa samples from patients were obtained with informed consent (Taipei Medical University-Wan Fang Hospital Institutional Review Board No. 99049). TMAs were constructed using a manual tissue-arraying instrument (Beecher Instruments, Sun Prairie, WI, USA). Briefly, carcinoma areas were manually punched, and duplicate tissue cores measuring 2.5 mm in diameter were inserted into recipient paraffin blocks. Sections measuring 5 μm in thickness were cut and transferred to glass slides. The presence of tumor tissue was further verified on a hematoxylin and eosin (H and E)-stained section.

4.3. Immunohistochemical (IHC) Staining

In brief, tissue microarray (TMA) sections were deparaffinized and immersed in 10 mM sodium citrate buffer (pH 6.0) in a microwave oven twice for 5 min to enhance antigen retrieval. After washing, slides were incubated with 0.3% H_2O_2 in methanol to quench the endogenous peroxidase activity. Slides were washed with phosphate-buffered saline (PBS) and incubated with anti-p-Akt (rabbit polyclonal antibody, Santa Cruz Biotechnology, Santa Cruz, CA, USA), anti-Snail (monoclonal mouse anti-Snail antibody, Biorbyt, Cambridge, UK), and appropriate negative control antibodies for 2 h at room temperature. After washing in PBS, slides were developed with a VECTASTAIN® ABC (avidin-biotin complex) peroxidase kit (Vector Laboratories, Burlingame, CA, USA) and a 3,3,9-diaminobenzidine (DAB) peroxidase substrate kit (Vector Laboratories) according to the manufacturer's instructions. All specimens were stained with H and E, which was used as a light counterstain.

4.4. Scoring of Immunoexpression

IHC results of p-Akt and Snail were classified into two groups according to the intensity and extent of staining. The intensity was scored semi-quantitatively as 0, negative; 1 point, weakly positive;

2 points, moderately positive; or 3 points, strongly positive. To determine the extent of Snail expression, 1000 consecutive malignant cells were counted in the area of the strongest staining. Numbers of cells with positive cytoplasmic staining for p-Akt and positive cytoplasmic and nuclear staining for Snail were recorded. The extent of p-Akt and Snail staining was semi-quantitatively scored as 0, positive in <1% of cells; 1 point, positive in 1%–25% of cells; 2 points, positive in 25%–50% of cells; 3 points, positive in 50%–75% of cells; or 4 points, positive in 75%–100% of cells. We then developed a p-Akt or Snail image score as previously described [6] by multiplying the intensity score (0–3 points) by the extent score (0–4 points) to represent the expression of p-Akt or Snail in cancer tissues. Low and high expression levels of p-Akt or Snail were respectively defined as 0–6 and 8–12 points. All sections were independently scored by the authors.

4.5. Statistical Analysis

SPSS 17.0 statistical software (SPSS, Chicago, IL, USA) was used for all statistical analyses. Differences in the clinicopathological features and Akt image scores of the tumors were assessed using paired *t*-tests for continuous and categorical variables. A Cox proportional hazards regression model was used for a univariate analysis when assessing predictors of biochemical progression. The Kaplan-Meier method was used to compare the time to recurrence among the groups. The diagnostic value of potential biomarkers as predictors of biochemical failure was evaluated with receiver-operator characteristic (ROC) curves. The area under the ROC curve (AUC) was determined from the plot of sensitivity versus 1–specificity (true positive rate versus false positive rate) and is a measure of the predictability of a test. Statistical significance was defined at $p < 0.05$.

5. Conclusions

Our data demonstrate, for the first time, that p-Akt expression is highly correlated with Snail expression in a Taiwanese population with primary localized PCa. We also documented that p-Akt exerts its tumor-promoting role because of its associations with various aggressive clinicopathological characteristics and BCR in men with clinically-localized PCa. Our results highlight that, in patients with clinically-localized PCa, and a high p-Akt image score in cancer tissues, adjuvant radiotherapy or hormone therapy might be suggested to prevent early BCR. However, larger prospective cohorts and experimental studies are needed for comprehensive functional validation and better understanding of the clinical significance of p-Akt and Snail expression in PCa.

Acknowledgments: This study was supported by grant numbers DOH-TD-B-111-003 and DOH102-TD-C-111-008 from Taipei Medical University and 105TMU-WFH-04 from Wan Fang Hospital, Taipei Medical University.

Author Contributions: Yu-Ching Wen, Kuo-Tai Hua, and Ming-Hsien Chien conceived and designed the experiments, contributed materials, and analyzed the data; Wei-Yu Chen and Chi-Long Chen performed the IHC experiments; Yen-Nien Liu contributed analytical tools; Ming-Hsien Chien, Yu-Ching Wen, and Wei-Jiunn Lee contributed reagents and wrote the paper.

Abbreviations

BPH	Benign prostatic hyperplasia
BCR	Biochemical recurrence
EMT	Epithelial-mesenchymal transition
PCa	Prostate cancer
PI3K	Phosphatidylinositol 3'-kinase
PSA	Prostate-specific antigen
RP	Radical prostatectomy
TMA	Tissue microarrays

References

1. Ferlay, J.; Soerjomataram, I.; Dikshit, R.; Eser, S.; Mathers, C.; Rebelo, M.; Parkin, D.M.; Forman, D.; Bray, F. Cancer incidence and mortality worldwide: Sources, methods and major patterns in GLOBOCAN 2012. *Int. J. Cancer* **2015**, *136*, E359–E386. [CrossRef] [PubMed]
2. Stephenson, A.J.; Scardino, P.T.; Eastham, J.A.; Bianco, F.J., Jr.; Dotan, Z.A.; Fearn, P.A.; Kattan, M.W. Preoperative nomogram predicting the 10-year probability of prostate cancer recurrence after radical prostatectomy. *J. Natl. Cancer Inst.* **2006**, *98*, 715–717. [CrossRef] [PubMed]
3. Hull, G.W.; Rabbani, F.; Abbas, F.; Wheeler, T.M.; Kattan, M.W.; Scardino, P.T. Cancer control with radical prostatectomy alone in 1000 consecutive patients. *J. Urol.* **2002**, *167*, 528–534. [CrossRef]
4. Stephenson, A.J.; Scardino, P.T.; Eastham, J.A.; Bianco, F.J., Jr.; Dotan, Z.A.; DiBlasio, C.J.; Reuther, A.; Klein, E.A.; Kattan, M.W. Postoperative nomogram predicting the 10-year probability of prostate cancer recurrence after radical prostatectomy. *J. Clin. Oncol.* **2005**, *23*, 7005–7012. [CrossRef] [PubMed]
5. Kotb, A.F.; Elabbady, A.A. Prognostic factors for the development of biochemical recurrence after radical prostatectomy. *Prostate Cancer* **2011**, *2011*, 485189. [CrossRef] [PubMed]
6. Wen, Y.C.; Chen, W.Y.; Lee, W.J.; Yang, S.F.; Lee, L.M.; Chien, M.H. Snail as a potential marker for predicting the recurrence of prostate cancer in patients at stage T2 after radical prostatectomy. *Clin. Chim. Acta* **2014**, *431*, 169–173. [CrossRef] [PubMed]
7. Wang, H.; Wang, H.S.; Zhou, B.H.; Li, C.L.; Zhang, F.; Wang, X.F.; Zhang, G.; Bu, X.Z.; Cai, S.H.; Du, J. Epithelial-mesenchymal transition (EMT) induced by TNF-α requires AKT/GSK-3β-mediated stabilization of snail in colorectal cancer. *PLoS ONE* **2013**, *8*, e56664. [CrossRef] [PubMed]
8. Grille, S.J.; Bellacosa, A.; Upson, J.; Klein-Szanto, A.J.; van Roy, F.; Lee-Kwon, W.; Donowitz, M.; Tsichlis, P.N.; Larue, L. The protein kinase Akt induces epithelial mesenchymal transition and promotes enhanced motility and invasiveness of squamous cell carcinoma lines. *Cancer Res.* **2003**, *63*, 2172–2178. [PubMed]
9. Liu, Z.C.; Wang, H.S.; Zhang, G.; Liu, H.; Chen, X.H.; Zhang, F.; Chen, D.Y.; Cai, S.H.; Du, J. AKT/GSK-3β regulates stability and transcription of snail which is crucial for bFGF-induced epithelial-mesenchymal transition of prostate cancer cells. *Biochim. Biophys. Acta* **2014**, *1840*, 3096–3105. [CrossRef] [PubMed]
10. Ayala, G.; Thompson, T.; Yang, G.; Frolov, A.; Li, R.; Scardino, P.; Ohori, M.; Wheeler, T.; Harper, W. High levels of phosphorylated form of Akt-1 in prostate cancer and non-neoplastic prostate tissues are strong predictors of biochemical recurrence. *Clin. Cancer Res.* **2004**, *10*, 6572–6578. [CrossRef] [PubMed]
11. Malik, S.N.; Brattain, M.; Ghosh, P.M.; Troyer, D.A.; Prihoda, T.; Bedolla, R.; Kreisberg, J.I. Immunohistochemical demonstration of phospho-Akt in high Gleason grade prostate cancer. *Clin. Cancer Res.* **2002**, *8*, 1168–1171. [PubMed]
12. Ghosh, P.M.; Malik, S.N.; Bedolla, R.G.; Wang, Y.; Mikhailova, M.; Prihoda, T.J.; Troyer, D.A.; Kreisberg, J.I. Signal transduction pathways in androgen-dependent and -independent prostate cancer cell proliferation. *Endocr. Relat. Cancer* **2005**, *12*, 119–134. [CrossRef] [PubMed]
13. Bedolla, R.; Prihoda, T.J.; Kreisberg, J.I.; Malik, S.N.; Krishnegowda, N.K.; Troyer, D.A.; Ghosh, P.M. Determining risk of biochemical recurrence in prostate cancer by immunohistochemical detection of PTEN expression and Akt activation. *Clin. Cancer Res.* **2007**, *13*, 3860–3867. [CrossRef] [PubMed]
14. Wang, H.; Fang, R.; Wang, X.F.; Zhang, F.; Chen, D.Y.; Zhou, B.; Wang, H.S.; Cai, S.H.; Du, J. Stabilization of Snail through AKT/GSK-3β signaling pathway is required for TNF-α-induced epithelial-mesenchymal transition in prostate cancer PC3 cells. *Eur. J. Pharmacol.* **2013**, *714*, 48–55. [CrossRef] [PubMed]
15. Siegel, R.L.; Miller, K.D.; Jemal, A. Cancer statistics, 2015. *CA Cancer J. Clin.* **2015**, *65*, 5–29. [CrossRef] [PubMed]
16. Kattan, M.W. Nomograms are superior to staging and risk grouping systems for identifying high-risk patients: preoperative application in prostate cancer. *Curr. Opin. Urol.* **2003**, *13*, 111–116. [CrossRef] [PubMed]
17. Chun, F.K.; Steuber, T.; Erbersdobler, A.; Currlin, E.; Walz, J.; Schlomm, T.; Haese, A.; Heinzer, H.; McCormack, M.; Huland, H.; et al. Development and internal validation of a nomogram predicting the probability of prostate cancer Gleason sum upgrading between biopsy and radical prostatectomy pathology. *Eur. Urol.* **2006**, *49*, 820–826. [CrossRef] [PubMed]
18. Matuszak, E.A.; Kyprianou, N. Androgen regulation of epithelial-mesenchymal transition in prostate tumorigenesis. *Expert Rev. Endocrinol. Metab.* **2011**, *6*, 469–482. [CrossRef] [PubMed]

19. Larue, L.; Bellacosa, A. Epithelial-mesenchymal transition in development and cancer: Role of phosphatidylinositol 3′ kinase/AKT pathways. *Oncogene* **2005**, *24*, 7443–7454. [CrossRef] [PubMed]
20. Peinado, H.; Olmeda, D.; Cano, A. Snail, Zeb and bHLH factors in tumour progression: An alliance against the epithelial phenotype? *Nat. Rev. Cancer* **2007**, *7*, 415–428. [CrossRef] [PubMed]
21. Julien, S.; Puig, I.; Caretti, E.; Bonaventure, J.; Nelles, L.; van Roy, F.; Dargemont, C.; de Herreros, A.G.; Bellacosa, A.; Larue, L. Activation of NF-κB by Akt upregulates Snail expression and induces epithelium mesenchyme transition. *Oncogene* **2007**, *26*, 7445–7456. [CrossRef] [PubMed]
22. Alessi, D.R.; Cohen, P. Mechanism of activation and function of protein kinase B. *Curr. Opin. Genet. Dev.* **1998**, *8*, 55–62. [CrossRef]
23. Graff, J.R.; Konicek, B.W.; McNulty, A.M.; Wang, Z.; Houck, K.; Allen, S.; Paul, J.D.; Hbaiu, A.; Goode, R.G.; Sandusky, G.E.; et al. Increased AKT activity contributes to prostate cancer progression by dramatically accelerating prostate tumor growth and diminishing p27Kip1 expression. *J. Biol. Chem.* **2000**, *275*, 24500–24505. [CrossRef] [PubMed]
24. Graff, J.R. Emerging targets in the AKT pathway for treatment of androgen-independent prostatic adenocarcinoma. *Expert Opin. Ther. Targets* **2002**, *6*, 103–113. [CrossRef] [PubMed]
25. Datta, S.R.; Dudek, H.; Tao, X.; Masters, S.; Fu, H.; Gotoh, Y.; Greenberg, M.E. Akt phosphorylation of BAD couples survival signals to the cell-intrinsic death machinery. *Cell* **1997**, *91*, 231–241. [CrossRef]
26. Murillo, H.; Huang, H.; Schmidt, L.J.; Smith, D.I.; Tindall, D.J. Role of PI3K signaling in survival and progression of LNCaP prostate cancer cells to the androgen refractory state. *Endocrinology* **2001**, *142*, 4795–4805. [CrossRef] [PubMed]
27. Le Page, C.; Koumakpayi, I.H.; Alam-Fahmy, M.; Mes-Masson, A.M.; Saad, F. Expression and localisation of Akt-1, Akt-2 and Akt-3 correlate with clinical outcome of prostate cancer patients. *Br. J. Cancer* **2006**, *94*, 1906–1912. [CrossRef] [PubMed]
28. Liao, Y.; Grobholz, R.; Abel, U.; Trojan, L.; Michel, M.S.; Angel, P.; Mayer, D. Increase of AKT/PKB expression correlates with Gleason pattern in human prostate cancer. *Int. J. Cancer* **2003**, *107*, 676–680. [CrossRef] [PubMed]
29. Kreisberg, J.I.; Malik, S.N.; Prihoda, T.J.; Bedolla, R.G.; Troyer, D.A.; Kreisberg, S.; Ghosh, P.M. Phosphorylation of Akt (Ser473) is an excellent predictor of poor clinical outcome in prostate cancer. *Cancer Res.* **2004**, *64*, 5232–5236. [CrossRef] [PubMed]
30. Koh, H.; Maru, N.; Muramoto, M.; Wheeler, T.M.; Scardino, P.T.; Ohori, M. The 1992 TNM classification of T2 prostate cancer predicts pathologic stage and prognosis better than the revised 1997 classification. *Nihon Hinyokika Gakkai Zasshi* **2002**, *93*, 595–601. [CrossRef] [PubMed]
31. Rice, K.R.; Furusato, B.; Chen, Y.; McLeod, D.G.; Sesterhenn, I.A.; Brassell, S.A. Clinicopathological behavior of single focus prostate adenocarcinoma. *J. Urol.* **2009**, *182*, 2689–2694. [CrossRef] [PubMed]
32. Masterson, T.A.; Cheng, L.; Mehan, R.M.; Koch, M.O. Tumor focality does not predict biochemical recurrence after radical prostatectomy in men with clinically localized prostate cancer. *J. Urol.* **2011**, *186*, 506–510. [CrossRef] [PubMed]
33. Freedland, S.J.; Sutter, M.E.; Dorey, F.; Aronson, W.J. Defining the ideal cutpoint for determining PSA recurrence after radical prostatectomy: Prostate-specific antigen. *Urology* **2003**, *61*, 365–369. [CrossRef]

5

Current Stem Cell Biomarkers and their Functional Mechanisms in Prostate Cancer

Kaile Zhang [1,2,†], Shukui Zhou [1,†], Leilei Wang [3], Jianlong Wang [4], Qingsong Zou [1], Weixin Zhao [2], Qiang Fu [1,*] and Xiaolan Fang [5,*,‡]

1 The Department of Urology, Affiliated Sixth People's Hospital, Shanghai JiaoTong University, Shanghai 200233, China; great_z0313@126.com (K.Z.); 2005507098@163.com (S.Z.); zou_qingsong@126.com (Q.Z.)
2 Wake Forest Institute for Regenerative Medicine, Winston-Salem, NC 27101, USA; wezhao@wakehealth.edu
3 VIP Department of Beijing Hospital, Beijing 100730, China; luckyleileiaaa@sina.com
4 Urology Department of Beijing Hospital, Beijing 100730, China; wjlspplaaa@sina.com
5 Department of Cancer Biology, Wake Forest University School of Medicine, Wake Forest Institute for Regenerative Medicine, Winston-Salem, NC 27101, USA
* Correspondence: jamesqfu@aliyun.com (Q.F.); afang@nygenome.org (X.F.)

† These authors contributed equally to this work.
‡ Current address: New York Genome Center, 101 Avenue of the Americas, New York, NY 10013, USA.

Academic Editor: Carsten Stephan

Abstract: Currently there is little effective treatment available for castration resistant prostate cancer, which is responsible for the majority of prostate cancer related deaths. Emerging evidence suggested that cancer stem cells might play an important role in resistance to traditional cancer therapies, and the studies of cancer stem cells (including specific isolation and targeting on those cells) might benefit the discovery of novel treatment of prostate cancer, especially castration resistant disease. In this review, we summarized major biomarkers for prostate cancer stem cells, as well as their functional mechanisms and potential application in clinical diagnosis and treatment of patients.

Keywords: prostate cancer; cancer stem cell; stem cell biomarker

1. Introduction

Prostate cancer (PCa) is the most common non-skin cancer in American men [1,2]. Standard PCa treatment includes radical prostatectomy, radiotherapy, chemotherapy and castration (either by drug or by surgery, mainly for androgen sensitive PCa), as well as immunotherapy and palliative therapy (mainly for castration resistant PCa (CRPC)). CRPC is responsible for majority of the PCa-related deaths [3], and currently there are two major hypotheses of CRPC carcinogenesis, the adaptive mechanism and the selective mechanism [4]. The adaptive mechanism suggests gene mutations in PCa cells (e.g., mutations of androgen receptor (AR)), dysregulated expression of genes, etc., contribute to CRPC development [5]. The selective mechanism, which is emerged in the last few decades, suggests that pre-existing castration-resistant subclones in primary PCa tissues and cancer stem cell selection dominates CRPC development (Figure 1) [6–8]. Recently, it has been suggested that stem-cell directed differentiation therapy could promote differentiation of cancer stem cells and sensitize them to anticancer drugs (such as synergistic androgen signaling blocking agents) [9].

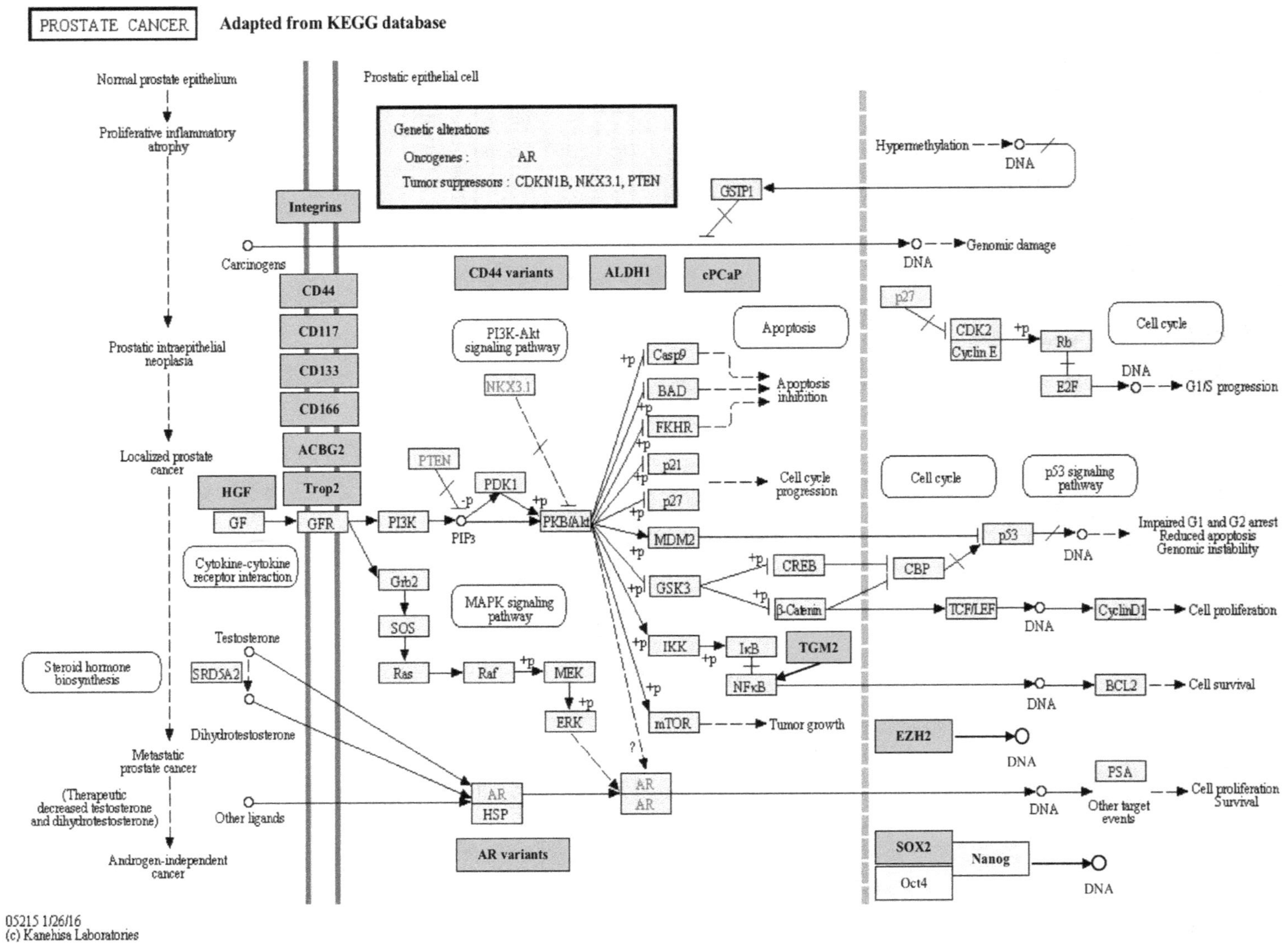

Figure 1. The mechanism and pathway map of the prostate cancer (modified based on KEGG database). Solid line between genes/molecules indicates direct regulation, while dashed lines indicates possible indirect regulation. Circle indicates a group of similar molecules (instead of a specific one). Biomarkers discussed in this review are highlighted in orange and in bold font, related molecules that are newly discovered are in yellow. Classic biomarkers included in KEGG prostate cancer pathway are highlighted in green. Key regulators in classical pathways involved in PCa are displayed in red (e.g., NKX3.1, PTEN, AR).

Cancer stem cells (CSCs) were defined as cells with capacity of self-renewal and proliferation in cancer tissue [8]. Over years, scientists have been arguing about the origin of cancer stem cells. CSCs were suggested to originate from mutated normal stem cells, from mutated progenitor cells in the process of differentiation which re-gains the characteristics of stem cells, or from mature cells that re-acquired self-renewal ability [10]. Various cell surface markers were used to isolate CSCs, whose proliferative potential was verified by in vitro andin vivo assays (Tables 1 and 2). This review summarizes recent research progress of current stem cell markers in PCa.

Table 1. Summary of prostate cancer stem cell biomarkers based on location and function.

Biomarker	Transmembrane Protein	Glycoprotein	Enzyme	Transcription Factor	Extracellular Protein	mRNA
Integrins	Yes	-	-	-	-	-
CD44	Yes	-	-	-	-	-
CD133	Yes	Yes	-	-	-	-
CD166	Yes	-	-	-	-	-
Trop2	Yes	Yes	-	-	-	-
CD117	Yes	-	Yes	-	-	-
ALDH1	-	-	-	Yes	-	-
ABCG2	Yes	-	-	-	-	-
SOX2	-	-	-	Yes	-	-
EZH2	-	-	Yes	-	-	-
cPAcP	-	-	Yes	-	-	-
AR splice variants	-	-	-	-	-	Yes
HGF	-	-	-	-	Yes	-
TGM2	-	-	Yes	-	-	-

Trop2, tumor-associated calcium signal transducer 2; ALDH1, aldehyde dehydrogenase 1; ABCG2, ATP binding membrane transporters; cPAcP, cellular prostatic acid phosphatase; HGF, hepatocyte growth factor; TGM2, transglutaminase II; SOX2, SRY-box 2; EZH2, enhancer of zeste 2 polycomb repressive complex 2 subunit.

Table 2. Summary of verifying studies and possible pathways of prostate cancer stem cell biomarkers.

Markers	PCa Cell Lines	Primary PCa Tissues	Mouse Models	Possible Involved Pathway in PCa
Integrins	Yes	Yes	-	-
CD44	Yes	Yes	-	-
CD133	Yes	Yes	-	-
CD166	-	-	Yes	-
Trop2	-	-	Yes	-
CD117	-	-	Yes	-
ALDH1	Yes	-	-	-
ABCG2	Yes	Yes	-	-
SOX2	-	Yes	-	-
EZH2	-	Yes	-	-
cPAcP	Yes	-	-	-
AR splice variants	Yes	-	-	AR
HGF	Yes	-	-	AR
TGM2	Yes	-	-	NF-κB

PCa, Prostate cancer.

2. Integrins

Integrins are a family of transmembrane receptors known to participate in cell-cell adhesion and cell-surface mediated signaling, serving as bridges for cell-cell and cell-extracellular matrix (ECM) interactions [11]. Integrin could interact with specific ligands to transfer signals through cell-cell or cell-ECM interactions and stimulate expression of downstream target genes. Integrins were generally overexpressed in PCa [12,13]. In PCa, expression of α2-integrin and EZH2 is observed in a small fraction of cancer cells, which is supportive for their role as stem cell marker [14]. α2β1 integrin plays an important role in epithelia-stroma interaction, which is suggested to contribute to selective bone metastasis [12]. In the meantime, it could be a new marker to screen for prostate stem cells. Collins et al. [15] has discovered that the prostate stem cells expressing α2β1 integrin locate at basal epithelial layer. Approximately 1% of basal cells examined by confocal microscopy were integrin positive, and these cells could be isolated directly from the tissue on the basis of rapid adhesion to type I collagen. This isolated cell population displays basal cell phenotype, marked by expression of CK5 and CK14 and lack of expression of differentiation-specific markers (such as prostate specific antigen (PSA) and prostatic acid phosphatase (PAP)). These prostate stem cells could be cultivated in vitro and display much greater capability to form colonies in vitro (comparing to total basal cell population). When α2β1 overexpressing cells and stromal cells were transplanted subcutaneously into nude mouse, they could form structure of normal prostate gland prostate-specific differentiation [15].

Microarray experiments performed by several independent groups found that Integrin-α6 (also known as CD49f) is consistently overexpressed in hematopoietic, neural, and embryonic stem cells, and it is suggested as an effective cell stemness marker [16]. It has been used for characterization of prostatic progenitor cells [17,18], and was suggested as an emerging biomarker for PCa evaluation [14,19,20].

3. CD44

CD44 is a single-pass type I transmembrane protein and an important cellular adhesion molecule related to signaling to extracellular matrix. CD44 was considered as a marker of cancer stem cells from many organs including prostate [21–23]. It was located extensively on cell membrane and is important for cell adhesion and signal transduction. It was reported that CD44 positive cells from primary prostatic tumor tissues possess cell stemness [24]. Molecular studies demonstrated that $CD44^+$ PCa cells retain certain intrinsic properties of progenitor cells [25]. $CD44^+$ cells express high levels of stemness genes including *Oct-3/4*, *Bmi*, β-catenin and Smoothened (*SMO*) [2,26,27]. Kasper et al. discovered that in PCa cells (such as LNCaP, DU145 and PC3), CD44 positive cells had much greater proliferative capability than CD44 negative cells [28]. Van et al. isolated the DU145 cells from $CD44^+$ and $CD44^-$ Cells and tested the gene expression of stem cells by RT-PCR. Low expression of luminal cell markers (e.g., CK18) and AR were observed in $CD44^+$ cells, whereas the genes highly related to stem cell proliferation and differentiation were overexpressed [29]. Recently, CD44 expression level was reported to be correlated with PCa grade in prostate biopsy samples [30], and proteomics analysis showed that $CD44^+$ cells had positive correlation with genes related to cancer proliferation and metastasis [31]. However, Ugolkov discovered that expression of CD44 and Oct4 were observed in large populations of benign and malignant cells in the prostate, which is somewhat contradictory to the definition of stem cells as a small fraction of the total cell population [32]. Their results suggested that combined expression of embryonic stem cell markers EZH2 and SOX2 might be used to identify potential cancer stem cells as a minor (<10%) subgroup in $CD44^+$ prostatic adenocarcinoma cells [32].

Recently, quite a few thorough analyses have been done on CD44 isoforms that are generated through alternative splicing of CD44 precursor mRNA. Those CD44 variants function distinctly in PCa and might serve as independent markers comparing to total CD44 expression level. For example, CD44v2 correlated with a better recurrence-free survival rate in PCa patients and is underexpressed in metastatic PCa cell lines [33]. Another well-studied isoform is CD44v6, which is associated with PCa proliferation, invasion, adhesion, metastasis, chemo-/radioresistance, and the induction of epithelial–mesenchymal transition (EMT) as well as the activation PI3K/Akt/mTOR and Wnt signaling pathways, and CD44v6 expression was closely associated with conventional prognostic factors and is identified as significant predictor for biochemical recurrence in PCa [34,35]. CD44v7–10 were overexpressed in PCa, and knock-down of CD44v7–10 by RNAi would significantly decrease invasion and migration in PCa cells [36].

Taken together, those results demonstrated CD44 RNA isoforms, but not total CD44 protein, might serve as specific marker for prostate cancer stem cells, though total CD44 protein level might still serve as a stem cell marker for other types of cancers [29].

4. CD133

CD133 is a glycoprotein with five transmembrane domains, generally expressed in various stem cells and endothelial progenitor cells but not in mature endothelial cells [37]. CD133 has been widely used, usually in combination with other stem cell markers such as CD44 and $\alpha 2\beta 1$ integrin, to isolate cancer stem cells from prostate tumors with different Gleason grade, including cells from both primary and metastatic lesions [38–41]. Approximately 0.1% of cells in any prostate tumor displayed this phenotype, though there was no correlation between the number of $CD44^{+}/\alpha 2\beta 1hi/CD133^{+}$ cells and tumor grade [23]. In normal prostate tissues, CD133 expression was observed in both basal and luminal cells [42]. Although its expression in normal prostate tissue is pretty low, CD133 is usually overexpressed in inflammation cell population [43].

Prostatic basal cells could be enriched based on $\alpha 2\beta 1$ integrin (hi) expression and further enriched for stem cells using CD133 in non-tumorigenic BPH-1 cells [44]. It is demonstrated that the tumorigenic potential did not reside in the $CD133^{+}$ stem cells but was consistently observed in the $CD133^{-}$ population [45]. These data confirmed that benign basal cells include cells of origin of prostate cancer and suggested that proliferative $CD133^{-}$ basal cells are more susceptible to tumorigenesis compared to the $CD133^{+}$-enriched stem cells. These findings challenged the current dogma that normal stem cells and cells of origin of cancer are the same cell type(s) [45]. Intensive studies need to be done to learn more about the role of CD133 in PCa origination.

5. ALDH1

ALDH1 was suggested as a stem cell marker for both normal and tumor tissues [46]. As a cytoplasmic enzyme, ALDH1 has multiple intracellular aldehydes which can be converted into carboxylic acids, and could be involved in intracellular degradation of cell toxic substances [47]. ALDH1 expression was reported to be correlated with tumor grade and prognosis in PCa patients [48]. Burger et al. [49] found that cells with high ALDH enzymatic activity have greater in vitro proliferative potential than cells with low ALDH activity. Similar results were observed in an in vivo prostate reconstitution assay [49]. Thus, ALDH enzymatic activity might be used as a functional marker of prostate stem/progenitor cells and allow for simple, efficient isolation of cells with primitive features. ALDH $\alpha 2+/\alpha 6+/\alpha V + CD44^{+}$ cells also displayed high colonization in vitro and highly invasive tumorigenesis and aggressive metastasis characteristics in vivo [50]. p63 cytoplasmic aberrance is associated with high ALDH1A1 expression, and it was found that cytoplasmic p63 levels were significantly associated with the frequency of proliferating cells and cells undergoing apoptosis in prostate cancers [51]. These components are suggested to have an important role in prostate cancer progression and may be used as a panel of molecular markers [52].

The aldehyde dehydrogenase enzymes are likely to protect stem cells by detoxification of cell toxic compounds, which indicates that ALDH1 might prevent prostate cancer stem cells from conventional chemotherapy attack, while effective inhibition of ALDH1 could enhance the chemotherapy efficiency. Thus, ALDH1 could not only be used as a prostate cancer stem cell marker for prognosis, but also as a potential drug target in cancer treatment.

6. ATP Binding Membrane Transporters (ABCG2, Also Known as Breast Cancer Resistant Protein or BCRP)

Studies have shown that prostate cancer contains side population cells (SP cells), which could be isolated by flow cytometry techniques based on behavioral characteristics of stem cells. SP cells have stem cell properties that are exclusively mediated by ABCG2. As a result, ABCG2 is considered as a marker of SP cells, as well as a cancer stem cell marker.

ABCG2 is ATP binding membrane transporters, and is related to prostate cancer multi-drug resistance [10]. After castration, ABCG2+/AR− prostate cancer stem cells could be isolated from prostate cancer tissues, and it is suggested that ABCG2 expression might protect prostate cancer stem cells from castration, chemotherapy and hypoxic environment. ABCG2 has been suggested as a biomarker for treatments targeting on prostate cancer stem cells [53]. Interestingly, Patrswala et al. [54] found that ABCG2(+) cells could produce ABCG2(−) cells, and both types of cells have similar tumorigenicity and colony formation ability. 30% of human cancer cell lines (and more in the bone marrow) and xenografts contain 0.04% to 0.20% of SP cells (low but detectable), yet most of the primary tumor cells have only a very small portion of the SP cells, almost impossible to detect [55,56]. Giving the evidence that non-recurrent PCa samples presented relatively lower level of ABCG2, compared to both normal tissue and recurrent samples, it might be associated with chemo-sensitivity [57]. Whether ABCG2 could be used as a specific biomarker in PCa diagnosis and prognosis is still unclear and requires further research.

7. SOX2 and EZH2

SOX2 and EZH2 are essential for the development of human embryonic stem cells. SOX2 is a transcription factor and plays a key role in maintaining undifferentiated status and keeping self-renewal ability of embryonic stem cells [58]. EZH2 is critical for embryonic stem cells rebuilding and embryonic development. Studies show that they play a key role in prostate cancer stem cells [32]. Recently, SOX2 and EZH2 are also suggested as markers in malignant glioma patients [59]. Ugolkov et al. [32] analyzed expression of CD44, CD133, Oct4, SOX2 and EZH2 in benign prostate tissues, high grade prostatic intraepithelial neoplasia (HGPIN) and PCa tissues, and found that EZH2 and SOX2 were expressed in <10% of benign prostate tissue, HGPINs and prostate cancer. In addition, 82% (27/33) of SOX2+ prostate cancer cases were EZH2+ type, and 100% (33/33) of cases were $CD44^+$. On the other hand, CD44 was found in 97% of benign prostate and HGPIN cases, and in 72% of prostate cancer cases. CD133 was found in only a small portion of PCa tissues (6%, 4/67). Oct4 expression was found to be closely correlated with benign and HGPIN, but not with PCa. It is believed that CD44 and Oct4 were expressed in most of benign and malignant prostate cells, which is not likely to be representative for a very small proportion of cancer cells (such as cancer stem cells).

8. CD166

CD166 is a newly discovered molecular surface marker of prostate cancer stem cells [60]. CD166 belongs to the Ig family of type I transmembrane proteins, which mediate cell-cell interactions, and have been used as prognostic markers for a variety of cancers [1]. CD166 was reported to enrich sphere-forming activity of WT LSC (hi) and Pten null LSC (hi), and enhance the sphere-forming ability of benign primary human prostate cells in vitro and induce the formation of tubule-like structures in vivo [60]. CD166 could be used to identify and isolate human, murine prostate cancer stem cells and hormone refractory prostate cancer [61]. CD166 protein level is upregulated in human PCa, especially in CRPC patients. Although genetic deletion of murine CD166 in the Pten null PCa model does not interfere with sphere formation or block prostate cancer progression and CRPC development, the presence of CD166 on prostate stem/progenitors and castration resistant sub-population of cells suggest that it could be a surface marker of cell stemness. It could be a potential therapeutic target for prostate cancer therapies, as reduced expression of CD166 might be able to interfere or reverse prostate cancer metastasis.

9. cPAcP

cPAcP is a prostate specific differentiation antigen. In PCa cells, decreased cPAcP expression is associated with androgen-independent cell proliferation and tumorigenicity as seen in advanced hormone-refractory prostate carcinomas [62]. It was demonstrated that HDAC inhibitor treatment could result in increased cPAcP protein level in cPAcP positive cells, increase androgen responsiveness, and exhibit higher inhibitory activities on AR/cPAcP-positive PCa cells than on AR/cPAcP-negative PCa cells. These data indicate that cPAcP has potential clinical importance serving as a useful biomarker in the identification of PCa patient sub-population suitable for HDAC inhibitor treatment [63,64].

10. Hepatocyte Growth Factor

It was found that prostate cancer stem-like cells (CSCs)/cancer initiating cells (CICs) express hepatocyte growth factor (HGF) and that the HGF/c-MET proto-oncogene product (c-MET) signal has a role in the maintenance of prostate CSCs/CICs in an autocrine fashion. Immunohistochemical staining of HGF was compared to biochemical recurrence after radical prostatectomy, and patients with PCa tumors exhibiting HGF positivity of 5% or more had a significantly shorter biochemical recurrence-free period than that of patients whose tumor HGF positivity was less than 5% ($p = 0.001$). In multivariate Cox regression, preoperative PSA and HGF positivity had the potential to be independent predictors of biochemical recurrence following prostatectomy [65].

11. Tumor-Associated Calcium Signal Transducer 2

Tumor-associated calcium signal transducer 2 (also known as Trop2) is a type I membrane glycoprotein which transduces intracellular calcium signal and acts as a cell surface receptor [66,67]. Trop2 is highly expressed in epithelial related cancers, and its protein level often correlates with poor prognosis [68–73]. Trop2 positive cells could be identified as a subpopulation of prostate basal cells with stem cell characteristics, and it has been used as an effective marker for isolation of basal prostate progenitor cells [74–76]. In prostate cancer, scientists discovered that Trop2 regulate cancer cell proliferation, self-renewal, cell-cell adhesion and metastasis through β-catenin and β1-integrin signaling pathways [77–79]. Interestingly, Trop2 expression in prostate cancer cells was regulated by energy restriction, glucose deprivation and methylation [80–82], making it a potential drug target in cancer treatment. Moreover, anti-Trop2 bispecific antibody was approved to effectively lead pre-targeted immunoPET and radioimmunotherapy of PCa in preclinical models, which significantly increased PCa related survival [83,84].

12. CD117

CD117 (also known as c-Kit) is a receptor tyrosine kinase protein, and has been used as an important cell surface marker to identify hematopoietic progenitors in bone marrow [85–87]. CD117 overexpression was observed in several types of solid tumors including prostate [88,89], and is correlated with the capacity of cell self-renewal and cancer progression [90,91]. Circulating CD117 positive cell percentage is correlated with cancer progression and PSA values in advanced PCa [92]. CD117 could be activated by its ligand, Stem Cell Factor (SCF), to promote bone marrow cell migration, tumor dissemination and potential bone metastasis [91–94].

13. AR Splice Variants

AR splice variants were found to promote EMT as well as induce the expression of stem cell signature genes [95]. Over 10 different AR splice variants were discovered in PCa cell lines, PCa xenografts and human patient samples, and a few of them were dissected to understand their functions in cancer progression [96–103]. More importantly, AR splice variants, such as AR-V7, were suggested to contribute to the drug resistance after suppression of AR signaling, especially in CRPCs [104,105]. High level of AR-V7 was observed in CRPC specimen, but rarely in hormone-naïve specimen [102]. It was suggested that transition from negative to positive status of AR-V7 might reflect the selective pressures on tumor, which makes it a dynamic marker for PCa diagnosis based on liquid biopsy samples, such as circulating tumor cells (CTC) [106].

14. TGM2

Transglutaminases are enzymes that catalyze the crosslinking of proteins by epsilon-γ glutamyl lysine isopeptide bonds. While the primary structure of transglutaminases is not conserved, they all have the same amino acid sequence at their active sites and their activity is calcium-dependent. The protein encoded by this gene acts as a monomer, is induced by retinoic acid, and appears to be involved in apoptosis. TGM2 expression is shown to negatively regulate AR expression and to attenuate androgen sensitivity of prostate cancer cells [107]. TGM2 activation of NF-κB expression induces NF-κB binding to DNA elements in the AR gene to reduce AR gene expression, and triggers epithelial–mesenchymal transition [107]. This suggests that TGM2-regulated inflammatory signaling may contribute to the androgen dependence of prostate cancer cells [107]. Thus, TGM2 is concluded as a cancer stem cell survival factor in various types of cancers, including prostate cancer [108].

15. Conclusions

Studies of prostate cancer stem cells have gained much progress in the past few years and numerous potential approaches were discussed for novel PCa treatment [109,110]. This review summarizes the major intracellular PCa stem cell biomarkers, including a few novel markers discovered recently. The normal or pathological process and potential drug response reflected by those biomarkers were discussed, which might help with early diagnosis, prevention, drug target identification, drug response evaluation and so on. With the progress in study of circulating biomarkers, we expect that more candidates would be identified to facilitate PCa biopsies, especially those soluble markers (circulating tumor cells (CTCs), circulating tumor nucleic acid (ctNAs), miRNA, lncRNA, exosomes, etc.) for liquid biopsies.

Acknowledgments: This work is supported by NIH grant CA079448 to Xiaolan Fang.

References

1. Siegel, R.; Ma, J.; Zou, Z.; Jemal, A. Cancer statistics, 2014. *CA Cancer J. Clin.* **2014**, *64*, 9–29. [CrossRef] [PubMed]
2. Monsef, N.; Soller, M.; Isaksson, M.; Abrahamsson, P.A.; Panagopoulos, I. The expression of pluripotency marker Oct 3/4 in prostate cancer and benign prostate hyperplasia. *Prostate* **2009**, *69*, 909–916. [CrossRef] [PubMed]
3. Attard, G.; Parker, C.; Eeles, R.A.; Schroder, F.; Tomlins, S.A.; Tannock, I.; Drake, C.G.; de Bono, J.S. Prostate Cancer. *Lancet* **2016**, *387*, 70–82. [CrossRef]
4. Zong, Y.; Goldstein, A.S. Adaptation or selection—Mechanisms of castration-resistant prostate cancer. *Nat. Rev. Urol.* **2013**, *10*, 90–98. [CrossRef] [PubMed]
5. Isaacs, J.T.; Coffey, D.S. Adaptation versus selection as the mechanism responsible for the relapse of prostatic cancer to androgen ablation therapy as studied in the Dunning R-3327-H adenocarcinoma. *Cancer Res.* **1981**, *41*, 5070–5075. [PubMed]
6. Blum, R.; Gupta, R.; Burger, P.E.; Ontiveros, C.S.; Salm, S.N.; Xiong, X.; Kamb, A.; Wesche, H.; Marshall, L.; Cutler, G.; et al. Molecular signatures of prostate stem cells reveal novel signaling pathways and provide insights into prostate cancer. *PLoS ONE* **2009**, *4*, e5722. [CrossRef] [PubMed]
7. Lang, S.H.; Frame, F.M.; Collins, A.T. Prostate cancer stem cells. *J. Pathol.* **2009**, *217*, 299–306. [CrossRef] [PubMed]
8. Chen, X.; Rycaj, K.; Liu, X.; Tang, D.G. New insights into prostate cancer stem cells. *Cell Cycle* **2013**, *12*, 579–586. [CrossRef] [PubMed]
9. Rane, J.K.; Pellacani, D.; Maitland, N.J. Advanced prostate cancer—A case for adjuvant differentiation therapy. *Nat. Rev. Urol.* **2012**, *9*, 595–602. [CrossRef] [PubMed]
10. Castillo, V.; Valenzuela, R.; Huidobro, C.; Contreras, H.R.; Castellon, E.A. Functional characteristics of cancer stem cells and their role in drug resistance of prostate cancer. *Int. J. Oncol.* **2014**, *45*, 985–994. [CrossRef] [PubMed]

11. McMillen, P.; Holley, S.A. Integration of cell–cell and cell–ECM adhesion in vertebrate morphogenesis. *Curr. Opin. Cell Biol.* **2015**, *36*, 48–53. [CrossRef] [PubMed]
12. Van Slambrouck, S.; Groux-Degroote, S.; Krzewinski-Recchi, M.A.; Cazet, A.; Delannoy, P.; Steelant, W.F. Carbohydrate-to-carbohydrate interactions between α2,3-linked sialic acids on α2 integrin subunits and asialo-GM1 underlie the bone metastatic behaviour of LNCAP-derivative C4-2B prostate cancer cells. *Biosci. Rep.* **2014**, *34*. [CrossRef] [PubMed]
13. Dedhar, S.; Saulnier, R.; Nagle, R.; Overall, C.M. Specific alterations in the expression of α3β1 and α6β4 integrins in highly invasive and metastatic variants of human prostate carcinoma cells selected by in vitro invasion through reconstituted basement membrane. *Clin. Exp. Metastasis* **1993**, *11*, 391–400. [CrossRef] [PubMed]
14. Hoogland, A.M.; Verhoef, E.I.; Roobol, M.J.; Schroder, F.H.; Wildhagen, M.F.; van der Kwast, T.H.; Jenster, G.; van Leenders, G.J. Validation of stem cell markers in clinical prostate cancer: α 6-integrin is predictive for non-aggressive disease. *Prostate* **2014**, *74*, 488–496. [CrossRef] [PubMed]
15. Collins, A.T.; Habib, F.K.; Maitland, N.J.; Neal, D.E. Identification and isolation of human prostate epithelial stem cells based on $\alpha_2\beta_1$-integrin expression. *J. Cell Sci.* **2001**, *114*, 3865–3872. [PubMed]
16. Fortunel, N.O.; Otu, H.H.; Ng, H.-H.; Chen, J.; Mu, X.; Chevassut, T.; Li, X.; Joseph, M.; Bailey, C.; Hatzfeld, J.A.; et al. Comment on "'Stemness': Transcriptional Profiling of Embryonic and Adult Stem Cells" and "A Stem Cell Molecular Signature" (I). *Science* **2003**, *302*, 393. [CrossRef] [PubMed]
17. Barclay, W.W.; Axanova, L.S.; Chen, W.; Romero, L.; Maund, S.L.; Soker, S.; Lees, C.J.; Cramer, S.D. Characterization of Adult Prostatic Progenitor/Stem Cells Exhibiting Self-Renewal and Multilineage Differentiation. *Stem Cells* **2008**, *26*, 600–610. [CrossRef] [PubMed]
18. Lawson, D.A.; Xin, L.; Lukacs, R.U.; Cheng, D.; Witte, O.N. Isolation and functional characterization of murine prostate stem cells. *Proc. Natl. Acad. Sci. USA* **2007**, *104*, 181–186. [CrossRef] [PubMed]
19. Marthick, J.R.; Dickinson, J.L. Emerging Putative Biomarkers: The Role of α 2 and 6 Integrins in Susceptibility, Treatment, and Prognosis. *Prostate Cancer* **2012**, *2012*, 298732. [CrossRef] [PubMed]
20. Finetti, F.; Terzuoli, E.; Giachetti, A.; Santi, R.; Villari, D.; Hanaka, H.; Radmark, O.; Ziche, M.; Donnini, S. mPGES-1 in prostate cancer controls stemness and amplifies epidermal growth factor receptor-driven oncogenicity. *Endocr. Relat. Cancer* **2015**, *22*, 665–678. [CrossRef] [PubMed]
21. Lokeshwar, B.L.; Lokeshwar, V.B.; Block, N.L. Expression of CD44 in prostate cancer cells: Association with cell proliferation and invasive potential. *Anticancer Res.* **1995**, *15*, 1191–1198. [PubMed]
22. Liu, A.Y. Expression of CD44 in prostate cancer cells. *Cancer Lett.* **1994**, *76*, 63–69. [CrossRef]
23. Collins, A.T.; Berry, P.A.; Hyde, C.; Stower, M.J.; Maitland, N.J. Prospective identification of tumorigenic prostate cancer stem cells. *Cancer Res.* **2005**, *65*, 10946–10951. [CrossRef] [PubMed]
24. Ajani, J.A.; Song, S.; Hochster, H.S.; Steinberg, I.B. Cancer stem cells: The promise and the potential. *Semin. Oncol.* **2015**, *42* (Suppl. S1), S3–S17. [CrossRef] [PubMed]
25. Wang, L.; Huang, X.; Zheng, X.; Wang, X.; Li, S.; Zhang, L.; Yang, Z.; Xia, Z. Enrichment of prostate cancer stem-like cells from human prostate cancer cell lines by culture in serum-free medium and chemoradiotherapy. *Int. J. Biol. Sci.* **2013**, *9*, 472–479. [CrossRef] [PubMed]
26. Yu, J.; Lu, Y.; Cui, D.; Li, E.; Zhu, Y.; Zhao, Y.; Zhao, F.; Xia, S. miR-200b suppresses cell proliferation, migration and enhances chemosensitivity in prostate cancer by regulating Bmi-1. *Oncol. Rep.* **2014**, *31*, 910–918. [PubMed]
27. Ibuki, N.; Ghaffari, M.; Pandey, M.; Iu, I.; Fazli, L.; Kashiwagi, M.; Tojo, H.; Nakanishi, O.; Gleave, M.E.; Cox, M.E. TAK-441, a novel investigational smoothened antagonist, delays castration-resistant progression in prostate cancer by disrupting paracrine hedgehog signaling. *Int. J. Cancer.* **2013**, *133*, 1955–1966. [CrossRef] [PubMed]
28. Kasper, S. Identification, characterization, and biological relevance of prostate cancer stem cells from clinical specimens. *Urol. Oncol.* **2009**, *27*, 301–303. [CrossRef] [PubMed]
29. Van Leenders, G.J.; Schalken, J.A. Stem cell differentiation within the human prostate epithelium: Implications for prostate carcinogenesis. *BJU Int.* **2001**, *88* (Suppl. S2), 35–42. [CrossRef] [PubMed]
30. Korski, K.; Malicka-Durczak, A.; Breborowicz, J. Expression of stem cell marker CD44 in prostate cancer biopsies predicts cancer grade in radical prostatectomy specimens. *Pol. J. Pathol.* **2014**, *65*, 291–295. [CrossRef] [PubMed]

31. Liu, C.; Kelnar, K.; Liu, B.; Chen, X.; Calhoun-Davis, T.; Li, H.; Patrawala, L.; Yan, H.; Jeter, C.; Honorio, S.; et al. The microRNA miR-34a inhibits prostate cancer stem cells and metastasis by directly repressing CD44. *Nat. Med.* **2011**, *17*, 211–215. [CrossRef] [PubMed]
32. Ugolkov, A.V.; Eisengart, L.J.; Luan, C.; Yang, X.J. Expression analysis of putative stem cell markers in human benign and malignant prostate. *Prostate* **2011**, *71*, 18–25. [CrossRef] [PubMed]
33. Moura, C.M.; Pontes, J.; Reis, S.T.; Viana, N.I.; Morais, D.R.; Dip, N.; Katz, B.; Srougi, M.; Leite, K.R.M. Expression profile of standard and variants forms of CD44 related to prostate cancer behavior. *Int. J. Biol. Markers* **2015**, *30*, e49–e55. [CrossRef] [PubMed]
34. Tei, H.; Miyake, H.; Harada, K.-I.; Fujisawa, M. Expression profile of CD44s, CD44v6, and CD44v10 in localized prostate cancer: Effect on prognostic outcomes following radical prostatectomy. *Urol. Oncol. Semin. Orig. Investig.* **2014**, *32*, 694–700. [CrossRef] [PubMed]
35. Ni, J.; Cozzi, P.J.; Hao, J.L.; Beretov, J.; Chang, L.; Duan, W.; Shigdar, S.; Delprado, W.J.; Graham, P.H.; Bucci, J.; et al. CD44 variant 6 is associated with prostate cancer metastasis and chemo-/radioresistance. *Prostate* **2014**, *74*, 602–617. [CrossRef] [PubMed]
36. Yang, K.; Tang, Y.; Habermehl, G.K.; Iczkowski, K.A. Stable alterations of CD44 isoform expression in prostate cancer cells decrease invasion and growth and alter ligand binding and chemosensitivity. *BMC Cancer* **2010**, *10*, 16. [CrossRef] [PubMed]
37. Choy, W.; Nagasawa, D.T.; Trang, A.; Thill, K.; Spasic, M.; Yang, I. CD133 as a marker for regulation and potential for targeted therapies in glioblastoma multiforme. *Neurosurg. Clin. N. Am.* **2012**, *23*, 391–405. [CrossRef] [PubMed]
38. Islam, F.; Gopalan, V.; Wahab, R.; Smith, R.A.; Lam, A.K. Cancer stem cells in oesophageal squamous cell carcinoma: Identification, prognostic and treatment perspectives. *Crit. Rev. Oncol./Hematol.* **2015**, *96*, 9–19. [CrossRef] [PubMed]
39. Zhou, Q.; Chen, A.; Song, H.; Tao, J.; Yang, H.; Zuo, M. Prognostic value of cancer stem cell marker CD133 in ovarian cancer: A meta-analysis. *Int. J. Clin. Exp. Med.* **2015**, *8*, 3080–3088. [PubMed]
40. Han, G.W.; Yi, S.H. Prostate stem cells: An update. *Zhonghua Nan Ke Xue* **2014**, *20*, 460–463. [PubMed]
41. Zenzmaier, C.; Untergasser, G.; Berger, P. Aging of the prostate epithelial stem/progenitor cell. *Exp. Gerontol.* **2008**, *43*, 981–985. [CrossRef] [PubMed]
42. Missol-Kolka, E.; Karbanova, J.; Janich, P.; Haase, M.; Fargeas, C.A.; Huttner, W.B.; Corbeil, D. Prominin-1 (CD133) is not restricted to stem cells located in the basal compartment of murine and human prostate. *Prostate* **2011**, *71*, 254–267. [CrossRef] [PubMed]
43. Hsu, W.T.; Jui, H.Y.; Huang, Y.H.; Su, M.Y.; Wu, Y.W.; Tseng, W.Y.; Hsu, M.C.; Chiang, B.L.; Wu, K.K.; Lee, C.M. CXCR4 Antagonist TG-0054 Mobilizes Mesenchymal Stem Cells, Attenuates Inflammation, and Preserves Cardiac Systolic Function in a Porcine Model of Myocardial Infarction. *Cell Transplant.* **2015**, *24*, 1313–1328. [CrossRef] [PubMed]
44. Trerotola, M.; Rathore, S.; Goel, H.L.; Li, J.; Alberti, S.; Piantelli, M.; Adams, D.; Jiang, Z.; Languino, L.R. CD133, Trop-2 and $\alpha 2\beta 1$ integrin surface receptors as markers of putative human prostate cancer stem cells. *Am. J. Transl. Res.* **2010**, *2*, 135–144. [PubMed]
45. Taylor, R.A.; Toivanen, R.; Frydenberg, M.; Pedersen, J.; Harewood, L.; Australian Prostate Cancer Bioresource; Collins, A.T.; Maitland, N.J.; Risbridger, G.P. Human epithelial basal cells are cells of origin of prostate cancer, independent of CD133 status. *Stem Cells* **2012**, *30*, 1087–1096. [CrossRef] [PubMed]
46. Liu, J.F.; Xia, P.; Hu, W.Q.; Wang, D.; Xu, X.Y. Aldehyde dehydrogenase 1 expression correlates with clinicopathologic features of patients with breast cancer: A meta-analysis. *Int. J. Clinl. Exp. Med.* **2015**, *8*, 8425–8432.
47. Schnier, J.B.; Kaur, G.; Kaiser, A.; Stinson, S.F.; Sausville, E.A.; Gardner, J.; Nishi, K.; Bradbury, E.M.; Senderowicz, A.M. Identification of cytosolic aldehyde dehydrogenase 1 from non-small cell lung carcinomas as a flavopiridol-binding protein. *FEBS Lett.* **1999**, *454*, 100–104. [CrossRef]
48. Li, T.; Su, Y.; Mei, Y.; Leng, Q.; Leng, B.; Liu, Z.; Stass, S.A.; Jiang, F. ALDH1A1 is a marker for malignant prostate stem cells and predictor of prostate cancer patients' outcome. *Lab. Investig. J. Tech. Methods Pathol.* **2010**, *90*, 234–244. [CrossRef] [PubMed]
49. Burger, P.E.; Gupta, R.; Xiong, X.; Ontiveros, C.S.; Salm, S.N.; Moscatelli, D.; Wilson, E.L. High aldehyde dehydrogenase activity: A novel functional marker of murine prostate stem/progenitor cells. *Stem Cells* **2009**, *27*, 2220–2228. [CrossRef] [PubMed]

50. Wang, G.; Wang, Z.; Sarkar, F.H.; Wei, W. Targeting prostate cancer stem cells for cancer therapy. *Discov. Med.* **2012**, *13*, 135–142. [PubMed]
51. Gangavarapu, K.J.; Azabdaftari, G.; Morrison, C.D.; Miller, A.; Foster, B.A.; Huss, W.J. Aldehyde dehydrogenase and ATP binding cassette transporter G2 (ABCG2) functional assays isolate different populations of prostate stem cells where ABCG2 function selects for cells with increased stem cell activity. *Stem Cell Res. Ther.* **2013**, *4*, 132. [CrossRef] [PubMed]
52. Ferronika, P.; Triningsih, F.X.; Ghozali, A.; Moeljono, A.; Rahmayanti, S.; Shadrina, A.N.; Naim, A.E.; Wudexi, I.; Arnurisa, A.M.; Nanwani, S.T.; et al. p63 cytoplasmic aberrance is associated with high prostate cancer stem cell expression. *Asian Pac. J. Cancer Prev. (APJCP)* **2012**, *13*, 1943–1948. [CrossRef] [PubMed]
53. An, Y.; Ongkeko, W.M. ABCG2: The key to chemoresistance in cancer stem cells? *Expert Opin. Drug Metab. Toxicol.* **2009**, *5*, 1529–1542. [CrossRef] [PubMed]
54. Patrawala, L.; Calhoun, T.; Schneider-Broussard, R.; Zhou, J.; Claypool, K.; Tang, D.G. Side population is enriched in tumorigenic, stem-like cancer cells, whereas $ABCG2^+$ and $ABCG2^-$ cancer cells are similarly tumorigenic. *Cancer Res.* **2005**, *65*, 6207–6219. [CrossRef] [PubMed]
55. Kim, H.A.; Kim, M.C.; Kim, N.Y.; Kim, Y. Inhibition of hedgehog signaling reduces the side population in human malignant mesothelioma cell lines. *Cancer Gene Ther.* **2015**, *22*, 387–395. [CrossRef] [PubMed]
56. Gao, G.; Sun, Z.; Wenyong, L.; Dongxia, Y.; Zhao, R.; Zhang, X. A preliminary study of side population cells in human gastric cancer cell line HGC-27. *Ann. Transplant. Q. Pol. Transplant. Soc.* **2015**, *20*, 147–153.
57. Guzel, E.; Karatas, O.F.; Duz, M.B.; Solak, M.; Ittmann, M.; Ozen, M. Differential expression of stem cell markers and ABCG2 in recurrent prostate cancer. *Prostate* **2014**, *74*, 1498–1505. [CrossRef] [PubMed]
58. Fu, T.Y.; Hsieh, I.C.; Cheng, J.T.; Tsai, M.H.; Hou, Y.Y.; Lee, J.H.; Liou, H.H.; Huang, S.F.; Chen, H.C.; Yen, L.M.; et al. Association of OCT4, SOX2, and NANOG expression with oral squamous cell carcinoma progression. *J. Oral Pathol. Med.* **2015**, *45*, 89–95. [CrossRef] [PubMed]
59. Li, A.M.; Dunham, C.; Tabori, U.; Carret, A.S.; McNeely, P.D.; Johnston, D.; Lafay-Cousin, L.; Wilson, B.; Eisenstat, D.D.; Jabado, N.; et al. EZH2 expression is a prognostic factor in childhood intracranial ependymoma: A Canadian Pediatric Brain Tumor Consortium study. *Cancer* **2015**, *121*, 1499–1507. [CrossRef] [PubMed]
60. Jiao, J.; Hindoyan, A.; Wang, S.; Tran, L.M.; Goldstein, A.S.; Lawson, D.; Chen, D.; Li, Y.; Guo, C.; Zhang, B.; et al. Identification of CD166 as a surface marker for enriching prostate stem/progenitor and cancer initiating cells. *PLoS ONE* **2012**, *7*, e42564. [CrossRef] [PubMed]
61. Rowehl, R.A.; Crawford, H.; Dufour, A.; Ju, J.; Botchkina, G.I. Genomic analysis of prostate cancer stem cells isolated from a highly metastatic cell line. *Cancer Genom. Proteom.* **2008**, *5*, 301–310.
62. Chuang, T.-D.; Chen, S.-J.; Lin, F.-F.; Veeramani, S.; Kumar, S.; Batra, S.K.; Tu, Y.; Lin, M.-F. Human Prostatic Acid Phosphatase, an Authentic Tyrosine Phosphatase, Dephosphorylates ErbB-2 and Regulates Prostate Cancer Cell Growth. *J. Biol. Chem.* **2010**, *285*, 23598–23606. [CrossRef] [PubMed]
63. Chou, Y.W.; Lin, F.F.; Muniyan, S.; Lin, F.C.; Chen, C.S.; Wang, J.; Huang, C.C.; Lin, M.F. Cellular prostatic acid phosphatase (cPAcP) serves as a useful biomarker of histone deacetylase (HDAC) inhibitors in prostate cancer cell growth suppression. *Cell Biosci.* **2015**, *5*, 38. [CrossRef] [PubMed]
64. Chou, Y.W.; Chaturvedi, N.K.; Ouyang, S.; Lin, F.F.; Kaushik, D.; Wang, J.; Kim, I.; Lin, M.F. Histone deacetylase inhibitor valproic acid suppresses the growth and increases the androgen responsiveness of prostate cancer cells. *Cancer Lett.* **2011**, *311*, 177–186. [CrossRef] [PubMed]
65. Nishida, S.; Hirohashi, Y.; Torigoe, T.; Nojima, M.; Inoue, R.; Kitamura, H.; Tanaka, T.; Asanuma, H.; Sato, N.; Masumori, N. Expression of hepatocyte growth factor in prostate cancer may indicate a biochemical recurrence after radical prostatectomy. *Anticancer Res.* **2015**, *35*, 413–418. [CrossRef]
66. Fornaro, M.; Dell'Arciprete, R.; Stella, M.; Bucci, C.; Nutini, M.; Capri, M.G.; Alberti, S. Cloning of the gene encoding Trop-2, a cell-surface glycoprotein expressed by human carcinomas. *Int. J. Cancer* **1995**, *62*, 610–618. [CrossRef] [PubMed]
67. Ripani, E.; Sacchetti, A.; Corda, D.; Alberti, S. Human Trop-2 is a tumor-associated calcium signal transducer. *Int. J. Cancer* **1998**, *76*, 671–676. [CrossRef]
68. Mühlmann, G.; Spizzo, G.; Gostner, J.; Zitt, M.; Maier, H.; Moser, P.; Gastl, G.; Müller, H.M.; Margreiter, R.; Öfner, D.; et al. TROP2 expression as prognostic marker for gastric carcinoma. *J. Clin. Pathol.* **2009**, *62*, 152–158. [CrossRef] [PubMed]

69. Fang, Y.J.; Lu, Z.H.; Wang, G.Q.; Pan, Z.Z.; Zhou, Z.W.; Yun, J.P.; Zhang, M.F.; Wan, D.S. Elevated expressions of MMP7, TROP2, and survivin are associated with survival, disease recurrence, and liver metastasis of colon cancer. *Int. J. Colorectal. Dis.* **2009**, *24*, 875–884. [CrossRef] [PubMed]
70. Nakashima, K.; Shimada, H.; Ochiai, T.; Kuboshima, M.; Kuroiwa, N.; Okazumi, S.; Matsubara, H.; Nomura, F.; Takiguchi, M.; Hiwasa, T. Serological identification of TROP2 by recombinant cDNA expression cloning using sera of patients with esophageal squamous cell carcinoma. *Int. J. Cancer* **2004**, *112*, 1029–1035. [CrossRef] [PubMed]
71. Ohmachi, T.; Tanaka, F.; Mimori, K.; Inoue, H.; Yanaga, K.; Mori, M. Clinical Significance of TROP2 Expression in Colorectal Cancer. *Clin. Cancer Res.* **2006**, *12*, 3057–3063. [CrossRef] [PubMed]
72. Fong, D.; Moser, P.; Krammel, C.; Gostner, J.M.; Margreiter, R.; Mitterer, M.; Gastl, G.; Spizzo, G. High expression of TROP2 correlates with poor prognosis in pancreatic cancer. *Br. J. Cancer* **2008**, *99*, 1290–1295. [CrossRef] [PubMed]
73. Köbel, M.; Kalloger, S.E.; Boyd, N.; McKinney, S.; Mehl, E.; Palmer, C.; Leung, S.; Bowen, N.J.; Ionescu, D.N.; Rajput, A.; et al. Ovarian carcinoma subtypes are different diseases: Implications for biomarker studies. *PLoS Med.* **2008**, *5*, e232. [CrossRef] [PubMed]
74. Höfner, T.; Eisen, C.; Klein, C.; Rigo-Watermeier, T.; Goeppinger, S.M.; Jauch, A.; Schoell, B.; Vogel, V.; Noll, E.; Weichert, W.; et al. Defined Conditions for the Isolation and Expansion of Basal Prostate Progenitor Cells of Mouse and Human Origin. *Stem Cell Rep.* **2015**, *4*, 503–518. [CrossRef] [PubMed]
75. Goldstein, A.S.; Lawson, D.A.; Cheng, D.; Sun, W.; Garraway, I.P.; Witte, O.N. Trop2 identifies a subpopulation of murine and human prostate basal cells with stem cell characteristics. *Proc. Natl. Acad. Sci. USA* **2008**, *105*, 20882–20887. [CrossRef] [PubMed]
76. Fedr, R.; Pernicová, Z.; Slabáková, E.; Straková, N.; Bouchal, J.; Grepl, M.; Kozubík, A.; Souček, K. Automatic cell cloning assay for determining the clonogenic capacity of cancer and cancer stem-like cells. *Cytom. A* **2013**, *83*, 472–482. [CrossRef] [PubMed]
77. Stoyanova, T.; Goldstein, A.S.; Cai, H.; Drake, J.M.; Huang, J.; Witte, O.N. Regulated proteolysis of Trop2 drives epithelial hyperplasia and stem cell self-renewal via β-catenin signaling. *Genes Dev.* **2012**, *26*, 2271–2285. [CrossRef] [PubMed]
78. Trerotola, M.; Jernigan, D.L.; Liu, Q.; Siddiqui, J.; Fatatis, A.; Languino, L.R. Trop-2 promotes prostate cancer metastasis by modulating β_1 integrin functions. *Cancer Res.* **2013**, *73*, 3155–3167. [CrossRef] [PubMed]
79. Trerotola, M.; Li, J.; Alberti, S.; Languino, L.R. Trop-2 inhibits prostate cancer cell adhesion to fibronectin through the β1 integrin-RACK1 axis. *J. Cell. Physiol.* **2012**, *227*, 3670–3677. [CrossRef] [PubMed]
80. Ibragimova, I.; de Cáceres, I.I.; Hoffman, A.M.; Potapova, A.; Dulaimi, E.; Al-Saleem, T.; Hudes, G.R.; Ochs, M.F.; Cairns, P. Global Reactivation of Epigenetically Silenced Genes in Prostate Cancer. *Cancer Prev. Res.* **2010**, *3*, 1084–1092. [CrossRef] [PubMed]
81. Jerónimo, C.; Esteller, M. DNA Methylation Markers for Prostate Cancer with a Stem Cell Twist. *Cancer Prev. Res.* **2010**, *3*, 1053–1055. [CrossRef] [PubMed]
82. Lin, H.-Y.; Kuo, Y.-C.; Weng, Y.-I.; Lai, I.L.; Huang, T.H.M.; Lin, S.-P.; Niu, D.-M.; Chen, C.-S. Activation of Silenced Tumor Suppressor Genes in Prostate Cancer Cells by a Novel Energy Restriction-Mimetic Agent. *Prostate* **2012**, *72*. [CrossRef] [PubMed]
83. Van Rij, C.M.; Frielink, C.; Goldenberg, D.M.; Sharkey, R.M.; Lutje, S.; McBride, W.J.; Oyen, W.J.; Boerman, O.C. Pretargeted Radioimmunotherapy of Prostate Cancer with an Anti-TROP-2× Anti-HSG Bispecific Antibody and a ^{177}Lu-Labeled Peptide. *Cancer Biother. Radiopharm.* **2014**, *29*, 323–329. [CrossRef] [PubMed]
84. Van Rij, C.M.; Lutje, S.; Frielink, C.; Sharkey, R.M.; Goldenberg, D.M.; Franssen, G.M.; McBride, W.J.; Rossi, E.A.; Oyen, W.J.; Boerman, O.C. Pretargeted immuno-PET and radioimmunotherapy of prostate cancer with an anti-TROP-2× anti-HSG bispecific antibody. *Eur. J. Nucl. Med. Mol. Imaging* **2013**, *40*, 1377–1383. [CrossRef] [PubMed]
85. Yarden, Y.; Kuang, W.J.; Yang-Feng, T.; Coussens, L.; Munemitsu, S.; Dull, T.J.; Chen, E.; Schlessinger, J.; Francke, U.; Ullrich, A. Human proto-oncogene c-kit: A new cell surface receptor tyrosine kinase for an unidentified ligand. *EMBO J.* **1987**, *6*, 3341–3351. [PubMed]
86. Matthews, W.; Jordan, C.T.; Wiegand, G.W.; Pardoll, D.; Lemischka, I.R. A receptor tyrosine kinase specific to hematopoietic stem and progenitor cell-enriched populations. *Cell* **1991**, *65*, 1143–1152. [CrossRef]

87. Broxmeyer, H.E.; Maze, R.; Miyazawa, K.; Carow, C.; Hendrie, P.C.; Cooper, S.; Hangoc, G.; Vadhan-Raj, S.; Lu, L. The kit receptor and its ligand, steel factor, as regulators of hemopoiesis. *Cancer Cells* **1991**, *3*, 480–487. [PubMed]
88. Chi, P.; Chen, Y.; Zhang, L.; Guo, X.; Wongvipat, J.; Shamu, T.; Fletcher, J.A.; Dewell, S.; Maki, R.G.; Zheng, D.; et al. ETV1 is a lineage-specific survival factor in GIST and cooperates with KIT in oncogenesis. *Nature* **2010**, *467*, 849–853. [CrossRef] [PubMed]
89. Di Lorenzo, G.; Autorino, R.; D'Armiento, F.P.; Mignogna, C.; de Laurentiis, M.; de Sio, M.; D'Armiento, M.; Damiano, R.; Vecchio, G.; de Placido, S. Expression of proto-oncogene c-kit in high risk prostate cancer. *Eur. J. Surg. Oncol.* **2004**, *30*, 987–992. [CrossRef] [PubMed]
90. Leong, K.G.; Wang, B.E.; Johnson, L.; Gao, W.Q. Generation of a prostate from a single adult stem cell. *Nature* **2008**, *456*, 804–808. [CrossRef] [PubMed]
91. Wiesner, C.; Nabha, S.M.; Dos Santos, E.B.; Yamamoto, H.; Meng, H.; Melchior, S.W.; Bittinger, F.; Thüroff, J.W.; Vessella, R.L.; Cher, M.L.; et al. C-Kit and Its Ligand Stem Cell Factor: Potential Contribution to Prostate Cancer Bone Metastasis. *Neoplasia* **2008**, *10*, 996–1003. [CrossRef] [PubMed]
92. Kerr, B.A.; Miocinovic, R.; Smith, A.K.; West, X.Z.; Watts, K.E.; Alzayed, A.W.; Klink, J.C.; Mir, M.C.; Sturey, T.; Hansel, D.E.; et al. $CD117^+$ cells in the circulation are predictive of advanced prostate cancer. *Oncotarget* **2015**, *6*, 1889–1897. [CrossRef] [PubMed]
93. Okumura, N.; Tsuji, K.; Ebihara, Y.; Tanaka, I.; Sawai, N.; Koike, K.; Komiyama, A.; Nakahata, T. Chemotactic and chemokinetic activities of stem cell factor on murine hematopoietic progenitor cells. *Blood* **1996**, *87*, 4100–4108. [PubMed]
94. Blume-Jensen, P.; Claesson-Welsh, L.; Siegbahn, A.; Zsebo, K.M.; Westermark, B.; Heldin, C.H. Activation of the human c-kit product by ligand-induced dimerization mediates circular actin reorganization and chemotaxis. *EMBO J.* **1991**, *10*, 4121–4128. [PubMed]
95. Kong, D.; Sethi, S.; Li, Y.; Chen, W.; Sakr, W.A.; Heath, E.; Sarkar, F.H. Androgen receptor splice variants contribute to prostate cancer aggressiveness through induction of EMT and expression of stem cell marker genes. *Prostate* **2015**, *75*, 161–174. [CrossRef] [PubMed]
96. Guo, Z.; Yang, X.; Sun, F.; Jiang, R.; Linn, D.E.; Chen, H.; Chen, H.; Kong, X.; Melamed, J.; Tepper, C.G.; et al. A novel androgen receptor splice variant is up-regulated during prostate cancer progression and promotes androgen depletion–resistant growth. *Cancer Res.* **2009**, *69*, 2305–2313. [CrossRef] [PubMed]
97. Marcias, G.; Erdmann, E.; Lapouge, G.; Siebert, C.; Barthélémy, P.; Duclos, B.; Bergerat, J.-P.; Céraline, J.; Kurtz, J.-E. Identification of novel truncated androgen receptor (AR) mutants including unreported pre-mRNA splicing variants in the 22Rv1 hormone-refractory prostate cancer (PCa) cell line. *Hum. Mutat.* **2010**, *31*, 74–80. [CrossRef] [PubMed]
98. Sun, S.; Sprenger, C.C.T.; Vessella, R.L.; Haugk, K.; Soriano, K.; Mostaghel, E.A.; Page, S.T.; Coleman, I.M.; Nguyen, H.M.; Sun, H.; et al. Castration resistance in human prostate cancer is conferred by a frequently occurring androgen receptor splice variant. *J. Clin. Investig.* **2010**, *120*, 2715–2730. [CrossRef] [PubMed]
99. Hu, R.; Isaacs, W.B.; Luo, J. A snapshot of the expression signature of androgen receptor splicing variants and their distinctive transcriptional activities. *Prostate* **2011**, *71*, 1656–1667. [CrossRef] [PubMed]
100. Watson, P.A.; Chen, Y.F.; Balbas, M.D.; Wongvipat, J.; Socci, N.D.; Viale, A.; Kim, K.; Sawyers, C.L. Constitutively active androgen receptor splice variants expressed in castration-resistant prostate cancer require full-length androgen receptor. *Proc. Natl. Acad. Sci. USA* **2010**, *107*, 16759–16765. [CrossRef] [PubMed]
101. Dehm, S.M.; Schmidt, L.J.; Heemers, H.V.; Vessella, R.L.; Tindall, D.J. Splicing of a Novel Androgen Receptor Exon Generates a Constitutively Active Androgen Receptor that Mediates Prostate Cancer Therapy Resistance. *Cancer Res.* **2008**, *68*, 5469–5477. [CrossRef] [PubMed]
102. Hu, R.; Dunn, T.A.; Wei, S.; Isharwal, S.; Veltri, R.W.; Humphreys, E.; Han, M.; Partin, A.W.; Vessella, R.L.; Isaacs, W.B.; et al. Ligand-Independent Androgen Receptor Variants Derived from Splicing of Cryptic Exons Signify Hormone-Refractory Prostate Cancer. *Cancer Res.* **2009**, *69*, 16–22. [CrossRef] [PubMed]
103. Dehm, S.M.; Tindall, D.J. Alternatively spliced androgen receptor variants. *Endocr. Relat. Cancer* **2011**, *18*, R183–R196. [CrossRef] [PubMed]
104. Nakazawa, M.; Antonarakis, E.; Luo, J. Androgen Receptor Splice Variants in the Era of Enzalutamide and Abiraterone. *Horm. Cancer* **2014**, *5*, 265–273. [CrossRef] [PubMed]

105. Onstenk, W.; Sieuwerts, A.M.; Kraan, J.; van, M.; Nieuweboer, A.J.M.; Mathijssen, R.H.J.; Hamberg, P.; Meulenbeld, H.J.; de Laere, B.; Dirix, L.Y.; et al. Efficacy of cabazitaxel in castration-resistant prostate cancer is independent of the presence of AR-V7 in circulating tumor cells. *Eur. Urol.* **2015**, *68*, 939–945. [CrossRef] [PubMed]
106. Nakazawa, M.; Lu, C.; Chen, Y.; Paller, C.J.; Carducci, M.A.; Eisenberger, M.A.; Luo, J.; Antonarakis, E.S. Serial blood-based analysis of AR-V7 in men with advanced prostate cancer. *Ann. Oncol.* **2015**. [CrossRef] [PubMed]
107. Han, A.L.; Kumar, S.; Fok, J.Y.; Tyagi, A.K.; Mehta, K. Tissue transglutaminase expression promotes castration-resistant phenotype and transcriptional repression of androgen receptor. *Eur. J. Cancer* **2014**, *50*, 1685–1696. [CrossRef] [PubMed]
108. Eckert, R.L.; Fisher, M.L.; Grun, D.; Adhikary, G.; Xu, W.; Kerr, C. Transglutaminase is a tumor cell and cancer stem cell survival factor. *Mol. Carcinog.* **2015**, *54*, 947–958. [CrossRef] [PubMed]
109. Mayer, M.J.; Klotz, L.H.; Venkateswaran, V. Metformin and prostate cancer stem cells: A novel therapeutic target. *Prostate Cancer Prostatic Dis.* **2015**, *18*, 303–309. [CrossRef] [PubMed]
110. Yu, V.Y.; Nguyen, D.; Pajonk, F.; Kupelian, P.; Kaprealian, T.; Selch, M.; Low, D.A.; Sheng, K. Incorporating cancer stem cells in radiation therapy treatment response modeling and the implication in glioblastoma multiforme treatment resistance. *Int. J. Radiat. Oncol. Biol. Phys.* **2015**, *91*, 866–875. [CrossRef] [PubMed]

6

Prostate Specific Antigen (PSA) as Predicting Marker for Clinical Outcome and Evaluation of Early Toxicity Rate after High-Dose Rate Brachytherapy (HDR-BT) in Combination with Additional External Beam Radiation Therapy (EBRT) for High Risk Prostate Cancer

Thorsten H. Ecke [1,*], Hui-Juan Huang-Tiel [2], Klaus Golka [3], Silvia Selinski [3], Berit Christine Geis [3], Stephan Koswig [4], Katrin Bathe [4], Steffen Hallmann [1] and Holger Gerullis [5]

1 Department of Urology, HELIOS Hospital, D-15526 Bad Saarow, Germany; steffen.hallmann@helios-kliniken.de
2 Department of Neurology/Emergency Unit, Vivantes Hospital Spandau, D-13585 Berlin, Germany; h.huang-tiel@t-online.de
3 Leibniz Research Centre for Working Environment and Human Factors IfADo, D-44139 Dortmund, Germany; golka@ifado.de (K.G.); selinski@ifado.de (S.S.); berit.geis@tu-dortmund.de (B.C.G.)
4 Department of Radio-Oncology, HELIOS Hospital, D-15525 Bad Saarow, Germany; stephan.koswig@helios-kliniken.de (S.K.); katrin.bathe@helios-kliniken.de (K.B.)
5 School of Medicine and Health Sciences Carl von Ossietzky, University Oldenburg, D-26133 Oldenburg, Germany; holger.gerullis@gmx.net
* Correspondence: thorsten.ecke@helios-kliniken.de

Academic Editor: Carsten Stephan

Abstract: High-dose-rate brachytherapy (HDR-BT) with external beam radiation therapy (EBRT) is a common treatment option for locally advanced prostate cancer (PCa). Seventy-nine male patients (median age 71 years, range 50 to 79) with high-risk PCa underwent HDR-BT following EBRT between December 2009 and January 2016 with a median follow-up of 21 months. HDR-BT was administered in two treatment sessions (one week interval) with 9 Gy per fraction using a planning system and the Ir192 treatment unit GammaMed Plus iX. EBRT was performed with CT-based 3D-conformal treatment planning with a total dose administration of 50.4 Gy with 1.8 Gy per fraction and five fractions per week. Follow-up for all patients was organized one, three, and five years after radiation therapy to evaluate early and late toxicity side effects, metastases, local recurrence, and prostate-specific antigen (PSA) value measured in ng/mL. The evaluated data included age, PSA at time of diagnosis, PSA density, BMI (body mass index), Gleason score, D'Amico risk classification for PCa, digital rectal examination (DRE), PSA value after one/three/five year(s) follow-up (FU), time of follow-up, TNM classification, prostate volume, and early toxicity rates. Early toxicity rates were 8.86% for gastrointestinal, and 6.33% for genitourinary side effects. Of all treated patients, 84.81% had no side effects. All reported complications in early toxicity were grade 1. PSA density at time of diagnosis ($p = 0.009$), PSA on date of first HDR-BT ($p = 0.033$), and PSA on date of first follow-up after one year ($p = 0.025$) have statistical significance on a higher risk to get a local recurrence during follow-up. HDR-BT in combination with additional EBRT in the presented design for high-risk PCa results in high biochemical control rates with minimal side-effects. PSA is a negative predictive biomarker for local recurrence during follow-up. A longer follow-up is needed to assess long-term outcome and toxicities.

Keywords: PSA; toxicity; HDR brachytherapy; prostate cancer

---

1. Introduction

High-dose-rate brachytherapy (HDR-BT) with additional external-beam radiation therapy (EBRT) is an important therapeutic option for men diagnosed with clinically localized and locally advanced high-risk prostate cancer (PCa) [1–3].

Regarding the actual European guidelines for the treatment of patients with intermediate- and high-risk PCa, a life expectancy of at least 10 years should be mandatory for treatments like radical prostatectomy (RP) or radiation therapy. Nevertheless, until now, there are no randomized clinical trials that compare the oncological outcome of HDR-BT vs. RP [4]. In general, there are not much data available regarding the oncological outcome of HDR-BT [5,6]. Especially, HDR-BT in combination with EBRT seems better than EBRT alone, with respect to biochemical recurrence (BCR)-free survival rates and aspects of quality of life [5,7]. PCa cells seem to have a low α/β ratio. This encourages the use of HDR-BT, where higher doses per fraction can be performed, therefore making it one of the most efficient interventions of hypofractionated radiotherapy. Most reported series combining HDR-BT and EBRT describe impressive results for the treatment of intermediate and high-risk PCa [8–10].

It has been reported by Schiffmann et al. that additional androgen deprivation therapy (ADT) shows higher BCR-free survival rates [11]. In this study, we focused on patients with intermediate- and high-risk PCa that were treated with HDR-BT plus ERBT plus ADT regarding complication rates and oncological outcome. It is difficult to determine an early treatment failure after therapy based on prostate-specific antigen (PSA) fluctuation and a potential benign PSA-rebound phenomenon [12]. In other studies, a benign PSA-rebound rate of up to 30% was described within the first 36 months after treatment [12–14]. The aim of this study was to determine early toxicity rates and the influence of PSA as a predictive marker of clinical outcome.

2. Results

The parameters age, IPSS, PSA (ng/mL) at time of diagnosis, PSA density, BMI, Gleason score, D'Amico risk classification for PCa, PSA value after one year FU, and time of FU are shown in Table 1. In that table, for all main clinical parameters, minimum, median, mean, maximum, standard deviation (SD), and 10%, 25%, 75%, and 90% intervals have been calculated. The median follow up time in our study was 21 months (6–80 months). In total, 8 out of 79 patients (10%) reached a FU time of more than five years. The frequencies of all important clinical parameters—PSA at time of diagnosis, Gleason score, T staging, and D'Amico risk classification for PCa—are detailed in Tables 2–5. Of the study cohort, 64.5% had an initial PSA value of more than 10 ng/mL, the Gleason score of more than 90% of the patients was $\geq$7, more than 80% of the patients had a clinical T staging of 3 (positive digital rectal examination and/or positive for tumor in transrectal ultrasound examination). According to the D'Amico risk classification for PCa, more than 90% are classified to risk group 3. In conclusion, all patients in that study for HDR-Brachytherapy treatment are high-risk PCa patients.

Table 1. Main clinical parameters. BMI: body mass index; FU: follow-up; IPSS: international prostate symptom score; PSA: prostate-specific antigen.

Parameter	Min	10%	25%	Median	Mean	75%	90%	Max	SD
Age	50.000	59.800	66.000	71.000	69.241	74.000	76.000	79.000	6.622
IPSS	0.000	2.000	3.000	5.500	6.271	9.000	11.100	19.000	4.426
PSA Diagnosis	1.360	4.464	7.045	14.550	22.345	24.995	44.736	226.000	29.506
PSA Density	0.053	0.126	0.250	0.463	0.764	0.828	1.760	4.969	0.924
BMI	20.761	23.397	25.282	27.099	27.385	28.572	31.760	44.379	3.713
Gleason Score	6.000	7.000	7.000	7.000	7.354	8.000	9.000	9.000	0.848
D'Amico	2.000	3.000	3.000	3.000	2.962	3.000	3.000	3.000	0.192
PSA FU 1a	0.000	0.010	0.030	0.040	0.167	0.165	0.304	2.300	0.357
time FU	6.000	8.800	11.000	21.000	26.620	35.500	57.400	80.000	18.912

Table 2. Frequency of important clinical parameters for the study cohort. Pre-treatment PSA value.

PSA Diagnosis	*N*	%
PSA < 10	28	35.44
10 ≤ PSA < 20	22	27.85
PSA ≥ 20	29	36.71
Total	79	100.00

Table 3. Frequency of important clinical parameters for the study cohort. Gleason Score.

Gleason Score	*N*	%
6	7	8.86
7	49	62.03
8	11	13.92
9	12	15.19
Total	79	100.00

Table 4. Frequency of important clinical parameters for the study cohort. Clinical T Stage.

T Stage	*N*	%
2a	1	1.27
2b	5	6.33
2c	7	8.86
3	66	83.54
Total	79	100.00

Table 5. Frequency of important clinical parameters for the study cohort. D'Amico risk classification for PCa.

D'Amico	*N*	%
1	0	0
2	3	3.80
3	76	96.20
Total	79	100.00

During follow-up, one patient (1.27%) died due to progressive disease and bone metastases 63 months after initial diagnosis of PCa. This patient was also the only one with the detection of metastases. In total, a local recurrence was detectable in three patients (3.80%).

Another focus of that study report is the description of side effects regarding early toxicity rates of the demonstrated treatment. Of all treated patients, 84.81% had no side effects. All reported complications in early toxicity were grade 1. The most reported side effects were anal pain (5.06%), symptomatic proctitis (1.27%), and diarrhea (2.53%) for the gastro-intestinal tract; high urinary frequency (3.80%), and urgency (2.53%) were the most complained side effects for the urinary tract. All complications are shown in Table 6.

After descriptive analyses of the documented data, we focused on the influence of PSA value while follow-up for local recurrence, metastases, and/or death. As only one patient died during follow-up, no statistical significance was calculable. However, the presence of local recurrence ($n = 3$) was used for the evaluation of PSA for risk assessment. Table 7 shows the p-value of all important parameters during follow-up regarding the influence on the presence of local recurrence. We could show that PSA density at time of diagnosis ($p = 0.009$), PSA on date of first HDR-BT ($p = 0.033$), and PSA on date of first follow-up after one year ($p = 0.025$) have statistical significance on a higher risk of having a local recurrence during follow-up. We found no statistical significance for Gleason score ($p = 0.463$) or D'Amico risk classification ($p = 0.995$).

Table 6. Early toxicity rates after radiation therapy.

Side Effects	N	%
None	67	84.81
Intestinal		
Pain	4	5.06
Proctitis	1	1.27
Diarrhea	2	2.53
Hemorhage	0	0
Genitourinary		
Frequency	3	3.80
Urgency	2	2.53
Incontinence	0	0
Hematuria	0	0
Renetntion	0	0
Pain	0	0
Total	79	100.00

Table 7. *p*-Value for relevant parameters regarding local recurrence during follow-up.

Variable	OR	2.5%	97.5%	*p*-Value
BMI	1.035	0.778	1.376	0.814
Age	0.876	0.755	1.016	0.080
IPSS	0.401	0.145	1.104	0.077
PSA pre-therapeutic	1.011	0.990	1.033	0.311
PSA density	3.102	1.331	7.228	*0.009*
No. of lymphnodes	0.973	0.795	1.190	0.789
PSA Lymphadenectomy	1.004	0.997	1.032	0.758
PSA HDR1	1.123	1.009	1.250	*0.033*
PSA HDR2	1.095	0.985	1.217	0.093
PSA FU 1a	8.022	1.306	49.287	*0.025*
PSA FU 3a	1.977	0.258	15.134	0.511
PSA FU 5a	4.204	0.422	41.914	0.221

HDR: high dose rate. Statistical significance is written in *italics*.

3. Discussion

HDR brachytherapy is one of the minimally invasive techniques of delivering conformal hypofractionated radiotherapy with steep fall-off of dose beyond the prostate gland. The prostate gland lays very close to critical normal tissues—the anterior rectum wall, urethra, and bladder neck. Because of that biological fact, HDR-BT is ideal for the treatment of PCa [15]. Many groups have shown that HDR-BT boost in combination with EBRT provides better results compared to EBRT alone [2,3]. Moreover, brachytherapy boost has the convenience of decreasing total treatment time, leading to decreased traveling time and expenses.

In the published data describing the experience of HDR-BT boost in combination with EBRT, various fractionation schedules have been used: 15 Gy in three fractions, 11–22 Gy in two fractions, and 12–15 Gy in one fraction. All of them had excellent results, so the Groupe Européen de Curiethérapie—European Society Therapy Radiation Oncology (GECESTRO) and the American Brachytherapy Society (ABS) do not recommend one fractionation schedule over another [16–18]. In this study, all patients were treated with two fractions of 9 Gy each following EBRT as reported above. In our cohort, 84.8% of the treated patients had no side effects. All reported side effects were defined as acute toxicity grade 1; most relevant were pain (5.06%), proctitis (1.27%), and diarrhea (2.53%) as intestinal; and frequency (3.8%) and urgency (2.53%) as genitourinary side effects. None of the patients developed acute GU or GI morbidity higher than Grade 2.

Hoskin et al. [19] reported about early ≥Grade 3 GU and GI morbidity was 3%–7% and 0%, respectively. Late Grade 3 GU toxicity was 3%–16% with no late Grade 3 or 4 GU or GI toxicity. Barkati et al. [20] reported 88% and 85% three-year and five-year biochemical control rates, respectively. They reported all acute GU toxicity as Grade 1. Chronic Grade 3 urinary toxicity was <10% with no Grade 4 toxicity seen.

4. Materials and Methods

4.1. Subjects

In this retrospective study, we report on 79 male patients (median age 71 years, range 50 to 79) who were treated between December 2009 and January 2016 at the Department of Urology and the Department of Radio-Oncology of HELIOS Hospital Bad Saarow, Germany. All patients selected for that treatment have been classified as intermediate and high-risk PCa patients.

4.2. Study Design

All included patients ($n = 79$) underwent HDR-BT after informed patient consent at the time of their treatment. Digital rectal examination, PSA, computerized tomography (CT), and a Technecium-99 bone scan was mandatory. Risk stratification was done as per the National Comprehensive Cancer Network (NCCN), which defines low-risk as PSA ≤ 10 ng/mL, T1c-T2 and a Gleason score (GS) ≤ 6; intermediate risk as PSA 10–20 ng/mL or GS 7; and high risk as a PSA > 20 ng/mL, T3, or GS 8–10. PSA measurements were performed with ElektroChemiLumineszenzImmonoAssay (ELCIA) by Roche Diagnostics GmbH, in accordance with WHO standards. We evaluated and documented the D'Amico risk stratification for PCa for each patient. Exclusion criteria were surgically positive lymph node metastases, distant metastasis, and prior pelvic radiotherapy. Patients with bladder outlet obstruction, patients who already had transurethral operations, and patients with a prostate volume of more than 100 cm^3 were also excluded. All patients had neoadjuvant and adjuvant androgen deprivation therapy (ADT) for at least two years starting after laparoscopic pelvic lymphadenectomy.

HDR-BT was administered before EBRT, based on transrectal ultrasound imaging, using a planning system and the Ir192 treatment unit GammaMed Plus iX (by Varian). HDR-BT was administered in two treatment sessions (one week interval) with 9 Gy per fraction. Overall, 18 Gy was applied to the prostate plus 2 mm margin. The maximal dose for the urethra and rectal wall was 8.0 and 5.0 Gy, respectively.

The HDR-BT procedure was done under general anesthesia. The patient was placed in the lithotomy position, a square lightweight template having a 5 mm grid array was fixed on a stepper stand on which a transrectal ultrasound machine (TRUS) was mounted, and the template was jammed against the perineal skin. There was a grid faceplate fixed onto the template, corresponding to the grid of the TRUS for accurate placement of the ProGuide needles. Under TRUS guidance, metallic trocars were inserted transperineally through the holes in the template to ascertain the position in the prostate as published before by Deger et al. [21]. Seven to twenty needles were inserted into the prostate, then the trocars were removed and replaced by the 6F ProGuide plastic needles in the same position. We always started with the peripheral and anterior needles, and then moved towards the center. As far as possible, the needles were placed at 1 cm intervals. No needles were placed within 7 mm of the urethra, in order to have control over the urethral dose. The needles were pushed beyond the prostate base, and the posterior needles were placed 2–3 mm anterior to the anterior wall of the rectum to avoid overdosing the rectum.

The planning target volume (PTV) was contoured by the radiation oncologist on each ultrasound slice and included the prostate with a 3 mm margin all around, except posteriorly, where no margin was given to avoid overdosing the anterior rectal wall. Superiorly, a margin of 5–7 mm was given to compensate for any post-implant edema and inadvertent caudal movement of the catheters in between the fractions. The PTV constraints were D90 (dose delivered to 90% of PTV) ≥ 97%, V95 ≥ 100%, and V150 $\leq$ 35%. Isodoses in transrectal ultrasound image are shown in Figure 1. A three-dimensional image with simulation of radiation is shown in Figure 2.

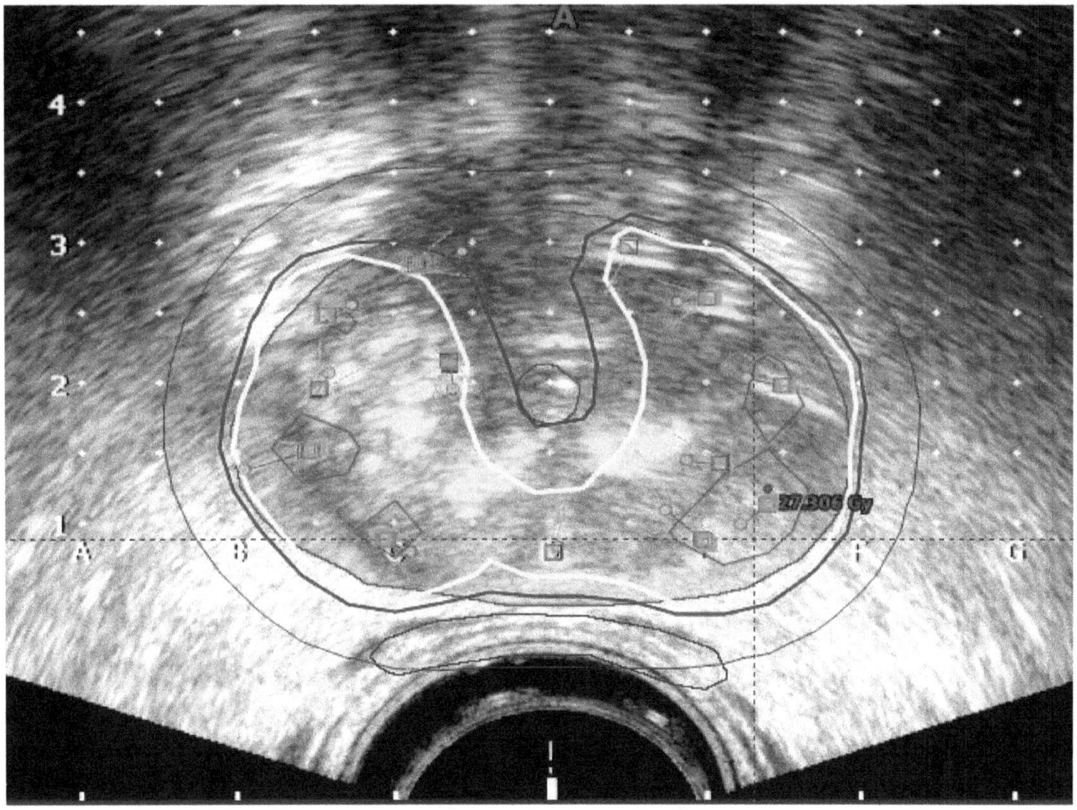

Figure 1. Isodoses in transrectal ultrasound image (red: 15 Gy; yellow: 9 Gy; blue: 8 Gy; brown: 5 Gy).

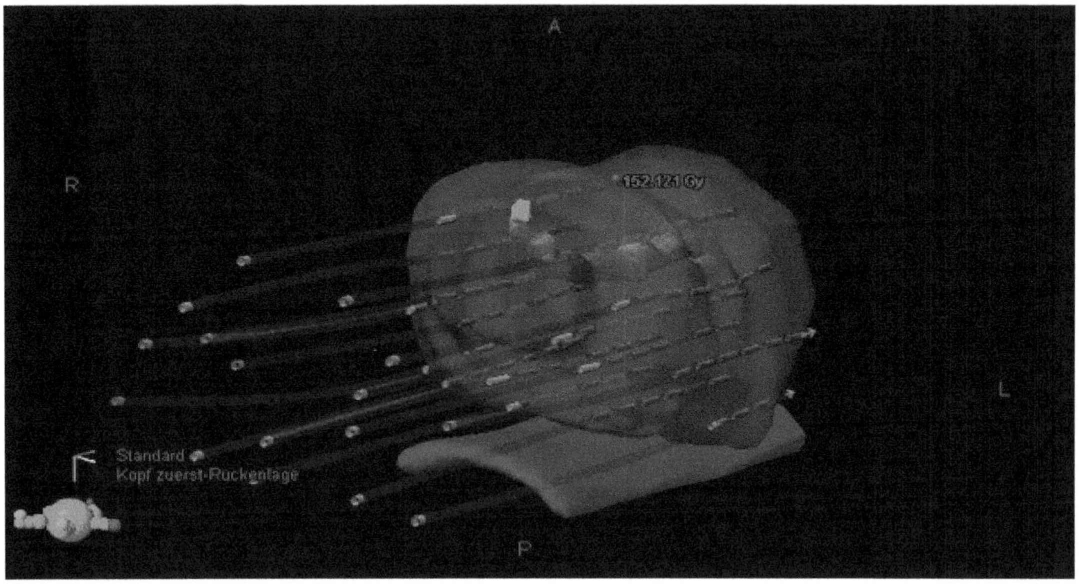

Figure 2. Three-dimensional image with simulation of radiation (red: prostate, green: urethra, blue: rectum, dark green: needle positions).

EBRT started a week after HDR-BT. EBRT was performed according to the standardized protocol with CT-based 3D-conformal treatment planning. The clinical target volume included prostate, the periprostatic region, and the basis of seminal vesicles; the planning target volume included the CTV (clinical target volume) and a margin—margin of 0.6 cm (posterior) and 1.0 cm in all other directions. The reference dose is defined in accordance with the International Commission on Radiation Units and Measurements report 50/63. All patients were irradiated in a supine position with a CT-planed IMRT/VMAT-technique (intensitivity modulated radiotherapy/volume modulated arc therapy) with 6 MV megavoltage photons (Varian, CClinac DHX, PaloAlto, CA, USA). A total dose of 50.4 Gy with 1.8 Gy per fraction and five fractions per week was administered.

Follow-up for all patients was organized one, three, and five years after radiation therapy in the department of Radiooncology to evaluate early and late toxicity side effects, metastases, local recurrence, and PSA value.

4.3. Evaluated Data

The evaluated data included the parameters age, PSA (ng/mL) at time of diagnosis, PSA density, body mass index (BMI), Gleason score, D'Amico risk classification for PCa, digital rectal examination (DRE), PSA value after one/three/five year(s) follow-up (FU), time of follow up, TNM classification, prostate volume, and early toxicity in follow-up. Pretreatment international prostate symptom score (IPSS), uroflow, and rest urine after voiding were also documented. All relevant dates were documented: date of birth, date of death, date of diagnosis, date of lymphadenectomy, date of ADT, date of HDR-BT, and date of follow-up after one, three, and five years.

A radiation oncologist and a urologist performed the follow-up evaluations, including digital rectal examinations and PSA level during follow-up scheme one, three, and five years after initial treatment. PSA failure was defined in terms of the American Society for Therapeutic Radiology and Oncology Consensus Panel recommendations [22]. Acute toxicities were scored according to the Common Terminology Criteria for Adverse Events, Version 4.0 (CTCAE v4.3), by the National Cancer Institute (Common Terminology Criteria for Adverse Events, Version 4.0. Available online: http://evs.nci.nih.gov/ftp1/CTCAE/CTCAE_4.03_2010-06-14_QuickReference_8.5x11.pdf). Acute toxicity was defined as symptoms that were observed during or after treatment and had been completely resolved 6 months after treatment. Following a strict plan for FU, all treated patients were investigated after six months, one, three and five years. Besides clinical investigation including DRE, an interview with a focus on acute toxicities following the Common Terminology Criteria for Adverse Events as written above was included.

4.4. Statistical Analysis

Bravais–Pearson correlation coefficients were estimated for pairs of variables. Odds ratios (OR), 95% confidence intervals (95% CI), and *p*-values of the Wald test were estimated using unadjusted logistic regression for local recurrence as dependent variable.

The level of significance was $\alpha = 0.05$. All tests and calculations were performed using the software R, version 3.1.2 (R Development Core Team 2014).

In our group, we could show that PSA density at time of diagnosis ($p = 0.009$), PSA on date of first HDR-BT ($p = 0.033$), and PSA on date of first follow-up after one year ($p = 0.025$) have statistical significance with respect to a higher risk of having a local recurrence during follow-up, but not age, Gleason score, or clinical stage. Concerning the number of patients ($n = 79$ in total), we are in average position compared to others and in a good position for a single-center study. Though the series of Yoshiaka et al. performed a monotherapeutic HDR-BT, they found the initial PSA level to be a significant prognostic factor ($p = 0.029$) along with younger age ($p = 0.019$) [23].

In the data published by Hoskin et al., Zwahlen et al., and Kestin et al. [3,5,8,24], they could show a better biological recurrence-free survival after HDR-BT in combination with EBRT, compared to EBRT alone. Combination of both modalities may also improve overall survival (OS) [25]. An explanation could be the high radiation dose that can be prescribed when HDR-BT is combined with EBRT.

Deger et al. [26] presented data of 422 patients with localized PCa treated between 1992 and 2001 with HDR-BT and 3DRT. As also performed in our treatment protocol, all patients underwent laparoscopic pelvic lymph node dissection to have an exact pathological lymph node staging and to be sure to exclude patients with lymphatic involvement. The biological non-evidence of disease (bNED) according to risk group were 100% for low risk, 75% for intermediate risk, and 60% for high risk at 5 years. Five-year bNEDs were 81% in the low risk, 65% in the intermediate risk, and 59% in the high risk group. Five-year OS and bNED were 87% and 94%, respectively. The authors also observed that initial PSA value, risk group, and age were significantly related to bNED. In contrast to our results, we found no statistical significance for D'Amico risk classification ($p = 0.995$) or Gleason score ($p = 0.463$). This could be caused by the fact that the presented cohort consists mainly of patients with high risk PCa and also high Gleason scores.

Most studies of radiotherapy in PCa focus on two points: not only the effectiveness of the treatment, but also its tolerance. However, due to different classifications of radiation reactions, it seems to be difficult to compare the toxicity rates.

There are still different opinions about the use of ADT for patients with intermediate- and high-risk PCa. Martinez et al. [27] published with a large number of patients ($n = 1260$) treated with pelvic RT and HDR-BT. The first group was treated with additional ADT up to six months prior to radiation, and the second group was not. The results for OS, disease free survival (DFS), and bNED have been similar. They observed that additional ADT did not confer a therapeutic advantage, but only side effects and cost. No statistically significant benefit on bNED rates with the use of additional ADT could be shown in any of the groups in that study.

The main limitation of this study is the relatively small number of patients and the short follow-up time regarding the influence on cancer-specific survival, overall survival, and biochemical relapse. Our study adds to the already existing evidence for the effectiveness of HDR-BT combined with EBRT for high-risk PCa.

In conclusion, this study demonstrates that HDR-BT combined with EBRT is effective in the radical radiotherapy of intermediate- and high-risk localized and locally advanced PCa. A longer follow-up is needed to assess long-term outcome and toxicities.

5. Conclusions

HDR-BT in combination with additional EBRT in the presented design for local advanced and high-risk PCa results in high biochemical control rates with minimal side-effects. PSA is a negative predictive biomarker for local recurrence during follow-up.

Author Contributions: Thorsten H. Ecke was mainly collecting data, writing the manuscript and performing the treatment as urologist. Hui-Juan Huang-Tiel was involved in collecting data and writing the manuscript. Klaus Golka, Silvia Selinski and Berit Christine Geis were mainly involved in performance of statistics. Stephan Koswig and Katrin Bathe were performing the treatment as radio-oncologists and collecting data. Steffen Hallmann was involved in writing the manuscript and making treatment decisions. Holger Gerullis was supervisor of writing the manuscript.

References

1. Heidenreich, A.; Bastian, P.J.; Bellmunt, J.; Bolla, M.; Joniau, S.; van der Kwast, T.; Mason, M.; Matveev, V.; Wiegel, T.; Zattoni, F.; et al. Eau guidelines on prostate cancer. Part 1: Screening, diagnosis, and local treatment with curative intent-update 2013. *Eur. Urol.* **2014**, *65*, 124–137. [CrossRef] [PubMed]
2. Sathya, J.R.; Davis, I.R.; Julian, J.A.; Guo, Q.; Daya, D.; Dayes, I.S.; Lukka, H.R.; Levine, M. Randomized trial comparing iridium implant plus external-beam radiation therapy with external-beam radiation therapy alone in node-negative locally advanced cancer of the prostate. *J. Clin. Oncol.* **2005**, *23*, 1192–1199. [CrossRef] [PubMed]

3. Hoskin, P.J.; Rojas, A.M.; Bownes, P.J.; Lowe, G.J.; Ostler, P.J.; Bryant, L. Randomised trial of external beam radiotherapy alone or combined with high-dose-rate brachytherapy boost for localised prostate cancer. *Radiother. Oncol.* **2012**, *103*, 217–222. [CrossRef] [PubMed]
4. Crook, J.M.; Gomez-Iturriaga, A.; Wallace, K.; Ma, C.; Fung, S.; Alibhai, S.; Jewett, M.; Fleshner, N. Comparison of health-related quality of life 5 years after spirit: Surgical prostatectomy versus interstitial radiation intervention trial. *J. Clin. Oncol.* **2011**, *29*, 362–368. [CrossRef] [PubMed]
5. Hoskin, P.J.; Motohashi, K.; Bownes, P.; Bryant, L.; Ostler, P. High dose rate brachytherapy in combination with external beam radiotherapy in the radical treatment of prostate cancer: Initial results of a randomised phase three trial. *Radiother. Oncol.* **2007**, *84*, 114–120. [CrossRef] [PubMed]
6. Galalae, R.M.; Zakikhany, N.H.; Geiger, F.; Siebert, F.A.; Bockelmann, G.; Schultze, J.; Kimmig, B. The 15-year outcomes of high-dose-rate brachytherapy for radical dose escalation in patients with prostate cancer—A benchmark for high-tech external beam radiotherapy alone? *Brachytherapy* **2014**, *13*, 117–122. [CrossRef] [PubMed]
7. Vordermark, D.; Wulf, J.; Markert, K.; Baier, K.; Kolbl, O.; Beckmann, G.; Bratengeier, K.; Noe, M.; Schon, G.; Flentje, M. 3-D conformal treatment of prostate cancer to 74 Gy vs. High-dose-rate brachytherapy boost: A cross-sectional quality-of-life survey. *Acta Oncol.* **2006**, *45*, 708–716. [CrossRef] [PubMed]
8. Zwahlen, D.R.; Andrianopoulos, N.; Matheson, B.; Duchesne, G.M.; Millar, J.L. High-dose-rate brachytherapy in combination with conformal external beam radiotherapy in the treatment of prostate cancer. *Brachytherapy* **2010**, *9*, 27–35. [CrossRef] [PubMed]
9. Kaprealian, T.; Weinberg, V.; Speight, J.L.; Gottschalk, A.R.; Roach, M., 3rd; Shinohara, K.; Hsu, I.C. High-dose-rate brachytherapy boost for prostate cancer: Comparison of two different fractionation schemes. *Int. J. Radiat. Oncol. Biol. Phys.* **2012**, *82*, 222–227. [CrossRef] [PubMed]
10. Wilder, R.B.; Barme, G.A.; Gilbert, R.F.; Holevas, R.E.; Kobashi, L.I.; Reed, R.R.; Solomon, R.S.; Walter, N.L.; Chittenden, L.; Mesa, A.V.; et al. Preliminary results in prostate cancer patients treated with high-dose-rate brachytherapy and intensity modulated radiation therapy (IMRT) vs. IMRT alone. *Brachytherapy* **2010**, *9*, 341–348. [CrossRef] [PubMed]
11. Schiffmann, J.; Lesmana, H.; Tennstedt, P.; Beyer, B.; Boehm, K.; Platz, V.; Tilki, D.; Salomon, G.; Petersen, C.; Krull, A.; et al. Additional androgen deprivation makes the difference: Biochemical recurrence-free survival in prostate cancer patients after hdr brachytherapy and external beam radiotherapy. *Strahlenther. Onkol.* **2015**, *191*, 330–337. [CrossRef] [PubMed]
12. Stephenson, A.J.; Eastham, J.A. Role of salvage radical prostatectomy for recurrent prostate cancer after radiation therapy. *J. Clin. Oncol.* **2005**, *23*, 8198–8203. [CrossRef] [PubMed]
13. Hanlon, A.L.; Pinover, W.H.; Horwitz, E.M.; Hanks, G.E. Patterns and fate of PSA bouncing following 3D-CRT. *Int. J. Radiat. Oncol. Biol. Phys.* **2001**, *50*, 845–849. [CrossRef]
14. Rosser, C.J.; Kuban, D.A.; Levy, L.B.; Chichakli, R.; Pollack, A.; Lee, A.K.; Pisters, L.L. Prostate specific antigen bounce phenomenon after external beam radiation for clinically localized prostate cancer. *J. Urol.* **2002**, *168*, 2001–2005. [CrossRef]
15. Pellizzon, A.C.; Nadalin, W.; Salvajoli, J.V.; Fogaroli, R.C.; Novaes, P.E.; Maia, M.A.; Ferrigno, R. Results of high dose rate afterloading brachytherapy boost to conventional external beam radiation therapy for initial and locally advanced prostate cancer. *Radiother. Oncol.* **2003**, *66*, 167–172. [CrossRef]
16. Roach, M., III; Hanks, G.; Thames, H., Jr.; Schellhammer, P.; Shipley, W.U.; Sokol, G.H.; Sandler, H. Defining biochemical failure following radiotherapy with or without hormonal therapy in men with clinically localized prostate cancer: Recommendations of the RTOG-ASTRO phoenix consensus conference. *Int. J. Radiat. Oncol. Biol. Phys.* **2006**, *65*, 965–974. [CrossRef] [PubMed]
17. Yamada, Y.; Rogers, L.; Demanes, D.J.; Morton, G.; Prestidge, B.R.; Pouliot, J.; Cohen, G.N.; Zaider, M.; Ghilezan, M.; Hsu, I.C. American brachytherapy society consensus guidelines for high-dose-rate prostate brachytherapy. *Brachytherapy* **2012**, *11*, 20–32. [CrossRef] [PubMed]
18. Hoskin, P.J.; Colombo, A.; Henry, A.; Niehoff, P.; Paulsen Hellebust, T.; Siebert, F.A.; Kovacs, G. GEC/ESTRO recommendations on high dose rate afterloading brachytherapy for localised prostate cancer: An update. *Radiother. Oncol.* **2013**, *107*, 325–332. [CrossRef] [PubMed]
19. Hoskin, P.; Rojas, A.; Lowe, G.; Bryant, L.; Ostler, P.; Hughes, R.; Milner, J.; Cladd, H. High-dose-rate brachytherapy alone for localized prostate cancer in patients at moderate or high risk of biochemical recurrence. *Int. J. Radiat. Oncol. Biol. Phys.* **2012**, *82*, 1376–1384. [CrossRef] [PubMed]

20. Barkati, M.; Williams, S.G.; Foroudi, F.; Tai, K.H.; Chander, S.; van Dyk, S.; See, A.; Duchesne, G.M. High-dose-rate brachytherapy as a monotherapy for favorable-risk prostate cancer: A phase II trial. *Int. J. Radiat. Oncol. Biol. Phys.* **2012**, *82*, 1889–1896. [CrossRef] [PubMed]
21. Deger, S.; Dinges, S.; Roigas, J.; Schnorr, D.; Turk, I.; Budach, V.; Hinkelbein, W.; Loening, S.A. High-dose rate iridium192 afterloading therapy in combination with external beam irradiation for localized prostate cancer. *Tech. Urol.* **1997**, *3*, 190–194. [PubMed]
22. Consensus statement: Guidelines for PSA following radiation therapy. American society for therapeutic radiology and oncology consensus panel. *Int. J. Radiat. Oncol. Biol. Phys.* **1997**, *37*, 1035–1041.
23. Yoshioka, Y.; Konishi, K.; Sumida, I.; Takahashi, Y.; Isohashi, F.; Ogata, T.; Koizumi, M.; Yamazaki, H.; Nonomura, N.; Okuyama, A.; et al. Monotherapeutic high-dose-rate brachytherapy for prostate cancer: Five-year results of an extreme hypofractionation regimen with 54 Gy in nine fractions. *Int. J. Radiat. Oncol. Biol. Phys.* **2011**, *80*, 469–475. [CrossRef] [PubMed]
24. Kestin, L.L.; Martinez, A.A.; Stromberg, J.S.; Edmundson, G.K.; Gustafson, G.S.; Brabbins, D.S.; Chen, P.Y.; Vicini, F.A. Matched-pair analysis of conformal high-dose-rate brachytherapy boost versus external-beam radiation therapy alone for locally advanced prostate cancer. *J. Clin. Oncol.* **2000**, *18*, 2869–2880. [PubMed]
25. Pieters, B.R.; de Back, D.Z.; Koning, C.C.; Zwinderman, A.H. Comparison of three radiotherapy modalities on biochemical control and overall survival for the treatment of prostate cancer: A systematic review. *Radiother. Oncol.* **2009**, *93*, 168–173. [CrossRef] [PubMed]
26. Deger, S.; Boehmer, D.; Roigas, J.; Schink, T.; Wernecke, K.D.; Wiegel, T.; Hinkelbein, W.; Budach, V.; Loening, S.A. High dose rate (HDR) brachytherapy with conformal radiation therapy for localized prostate cancer. *Eur. Urol.* **2005**, *47*, 441–448. [CrossRef] [PubMed]
27. Martinez, A.A.; Demanes, D.J.; Galalae, R.; Vargas, C.; Bertermann, H.; Rodriguez, R.; Gustafson, G.; Altieri, G.; Gonzalez, J. Lack of benefit from a short course of androgen deprivation for unfavorable prostate cancer patients treated with an accelerated hypofractionated regime. *Int. J. Radiat. Oncol. Biol. Phys.* **2005**, *62*, 1322–1331. [CrossRef] [PubMed]

Neuroendocrine Differentiation in Metastatic Conventional Prostate Cancer is Significantly Increased in Lymph Node Metastases Compared to the Primary Tumors

Vera Genitsch [1], Inti Zlobec [1], Roland Seiler [2], George N. Thalmann [2] and Achim Fleischmann [1,*]

1 Institute of Pathology, University of Bern, Bern 3008, Switzerland; vera.genitsch@pathology.unibe.ch (V.G.); inti.zlobec@pathology.unibe.ch (I.Z.)

2 Department of Urology, University of Bern, Bern 3010, Switzerland; roland.seiler@insel.ch (R.S.); george.thalmann@insel.ch (G.N.T.)

* Correspondence: achim.fleischmann@stgag.ch

Abstract: Neuroendocrine serum markers released from prostate cancers have been proposed for monitoring disease and predicting survival. However, neuroendocrine differentiation (NED) in various tissue compartments of metastatic prostate cancer is poorly described and its correlation with specific tumor features is unclear. NED was determined by Chromogranin A expression on immunostains from a tissue microarray of 119 nodal positive, hormone treatment-naïve prostate cancer patients who underwent radical prostatectomy and extended lymphadenectomy. NED in the primary cancer and in the metastases was correlated with tumor features and survival. The mean percentage of NED cells increased significantly ($p < 0.001$) from normal prostate glands (0.4%), to primary prostate cancer (1.0%) and nodal metastases (2.6%). In primary tumors and nodal metastases, tumor areas with higher Gleason patterns tended to display a higher NED, although no significance was reached. The same was observed in patients with a larger primary tumor volume and higher total size and number of metastases. NED neither in the primary tumors nor in the metastases predicted outcome significantly. Our data suggest that (a) increasing levels of neuroendocrine serum markers in the course of prostate cancer might primarily derive from a poorly differentiated metastatic tumor component; and (b) NED in conventional hormone-naïve prostate cancers is not significantly linked to adverse tumor features.

Keywords: prostate cancer; lymph node metastases; neuroendocrine; chromogranin A; prognosis

1. Introduction

The current World Health Organization (WHO) classification of prostate neoplasms with neuroendocrine (NE) differentiation (NED) comprises of: (1) adenocarcinomas with NED; (2) well-differentiated NE tumors (carcinoid); (3) small-cell NE carcinomas; and (4) large cell NE carcinomas [1]. While the last three entities are exceedingly rare, the first occurs frequently. In 10–100% of the conventional adenocarcinomas, NED can be demonstrated immunohistochemically in the form of scattered NE cancer cells, depending on the number of slides evaluated and the number of antibodies used [1].

NE cells in prostate cancer most likely emerge from the secretory prostate cancer cells by trans-differentiation [2–4]. Each NE cell may store a single, or a mix of neuropeptides in cytoplasmic granules, including Chromogranin A, the most frequently detected and most intensely studied NE product in prostate tissue [5], serotonin, somatostatin and bombesin [6]. The exact biological function of neuropeptides in prostate cancer is largely unknown; however, data indicate that they may stimulate growth, differentiation and secretory processes [5,7]. While small and large cell NE carcinomas are particularly aggressive [8], the prognostic significance of NE cells in conventional adenocarcinomas of the prostate is still controversial [4,9,10]. Importantly, neuropeptides released from the NE prostate cancer cells may appear in the circulation [6]. These serum markers have recently attracted considerable attention for their ability to monitor disease [6,11] and predict survival [12,13]. NE serum markers have been suggested as beneficial surrogates for tumor burden [6] and mirror prostate cancer progression when raising. In line with this, serum levels of Chromogranin A are significantly higher in metastatic compared to non-metastatic prostate cancers [14]. However, despite this interest in NE serum markers, little is known about the distribution of their source, which are the NE tumor cells, in the various growth patterns and in the metastases of prostate cancer. In this study, we more accurately describe the extent of NED in the different tissue compartments of metastasizing prostate cancer, and determine its correlations with different tumor features and survival.

2. Results

2.1. Patient Characteristics and Expression of Chromogranin A in Benign Prostate, Primary Tumors and Lymph Node Metastases Considering the Gleason Patterns

The patient, prostatectomy and lymphadenectomy characteristics are specified in Table 1. A higher proportion of 92% of primary tumors displayed any positivity for Chromogranin A compared to lymph node metastases with a positive expression in 77%. When the density of NE cancer cells was recorded, a progressive and significant increase in expression from non-neoplastic prostate glands (0.4% mean of Chromogranin A positive cells) to primary tumors (1.0%) and lymph node metastases (2.6%; $p < 0.001$) was noted for Chromogranin A (Figure 1A).

A tendency for higher Chromogranin A expression in less-differentiated tumor areas (reflected by a higher Gleason pattern (GP)) was observed in the primary tumors (GP3: 0.8% mean of Chromogranin A positive cells; GP4: 1.0%; GP5: 1.4%; $p > 0.05$) and in the nodal metastases (GP3: 0.0%; GP4: 1.8%; GP5: 7.8%; P = NE), but no statistical significance was reached (Figure 1B).

Table 1. Characteristics of 119 nodal positive prostate cancer patients.

Patient Data (*n* = 119)	
Age (median, range) at surgery (years)	65 (45–75)
Follow-up (median, range) (years)	5.9 (0.1–15.2)
Patients with biochemical failure at last follow-up (*n*)	103
Patients dead of disease at last follow-up (*n*)	33
Patients dead at last follow-up (*n*)	40
Prostatectomy Data	
pT2 (*n*)	14
pT3a (*n*)	55
pT3b (*n*)	50
Prostate cancer volume (median, range) (cm^3)	12.6 (0.66–127)
Gleason score 6 (*n*)	12
Gleason score 7 (*n*)	63
Gleason score 8 (*n*)	21
Gleason score 9 (*n*)	23
Lymphadenectomy Data	
Evaluated nodes per patient (median, range) (*n*)	22 (9–68)
Positive nodes per patient (median, range) (*n*)	2 (1–24)

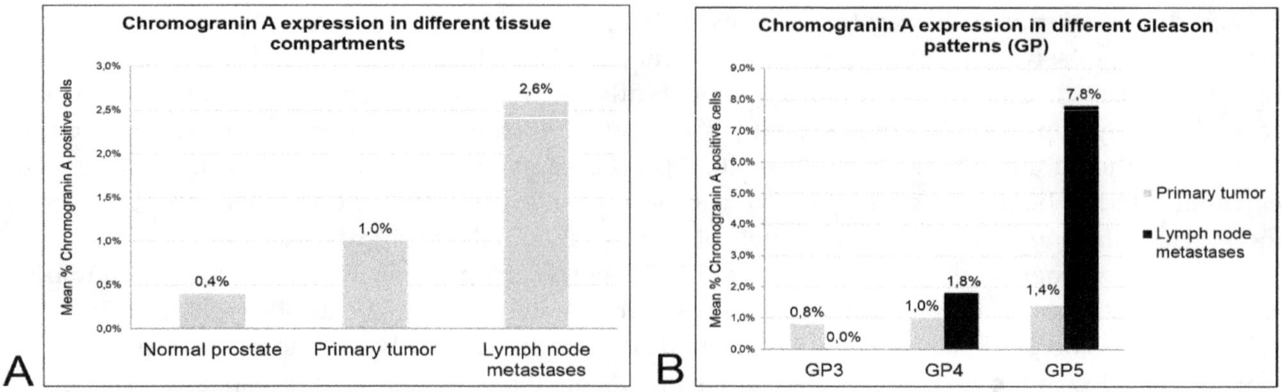

Figure 1. Mean density of Chromogranin A positive cells is significantly different between normal prostate glands, primary prostate cancer and matched lymph node metastases ((**A**) $p < 0.001$). The difference between the Gleason patterns is not significant ((**B**) $p > 0.05$).

2.2. *Correlations of Chromogranin A Expression in Primary Tumors and Lymph Node Metastases with Clinico-Pathological Tumor Characteristics and Survival*

Primary tumors with Chromogranin A expression were larger (mean 21.5 ± 24.9 cm^3 versus 18.0 ± 15.4 cm^3; $p = 0.821$) and the tumor burden of a Chromogranin A positive metastasizing component was higher for mean total size and number of metastases (36.4 ± 49.4 mm versus 19.4 ± 31.7 mm; $p = 0.458$ and 5.3 ± 6.9 versus 3.3 ± 3.4; $p = 0.279$) (Table 2); however, these differences were not statistically significant. Chromogranin A expression in primary tumors or lymph node metastases was not associated with categorical tumor characteristics as stage of the primary tumor. In univariate analysis, Chromogranin A expression in primary tumors or lymph node metastases did not significantly predict biochemical recurrence-free, cancer-specific, or overall survival (Figure 2). Only the total size of metastases independently predicted all three endpoints in a multivariate analysis (Table 3).

Table 2. Tumor features according to Chromogranin A expression.

CgA Expression	Parameters of the Primary Tumor (Mean ± SD)				Parameters of Nodal Metastases (Mean ± SD)			
	Age	*p*	Tumor volume (cm^3)	*p*	Total size (mm)	*p*	Total number	*p*
Primary Tumor								
CgA negative	64.4 ± 6.1	0.978	18.0 ± 15.4	0.821	19.6 ± 34.8	0.989	3.3 ± 3.8	0.813
CgA positive	64.3 ± 5.8		21.5 ± 24.9		17.2 ± 24.4		3.0 ± 3.3	
Nodal Metastases								
CgA negative	64.3 ± 5.9	0.027	19.1 ± 19.5	0.819	19.4 ± 31.7	0.458	3.3 ± 3.4	0.279
CgA positive	59.3 ± 6.3		18.9 ± 13.7		36.4 ± 49.4		5.3 ± 6.9	

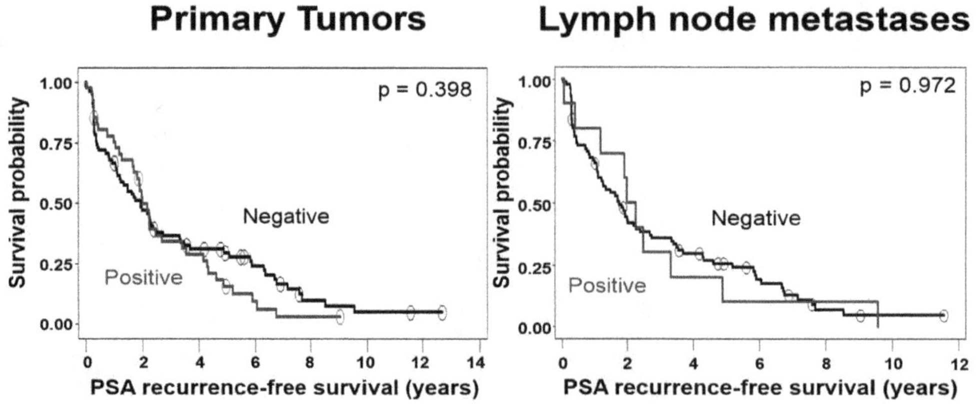

Figure 2. *Cont.*

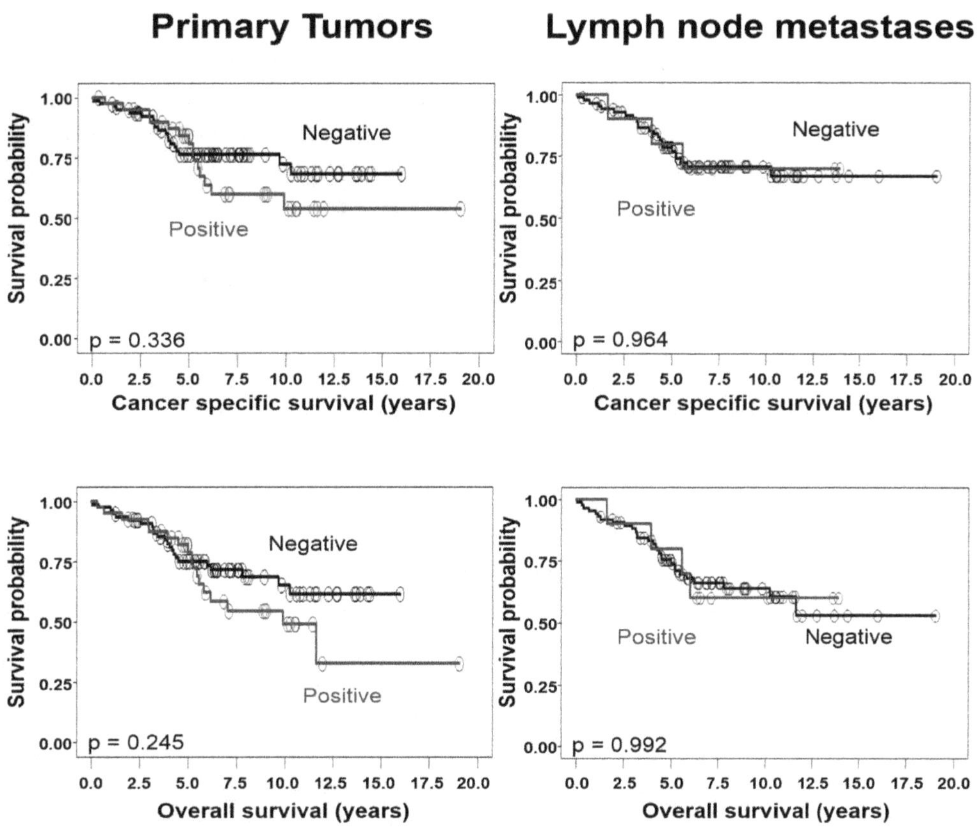

Figure 2. Chromogranin A expression in primary tumors and metastases is not significantly correlated with outcome.

Table 3. Multivariate analyses for the prognostic impact of Chromogranin A (CgA) expression in primary prostate cancer (upper half) and in lymph node metastases (lower half), after adjustment for total size of metastases and Gleason score of primary tumor: Only nodal tumor burden predicts survival independently. HR, hazard ratio; and CI, confidence interval.

Parameter	Cut-Off	Overall Survival		Disease-Specific Survival		Recurrence-Free Survival	
		HR (95% CI)	*p*	HR (95% CI)	*p*	HR (95% CI)	*p*
CgA in Primary Tumor	Positive Negative	1.0 1.65 (0.9–3.1)	0.132	1.0 1.54 (0.8–3.1)	0.241	1.0 1.1 (0.7–1.7)	0.66
Metastases size	<7.5 mm ≥7.5 mm	1.0 4.34 (2.0–9.6)	**<0.001**	1.0 4.12 (1.7–10.0)	**0.002**	1.0 1.58 (1.1–2.4)	**0.036**
Gleason score	6 to 8 9 to 10	1.0 1.23 (0.6–2.5)	0.571	1.0 1.41 (0.7–3.0)	0.375	1.0 1.57 (1.0–2.6)	0.074
CgA in Nodal Metastases	Positive Negative	1.0 0.73 (0.2–2.2)	0.571	1.0 0.65 (0.2–2.8)	0.5	1.0 0.69 (0.3–1.4)	0.327
Metastases size	<7.5 mm ≥7.5 mm	1.0 5.3 (2.0–14.1)	**<0.001**	1.0 6.44 (1.9–22.1)	**0.003**	1.0 1.58 (1.0–2.5)	0.063
Gleason score	6 to 8 9 to 10	1.0 1.43 (0.7–3.1)	0.365	1.0 1.75 (0.8–4.0)	1.88	1.0 1.62 (0.9–2.8)	0.082

3. Discussion

Only a few studies on prostate cancers have evaluated NED in metastatic tissues from lymph nodes and various other organs with immunohistochemistry [15–20]. Reported incidences for bone metastases were 19% [18] and 52% [16], those for lymph node metastases 12% [19], 37.5% [17] and 46% [16]. A wide range in the extent of NED in metastases was also noted in an autopsy series by Roudier et al. [20], specifically between patients, and also between different metastases of a single patient. In our series, NED in lymph node metastases was present in 77% of the patients. The metastases had a lower prevalence for NED positivity compared to the primary tumors, which showed NE differentiation in 92%. This decrease was consistent with the only two series on NED in surgically treated nodal positive prostate cancer reported by Bostwick et al. [17] and Quek et al. [19]. However, when considering not only the presence or absence of NED, but also the density of positive cells in primary tumors and metastases, we noticed a significant increase in NED in metastases when compared to primary tumors. Furthermore, NED increased in higher Gleason patterns in the primary tumors, and was even more striking in the metastases where tumor growths of Gleason pattern 5 showed the highest levels of NED among all evaluated cancer components. Our findings were consistent with reports on a positive correlation of the extent of NED and the Gleason score in primary tumors [21,22]. Together with the previously described correlation of Chromogranin A expression by the tumor tissue with its serum level [23], our data might suggest that elevated NE serum markers in metastatic prostate cancer [14] may primarily reflect the metastatic, frequently poorly differentiated tumor burden [24–26].

The presence of NED in our prostate cancer patients showed a tendency for association with adverse tumor characteristics. Patients with detected NED in primary tumors had larger tumors, and those with NED present in metastases had a greater nodal tumor burden, indicated by more metastases and greater total diameter of metastases when compared with patients without NED. Consistent with our data, Quek et al. [19] reported the association of high NED with an advanced tumor stage. Furthermore, NED in the primary tumors of our patients translated into long-term survival. After five years, the curves for disease-specific and overall survival segregate clearly indicated a poorer outcome for patients with NED when compared to those without NED. However, this was not significant, most likely due to the size of our cohort. Contrarily, survival curves based on NED in lymph node metastases intersected repeatedly. Only two other studies have evaluated NED in nodal positive prostate cancer patients treated by radical prostatectomy and bilateral lymphadenectomy. NED detected by Chromogranin A was not a risk factor in the study by Bostwick et al. [17], neither in the primary tumors nor in the metastases, whereas Queck et al. [19] reported significantly poorer median recurrence-free and overall survival for patients with high NED in the primary tumor and metastases, respectively, when compared to patients with low NED. However, survival curves were not presented in the latter study and other outcome measures were not significantly different.

Previous studies on NED in prostate cancer tissues assessed expression on large sections (for comprehensive review of the literature see Table 3 in Bostwick et al. [17]) and cancers were categorized as negative (absence of NE cells), or positive (presence of NE cells). While it was generally noticed that NED in prostate cancer is a very focal, dispersed phenomenon, reported incidences for NED varied between 24 and 98.5% [17]. This wide range was attributed to differences between the cohorts, sample types, types and extent of fixation, the antibodies used in determining the presence of malignant NE cells, variance in interpretation and, most importantly, a sampling error related to the focal and unequal distribution of NE cells in most tumors [27]. It is evident that the amount of tumor tissue evaluated may impact on reported prevalence in cases of only focally expressed biomarkers like NED. We determined NED in primary tumors and metastases by tissue microarray (TMA). This technology has also been considered to be useful for these focally expressed biomarkers in prostate cancer by a study comparing the expression of NE markers on whole tissue sections to a TMA [28]. Investigating these focally expressed biomarkers on large sections may have also been problematic as tissue slides from primary prostate cancer generally contain much greater amounts of tumor tissue than the usually scarce metastatic tissue that makes the comparison of incidences difficult. However, the use of a TMA certainly remains a limiting factor in our study. Finally, for a delicate biomarker like NED in prostate cancer, the size of the cohort may play a major role in detecting significant correlations between tumor features and survival. Our cohort was comparably large for surgically treated nodal positive prostate cancer and therefore allowed detection of a significant increase in NED in nodal metastases and trends between biomarker expression levels, tumor features and survival. However, it may have been too small to demonstrate these trends as significant.

4. Materials and Methods

4.1. Patients

In total, 119 consecutive prostate cancer patients without demonstrable metastases (physical and radiological examination), but with nodal metastases upon histological investigation of the lymphadenectomy specimens were studied. All patients had undergone standardized surgery at the Department of Urology, University of Bern between 1989 and 2006 with bilateral extended pelvic lymphadenectomy and radical prostatectomy as a single procedure. Follow-up was performed prospectively. Neoadjuvant therapy was not implemented and no adjuvant treatment, especially androgen deprivation, was suggested before symptomatic disease progression.

4.2. Surgical Technique of Lymphadenectomy

A bilateral pelvic lymphadenectomy was performed in all patients as previously described [29]. Summarized, lymph nodes were dissected along the external iliac vein down to the deep circumflex iliac vein and femoral canal, up to the bifurcation of the common iliac artery and the obturator fossa. Thereafter, the lymphatic tissue along the medial and lateral aspect of the internal iliac artery and vein was excised. Three tissue samples from each side were submitted separately for pathological examination. Frozen sections were not carried out.

4.3. Pathology

All specimens were processed at the Institute of Pathology, University of Bern [24,30]. The prostatectomies were completely embedded as described in references [24,30]. The following microscopic tumor characteristics were noted: type, Gleason score [31], tertiary Gleason pattern, tumor stage, and the percentage of prostate tissue area on the sections occupied by the tumor. NE tumors/carcinomas of the prostate were excluded. Tumor volume was estimated by multiplying the percentage of the specimen involved by cancer by the prostate volume.

The fatty tissue of lymphadenectomy specimens was dissolved in aceton after formalin fixation and all lymph nodes were entirely embedded. One section per paraffin block was stained with hematoxylin and eosin. The length and width of the metastatic deposits were measured. A Gleason score (primary and secondary pattern) and a tertiary Gleason pattern (if present), were determined based on the entire metastatic tissue.

All Gleason patterns present in the primary tumors and lymph node metastases were accurately marked for subsequent TMA construction. Staging was completed according to the 8th edition of the International Union Against Cancer (UICC) TNM Classification [32].

4.4. Tissue Microarray

For TMA construction, one 0.6 mm tissue core of benign prostatic tissue (peripheral zone) and every Gleason pattern present in primary tumors and matched lymph node metastases was retrieved from the paraffin blocks. The TMA contains overall 403 prostate tissue samples, 119 normal prostate tissues and 284 primary cancers (mean per patient, 3.3; range, 2–4; including 101, 112 and 71 samples from Gleason patterns 3, 4 and 5, respectively) and 167 lymph node metastases (mean per patient, 1.4; range, 1–3; including 35, 103 and 29 samples from Gleason patterns 3, 4 and 5, respectively). In the vast majority of primary tumors, all Gleason patterns sampled were present in the index tumor. Additional tissue from separate tumor foci was included only rarely, when a Gleason pattern not present in the index tumor was detected here. Although sampling from the primary tumor was more extensive, the relative tumor amount in the TMA was larger from the metastases due to their smaller volume.

4.5. *Immunohistochemistry*

Freshly cut TMA sections were pre-treated by steam with target retrieval solution, pH 9 (Dako, Glostrup, Denmark). For Chromogranin A detection, a monoclonal mouse antibody cocktail (clone LK2H10 + PHE5; Bicarta; Hamburg, Germany) was used at 1:500 antibody dilution. Bound primary antibodies were detected using the Envision Plus system (Dako, Glostrup, Denmark). Chromogranin A was expressed in the cytoplasm of the prostate cancer cells (Figure 3). The percentage of positive neoplastic cells was determined for every tissue sample.

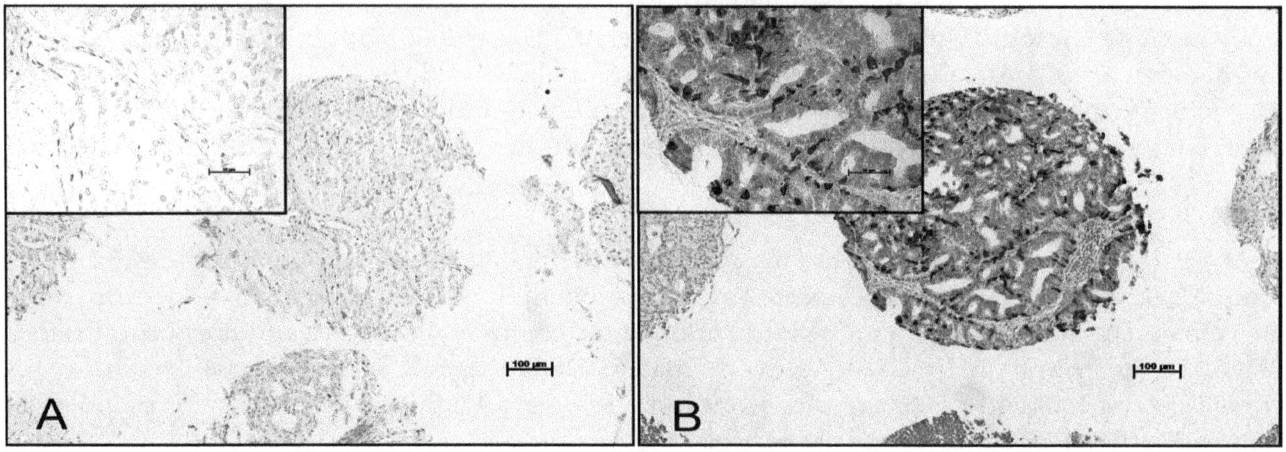

Figure 3. No Chromogranin A expression in (**A**) primary prostate cancer; and (**B**) high Chromogranin A expression in a lymph node metastasis.

4.6. *Statistical Analysis*

Chromogranin A expression in normal prostate, primary tumors and lymph node metastases was evaluated using the Wilcoxon Signed Rank test and the Friedman test for differences between Gleason pattern 3, 4 and 5 within primary carcinomas and nodal metastases. Chromogranin A expression was compared with normally distributed quantitative and categorical tumor attributes using Wilcoxon Signed Rank test and χ-Square test, respectively. Suitable cut-off values for positive (more than 0 positive cells) and negative (0 positive cells) Chromogranin A expression in primary tumors and lymph node metastases were defined using Receiver-operating characteristic curves [33]. Outcome was analyzed for Prostate-Specific Antigen (PSA) recurrence-free, cancer-specific and overall survival defined as the intervals from surgery to the date of biochemical recurrence (PSA failure defined as values >0.2 ng/mL), death from prostate carcinoma, and death from any cause, respectively. Patients without event for the respective endpoints were censored at the date of last follow-up. The above time-to-events were performed using log-rank test; p values < 0.05 were regarded as significant. The Cox proportional hazards model was used to identify independent prognostic factors for all three endpoints. Statistical analysis was made using SAS 9.2 (The SAS Institute, Cary, NC, USA).

5. Conclusions

Our data suggest that, firstly, increasing serum levels of neuroendocrine serum markers in prostate cancer primarily mirror growth of a poorly differentiated metastatic tumor component and, secondly, NED in early metastasizing, hormone-naïve prostate cancer is only weakly linked to adverse tumor features.

Acknowledgments: Project received funding from the Bernische Krebsliga and the Krebsliga Thurgau (Achim Fleischmann).

Author Contributions: Achim Fleischmann conceived and designed the experiments; Inti Zlobec performed the statistical analysis; Vera Genitsch, Roland Seiler, George N. Thalmann and Achim Fleischmann analyzed the data; Vera Genitsch and Achim Fleischmann wrote the paper; Roland Seiler and George N. Thalmann revised the manuscript for important intellectual content.

Abbreviations

NED	Neuroendocrine Differentiation
NE	Neuroendocrine
GP	Gleason Pattern
CgA	Chromogranin A
HR	Hazard Ratio
CI	Confidence Interval
TMA	Tissue Microarray
PSA	Prostate-Specific Antigen

References

1. Epstein, J.I.; Amin, M.B.; Evans, A.J.; Huang, J.; Rubin, M.A. Neuroendocrine tumours. In *WHO Classification of Tumours of the Urinary System and Male Genital Organs*; Moch, H., Humphrey, P.A., Ulbright, T.M., Reuter, V.E., Eds.; IARC: Lyon, France, 2016.
2. Bonkhoff, H.; Stein, U.; Remberger, K. Multidirectional differentiation in the normal, hyperplastic, and neoplastic human prostate: Simultaneous demonstration of cell-specific epithelial markers. *Hum. Pathol.* **1994**, *25*, 42–46. [CrossRef]
3. Yuan, T.C.; Veeramani, S.; Lin, M.F. Neuroendocrine-like prostate cancer cells: Neuroendocrine transdifferentiation of prostate adenocarcinoma cells. *Endocr. Relat. Cancer* **2007**, *14*, 531–547.
4. Priemer, D.S.; Montironi, R.; Wang, L.; Williamson, S.R.; Lopez-Beltran, A.; Cheng, L. Neuroendocrine tumors of the prostate: Emerging insights from molecular data and updates to the 2016 world health organization classification. *Endocr. Pathol.* **2016**, *27*, 123–135. [CrossRef] [PubMed]
5. Sciarra, A.; Cardi, A.; Dattilo, C.; Mariotti, G.; di Monaco, F.; di Silverio, F. New perspective in the management of neuroendocrine differentiation in prostate adenocarcinoma. *Int. J. Clin. Pract.* **2006**, *60*, 462–470. [CrossRef] [PubMed]
6. Komiya, A.; Suzuki, H.; Imamoto, T.; Kamiya, N.; Nihei, N.; Naya, Y.; Ichikawa, T.; Fuse, H. Neuroendocrine differentiation in the progression of prostate cancer. *Int. J. Urol.* **2008**, *16*, 37–44. [CrossRef] [PubMed]
7. Grigore, A.D.; Ben-Jacob, E.; Farach-Carson, M.C. Prostate cancer and neuroendocrine differentiation: More neuronal, less endocrine? *Front. Oncol.* **2015**, *5*, 37. [CrossRef] [PubMed]
8. Wang, H.T.; Yao, Y.H.; Li, B.G.; Tang, Y.; Chang, J.W.; Zhang, J. Neuroendocrine prostate cancer (NEPC) progressing from conventional prostatic adenocarcinoma: Factors associated with time to development of NEPC and survival from NEPC diagnosis—A systematic review and pooled analysis. *J. Clin. Oncol.* **2014**, *32*, 3383–3390. [PubMed]
9. Epstein, J.I.; Amin, M.B.; Beltran, H.; Lotan, T.L.; Mosquera, J.-M.; Reuter, V.E.; Robinson, B.D.; Troncoso, P.; Rubin, M.A. Proposed morphologic classification of prostate cancer with neuroendocrine differentiation. *Am. J. Surg. Pathol.* **2014**, *38*, 756–767. [CrossRef] [PubMed]
10. Berruti, A.; Vignani, F.; Russo, L.; Bertaglia, V.; Tullio, M.; Tucci, M.; Poggio, M.; Dogliotti, L. Prognostic role of neuroendocrine differentiation in prostate cancer, putting together the pieces of the puzzle. *Open Access J. Urol.* **2010**, *2*, 109–124. [CrossRef] [PubMed]
11. Appetecchia, M.; Meçule, A.; Pasimeni, G.; Iannucci, C.V.; de Carli, P.; Baldelli, R.; Barnabei, A.; Cigliana, G.; Sperduti, I.; Gallucci, M. Incidence of high Chromogranin A serum levels in patients with non metastatic prostate adenocarcinoma. *J. Exp. Clin. Cancer Res.* **2010**, *29*, 166. [CrossRef] [PubMed]
12. Burgio, S.L.; Conteduca, V.; Menna, C.; Carretta, E.; Rossi, L.; Bianchi, E.; Kopf, B.; Fabbri, F.; Amadori, D.; de Giorgi, U. Chromogranin A predicts outcome in prostate cancer patients treated with abiraterone. *Endocr. Relat. Cancer* **2014**, *21*, 487–493. [CrossRef] [PubMed]
13. Conteduca, V.; Burgio, S.L.; Menna, C.; Carretta, E.; Rossi, L.; Bianchi, E.; Masini, C.; Amadori, D.; de Giorgi, U. Chromogranin A is a potential prognostic marker in prostate cancer patients treated with enzalutamide. *Prostate* **2014**, *74*, 1691–1696. [CrossRef] [PubMed]

14. Sciarra, A.; di Silverio, F.; Autran, A.M.; Salciccia, S.; Gentilucci, A.; Alfarone, A.; Gentile, V. Distribution of high Chromogranin A serum levels in patients with nonmetastatic and metastatic prostate adenocarcinoma. *Urol. Int.* **2009**, *82*, 147–151. [CrossRef] [PubMed]
15. Aprikian, A.G.; Cordon-Cardo, C.; Fair, W.R.; Reuter, V.E. Characterization of neuroendocrine differentiation in human benign prostate and prostatic adenocarcinoma. *Cancer* **1993**, *71*, 3952–3965. [CrossRef]
16. Aprikian, A.G.; Cordon-Cardo, C.; Fair, W.R.; Zhang, Z.F.; Bazinet, M.; Hamdy, S.M.; Reuter, V.E. Neuroendocrine differentiation in metastatic prostatic adenocarcinoma. *J. Urol.* **1994**, *151*, 914–919.
17. Bostwick, D.G.; Qian, J.; Pacelli, A.; Zincke, H.; Blute, M.; Bergstralh, E.J.; Slezak, J.M.; Cheng, L. Neuroendocrine expression in node positive prostate cancer: Correlation with systemic progression and patient survival. *J. Urol.* **2002**, *168*, 1204–1211. [CrossRef]
18. Cheville, J.C.; Tindall, D.; Boelter, C.; Jenkins, R.; Lohse, C.M.; Pankratz, V.S.; Sebo, T.J.; Davis, B.; Blute, M.L. Metastatic prostate carcinoma to bone. *Cancer* **2002**, *95*, 1028–1036. [CrossRef] [PubMed]
19. Quek, M.L.; Daneshmand, S.; Rodrigo, S.; Cai, J.; Dorff, T.B.; Groshen, S.; Skinner, D.G.; Lieskovsky, G.; Pinski, J. Prognostic significance of neuroendocrine expression in lymph node-positive prostate cancer. *Urology* **2006**, *67*, 1247–1252. [CrossRef] [PubMed]
20. Roudier, M.P.; True, L.D.; Higano, C.S.; Vesselle, H.; Ellis, W.; Lange, P.; Vessella, R.L. Phenotypic heterogeneity of end-stage prostate carcinoma metastatic to bone. *Hum. Pathol.* **2003**, *34*, 646–653. [CrossRef]
21. McWilliam, L.J.; Manson, C.; George, N.J. Neuroendocrine differentiation and prognosis in prostatic adenocarcinoma. *Br. J. Urol.* **1997**, *80*, 287–290. [CrossRef] [PubMed]
22. Pruneri, G.; Galli, S.; Rossi, R.S.; Roncalli, M.; Coggi, G.; Ferrari, A.; Simonato, A.; Siccardi, A.G.; Carboni, N.; Buffa, R. Chromogranin A and B and secretogranin II in prostatic adenocarcinomas: Neuroendocrine expression in patients untreated and treated with androgen deprivation therapy. *Prostate* **1998**, *34*, 113–120.
23. Angelsen, A.; Syversen, U.; Haugen, O.A.; Stridsberg, M.; Mjølnerød, O.K.; Waldum, H.L. Neuroendocrine differentiation in carcinomas of the prostate: Do neuroendocrine serum markers reflect immunohistochemical findings? *Prostate* **1997**, *30*, 1–6. [CrossRef]
24. Fleischmann, A.; Schobinger, S.; Schumacher, M.; Thalmann, G.N.; Studer, U.E. Survival in surgically treated, nodal positive prostate cancer patients is predicted by histopathological characteristics of the primary tumor and its lymph node metastases. *Prostate* **2009**, *69*, 352–362. [CrossRef] [PubMed]
25. Brawn, P.N.; Speights, V.O. The dedifferentiation of metastatic prostate carcinoma. *Br. J. Cancer* **1989**, *59*, 85–88. [CrossRef] [PubMed]
26. Cheng, L.; Slezak, J.; Bergstralh, E.J.; Cheville, J.C.; Sweat, S.; Zincke, H.; Bostwick, D.G. Dedifferentiation in the metastatic progression of prostate carcinoma. *Cancer* **1999**, *86*, 657–663. [CrossRef]
27. Abrahamsson, P.A. Neuroendocrine differentiation in prostatic carcinoma. *Prostate* **1999**, *39*, 135–148.
28. Mucci, N.R.; Akdas, G.; Manely, S.; Rubin, M.A. Neuroendocrine expression in metastatic prostate cancer: Evaluation of high throughput tissue microarrays to detect heterogeneous protein expression. *Hum. Pathol.* **2000**, *31*, 406–414. [CrossRef] [PubMed]
29. Bader, P.; Burkhard, F.C.; Markwalder, R.; Studer, U.E. Disease progression and survival of patients with positive lymph nodes after radical prostatectomy. Is there a chance of cure? *J. Urol.* **2003**, *169*, 849–854.
30. Fleischmann, A.; Schobinger, S.; Markwalder, R.; Schumacher, M.; Burkhard, F.; Thalmann, G.N.; Studer, U.E. Prognostic factors in lymph node metastases of prostatic cancer patients: The size of the metastases but not extranodal extension independently predicts survival. *Histopathology* **2008**, *53*, 468–475. [CrossRef] [PubMed]
31. Epstein, J.I.; Helpap, B.; Algaba, F.; Humphrey, P.A.; Allsbrook, W.C.; Iczkowski, K.A.; Bastacky, S.; Lopez-Beltran, A.; Boccon-Gibod, L.; Montironi, R.; et al. Acinar adenocarcinoma. In *Pathology and Genetics of Tumours of the Urinary System and Male Genital Organs*; Eble, J.N., Sauter, G., Epstein, J.I., Sesterhenn, I.A., Eds.; IARC Press: Lyon, France, 2004.
32. Green, F.L. *TNM Classification of Malignant Tumors*; Bierley, J., Gospodarowicz, M.K., Wittekind, C., Eds.; Wiley-Blackwell: Oxford, UK, 2017.
33. Søreide, K. Receiver-operating characteristic curve analysis in diagnostic, prognostic and predictive biomarker research. *J. Clin. Pathol.* **2008**, *62*, 1–5. [CrossRef] [PubMed]

8

Comparative Study of Blood-Based Biomarkers, α2,3-Sialic Acid PSA and PHI, for High-Risk Prostate Cancer Detection

Montserrat Ferrer-Batallé [1,2,†], Esther Llop [1,2,†], Manel Ramírez [2,3], Rosa Núria Aleixandre [2,3], Marc Saez [4,5], Josep Comet [2,3], Rafael de Llorens [1,3,*] and Rosa Peracaula [1,3,*]

1 Biochemistry and Molecular Biology Unit, Department of Biology, University of Girona, 17003 Girona, Spain; montserrat.ferrer@udg.edu (M.F.-B.); esther.llop@udg.edu (E.L.)
2 Girona Biomedical Research Institute (IDIBGI), 17190 Salt (Girona), Spain; jramirez.girona.ics@gencat.cat (M.R.); rnaleixandre@infonegocio.com (R.N.A.); 28547jcb@comb.cat (J.C.)
3 Catalan Health Institute, University Hospital of Girona Dr. Josep Trueta, 17007 Girona, Spain
4 Research Group on Statistics, Econometrics and Health (GRECS), University of Girona, 17003 Girona, Spain; marc.saez@udg.edu
5 CIBER of Epidemiology and Public Health (CIBERESP), 28029 Madrid, Spain
* Correspondence: rafael.llorens@udg.edu (R.d.L.); rosa.peracaula@udg.edu (R.P.)

† These authors contributed equally to this work.

Academic Editor: Carsten Stephan

Abstract: Prostate Specific Antigen (PSA) is the most commonly used serum marker for prostate cancer (PCa), although it is not specific and sensitive enough to allow the differential diagnosis of the more aggressive tumors. For that, new diagnostic methods are being developed, such as PCA-3, PSA isoforms that have resulted in the 4K score or the Prostate Health Index (PHI), and PSA glycoforms. In the present study, we have compared the PHI with our recently developed PSA glycoform assay, based on the determination of the α2,3-sialic acid percentage of serum PSA (% α2,3-SA), in a cohort of 79 patients, which include 50 PCa of different grades and 29 benign prostate hyperplasia (BPH) patients. The % α2,3-SA could distinguish high-risk PCa patients from the rest of patients better than the PHI (area under the curve (AUC) of 0.971 vs. 0.840), although the PHI correlated better with the Gleason score than the % α2,3-SA. The combination of both markers increased the AUC up to 0.985 resulting in 100% sensitivity and 94.7% specificity to differentiate high-risk PCa from the other low and intermediate-risk PCa and BPH patients. These results suggest that both serum markers complement each other and offer an improved diagnostic tool to identify high-risk PCa, which is an important requirement for guiding treatment decisions.

Keywords: diagnosis; glycosylation; prostate cancer; prostate specific antigen; proPSA; PHI; α2,3-sialic acid

1. Introduction

Prostate cancer (PCa) is an important problem in public health and a major disease that affects men's health worldwide. It was the most commonly diagnosed male neoplasia in western countries and Japan last year. It is expected that around one of each six men will be diagnosed with PCa during his life. In addition, as the number of older people increase, the incidence of the disease will raise dramatically in the coming decades [1].

The serum marker Prostate Specific Antigen (PSA), adopted in the early 1990's, has been the widely used and preferred assay for prostate diseases, including PCa, with important levels of success, and represents the gold standard marker as an essential tool for urologists [1,2]. In addition, since PCa has a long natural history, the PSA assay predicts a prostate pathology decades before a confirmatory diagnostic [3]. This means that a majority of men diagnosed with PCa could be detected at early stages and with localized prostate cancer. Epidemiologic studies indicate an important and continuous decrease in prostate cancer mortality since the application of the PSA screening test [4].

However, the PSA test presents some limitations. It is organ specific but not cancer specific [5]. Serum PSA levels could also be elevated in benign prostate hyperplasia (BPH), prostatitis, and prostate manipulations (as DRE and bicycling), and cannot discriminate between aggressive and non-aggressive cancers. PSA assays present a high rate of false positives that leads to over-diagnosis, unnecessary biopsies, and over-treatments [6]. Actually only 25% of men biopsied after an elevated PSA level have PCa, and many of these cancers are slow growing, with no impact in the patient's life [7].

New non-invasive biomarkers with greater sensitivity and specificity that are capable of distinguishing aggressive tumors from indolent ones are required [5]. To improve the specificity of the PSA as a biomarker, different strategies using several PSA isoforms (ratio free PSA/total PSA, PSA density and velocity, proPSA forms, 4K score, and Prostate Health Index (PHI)) have been developed [7], recently including, PSA glycoforms [8–10].

Regarding proPSA forms, these were first identified in the serum of patients with prostate cancer in 1997 [11]. ProPSAs were preferentially elevated in the peripheral zone of prostatic tissue containing cancer, whilst remaining largely undetectable in the transitional zone of the prostate [12]. These proPSA forms comprised the complete sequence of inactive zymogen [−7]proPSA, and also shorter forms as [−5] [−4] and [−2]proPSA. [−2]proPSA was present in the sera of prostate cancer patients and it was a more specific serum marker that could improve a PSA assay. [−7] and [−5]proPSA did not give adequate results as biomarkers [13]. The interesting positive results of the [−2]proPSA detection moved Beckman & Coulter Inc. (Brea, CA, USA), in partnership with the NCI Early Detection Research Network, to develop a mathematical algorithm with [−2]proPSA, tPSA, and fPSA serum levels, the so called Prostate Health Index: $PHI = ([-2]proPSA/fPSA) \times \sqrt{tPSA}$ [14]. PHI received the FDA approval in 2012 [7]. Several works, including numerous international multicenter studies, have indicated that PHI score outperforms its individual components for the prediction of overall and high-grade prostate cancer [6,15–17]. PHI score has a high diagnostic accuracy rate and may be useful as a tumor marker in predicting patients harboring more aggressive disease. PHI also predicts the likelihood of progression during active surveillance. PHI score has been reported to correlate with PSA serum levels and Gleason scores. Nowadays, PHI has regulatory approval in more than 50 countries worldwide and is now being incorporated into prostate cancer guidelines for early prostate cancer detection and risk stratification [18]. However, others studies do not completely agree with these results and indicated that when the goal is to detect at least 95% of the aggressive tumors, PHI does not seem to be much more effective than the %fPSA and the PSA density [19].

To address the problem of the discovery of new non-invasive PCa markers that can predict PCa aggressiveness, several authors have determined the glycosylation pattern of PSA from healthy donors, PCa cancer cell lines, and PCa serum patients, and have shown specific changes in the PSA core fucosylation and sialylation levels in PCa patients [8,10,20–27]. In this regard, we have developed a methodology to quantify the ratio of core fucosylation of serum PSA and the percentage of α2,3-sialic acid of serum PSA and have shown a decrease in the content of core fucose and an increase in α2,3-sialic acid of PSA *N*-glycans in patients with high-risk PCa [9]. In particular, the percentage of α2,3-sialic acid of PSA was increased in the high-risk PCa patients compared with low or intermediate-risk PCa and BPH patients and gave an AUC of 0.971, with 85.7% sensitivity and 95.3% specificity. Interestingly, the percentage of α2,3-sialic acid of PSA also correlated with the Gleason score of PCa patients.

With the aim of searching for new serum markers that could assist in the identification of the aggressive prostate cancers, the present study compared the potential of PHI and the percentage of α2,3-sialic of PSA, alone and in combination, to identify high risk PCa cancer in a cohort of 79 patients' serum samples.

2. Results

2.1. Clinical and Pathological Characteristics of the Patients

A cohort of 79 serum samples containing 29 BPH and 50 PCa samples was used for the study of the two blood-based biomarkers, PHI and the percentage of α2,3-sialic of PSA. PCa staging was determined according to the International Union Against Cancer (IUAC) and patients were classified in high-risk ($N = 22$), intermediate-risk ($N = 21$) and low-risk ($N = 7$). Clinical data of the subjects included in this study are summarized in Table 1.

The seven low-risk PCa patients had tPSA levels below 10 ng/mL and Gleason scores ≤6. The 21 intermediate-risk PCa group comprised five patients with a Gleason score of six and clinical stage >pT2a; 15 patients with a Gleason score of seven and one subject presenting a focal Gleason score of eight. Their tPSA levels were between 3.73 and 12.42 ng/mL. The 22 high-risk PCa included 18 with a Gleason score ≥8, two with a Gleason score of seven and metastasis, and two other subjects with an undetermined Gleason score who also presented metastasis. Data corresponding to the age and total and free PSA values of all groups of patients are shown in Table 1.

Evaluation of the clinical outcome of the PCa patients showed a PCa recurrence one year after treatment of 0%, 4.8%, and 59% in the low, intermediate, and high-risk PCa groups respectively. Data of the five-year relapse-free survival was reported for all patients in the low-risk group being 100%. However, this information was not available for all patients in the other two groups. The five-year relapse-free survival was 95% for the intermediate-risk group corresponding to 20 out of the 21 patients, and it was 40% in the high-risk group corresponding to 15 out of the 22 patients.

2.2. Analysis of α2,3-Sialic Acid PSA in Serum Samples

For the analysis of percentage of α2,3-sialic acid PSA, 0.75 mL of each serum were required. First, the serum samples were treated with ethanolamine, in order to release PSA from its complex with α1-antichymotrypsin. Then, total PSA from the serum samples was immunoprecipitated and loaded into a SNA lectin column. This lectin chromatography, which binds to α2,6-sialylated glycoconjugates, allows for the separation of α2,3-sialylated from α2,6-sialylated PSA glycoforms [9]. After the lectin chromatography, free PSA in the unbound (α2,3-sialylated PSA) and bound fractions (α2,6-sialylated PSA) was measured, and from these data the percentage of fPSA in both fractions was calculated. The percentage of the unbound fraction corresponded to the percentage of α2,3-sialic acid PSA.

The potential of the percentage of α2,3-sialic acid PSA as a blood biomarker for aggressive PCa was assessed in the cohort of sera (29 BPH, seven low-risk, 21 intermediate-risk and 22 high-risk PCa). Three different PCa serum samples, containing different values of tPSA (12.87, 23.08, and 40.61 ng/mL) were repeatedly analyzed in the different batches of samples in order to calculate the inter-assay variation of the method that was lower than 12%.

The plot of the percentage of α2,3-sialylated PSA is represented against the concentration of the total PSA of each sample (Figure 1A) and in the four groups (Figure 1B). A significant increase of percentage of α2,3-sialylated PSA in the group of high-risk PCa patients (26.8–61.4%) compared with the other three groups, intermediate-risk PCa (12.7–35.5%; $p < 0.001$), low-risk PCa (12.3–29.9%; $p = 0.006$), and BPH (10.9–33.5%; $p < 0.001$) was shown. However, no significant differences were found between BPH and low and intermediate-risk PCa patients. The correlation of α2,3-sialylated PSA values of the samples with their corresponding tPSA levels was tested and resulted to be non-significant in any of the BPH and PCa groups. Both parameters were then independent, indicating that a high or a low percentage of α2,3-sialylated PSA could be found in sera with either low or high tPSA levels in any group of patients (Figure 1A).

Table 1. Clinical and pathological characteristics of the patients.

Pathology	Cases	N	PCa Recurrence, 1 Year	Gleason Score	N	Age Average	Range	tPSA ng/mL	±SD	Range	fPSA ng/mL	±SD	Range
BPH		29				63.24	44–76	7.59	2.39	3.89–14.47	1.26	0.53	0.30–2.28
PCa $N = 50$	Low-risk	7	0%	Gleason 5	1	84		2.45			0.27		
				Gleason 6	6	66.2	61–74	4.91	1.38	2.64–6.33	0.88	0.22	0.61–1.14
	Intermediate risk	21	4.8%	Gleason 6	5	56	47–75	5.79	3.73	3.73–12.42	0.53	0.33	0.19–0.97
				Gleason 7	15	65.2	46–78	6.61	1.84	5.13–10.39	0.65	0.29	0.58–1.36
				Gleason 8 focal	1	70		7.16			1.76		
	High-risk	22	59%	Gleason 7/metastasis	2	76	69–83	12.08	2.85	10.07–14.1	1.93	1.63	0.78–3.09
				Gleason 8	10	65.5	51–83	16.23	11.93	1.96–40.61	1.58	1.46	0.35–5.29
				Gleason 9	7	67.8	49–79	14.81	5.22	4.34–18.77	3.28	2.18	0.7–7.09
				Gleason 10	1	67		87.51			12.77		
				Gleason ND */metastasis	2	75	67–83	7.28	3.65	4.7–9.86	1.37	1.22	0.51–2.23

* ND: not determined; SD: Standard deviation.

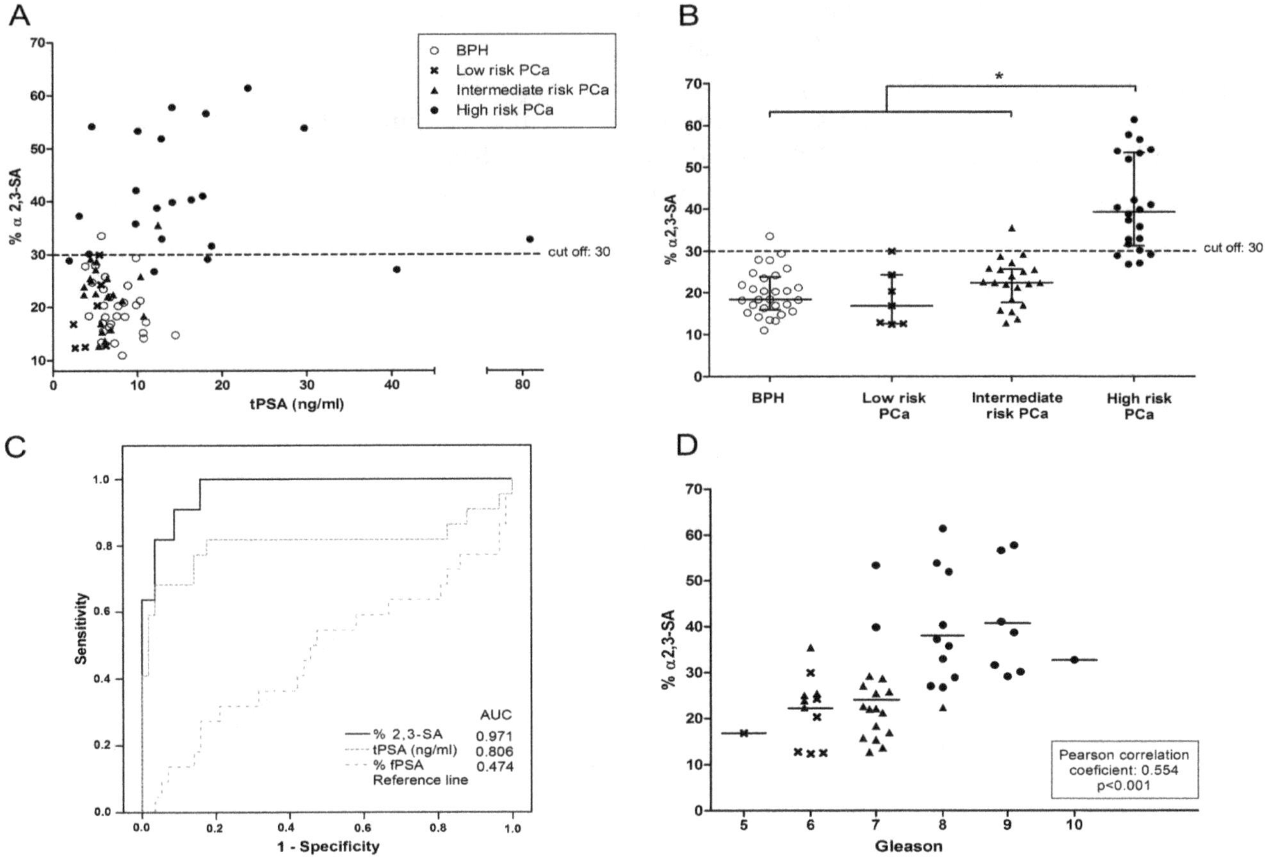

Figure 1. α2,3-SA percentage of Prostate Specific Antigen (PSA) (% α2,3-SA) of the cohort of 79 serum samples. Benign Prostate Hyperplasia (BPH) samples are represented with an open circle (o), low risk PCa with a cross (×), intermediate risk PCa with a filled triangle (▲) and high risk PCa with a filled circle (●). (**A**) Representation of % α2,3-SA against tPSA serum levels; dotted line (- - -) shows the cutoff value for discriminating high risk PCa samples from the other three groups; (**B**) Representation of % α2,3-SA against the pathology. The center line indicates the median, and the top and bottom lines, the 75th and 25th percentiles, respectively; (**C**) Representation of the Receiver operating characteristic (ROC) curves for % α2,3-SA, tPSA, and %fPSA; (**D**) Correlation plot of % α2,3-SA from the PCa serum samples with their Gleason score. The mean of % α2,3-SA of each Gleason score is shown with a horizontal line (-).

In order to compare the performance of PSA α2,3-sialic acid percentage with that of tPSA and the %fPSA values, the Receiver operating characteristic (ROC) curves of these three parameters were compared (Figure 1C). The ROC assay showed that % α2,3-sialic acid had the highest performance and could separate high-risk PCa patients from BPH, low, or intermediate-risk prostate cancers with 81.8% sensitivity and 96.5% specificity with a cutoff of 30%, resulting in an AUC of 0.97. In addition, this biomarker, which is based on the detection of specific PSA glycoforms, significantly correlated with the Gleason score of the tumor (correlation coefficient 0.554, $p < 0.001$) (Figure 1D), which highlights its potential as a marker for aggressive PCa.

2.3. Prostate Health Index (PHI) Score Analysis of Serum Samples

For this analysis, patients' sera were analyzed for total PSA (tPSA), free PSA (fPSA), and [−2]proPSA. Then the Prostate Health Index (PHI) score was calculated [$PHI = ([-2]proPSA\ /fPSA) \times \sqrt{tPSA}$]. This methodology was used to analyze the cohort of serum samples tested previously for α2,3-sialic acid percentage of PSA.

The plot of the PHI score is shown against the concentration of total serum PSA of each sample (Figure 2A) and in the four groups (Figure 2B). There was a significant increase of PHI score in the group of high-risk PCa patients compared with the other two groups, low-risk PCa ($p = 0.006$) and BPH ($p < 0.001$). The intermediate-risk PCa group showed also a significant increase of PHI compared with low-risk PCa ($p = 0.006$) and BPH ($p = 0.022$). No significant differences were found between high-risk PCa patients and intermediate-risk PCa neither between BPH and low-risk PCa patients.

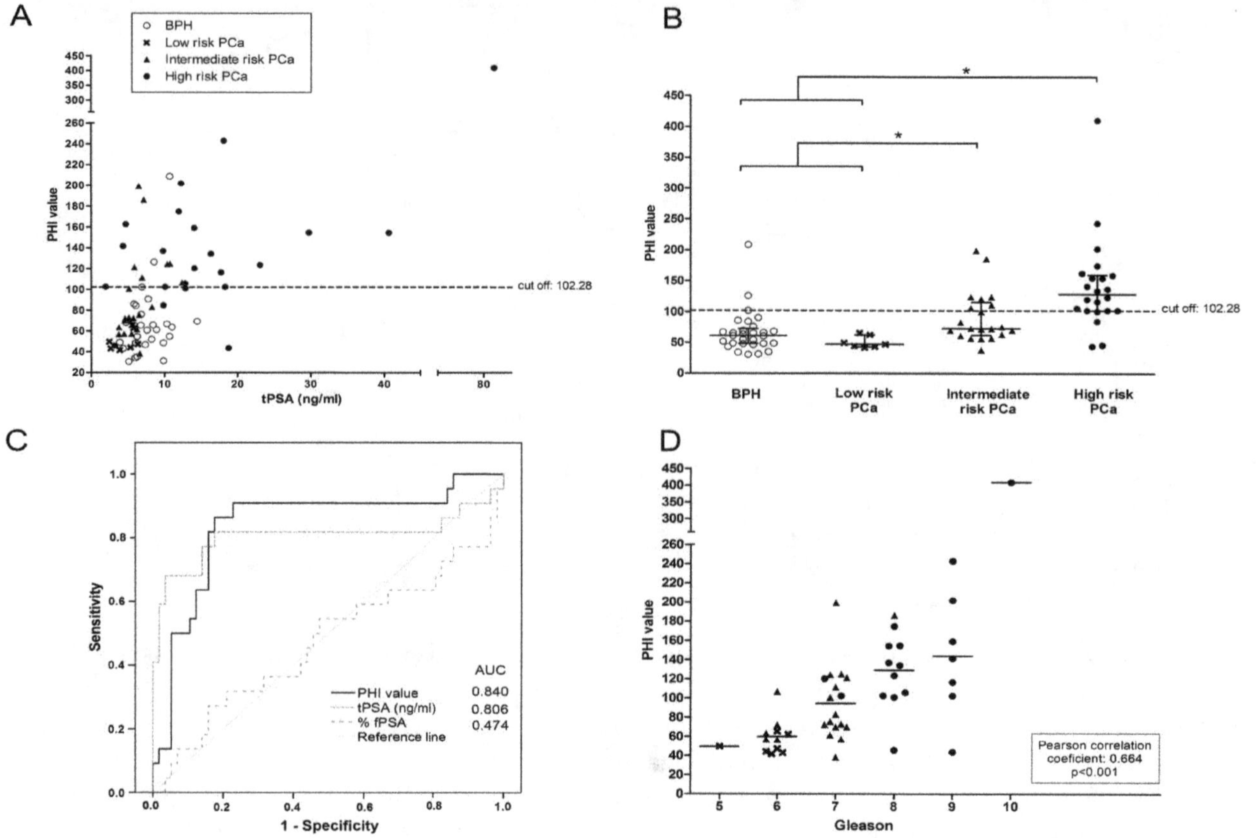

Figure 2. Prostate Health Index (PHI) values of the cohort of 79 serum samples. BPH samples are represented with an open circle (o), low risk PCa with a cross (×), intermediate risk PCa with a filled triangle (▲) and high risk PCa with a filled circle (●). (**A**) Representation of PHI value against tPSA serum levels; dotted line (- - -) shows the cutoff value for discriminating high risk PCa samples from the other three groups; (**B**) Representation of PHI value against the pathology. The center line indicates the median, and the top and bottom lines, the 75th and 25th percentiles, respectively; (**C**) Representation of the ROC curves for the PHI value, tPSA and %fPSA (**D**) Correlation plot of PHI value of the PCa samples with their Gleason score. The mean PHI value of each Gleason score is shown with a horizontal line (-).

PHI values correlated with the tPSA levels of the sample in the high-risk PCa group (correlation coefficient 0.758, $p < 0.001$), while there was no correlation for the other individual groups.

ROC analysis of the PHI score gave an AUC of 0.840 to discriminate high-risk PCa patients from the other groups, BPH and low- and intermediate-risk PCa. With a PHI cutoff of 102.28, the sensitivity was 81.8% and the specificity was 84.2%. The performance of the PHI score was higher than that of tPSA and %fPSA (Figure 2C). PHI score values showed a significant correlation with the Gleason score of the prostate tumor tissues (correlation coefficient of 0.664; $p < 0.001$) (Figure 2D).

Since PHI values of the high risk group were dependent on tPSA values, a subcohort of patients with tPSA levels lower than 13 ng/mL ($N = 67$, 28 BPH, seven low-risk, 21 intermediate-risk and 11 high-risk PCa) was evaluated. This subcohort reduced basically the number of high-risk PCa patients, which had high levels of tPSA. In this subcohort, there was no correlation of PHI values and tPSA levels within the high-risk group. The AUC of PHI in this subcohort for identifying high-risk PCa was 0.81, slightly lower than when analyzing the whole cohort.

When PHI was assayed to discriminate PCa from BPH, the AUC was of 0.735, sensitivity of 84% and specificity 45%, with a cutoff of 55.7. The diagnostic performance of PHI was higher than tPSA (AUC of 0.506) and %fPSA (AUC of 0.632), in agreement with bibliographic studies. In the subcohort of patients with tPSA levels lower than 13 ng/mL ($N = 67$, 28 BPH, seven low-risk, 21 intermediate-risk and 11 high-risk PCa), PHI performance for PCa diagnosing (AUC of 0.694) was still higher than tPSA (AUC of 0.382) and %fPSA (AUC of 0.630).

2.4. Combinatorial Analysis of PHI and α2,3-Sialic Acid PSA

In order to assess the performance of the combination of PHI and α2,3-sialic acid PSA, the R statistic package was used. The combination of both biomarkers showed a high performance to differentiate the high-risk PCa group from the other groups with an AUC of 0.985, much higher than PHI alone (Figure 3A,C). The combination of PHI and α2,3-sialic acid PSA also correlated with the Gleason score of the PCa patients and interestingly the two high-risk PCa patients with GS = 7 were classified correctly and were differentiated from 14 out of 15 patients of GS = 7 of the intermediate-risk PCa group (Figure 3B).

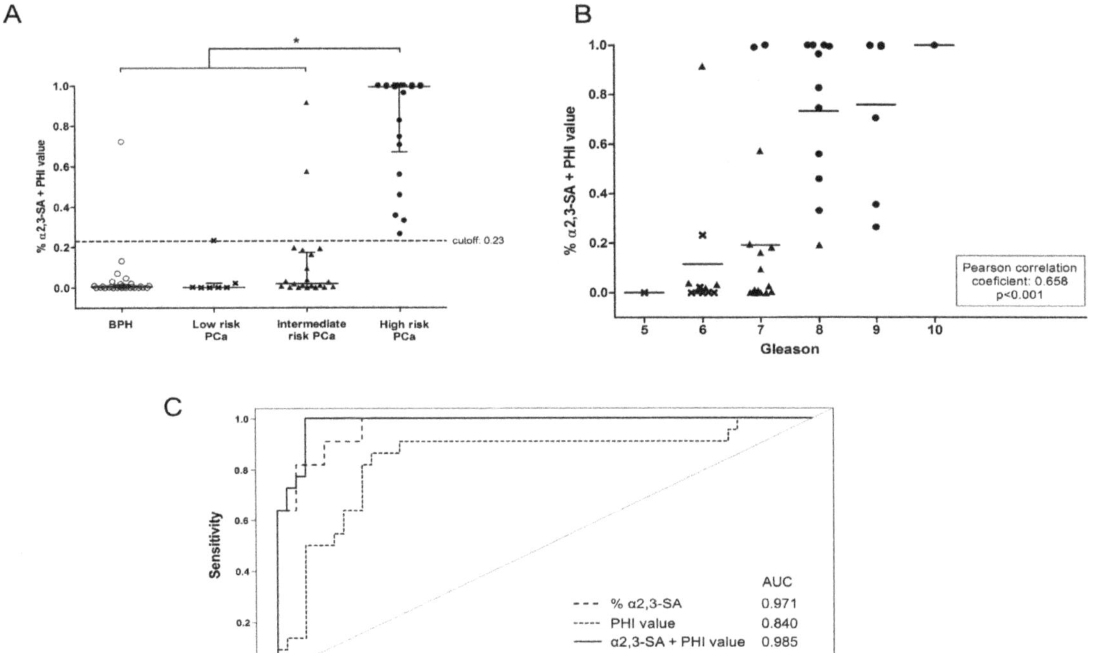

Figure 3. % α2,3-SA and PHI combination of the cohort of 79 serum samples. BPH samples are represented with an open circle (o), low risk PCa with a cross (×), intermediate risk PCa with a filled triangle (▲) and high risk PCa with a filled circle (●). (**A**) Representation of % α2,3-SA and PHI combination values against the pathology. The center line indicates the median, and the top and bottom lines, the 75th and 25th percentiles, respectively; dotted line (- - -) shows the cutoff value for discriminating high risk PCa samples from the other three groups; (**B**) Correlation plot of % α2,3-SA and PHI combination of the PCa samples with their Gleason score. The mean % α2,3-SA and PHI combination value of each Gleason score is shown with a horizontal line (-); (**C**) ROC curves for the diagnosis of high-risk PCa versus low- and intermediate-risk PCa and BPH. Diagnostic performance of % α2,3-SA and PHI combination (solid line) compared with PHI (dotted line) and % α2,3-SA (dashed line).

With the aim of implementing the combination of PHI and % α2,3-SA in clinics, an algorithm that includes both variables was developed. This consisted of a generalized lineal model (GLM) with a binomial response. After the introduction of PHI and α2,3-sialic acid percentage values, the GLM allowed to classify the patients as high-risk PCa with 100% sensitivity and 94.7% specificity. The cutoff for PHI score was 65.4 and for α2,3-sialic acid percentage of PSA was 29.94%. The model calculates the probability of a patient to be diagnosed as high-risk PCa or not (either low and intermediate-risk PCa or BPH). For a probability equal to, or higher than 23.2% (that corresponds to the point with maximum sensitivity and specificity) the patient will be classified as high-risk PCa with a sensitivity of 100% and a specificity of 94.7%. For a probability lower than 23.2% the patient will be classified either as a low- or intermediate-risk PCa, or a BPH. The probability for each patient is calculated with the following function using the patient values of PHI and α2,3-sialic acid percentage of PSA (% α2,3-SA), where β_0, β_1 and β_2 are parameters estimated by the model:

$$\mathrm{Prob(High-riskPCa)} = \frac{e^{(\beta_0+\beta_1 \mathrm{PHI}+\beta_2 \%\alpha 2,3-\mathrm{SA})}}{1+e^{(\beta_0+\beta_1 \mathrm{PHI}+\beta_2 \%\alpha 2,3-\mathrm{SA})}}.$$

3. Discussion

New generation of tumor markers for PCa diagnosis should be able to discriminate between patients with aggressive tumors and those without cancer or low aggressive tumors. Thus, the skills required for the new generation of markers of PCa are high sensitivity and specificity for aggressive tumors. This way, an unnecessary biopsy in men who do not have an aggressive or asymptomatic PCa could be avoided [19,28]. Early diagnosis of PCa frequently, involves the over-detection of non-aggressive tumors.

In the next future, PCa diagnosis and prognosis will probably depend on panels of biomarkers that will allow a more accurate prediction of PCa presence, stage and aggressiveness, so they will be key factors in a clinician making decisions. These markers could include serum non-invasive markers, as well as imaging markers, such as multi-parametric prostate magnetic resonance (mpMRI), which has also been proposed as a means to avoid the incidental detection of low-grade cancers [29–31].

PHI is a simple and affordable blood test that could be used as part of a multivariable approach to screening. In this sense, PHI has shown good performance for PCa diagnosis [16]. Our results are in agreement with the reported data and have shown that PHI identifies PCa from BPH with an AUC of 0.735 with higher performance than tPSA (AUC = 0.506) and %fPSA (AUC = 0.632). Since PHI has been recommended for PSA levels between 4–10 ng/mL, we examined PHI performance in the subcohort with levels of tPSA lower than 13 ng/mL and the AUC decreased to 0.694, but was still higher than tPSA (AUC = 0.382) and %fPSA (AUC = 0.630).

However, the performance of PHI in identifying high-risk PCa from the non-aggressive PCa and BPHs is much higher than for identifying PCa from BPH in both the whole cohort and the subcohort, which can be explained because PHI correlates with the Gleason score, as has also been described previously by other studies [32].

The potential of % α2,3-SA to identify high-risk PCa has been confirmed in this study. The AUC was 0.97 with a cutoff of 30%, as previously described. Interestingly, % α2,3-SA performance was not influenced by the tPSA levels of the samples, and had the same performance in the subcohort of tPSA levels lower than 13 ng/mL.

% α2,3-SA test identifies PSA glycoforms containing α2,3-sialic acid, which have been linked to PCa aggressiveness [9,10,33]. PHI score comprises other PSA isoforms linked to PCa, namely [−2]proPSA, fPSA and tPSA. In this work, we have assessed whether these different PSA forms could complement each other to better identify high-risk PCa. The combination of both markers, % α2,3-SA and PHI, has given the best performance to identify high-risk PCa, with an AUC of 0.985 (100% sensitivity, 94% specificity), although larger independent cohorts are required to validate these promising results. In this regard, the methodology to determine the percentage of α2,3-sialic acid of PSA is currently being implemented to make it more automated so that it could be used in a clinical setting.

These results highlight that the future of prostate cancer diagnosis might rely on the combination of a panel of markers based on PSA forms that can give accurate molecular diagnosis and staging and indicate the likelihood of aggressive behavior.

4. Materials and Methods

4.1. Serum Samples

The study population included 79 patients (29 BPH and 50 PCa) from Hospital Universitari Dr. Josep Trueta (Girona, Spain) between 2006 and 2013. The study was approved by the Hospital Ethics Committee (Refs. 169.06 and 023.10) and all patients provided written informed consent before being enrolled. Patients' sera were collected and stored at −80 °C. Urology and Pathology units from Hospital Universitari Dr. J. Trueta (Girona, Spain) performed the diagnosis using Transrectal Ultrasound-guided biopsy and/or adenomectomy/prostatectomy followed by pathological analysis.

The 29 BPH patients of the study (age range 44–76 years old) had a medical follow-up for a minimum of 2 years. 24 BPH patients had, at least, two negative biopsies with no evidence of high-grade Prostatic Intraepithelial Neoplasia (PIN). The 5 BPH left were subjected to prostate surgery (adenomectomy or prostate transurethral resection) and confirmed not to have prostate cancer by the Pathology Unit.

The 50 PCa patients of the study (age range 46–84 years old) were graded according to the Tumor-Node-Metastasis (TNM) classification following the general guidelines of the European Association of Urology. PCa patients were treatment naïve when serum samples were collected, except one PCa patient of the high-risk group, who was receiving hormonal therapy. High-risk PCa group comprised 22 patients with Gleason scores ≥8 (4 + 4) and/or with metastasis. The low-risk PCa group included 7 patients with Gleason scores of ≤6 (3 + 3), tPSA levels <10 ng/mL and clinical stage ≤pT2a. The group of intermediate-risk patients was comprised of 21 patients that did not meet the above criteria. They had Gleason scores of 7 (3 + 4 or 4 + 3) and 6 (3 + 3) and also included a patient with focal Gleason 8, tPSA levels <10 ng/mL and clinical stage pT2a considering his 10-year relapse-free survival.

The average of tPSA serum levels for BPH patients was 7.59 ng/mL (range, 3.89 to 14.47 ng/mL). The average of tPSA for the PCa groups was: 17.83 ng/ml (range, 1.96 to 87.51 ng/mL) for high-risk PCa patients, 6.44 ng/mL (range, 3.73 to 12.42 ng/mL) for intermediate-risk PCa patients, and 4.56 ng/mL (range, 2.45 to 6.33 ng/mL) for low-risk PCa patients.

4.2. Analysis of α2,3-Sialic Acid of Serum PSA

The determination of % α2,3-sialic acid of PSA was performed using a previously published method [9]. Briefly, ethanolamine 5 M was added to 0.75 mL of each serum sample to a final concentration of 1 M to release the PSA complexed to α1-antichymotrypsin. Total PSA was immunopurified using the Access Hybritech PSA assay Kit (Beckman Coulter, Brea, CA, USA). Amicon Ultra-0.5 3K Centrifugal Filter Devices (Millipore, Cork, Ireland) were used for desalting and concentrating the immunopurified tPSA samples up to a final volume of 40 μL. Samples were then applied to a lectin chromatography using *Sambucus nigra* (SNA)-agarose lectin (Vector Laboratories, Inc., Burlingame, CA, USA). Eluted unbound and bound chromatographic fractions were collected by centrifugation and quantification of free PSA of these fractions was performed using the Roche ELECSYS platform and used to determine the percentages of fPSA in the unbound fraction, corresponding to α2,3-sialic acid PSA, and in the bound fractions, which correspond to α2,6-sialic acid PSA.

4.3. Quantification of tPSA, fPSA and [−2]proPSA

Patient sera were analyzed for total PSA (tPSA), free PSA (fPSA), and [−2]proPSA on the Beckman Coulter Access 2 analyzer using WHO-standard-calibration. The Prostate Health Index (PHI) score was then calculated [PHI = ([−2]proPSA/fPSA) × $\sqrt{tPSA}$]. Assays kits used were: Hybritech total PSA assay kit (Beckman Coulter, Fullerton, CA, USA; cat. no. 37200; Lot no. 523610), Hybritech free PSA assay kit (Beckman Coulter, Fullerton, CA, USA; cat. no. 37210; Lot no. 570228) and Hybritech p2PSA assay kit (Beckman Coulter, Fullerton, CA, USA; cat. no. P090026; Lot no. 527739). Assays were performed according to the instructions of their manufacturer and calibration and control materials used in each assay where the ones recommended by the manufacturer.

4.4. Statistics

Statistical analyses of both PHI and % α2,3-SA as PCa biomarkers were performed using IBM SPSS Statistics 23 for Windows and graphics were generated with SPSS software and GraphPad Prism 5 (GraphPad Software, Inc., La Jolla, CA, USA).

Patients were classified into four groups (BPH, low-risk PCa, intermediate-risk PCa, and high-risk PCa) and Shapiro-Wilk and Levene's tests were used to assess the normality and homoscedasticity of variables. Differences of % α2,3-SA and PHI value between groups were analyzed using a Mann–Whitney *U* test. Receiver operating characteristic (ROC) curves were analyzed for tPSA, fPSA, % α2,3-SA, and PHI for distinguishing between high-risk PCa from the group of low-risk PCa, intermediate-risk PCa, and BPH, and also for distinguishing between PCa from BPH.

Bivariate regression (Pearson correlation) was used to analyze the correlation of % α2,3-SA and PHI with either the Gleason score or the tPSA levels.

To combine PHI and % α2,3-SA, a logistic regression was performed, in which the response variable corresponded to the probability that the event of interest was a high-risk PCa (variable taking the value 1) or the group comprising low- and intermediate-risk PCa and BPH (variable taking the value 0). An R statistical package was used to develop a generalized lineal model (GLM) with binomial response. The construction and the comparison of the AUC of the ROC curves were performed using the Epi [34,35] and pROC libraries [36].

In all these analyses, $p < 0.05$ was considered statistically significant.

Acknowledgments: This work was supported by the Spanish Ministerio de Economia y Competitividad (CDTI grant IDI20130186 and grant BIO 2015-66356-R), by the Generalitat de Catalunya, Spain (grant 2014 SGR 229), and by Roche Diagnostics (Barcelona, Spain). We thank Mireia Lopez-Siles for her support with GraphPad Prism 5.

Author Contributions: Rafael de Llorens and Rosa Peracaula conceived and designed the experiments; Montserrat Ferrer-Batallé, Esther Llop and Manel Ramírez performed the experiments; Montserrat Ferrer-Batallé, Esther Llop, Marc Saez, Josep Comet, Rafael de Llorens and Rosa Peracaula analyzed the data; Manel Ramírez and Rosa Núria Aleixandre contributed reagents/materials/analysis tools; Montserrat Ferrer-Batallé, Esther Llop, Rafael de Llorens and Rosa Peracaula wrote the paper. All of the authors read and approved the final manuscript.

Abbreviations

PCa	Prostate cancer
PSA	Prostate Specific Antigen
PHI	Prostate Health Index
BPH	Benign Prostate Hyperplasia
AUC	Area Under the Curve
% α2,3-SA	Percentage of α2,3 sialic acid of PSA
DRE	Digital rectal examination
tPSA	Total PSA
fPSA	Free PSA
FDA	Food and Drug Administration
%fPSA	Free-to-total prostate-specific antigen ratio
PIN	Prostatic Intraepithelial Neoplasia

TNM	Tumor-Node-Metastasis
ACT	α1-Antichymotrypsin
SNA	*Sambucus nigra* lectin
CV	Coefficient of variation
mpMRI	Multi-parametric magnetic resonance imaging

References

1. Shoag, J.E.; Schlegel, P.N.; Hu, J.C. Prostate-Specific Antigen Screening: Time to Change the Dominant Forces on the Pendulum. *J. Clin. Oncol.* **2016**. [CrossRef] [PubMed]
2. Schmid, M.; Trinh, Q.D.; Graefen, M.; Fisch, M.; Chun, F.K.; Hansen, J. The role of biomarkers in the assessment of prostate cancer risk prior to prostate biopsy: Which markers matter and how should they be used? *World J. Urol.* **2014**, *32*, 871–880. [CrossRef] [PubMed]
3. Sohn, E. Screening: Diagnostic dilemma. *Nature* **2015**, *528*, S120–S122. [CrossRef] [PubMed]
4. Roobol, M. Perspective: Enforce the clinical guidelines. *Nature* **2015**, *528*, S123. [CrossRef] [PubMed]
5. Heidegger, I.; Klocker, H.; Steiner, E.; Skradski, V.; Ladurner, M.; Pichler, R.; Schafer, G.; Horninger, W.; Bektic, J. [−2]proPSA is an early marker for prostate cancer aggressiveness. *Prostate Cancer Prostatic Dis.* **2014**, *17*, 70–74. [CrossRef] [PubMed]
6. Hatakeyama, S.; Yoneyama, T.; Tobisawa, Y.; Ohyama, C. Recent progress and perspectives on prostate cancer biomarkers. *Int. J. Clin. Oncol.* **2016**, *22*, 214–221. [CrossRef] [PubMed]
7. Crawford, E.D.; Denes, B.S.; Ventil, K.H.; Shore, N. Prostate cancer: Incorporating genomic biomarkers in prostate cancer decisions. *Clin. Pract.* **2014**, *11*, 605–612. [CrossRef]
8. Li, Q.K.; Chen, L.; Ao, M.H.; Chiu, J.H.; Zhang, Z.; Zhang, H.; Chan, D.W. Serum fucosylated prostate-specific antigen (PSA) improves the differentiation of aggressive from non-aggressive prostate cancers. *Theranostics* **2015**, *5*, 267–276. [CrossRef] [PubMed]
9. Llop, E.; Ferrer-Batallé, M.; Barrabés, S.; Guerrero, P.; Ramírez, M.; Saldova, R.; Rudd, P.; Aleixandre, R.; Comet, J.; de Llorens, R.; et al. Improvement of Prostate Cancer Diagnosis by Detecting PSA Glycosylation-Specific Changes. *Theranostics* **2016**, *6*, 1190–1204. [CrossRef] [PubMed]
10. Ishikawa, T.; Yoneyama, T.; Tobisawa, Y.; Hatakeyama, S.; Kurosawa, T.; Nakamura, K.; Narita, S.; Mitsuzuka, K.; Duivenvoorden, W.; Pinthus, J.H.; et al. An Automated Micro-Total Immunoassay System for Measuring Cancer-Associated α2,3-linked Sialyl *N*-Glycan-Carrying Prostate-Specific Antigen May Improve the Accuracy of Prostate Cancer Diagnosis. *Int. J. Mol. Sci.* **2017**, *18*, 470. [CrossRef] [PubMed]
11. Sartori, D.A.; Chan, D.W. Biomarkers in prostate cancer: What's new? *Curr. Opin. Oncol.* **2014**, *26*, 259–264. [CrossRef] [PubMed]
12. Mikolajczyk, S.D.; Millar, L.S.; Wang, T.J.; Rittenhouse, H.G.; Marks, L.S.; Song, W.; Wheeler, T.M.; Slawin, K.M. A precursor form of prostate-specific antigen is more highly elevated in prostate cancer compared with benign transition zone prostate tissue. *Cancer Res.* **2000**, *60*, 756–759. [PubMed]
13. Stephan, C.; Meyer, H.A.; Paul, E.M.; Kristiansen, G.; Loening, S.A.; Lein, M.; Jung, K. Serum (-5, -7) proPSA for distinguishing stage and grade of prostate cancer. *Anticancer Res.* **2007**, *27*, 1833–1836. [PubMed]
14. Hori, S.; Blanchet, J.S.; McLoughlin, J. From prostate-specific antigen (PSA) to precursor PSA (proPSA) isoforms: A review of the emerging role of proPSAs in the detection and management of early prostate cancer. *BJU Int.* **2013**, *112*, 717–728. [CrossRef] [PubMed]
15. Lazzeri, M.; Lughezzani, G.; Haese, A.; McNicholas, T.; de la Taille, A.; Buffi, N.M.; Cardone, P.; Hurle, R.; Casale, P.; Bini, V.; et al. Clinical performance of prostate health index in men with tPSA >10 ng/ml: Results from a multicentric European study. *Urol. Oncol.* **2016**, *34*, 415. [CrossRef] [PubMed]
16. Loeb, S.; Catalona, W.J. The Prostate Health Index: A new test for the detection of prostate cancer. *Ther. Adv. Urol.* **2014**, *6*, 74–77. [CrossRef] [PubMed]
17. Wang, W.; Wang, M.; Wang, L.; Adams, T.S.; Tian, Y.; Xu, J. Diagnostic ability of %p2PSA and prostate health index for aggressive prostate cancer: A meta-analysis. *Sci. Rep.* **2014**, *4*, 5012. [CrossRef] [PubMed]
18. Loeb, S. Time to replace prostate-specific antigen (PSA) with the Prostate Health Index (PHI)? Yet more evidence that the phi consistently outperforms PSA across diverse populations. *BJU Int.* **2015**, *115*, 500. [CrossRef] [PubMed]

19. Morote, J.; Celma, A.; Planas, J.; Placer, J.; Ferrer, R.; de Torres, I.; Pacciuci, R.; Olivan, M. Diagnostic accuracy of prostate health index to identify aggressive prostate cancer. An Institutional validation study. *Actas Urol. Esp.* **2016**, *40*, 378–385. [CrossRef] [PubMed]
20. Peracaula, R.; Tabares, G.; Royle, L.; Harvey, D.J.; Dwek, R.A.; Rudd, P.M.; de Llorens, R. Altered glycosylation pattern allows the distinction between prostate-specific antigen (PSA) from normal and tumor origins. *Glycobiology* **2003**, *13*, 457–470. [CrossRef] [PubMed]
21. Ohyama, C.; Hosono, M.; Nitta, K.; Oh-eda, M.; Yoshikawa, K.; Habuchi, T.; Arai, Y.; Fukuda, M. Carbohydrate structure and differential binding of prostate specific antigen to Maackia amurensis lectin between prostate cancer and benign prostate hypertrophy. *Glycobiology* **2004**, *14*, 671–679. [CrossRef] [PubMed]
22. Tabares, G.; Radcliffe, C.M.; Barrabes, S.; Ramirez, M.; Aleixandre, R.N.; Hoesel, W.; Dwek, R.A.; Rudd, P.M.; Peracaula, R.; de Llorens, R. Different glycan structures in prostate-specific antigen from prostate cancer sera in relation to seminal plasma PSA. *Glycobiology* **2006**, *16*, 132–145. [CrossRef] [PubMed]
23. Tajiri, M.; Ohyama, C.; Wada, Y. Oligosaccharide profiles of the prostate specific antigen in free and complexed forms from the prostate cancer patient serum and in seminal plasma: A glycopeptide approach. *Glycobiology* **2008**, *18*, 2–8. [CrossRef] [PubMed]
24. Meany, D.L.; Zhang, Z.; Sokoll, L.J.; Zhang, H.; Chan, D.W. Glycoproteomics for prostate cancer detection: Changes in serum PSA glycosylation patterns. *J. Proteom. Res.* **2009**, *8*, 613–619. [CrossRef] [PubMed]
25. Sarrats, A.; Saldova, R.; Comet, J.; O'Donoghue, N.; de Llorens, R.; Rudd, P.M.; Peracaula, R. Glycan characterization of PSA 2-DE subforms from serum and seminal plasma. *OMICS* **2010**, *14*, 465–474. [CrossRef] [PubMed]
26. Sarrats, A.; Comet, J.; Tabares, G.; Ramirez, M.; Aleixandre, R.N.; de Llorens, R.; Peracaula, R. Differential percentage of serum prostate-specific antigen subforms suggests a new way to improve prostate cancer diagnosis. *Prostate* **2010**, *70*, 1–9. [CrossRef] [PubMed]
27. Yoneyama, T.; Ohyama, C.; Hatakeyama, S.; Narita, S.; Habuchi, T.; Koie, T.; Mori, K.; Hidari, K.I.; Yamaguchi, M.; Suzuki, T.; et al. Measurement of aberrant glycosylation of prostate specific antigen can improve specificity in early detection of prostate cancer. *Biochem. Biophys. Res. Commun.* **2014**, *448*, 390–396.
28. Mohammed, A.A. Biomarkers in prostate cancer: New era and prospective. *Med. Oncol.* **2014**, *31*, 140.
29. Leapman, M.S.; Carroll, P.R. What is the best way not to treat prostate cancer? *Urol. Oncol.* **2017**, *35*, 42–50.
30. Vilanova, J.C.; Barcelo-Vidal, C.; Comet, J.; Boada, M.; Barcelo, J.; Ferrer, J.; Albanell, J. Usefulness of prebiopsy multifunctional and morphologic MRI combined with free-to-total prostate-specific antigen ratio in the detection of prostate cancer. *AJR Am. J. Roentgenol.* **2011**, *196*, W715–W722. [CrossRef] [PubMed]
31. Polascik, T.J.; Passoni, N.M.; Villers, A.; Choyke, P.L. Modernizing the diagnostic and decision-making pathway for prostate cancer. *Clin. Cancer Res.* **2014**, *20*, 6254–6257. [CrossRef] [PubMed]
32. Stephan, C.; Vincendeau, S.; Houlgatte, A.; Cammann, H.; Jung, K.; Semjonow, A. Multicenter evaluation of [-2]proprostate-specific antigen and the prostate health index for detecting prostate cancer. *Clin. Chem.* **2013**, *59*, 306–314. [CrossRef] [PubMed]
33. Kosanovic, M.M.; Jankovic, M.M. Sialylation and fucosylation of cancer-associated prostate specific antigen. *J. BUON* **2005**, *10*, 247–250. [PubMed]
34. Hills, M.; Cartensen, B.; Plummer, M. Follow-Up with the Epi Package. 2009. Available online: http://bendixcarstensen.com/Epi/Follow-up.pdf (accessed on 20 February 2017).
35. Cartensen, B.; Plummer, M.; Laara, E.; Hills, M. Epi: A Package for Statistical Analysis in Epidemiology, R Package Version 2.10. 2017. Available online: https://cran.r-project.org/web/packages/Epi/Epi.pdf (accessed on 20 February 2017).
36. Robin, X.; Turck, M.; Hainard, A.; Tiberti, N.; Lisacek, F.; Sanchez, J.C.; Müller, M.; Siegert, S. Display and Analyze ROC Curves, Package "pROC" Version 1.9.1. 2017. Available online: https://cran.r-project.org/web/packages/pROC/pROC.pdf (accessed on 20 February 2017).

Protease Expression Levels in Prostate Cancer Tissue can Explain Prostate Cancer-Associated Seminal Biomarkers—An Explorative Concept Study

Jochen Neuhaus [1,*,†], Eric Schiffer [2,†], Ferdinando Mannello [3], Lars-Christian Horn [4], Roman Ganzer [5] and Jens-Uwe Stolzenburg [5]

1 Department of Urology, Research Laboratory, University of Leipzig, Liebigstraße 19, 04103 Leipzig, Germany
2 Numares AG, Regensburg, Am BioPark 9, 93053 Regensburg, Germany; eric.schiffer@numares.com
3 Department of Biomolecular Sciences, University "Carlo Bo", Via O. Ubaldini 7, 61029 Urbino (PU), Italy; ferdinando.mannello@uniurb.it
4 Institute of Pathology, University Hospital Leipzig, Liebigstraße 24, 04103 Leipzig, Germany; Lars-Christian.Horn@uniklinik-leipzig.de
5 Department of Urology, University Hospital Leipzig, Liebigstraße 20, 04103 Leipzig, Germany; Roman.Ganzer@uniklinik-leipzig.de (R.G.); Jens-Uwe.Stolzenburg@uniklinik-leipzig.de (J.-U.S.)
* Correspondence: jochen.neuhaus@medizin.uni-leipzig.de
† These authors contributed equally to this work.

Academic Editor: Carsten Stephan

Abstract: Previously, we described prostate cancer (PCa) detection (83% sensitivity; 67% specificity) in seminal plasma by CE-MS/MS. Moreover, advanced disease was distinguished from organ-confined tumors with 80% sensitivity and 82% specificity. The discovered biomarkers were naturally occurring fragments of larger seminal proteins, predominantly semenogelin 1 and 2, representing endpoints of the ejaculate liquefaction. Here we identified proteases putatively involved in PCa specific protein cleavage, and examined gene expression and tissue protein levels, jointly with cell localization in normal prostate (nP), benign prostate hyperplasia (BPH), seminal vesicles and PCa using qPCR, Western blotting and confocal laser scanning microscopy. We found differential gene expression of chymase (CMA1), matrix metalloproteinases (MMP3, MMP7), and upregulation of MMP14 and tissue inhibitors (TIMP1 and TIMP2) in BPH. In contrast tissue protein levels of MMP14 were downregulated in PCa. MMP3/TIMP1 and MMP7/TIMP1 ratios were decreased in BPH. In seminal vesicles, we found low-level expression of most proteases and, interestingly, we also detected TIMP1 and low levels of TIMP2. We conclude that MMP3 and MMP7 activity is different in PCa compared to BPH due to fine regulation by their inhibitor TIMP1. Our findings support the concept of seminal plasma biomarkers as non-invasive tool for PCa detection and risk stratification.

Keywords: seminal plasma biomarkers; matrix metalloproteinase (MMP); tissue inhibitor of MMP (TIMP); qPCR; confocal laser scanning microscopy; Western blotting

1. Introduction

Prostate cancer (PCa) is the main gender-specific malignancy in men and prostate specific antigen (PSA) testing is the gold standard in PCa detection [1]. However, comprehensive PSA screening resulted in significant overdiagnosis and overtreatment [2] and in consequence PSA screening is recommended only for men aged 55 to 69 years by the AUA [3]. New PCa biomarkers are urgently needed to identify patients who may be candidates for curative intervention and guide clinical decisions [4].

Recently, seminal fluid has been acknowledged as a promising source of PCa related biomarkers as it directly reflects the pathological processes within the prostate [5]. The high biological variability of prostate cancer [6] necessitates a distinct and clearly defined set of biomarkers, rather than a single or a combination of few biomarkers for efficient description of the disease on a molecular level [7]. In a previous study, we defined distinct panels of small peptide biomarkers in seminal plasma by capillary electrophoresis mass spectrometry (CE-MS), which could be used for PCa detection and stratification [8]. The procedure distinguished PCa from benign prostate hyperplasia (BPH), chronic prostatitis (CP) and normal prostate (nP) with 83% sensitivity and 67% specificity (AUC 75%, $p < 0.0001$) in a small clinical validation cohort of 125 patients. A further set of biomarkers correctly identified advanced (≥pT3a) and organ-confined (<pT3a) tumors (AUC 83%, $p = 0.0055$) with 80% sensitivity and 82% specificity [8].

The discovered biomarkers were fragments of larger parental seminal proteins, such as *N*-acetyl lactosaminide β-1,3-*N*-acetyl glucosaminyl transferase, prostatic acid phosphatase, stabilin-2 and most dominantly semenogelin-1 and -2. Although the parental proteins were also detected earlier [9–11], the use of these naturally occurring fragments reflecting natural proteolytic liquefaction is a new concept.

There are mutual activation and inhibition mechanisms within the liquefaction cascade, which could lead to different downstream proteolytic cleavage patterns [12]. The investigation of these disease-associated proteinase networks [13] represents a challenging task to close the gap between the classical protein expression based biomarker concept and the hypothesis-free proteomic profiling concepts.

We suggest that seminal polypeptide panels may be the smoking gun that links the complex proteolytic alterations of seminal proteins to PCa providing novel insights into PCa biology with special emphasis on disease-associated proteolytic activities. The aim of this study was to identify potential proteinases and inhibitors involved in the formation of the specific seminal biomarkers.

2. Results

2.1. Sequence Analysis and Putative Proteolytic Cleavage Sites

Of the 141 seminal peptides discovered in our previous study, representing a total of 47 different parental proteins, almost 60% were fragments of semenogelin-1 or -2 (SEMG1 and SEMG2). Therefore, we focused our data base searches on SEMG1 and SEMG2 cleavage patterns. Using MEROPS database (Available online: http://merops.sanger.ac.uk/cgi-bin/specsearch.pl) we could assign SEMG1 (316–344) to kallikrein-3 (KLK3, PSA) cleavage at site 315 (peptide-SSIY//SQTE-peptide). Limiting searches from octa- to hexamere recognition (peptide-IY//SQ-peptide) resulted in chymase (CMA1) and cathepsin G (CTSG) as potential alternative proteinases (Table 1). In contrast, KLK3 activity may not account for biomarker SEMG2 (194–215) cleaved at position 193 (peptide-SQSS//YVLQ-peptide. Searching cleavage site 193 (peptide-SS//YV-peptide) revealed matrix metallopeptidase-3 (MMP3), -7 (MMP7), -13 (MMP13), -14 (MMP14) or -20 (MMP20) as potentially involved proteases (Table 1). KLK3 activity may also promote for cleavage between Q and T at position 197 (peptide-QVLQ//TEEL-peptide), resulting in biomarkers SEMG1 (198–215) and SEMG2 (198–215) (Table 1). Although KLK3 Q//T-cleavage is reported for SMG1 and SMG2 at position 235, position 197 remains inconclusive (see MEROPS database). KLK cleavage of SEMG1 and SEMG2 at position 194 (peptide-QSSY//VLQT-peptide) between Y and V, results in the observed non-marker fragments starting from position 195 (Table 1).

Table 1. Semenogelin derived seminal peptides and their putative proteolytic cleavage sites.

Peptide ID	PCa Biomarker	Peptide Sequence	Peptide Identification	Cleavage Site	Putative Protease
15331	Yes	YVLQTEELVVN KQQRETKNSHQ	SEMG2 (194-215)	SQSS//YVLQ	MMP3, MMP7, MMP13, MMP14, MMP20
1677	No	VLQTEELVA	SEMG1 (195-203)	QSSY//VLQT	KLK3
6925	No	VLQTEELVANKQQ	SEMG1 (195-207)	QSSY//VLQT	KLK3
7186	No	VLQTEELVVNKQQ	SEMG2 (195-207)	QSSY//VLQT	KLK3
10289	No	VLQTEELVANKQQRET	SEMG1 (195-210)	QSSY//VLQT	KLK3
11260	No	VLQTEELVVNKQQRETK	SEMG2 (195-211)	QSSY//VLQT	KLK3
11899	Yes	TEELVANKQQRETKNSHQ	SEMG1 (198-215)	YVLQ//TEEL	KLK3
12083	Yes	TEELVVNKQQRETKNSHQ	SEMG2 (198-215)	YVLQ//TEEL	KLK3
18990	Yes	SQTEEKAQGKSQKQI TIPSQEQEHSQKAN	SEMG1 (316-344)	SSIY//TEEL	KLK3, CMA1, CTSG

Peptide sequences including LC-MS/MS data have been recently published by our group [8]. ID: polypeptide identifier annotated by the structured query language (SQL) database (ID); known cleavage sites are indicated for semenogelin-1 (P04279, Swiss-Prot Acc.No.) and semenogelin-2 (Q02383) with their putative proteases, as supported by literature research of web databases: http://merops.sanger.ac.uk/, http://pmap.burnham.org/proteases and http://www.proteolysis.org/proteases.

2.2. *Gene Expression of Proteases in Human Prostate Samples*

Gene expression of KLK3, prostatic acid phosphatase (ACPP) and ACPP-V1 (isoform 1) was high, while matrix metalloproteinases MMP3, MMP7, MMP14 showed low abundance expression by qPCR (Figure 1). KLK3 showed a tendency of increased levels in BPH (Figure 1A). Significant higher transcript levels in BPH were found for MMP7, MMP14 and CMA1 compared to PCa (Figure 1C). Some of the low abundance genes (CTSG, MMP3) also showed a tendency for higher expression in BPH (Figure 1B). MMP13 and MMP20 were at the detection limits (data not shown).

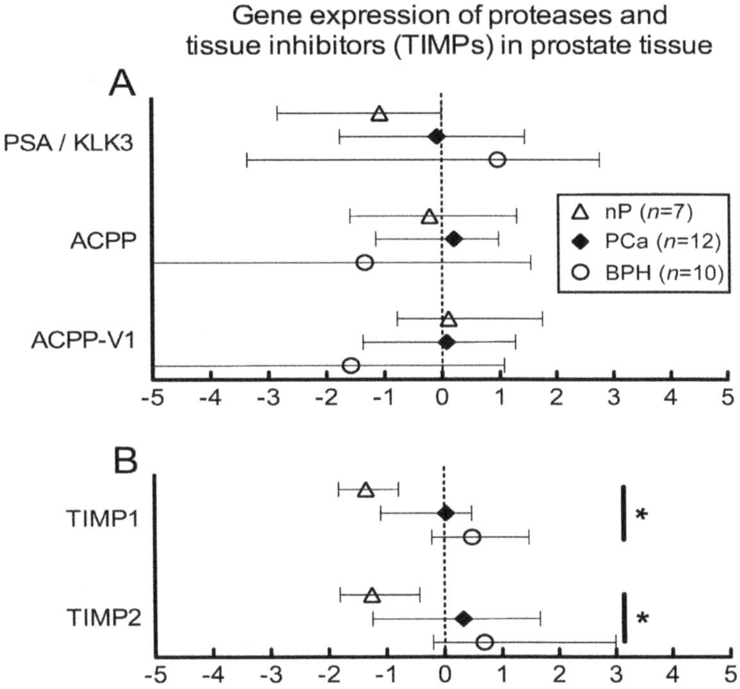

Figure 1. *Cont.*

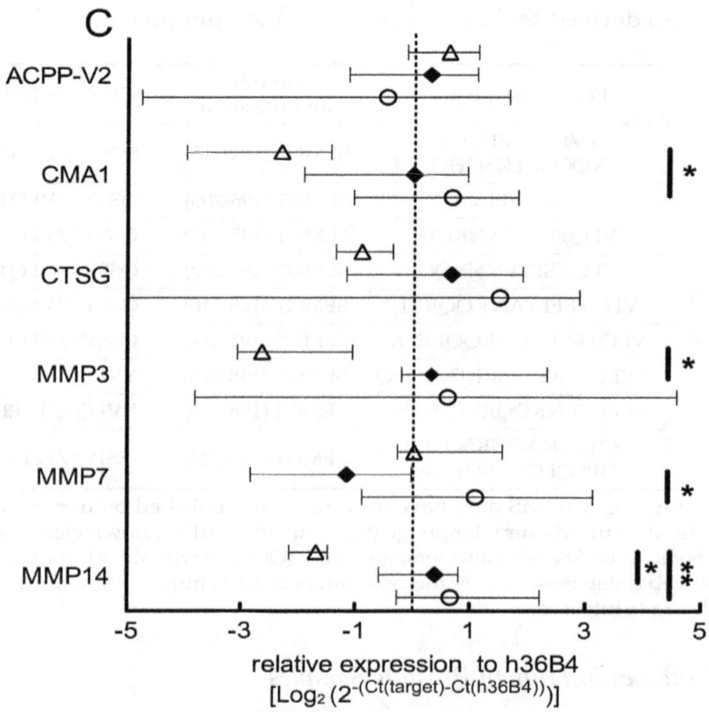

Figure 1. Gene expression analysis. (**A–C**) Expression levels compared to h36B4, global normalization; (**A**) High abundance genes (ratio > 1.0); KLK3 (PSA): kallikrein related peptidase 3; ACPP: total prostatic acid phosphatase; ACPP-V1: splice variant 1 (short secreted isoform of ACPP). The observed differences in mRNA levels between PCa ($n = 12$), benign prostatic hyperplasia (BPH) ($n = 10$) and normal Prostate (nP; $n = 7$) were not significant. However, range of KLK3 expression was much higher in BPH and PCa; (**B**) TIMP1 and TIMP2 expression was significantly different between BPH and nP samples; (**C**) Low abundance genes (ratio < 1.0); ACPP-V2: splice variant 2 (long intracellular isoform); CMA1: chymase 1, CTSG: cathepsin G, and MMP: matrix metalloproteinase. Differential expression levels were detected for CMA1, MMP3, MMP7 and MMP14. Symbols represent medians, whiskers indicate interquartile range. Global normalization; interquartile range: 25%–median–75%; significance: *Kruskal–Wallis* test and *Dunn's* multiple comparison test; * $p < 0.05$, ** $p < 0.01$).

2.3. Protein Levels of Proteinases in Human Prostate and Seminal Vesicles

Highest tissue levels were seen for KLK3 and ACPP-V1 by Western blotting (Figure 2A,B; lanes 1 and 2) and epithelial cells showed highest immunofluorescence in CLSM (Figure 3A,M and Figure 4A,B). Differences in total IF among groups were not significant (Figure 3M), except for TIMP1-IF ($p = 0.0368$) as were the calculated ratios: MMP3/TIMP1 ($p = 0.0119$) and MMP7/TIMP1 ($p = 0.0145$; Figure 3M). TIMP1-IF was especially high in epithelium and in interstitium of the prostate, comprising smooth muscle cells (orange labelling in Figure 3E) and interstitial cells (red labelling) in BPH, while being markedly diminished in epithelium and interstitial cells in PCa (Figure 3H). ACPP-V1 (short, secreted isoform of ACPP) showed significant lower immunofluorescence in grade 4 PCa (Figure 4B). Differences between MMP3-IF, MMP7-IF and TIMP2 were not significant (Figure 4C,D,I), whereas trends of lower TIMP2-IF compared to nP were evident in PCa-gp3 (Figure 4I). Total MMP14-IF was lower in PCa-gp3 ($p < 0.05$) and in PCa-gp4 (trend, not significant), and TIMP1-IF was significantly higher in epithelial cells of BPH compared to PCa-gp3 (Figure 4H).

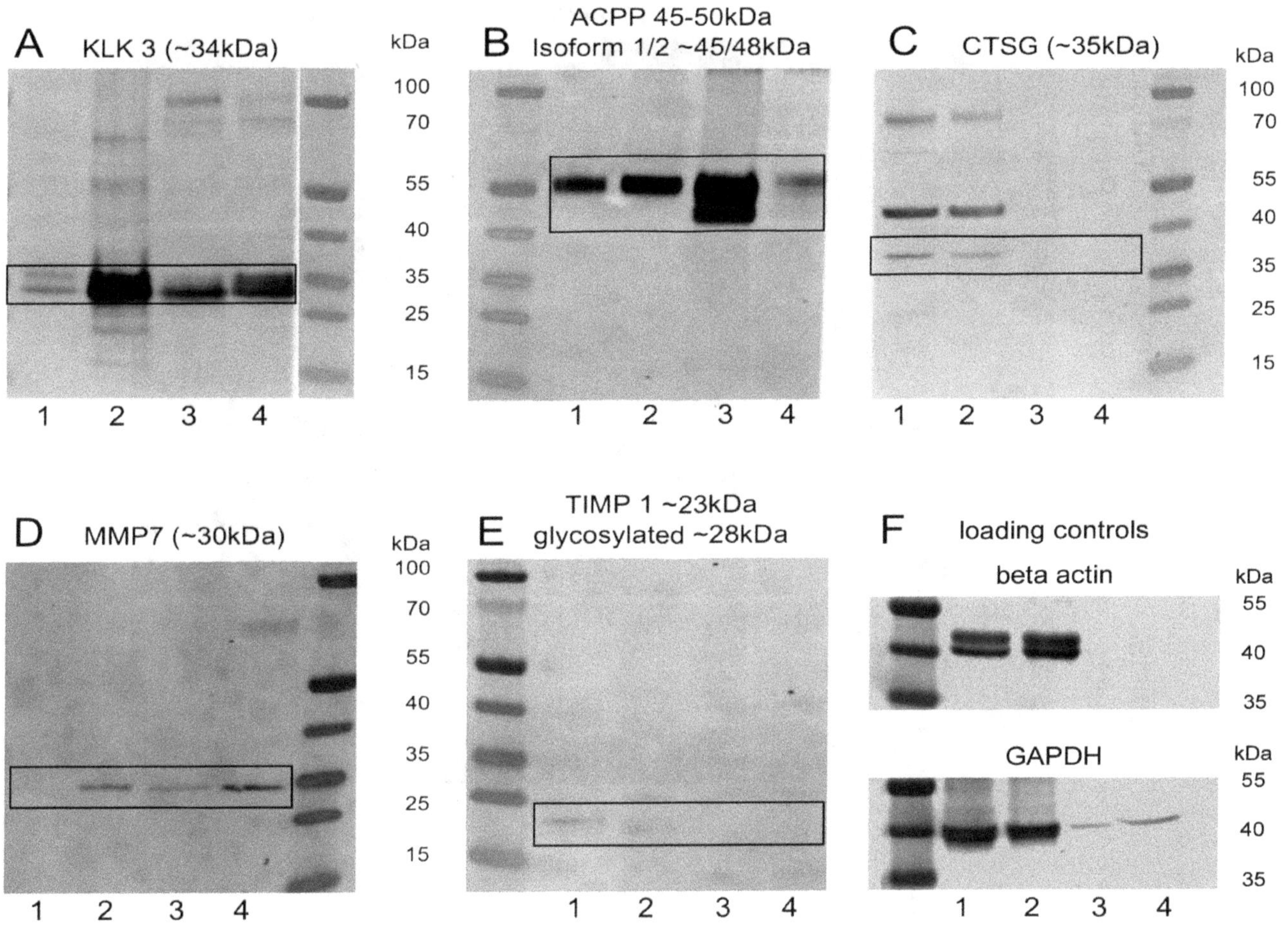

Figure 2. Western blot analysis of prostate and seminal plasma. KLK3 and ACPP were detected in high abundance in prostate tissue (**lanes 1, 2**) and seminal plasma (**lanes 3, 4**) at the predicted molecular weight of 34 and 50 kDa, respectively (**A**,**B**); occasionally multiple banding indicated isoforms or post-translational modification (glycosylation); CTSG was detected exclusively in prostate tissue showing three to four distinct bands at ~35, ~45; ~60 and ~80 kDa (**C**); MMP7 could be detected in prostate tissue and seminal plasma at ~30 kDa (**D**) and we found very low levels of TIMP1 (**E**). MMP14, MMP3, TIMP2 and CMA1 were negative in all examined samples (data not shown; $n = 4$ prostate; $n = 6$ seminal plasma); (**F**) loading controls; note negative staining for β actin in seminal.

CLSM clearly revealed the different contributions of the epithelial cells and smooth muscle cells to the observed alterations in total IF. Interestingly, KLK3-IF (=PSA) was not different between groups (Figure 4A). Also, MMP3-IF and MMP7-IF showed no differences (Figure 4E,F) whereas MMP14-IF was lower in PCa-gp3 than in nP (Figure 4G); and significant differences were detected for TIMP1-IF (Figure 4H). TIMP2-IF was low in PCa-gp3 but did not reach statistical significance (Figure 4I).

We calculated the specific MMP/TIMP ratios as a surrogate of MMP activity. We found that MMPs and TIMP2 were almost balanced in case of MMP3 and MMP7 (values around 1.0; data not shown), while TIMP1 was present in excess indicated by ratios < 1.0 (Figure 5A,B). In contrast, expression of MMP14 well exceeded TIMP2 in nP and PCa as indicated by ratios > 1.0 (Figure 5C), while expression in BPH was balanced.

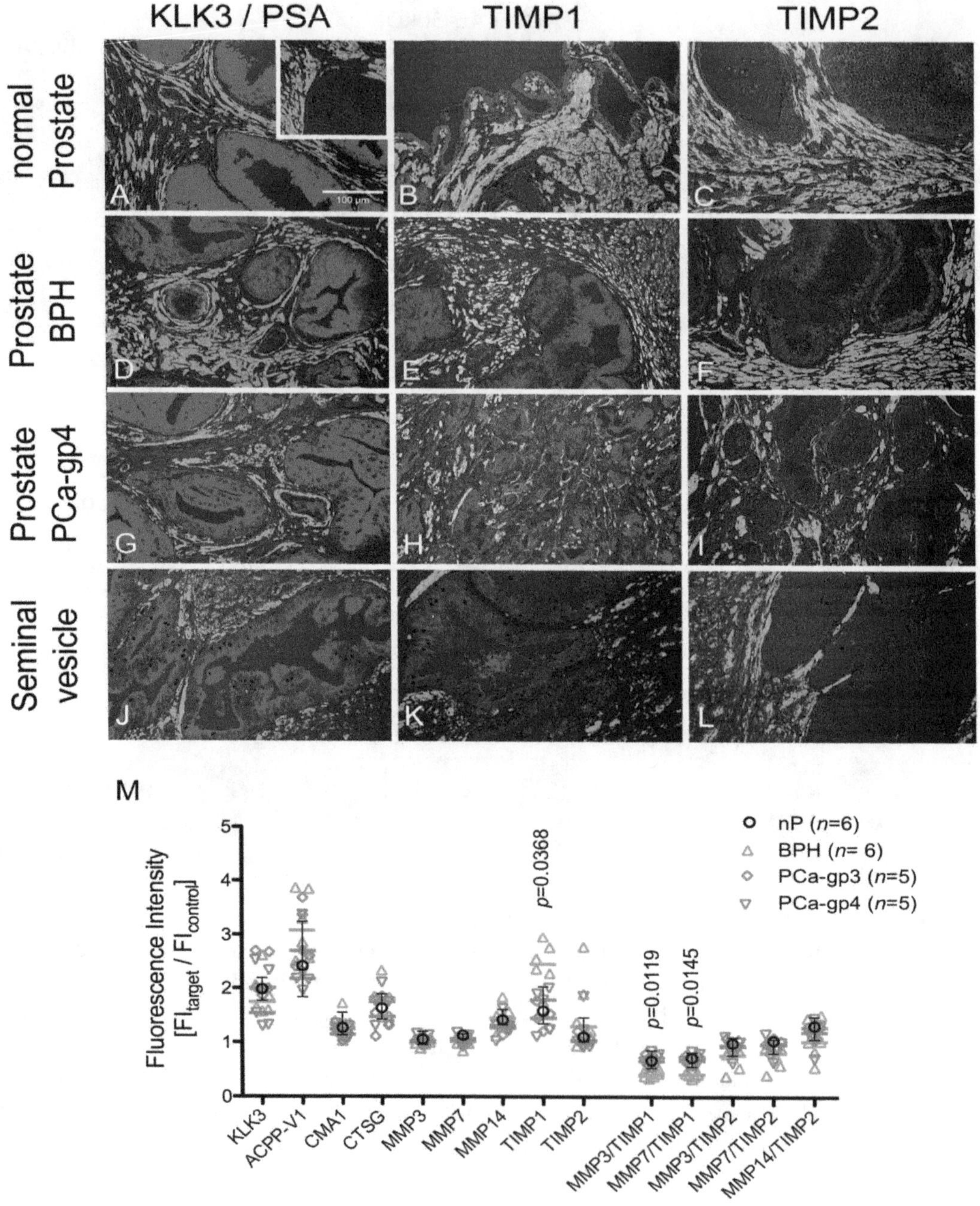

Figure 3. Protein expression analysis using confocal immunofluorescence imaging. Immunohistochemical tissue expression of selected proteases and tissue inhibitors of metalloproteinases. (**A–L**) Confocal images demonstrating tissue distribution of target proteins (red); alpha-smooth muscle cell actin (aSMCA; green). Phase contrast images are merged for tissue structure. Immunofluorescence (IF) of KLK3, TIMP1 and TIMP2 in normal prostate (**A–C**), BPH (**D–F**); PCa Gleason pattern 4 (PCa-gp4; **G–I**) and seminal vesicle (**J–L**). Note the marked upregulation of TIMP1 in BPH especially in SMC (**E**; orange colored cells) and the downregulation of TIMP1-IF in the smooth muscle cells of PCa-gp4 (**H**); TIMP2-IF is almost completely lost in PCa-gp4 tissue (**I**); KLK3-IF in seminal vesicle was low, TIMP1-IF moderate and TIMP2-IF was very low (**J–I**); Scale bar indicating 100 µm in (**A**) applies to all micrographs; staining control (inset in **A**); (**M**) Scatter plot of fluorescence intensities; lines indicate medians. Normal prostate (black symbols) are depicted as median with interquartile range. *p*-Values are based on nonparametric *Kruskal–Wallis* test.

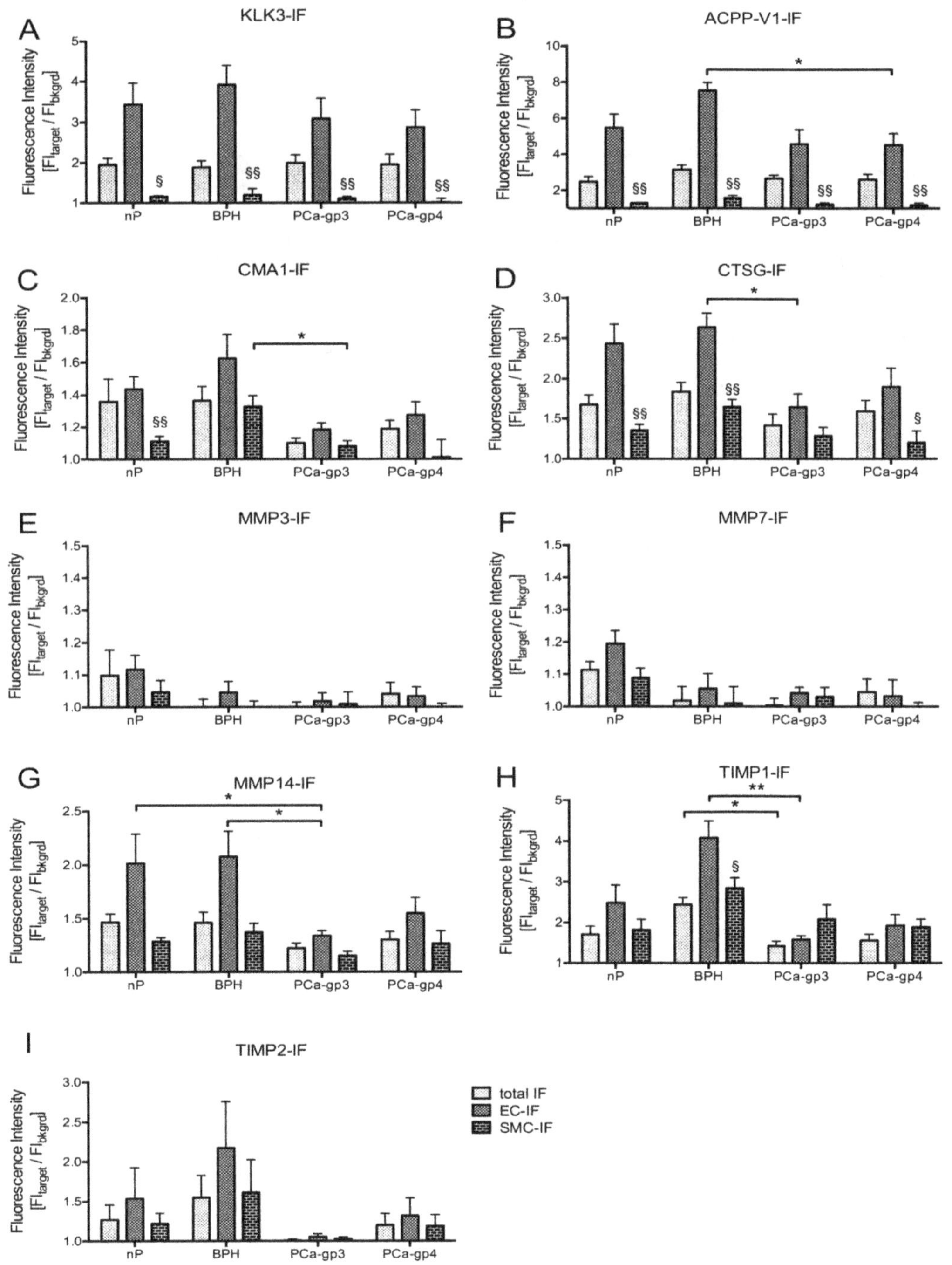

Figure 4. Cellular distribution in prostate tissue. Data (mean (SEM)) are presented as fluorescence intensity [$FI_{target}/FI_{control}$]; background fluorescence (bkgrd) = 1. Total fluorescence included complete tissue area omitting the lumen. Smooth muscle cells (SMC) were identified by anti-smooth muscle cell actin staining (green fluorescence, cf. Figure 2); epithelial cells (EC) area was delineated from DIC images. Note the differences in Y-axis scaling. Differences in fluorescence intensities were not significant for KLK3-IF (**A**), MMP3-IF (**E**), MMP7-IF (**F**) and TIMP2-IF (**I**). Note that the total-IF and SMC-IF is unaltered for ACPP-V1 (**B**), CMA1 (**C**) and CTSG (**D**) whereas epithelial (EC)-IF is significantly lower in PCa compared to BPH, indicating contribution of interstitial cells to total-IF. A comparable trend not reaching significance level ($p < 0.05$) is seen for MMP14 (**G**). In contrast, the significant reduction of TIMP1 total-IF is reflected by significant reduction of EC-IF (**H**). *Kruskal–Wallis* test with post-hoc Dunn's Multiple Comparison test as indicated by bars (* $p < 0.05$; ** $p < 0.01$); § indicates significant difference between EC and SMC; § $p < 0.05$; §§ $p < 0.01$.

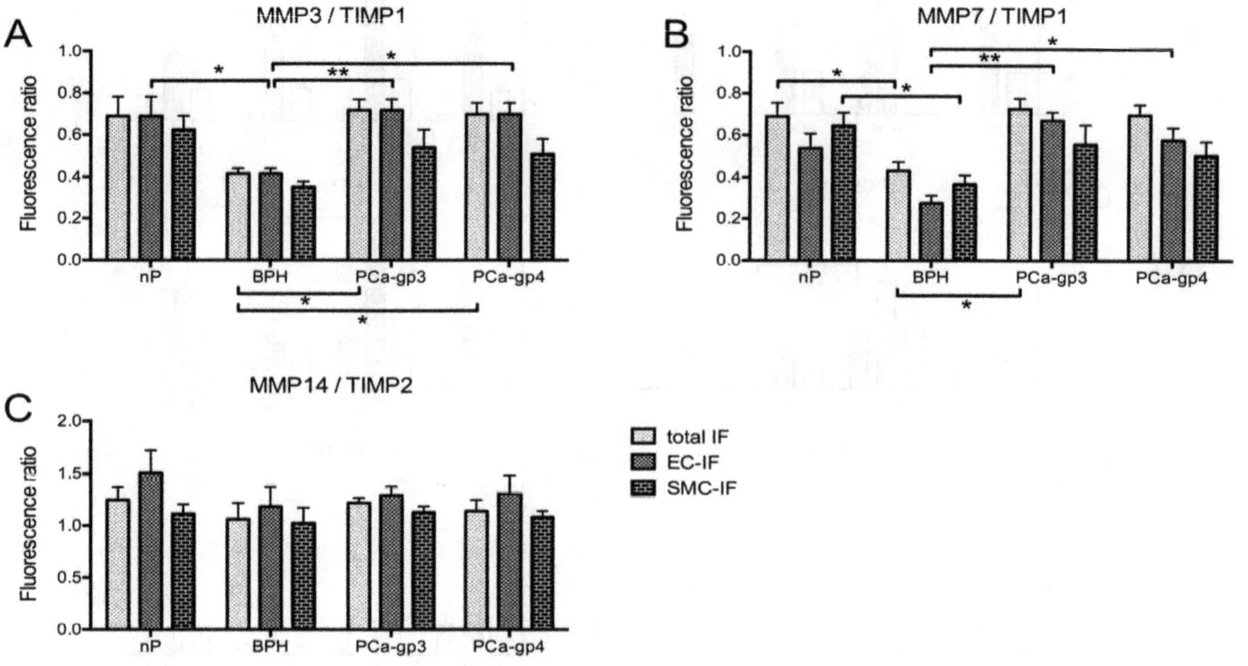

Figure 5. Cellular distribution of MMP/TIMP ratios. Ratios (mean (SEM)) were calculated from means of FI_{target}/FI_{bkgrd} of the respective MMP-TIMP pairs and presented as FI-ratio. Note that MMP14/TIMP2 ratios are >1.0 indicating excess of MMP14 (**C**), while MMP3/TIMP1 and MMP7/TIMP1 ratios are <1.0 indicating excess of TIMP1 (**A**,**B**). *Kruskal–Wallis* test with post-hoc *Dunn's* Multiple Comparison test as indicated by bars (* $p < 0.05$; ** $p < 0.01$); no significant differences were observed between EC and SMC.

To address the contribution of seminal vesicles in protease and inhibitor production, we also investigated seminal vesicles (SV) by CLSM and compared the expression to nP. We found no significant differences (*Mann–Whitney* test) but considerably lower IF for KLK3 and ACPP-V1 especially in epithelial cells (EC IF, Figure 6).

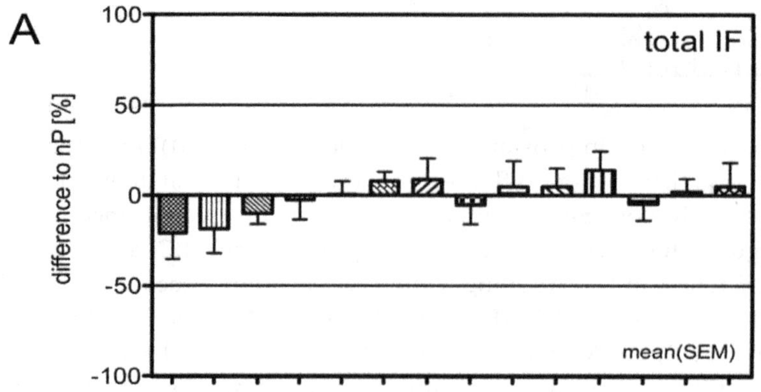

Figure 6. *Cont.*

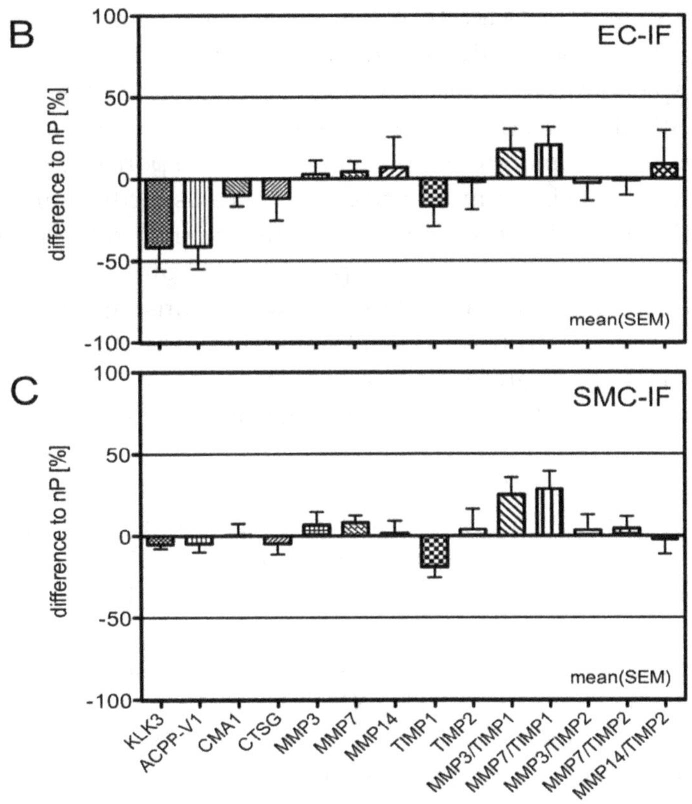

Figure 6. CLSM analysis in seminal vesicles (SV). (**A**–**C**) Immunofluorescence in SV (n = 6) was normalized to the IF in nP (n = 6). Parameter-free *Mann–Whitney* test detected no significant differences between expression levels in nP and SV, but considerably lower IF was found for KLK3 and ACPP-V1, especially in epithelial cells (EC, **B**).

3. Discussion

Based on our previous study, which defined small protein fragments within the seminal plasma as biomarker fingerprint of prostate carcinoma [8], we were interested in the molecular background of the production of these small peptides (≤20 kDa). We therefore explored the cellular expression of certain proteases and their specific inhibitors within the prostate and seminal vesicle tissues. Most of the small peptides that make up the biomarker pattern were derived from SEMG1 and SEMG2. Cleavage site analysis revealed, that the observed SEMG1 and SEMG2 derived biomarkers cannot be explained by KLK3 cleavage alone, implicating the presence of additional cleavage events. From the available sequence data and proteolytic cleavage site searches we hypothesized proteolysis schemes for SEMG1 and SEMG2 based on the involvement of KLK3, CMA1, CTSG, MMP3, MMP7, MMP13, MMP14 or MMP20 as well as the pleiotropic functions of TIMP1 and TIMP2 [14].

As major findings of our study we highlighted that biomarkers found in seminal fluids represent the endpoint of a complex liquefaction proteolytic cascade that involves matrix metalloproteinases MMP3, MMP7 and MMP14 particularly when associated with down-regulation of TIMP1. Downregulation of TIMP1 and TIMP2 has been found by in situ hybridization in the stroma of PCa with higher Gleason scores (GS 8–10) compared to tissue of low Gleason scores [15], supporting our immunohistochemical findings. MMPs are generally more active in advanced stages, caused either by upregulation of MMPs and/or downregulation of their specific TIMPs and MMP activity has been linked to metastasis [16]. MMPs can interfere with growth signals, inhibit apoptosis, and induce angiogenesis and lymphangiogenesis all promoting tumor progression and metastasis. However, MMPs may also possess nonproteolytic functions, like triggering cell migration by chemotaxis (MMP14/TIMP2-MMP2 complex) or interfering with the complement proteinase cascade by interaction with C1q [17]. In line with existing literature, we found significant downregulation of TIMP1 in PCa-gp3, while downregulation of TIMP2 did not reach significant levels. TIMP1- and TIMP2-levels were also lower in PCa-gp4 compared to BPH (Figure 4). In most cases, fluorescence intensity was significantly higher in epithelial cells (EC) than in interstitial smooth muscle cells (SMC), supporting the notion, that malignant transformation of epithelial cells is responsible for the altered protease and inhibitor levels. Further studies, using tumor or tumor stem cell specific markers are needed to analyze the subpopulations of epithelial cells and their contribution to the protease pattern [18].

Except for TIMP1 (Figures 3B and 4H) gene expression and protein expression was not correlated. This is in line with the finding that the concordance between transcript levels and protein expression is only 48–64% in prostate specific proteome [19]. We used immunofluorescence techniques to study cellular protein expression levels. Therefore, variations in the protein detection might be due to weak antibody staining in the case of MMPs complex formation with TIMP1 and TIMP2 [20] or due to epitope masking [21].

Our findings that MMP3/TIMP1 and MMP7/TIMP1 ratios were significantly lower in BPH compared to nP and PCa (Figure 5A,B) is in line with the significant higher transcript expression levels in BPH (Figure 1B) and the higher protein expression in confocal analysis (Figure 4H,I). In consequence, activity of those two MMPs would be lower in BPH tissue, resulting in less cleavage activity in seminal plasma as well.

Although western blotting analysis of seminal plasma consistently detected KLK3, ACPP and MMP7 (Figure 2, lanes 3,4), the detection of CTSG, CMA1, MMP3, MMP14, TIMP1 and TIMP2 failed in seminal plasma even though they were detectable in prostate tissue samples. These results could reflect the complexation of MMPs with TIMPs that may mask the antibody recognition site as discussed above. Concerning CTSG and CMA1, it is well known that seminal plasma contains several specific CTSG inhibitors [22,23] and several classes of proteinases (e.g., Metalloproteinases, serine and cysteine proteinases) may be able to activate and degrade CTSG and CMA1 [24,25].

In case of MMP14 discrepancies between gene expression (significantly up regulated in BPH and PCa compared to nP) and protein tissue levels (significantly down regulated in PCa, compared to nP and BPH) cannot be explained by complexation with TIMP2. Our findings indicate that cells of the prostate interstitium (included in "total IF" columns) have increased protein expression and may account for levelling the decrease in protein expression in epithelial cells (Figure 4). Additionally, it should be taken into account that the protein content within cells considerably depends on secretion rates and secretory status. Thus, especially high MMP14 secretion rates from epithelial cells in PCa might account for the low levels of MMP14-IF measured in PCa tissues (Figure 4G).

In addition, we investigated seminal vesicles as a source of proteases and inhibitors. We found low-level expression of most proteases and, interestingly, we also detected TIMP1 and low levels of TIMP2 in seminal vesicles (Figure 3K,L).

So far, TIMP1 has been detected only in bovine tissue [26]. To our best knowledge, this study is the first evidence for TIMP expression in human seminal vesicles. Of noteworthy, TIMPs play an independent role beyond MMP inhibition, e.g., inhibition of tumor growth, invasion and metastasis, growth factor-like activity, inhibition of angiogenesis and suppression of programmed cell death [27,28]. TIMPs have also been detected in seminal plasma and peculiar secretion by human seminal vesicles has been suggested [29,30].

Our findings suggest that the proteinase cocktail provided for semen liquefaction varies considerably between nP (60.71 $\pm$ 6.80 years; mean $\pm$ SD), BPH (70.30 $\pm$ 6.45 years) and PCa (65.17 $\pm$ 6.83 years). Significant alterations in TIMP1 expression strongly suggests that altered proteinase activities could lead to formation of seminal protein fragments and could be a candidate for prostate cancer biomarkers. Although we did not directly measure MMP activity, the observed increases in MMP/TIMP-ratios might indicate disruption/degradation of physiological extracellular matrix associated to tumor growth. Interestingly, MMP3/TIMP1 and MMP7/TIMP1 ratios were not different in nP and PCa, while they were significantly lower in BPH (Figure 5). As the prevalence of

BPH constantly rises with age affecting 50–70% in men in the 5th and 6th decade, respectively [31], it should be differentiated from PCa which occurs in the same age group. This view is supported by our previous study demonstrating the need of a two-step procedure using two different biomarker panels to reach accurate separation of groups: (1) 21PP for separation of PCa + BPH from CP + HC and (2) 5PP for final detection of PCa (PCa vs. BPH) [8].

At the moment the effect of alterations in single proteases cannot be clearly linked to the appearance of a specific cleavage product in seminal plasma due to unidentified co-players (e.g., endopeptidases) in the complex liquefaction cascade. However, elevated serum MMP7 levels were reported to be significantly associated with metastatic and advanced PCa and was therefore considered to be a biomarker candidate to detect metastatic PCa [32]. In addition, TIMP1 was found downregulated in adenocarcinoma compared to BPH [33] and loss of TIMP1 correlated with biochemical recurrence in patients with localized PCa [34]. These results are in line with our findings and support the idea of regulation of MMP activity by TIMPs as crucial event in PCa growth and progression.

The complex network of proteinases found in the seminal plasma during prostate diseases (Figure 7) seems to generate many small proteolytic protein fragments, which represent the prostate cancer microenvironment and may be useful for both understanding prostate biology and as potent novel PCa biomarkers.

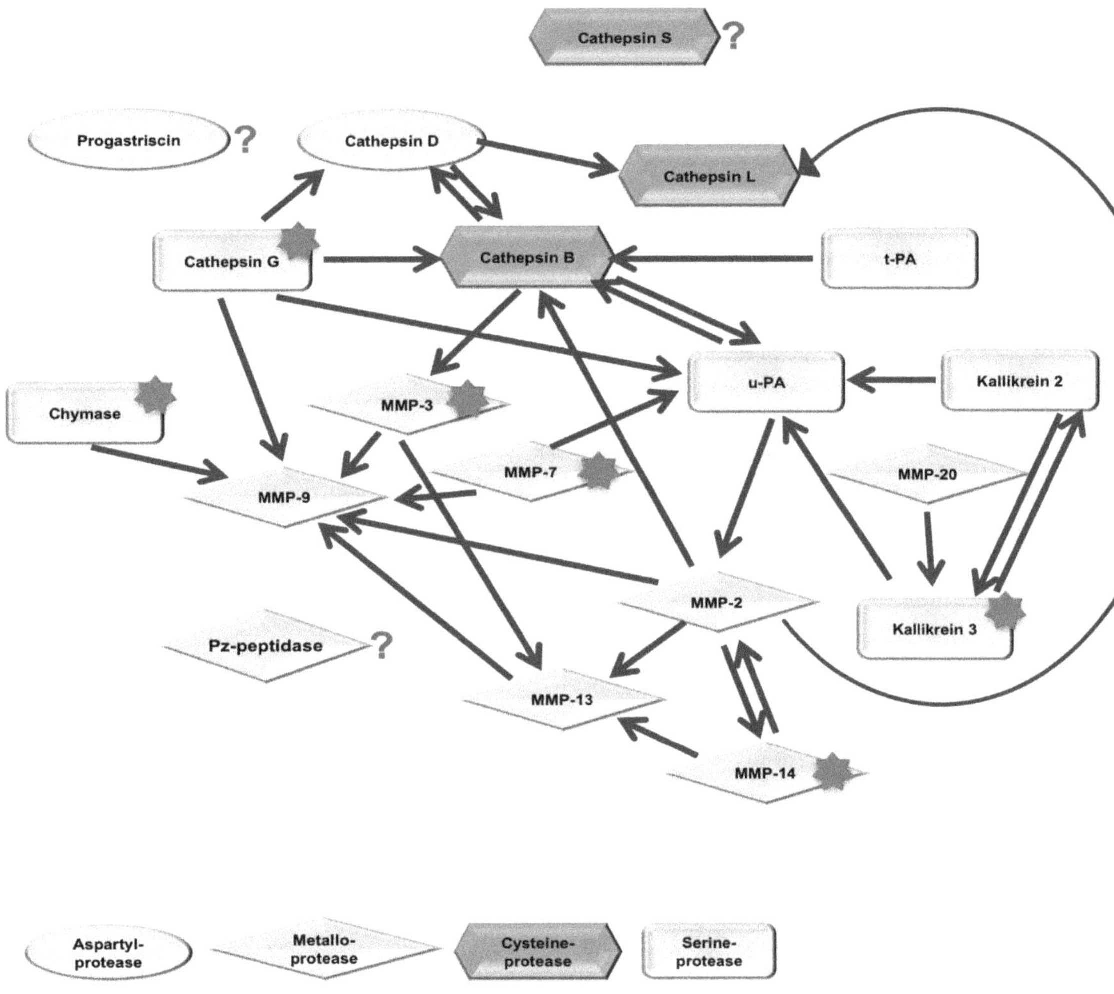

Figure 7. Proteolytic network in human seminal plasma. The role of some enzymes in liquefaction cascade is still obscure (?).

Semen liquefaction is the result of a complex proteolytic cascade involving different and multidirectional protease-protease interactions. Although the interactions involve proteinases from several families, at least three proteinases have been identified in seminal fluid with unknown direct/indirect interactions/functions with other protease classes (adaptation from reference data [13] and web databases: http://merops.sanger.ac.uk/, http://pmap.burnham.org/proteases; asterisks = proteinases with significant changes in MS/MS [8] and qPCR analyses (CMA1, MMP3, MMP7, MMP14, TIMP1, TIMP2; this study).

The major limitation of the present retrospective study was the restricted sample size. However, the aim of this study was to explore the role of MMP/TIMP network in prostate and seminal vesicles in the production of prostate cancer specific peptide patterns found in the seminal plasma. Future extended studies, including metastatic castration-resistant prostate cancer (CRPC) patients, are needed to validate this concept and to encourage the use of urine diagnostic markers as a tool for prostate cancer diagnosis and prognosis.

4. Material and Methods

4.1. Ethics Statement

The study was approved by the Ethics Committee of the University of Leipzig (Reg.No. 084-2009-20042009; 305-12-24092012) and was conducted according to the principles expressed in the Declaration of Helsinki. Written informed consent was obtained from all patients.

4.2. Quantitative Real-Time Polymerase Chain Reaction (qPCR)

We included samples from radical prostatectomies of patients with PCa (n = 12), transurethral resection of BPH (n = 10) and normal prostate tissue (nP; n = 7) after instantaneous section evaluation by our pathologist (LCH; Table 2).

Table 2. Characteristics of patients used for qPCR analysis.

Group	n	Age (Mean ± SD) (95% CI)	PSA [ng/mL] (95% CI)	Gleason Score	Histology
nP	7	60.71 ± 6.80 (54.43–67.00)	n.a.	n.a.	normal prostate
BPH	10	70.30 ± 6.447 (65.69–74.91)	n.a.	n.a.	BPH
PCa	12	65.17 ± 6.834 (60.82–69.51)	6.097 ± 1.868 (4.910–7.284)	≤6 (n = 6) 7 (n = 2) >7 (n = 4)	pT2a (n = 2) pT2c (n = 7) pT3a (n = 3)

Age was not significantly different between groups (p = 0.0556; *Kruskal–Wallis* test, *Dunn's* Multiple Comparison Test). PSA values were not available for nP and BPH patients (n.a.).

Total RNA was extracted from deep frozen tissue specimens using peqGOLD TriFast extraction kit (peQLab, Erlangen, Germany) according to the manufacturers protocol and transcribed into cDNA using the Maxima First Strand cDNA Synthesis Kit (Fermentas, St. Leon-Rot, Germany). Quantitative PCR was performed with the real-time PCR-System realplex2 Mastercycler (Eppendorf, Hamburg, Germany) using the SYBR-Green quantitative PCR Mastermix (Fermentas) and custom primers (MWG-Biotech, Ebersberg, Germany; Table 3). Human 36B4 (acidic ribosomal phosphoprotein P0) served as internal standard for normalization using the $2^{-\Delta\Delta Ct}$ method for relative quantification [35].

Table 3. Primer pairs used for qPCR analysis of the liquefaction cascade. KLK3 (PSA): kallikrein related peptidase 3; MMP: matrix metalloproteinase; CMA1: chymase 1; CTSG: cathepsin G; ACPP: prostatic acid phosphatase; h36B4: ribosomal protein P0 (housekeeping gene).

Gene	Acc. No.	Sequence (F) forward, (R) reverse	Binding to Exon
ACPP (both isoforms)	NM_001099.4	(F) 5′-cga agt ccc att gac acc tt-3′ (R) 5′-atc aaa gtc cgg tca acg tc-3′	2 4
ACPP-V1 (transcript variant 1)	NM_001099.4	(F) 5′-tgt gag tgg cct aca gat gg-3′ (R) 5′-tgt act gtc ttc agt acc ttg a-3′	9 10
ACPP-V2 (transcript variant 2)	NM_001134194.1	(F) 5′-gga ctc ctt cct ccc tat gc-3′ (R) 5′-agg caa cag caa aga tga cc-3′	9 11
PSA/KLK3	NM_001030047.1	(F) 5′-cat gct gtg aag gtc atg ga-3′ (R) 5′-agc aca cag cat gaa ctt gg-3′	3 4
MMP3	NM_002422.1	(F) 5′-gca gtt tgc tca gcc tat cc-3′ (R) 5′-gag tgt cgg agt cca gct tc-3′	1 2
MMP7	NM_002423.3	(F) 5′-gag tgc cag atg ttg cag aa-3′ (R) 5′-gcc aat cat gat gtc agc ag-3′	2 3
MMP13	NM_002427.3	(F) 5′-ttg agc tgg act cat tgt cg-3′ (R) 5′-gga gcc tct cag tca tgg ag-3′	1 2
MMP14	NM_004995.2	(F) 5′- caa gca ttg ggt gtt tga tg-3′ (R) 5′-tcc ctt ccc aga ctt tga tg-3′	8 9
MMP20	NM_004771.3	(F) 5′-ctc atc ctt tga cgc tgt ga-3′ (R) 5′-ctt cgt aag ctg cat cca ca-3′	6 7
CMA1	NM_001836.2	(F) 5′-tgc aag agg tga agc tga ga-3′ (R) 5′-gag att cgg gtg aag aca gc-3′	4 5
CTSG	NM_001911.2	(F) 5′-ata atc agc gga cca tcc ag-3′ (R) 5′-tgc cta tcc ctc tgc act ct-3′	3 4
h36B4	NM_002775.1	(F) 5′-ccg act cct ccg act ctt c-3′ (R) 5′-aac atg ctc aac atc tcc cc-3′	6 8

4.3. Protein Analysis by Indirect Immunofluorescence

We performed semi-quantitative analyses of the immunofluorescence (IF) and distribution of target proteins in tissue samples of normal prostate (n = 6), BPH (n = 6), seminal vesicles (n = 6) and PCa (n = 10; Table 4) using confocal laser scanning microscopy (CLSM).

Table 4. Characteristics of patients used for immunofluorescence analysis.

Group	*n*	Age (95% CI)	PSA [ng/mL] (95%CI)	Gleason Score	Histology
nP	6	62.17 ± 4.79 (57.14–67.20)	n.a.	n.a.	normal prostate
BPH	6	67.50 ± 5.93 (61.28–73.72)	n.a.	n.a.	BPH
PCa	10	61.50 ± 9.25 (54.88–68.12)	19.44 ± 12.62 (n = 8)	6 (n = 2) 7 (n = 8)	pT1c (n = 7) pT2c (n = 3)
SV	6	61.17 ± 8.68 (52.06–70.28)	11.41 ± 4.87 (n = 5)	6 (n = 2) 7 (n = 4)	normal, not infiltrated

Age was not significantly different between groups (p = 0.3997; *Kruskal–Wallis* test, *Dunn's* Multiple Comparison Test). PSA values were not available for nP and BPH patients (n.a.).

Seven micron thick paraffin sections of prostate biopsies and material from radical prostatectomies were deparaffinized, rehydrated and processed for antigen retrieval in 10 mM citrate buffer (pH 6.0, 100 °C) in a steamer (Braun, Kronberg, Germany). Slices were then washed in phosphate-buffered saline (pH 7.4) and transferred to Tris-buffered saline (50 mM TBS, pH 7.4). Following treatment with TBS (0.1% Triton X-100) for 10 min and blocking unspecific binding (TBS, 0.1% Triton X-100, 1% bovine serum albumin, 3% fat-free milk powder) for 15 min at room temperature, slices were incubated overnight in a cocktail of anti-alpha smooth muscle cell actin monoclonal mouse IgG2a antibody (1:2000) and target antibody in blocking buffer at 4 °C (Table 5).

Table 5. Antibodies used in indirect immunofluorescence (IF) and Western blotting (WB). Sources: [1] Acris Antibodies GmbH, Herford, Germany; [2] antibodies online, Aachen, Germany; [3] Santa Cruz Biotechnology Inc., Santa Cruz, CA, USA; [4] Proteintech Group Inc., Manchester, UK; [5] Histo-line Laboratories, Milan, Italy; [6] Abcam Inc., Cambridge, MA, USA; [7] QED Bioscience Inc., San Diego, CA, USA; [8] Novus Biologicals Europe, Abingdon, UK; [9] Sigma-Aldrich Chemie GmbH, Steinheim, Germany; [10] LI-COR Biosciences GmbH, Bad Homburg, Germany; Rb (rabbit); Ms (mouse); polyclonal (poly); monoclonal (mono).

Antigen/Primary Antibodies	Source	Type	Order-No.	Dilution
KLK3	1	Rb, poly	AP15748PU-S	1:200 (IF), 1:500 (WB)
CMA1	2	Rb, poly	ABIN679853	1:200 (IF), 1:400 (WB)
CTSG	2	Rb, poly	ABIN731843	1:200 (IF), 1:500 (WB)
MMP3	2	Rb, poly	ABIN668301	1:200 (IF)
MMP3	3	Ms, mono	sc-21732	1:500 (WB)
MMP7	2	Rb, poly	ABIN668451	1:200 (IF)
MMP7	4	Rb, poly	10374-2-AP	1:500 (WB)
MMP14	5	Rb, poly	29025	1:200 (IF)
MMP14	6	Rb, poly	ab3644	1:500 (WB)
ACPP-V1	2	Rb, poly	ABIN966903	1:80 (IF), 1:500 (WB)
TIMP1	7	Rb, poly	29022	1:200 (IF), 1:1000 (WB)
TIMP2	2	Rb, poly	ABIN373976	1:200
β Actin	8	Ms, mono	NB600-501	1:4000 (WB)
GAPDH	3	Ms, mono	sc-47724	1:1000 (WB)
alpha-smooth muscle actin	9	Ms, mono	A2547	1:2000
goat-anti Ms IRDye® 680RD	10	Goat IgG	926-68070	1:8000 (WB)
goat-anti Rb IRDye® 680RD	10	Goat IgG	926-68071	1:8000 (WB)

For visualization, the sections were incubated with Alexa Fluor® 488 goat-anti-mouse IgG2a and Alexa Fluor® 555 goat anti-rabbit antibodies (Invitrogen, Karlsruhe, Germany) at a dilution of 1:500 for 1 h at room temperature. For semi-quantitative analysis scans were acquired at a LSM5 Pascal (Carl Zeiss, Jena, Germany) using a Plan-Neofluar 20x/0.5 Objective (Carl Zeiss, Jena, Germany) at 488 and 543 nm excitation wavelengths. Pinholes were adjusted to give an optical slice of <5.0 μm. Hematoxylin/Eosin stained sections were evaluated by the pathologist and regions of defined histological grading were defined. Five images were taken randomly in corresponding immunofluorescence stained sections and analysed in ImageJ 1.49t (Rasband WS. ImageJ. U S National Institutes of Health, Bethesda, Maryland, USA, available online: http://rsb.info.nih.gov/ij/, 1997–2006) using self-written analysis tools. Data were transferred to Apache OpenOffice™ 3 (Apache Software Foundation, available online: https://www.apache.org) for calculations. Target mean fluorescence intensities were normalized to staining control (omission of primary antibody) fluorescence intensities.

4.4. SDS Page and Western Blotting

We used six samples of normal prostate tissue that was excised following radical resection of the prostate and examined by our pathologist (LCH) to ensure tumor-free samples. Seminal plasma samples were collected and stored in liquid nitrogen at −196 °C until use. For SDS-PAGE (sodium dodecyl sulphate polyacrylamide gel electrophoresis), prostate tissue specimens were thawed on ice and later extracted using 500 μL/100 mg 50 mmol/L Tris-HCL supplemented with 1% sodium dodecyl sulphate (SDS), 5 μL protease inhibitor cocktail (Sigma-Aldrich, Steinheim, Germany) and 5 μL phenylmethylsulfonylfluoride. The tissue was homogenized on ice using an Ultra Turrax T10 (Ika GmbH & Co., Staufen, Germany), further extracted for 1 h at 4°C and thereafter centrifuged at 500× *g* for 2 min at 4 °C. Protein concentration of the supernatant was determined by Pierce™ BCA Protein Assay Kit (Thermo Fischer Scientific, Rockford, IL, USA) using a NanoDrop 1000 spectrophotometer (PEQLAB Biotechnologie GmbH, Erlangen, Germany). Seminal plasma probes were thawed on ice and protein concentration was determined as indicated above. 30 or 50 μg protein was used per lane on NuPage Bis-Tris 4–12% gradient mini gels (Life Technologies, Darmstadt, Germany).

Western blotting was performed onto PVDF membranes according to supplier's protocol in a Bio-Rad Mini Trans-Blot® system (Bio-Rad Laboratories GmbH, München, Germany). Membranes were blocked for 1 h with 2% BSA (Carl Roth GmbH & Co. KG, Karlsruhe, Germany) followed by incubation with primary antibody incubation at 4 °C (Table 5). Anti-beta actin and anti-GAPDH antibodies were used as loading controls. For detection, we used goat-anti mouse IRDye 680 or goat-anti rabbit IRDye 680 secondary antibodies diluted at 1:8000 (LI-COR Biosciences GmbH, Bad Homburg, Germany). Blots were scanned using an Odyssey Infrared Imaging System (LI-COR).

4.5. Statistical Analysis

Statistics and graphing were done with Prism 5 (GraphPad Software Inc., La Jolla, CA, USA). Parameter free tests were used as indicated in the figure legends. All numbers are given as mean ± SEM (standard error of the mean), unless indicated otherwise.

5. Conclusions

We conclude that tissue levels of MMP3 and MMP7 (finely regulated by their inhibitors TIMP1 and TIMP2) are altered in PCa compared to benign prostatic hyperplasia, which is of special relevance in elderly men. These findings link tissue alterations to altered liquefaction cascade, indicating disease-related alterations in prostate tissue and hence in liquefaction cascade. For the first time, we present evidence for a contribution of seminal vesicles to the fine-tuning of the liquefaction protease network. Our findings thus support the concept of seminal plasma biomarkers as non-invasive tool for PCa detection and risk stratification in men aged 60–70 years.

Acknowledgments: The authors gratefully acknowledge the excellent technical support by Annett Weimann, Mandy Berndt-Paetz and Christine Kellner. We thank Vinodh Kumar Adithyaa Arthanareeswaran for language editing and proofreading of the manuscript.

Author Contributions: Conceived and designed the experiments: Jochen Neuhaus, Eric Schiffer. Performed the experiments: Jochen Neuhaus, Eric Schiffer, Ferdinando Mannello. Analyzed the data: Jochen Neuhaus, Eric Schiffer, Lars-Christian Horn. Contributed reagents/materials/analysis tools: Jens-Uwe Stolzenburg, Ferdinando Mannello. Wrote the manuscript: Jochen Neuhaus, Eric Schiffer, Ferdinando Mannello. Edited the manuscript: Jens-Uwe Stolzenburg, Roman Ganzer, Lars-Christian Horn.

References

1. Siegel, R.; Naishadham, D.; Jemal, A. Cancer statistics, 2013. *CA Cancer J. Clin.* **2013**, *63*, 11–30. [CrossRef] [PubMed]
2. Hugosson, J.; Carlsson, S.; Aus, G.; Bergdahl, S.; Khatami, A.; Lodding, P.; Pihl, C.G.; Stranne, J.; Holmberg, E.; Lilja, H. Mortality results from the Goteborg randomised population-based prostate-cancer screening trial. *Lancet Oncol.* **2010**' *11*, 725–732. [CrossRef]

3. Carter, H.B. American Urological Association (AUA) guideline on prostate cancer detection: Process and rationale. *BJU Int.* **2013**, *112*, 543–547. [CrossRef] [PubMed]
4. Prensner, J.R.; Rubin, M.A.; Wei, J.T.; Chinnaiyan, A.M. Beyond PSA: The next generation of prostate cancer biomarkers. *Sci. Transl. Med.* **2012**. [CrossRef] [PubMed]
5. Roberts, M.J.; Richards, R.S.; Gardiner, R.A.; Selth, L.A. Seminal fluid: A useful source of prostate cancer biomarkers? *Biomark. Med.* **2015**, *9*, 77–80. [CrossRef] [PubMed]
6. Rajan, P.; Elliott, D.J.; Robson, C.N.; Leung, H.Y. Alternative splicing and biological heterogeneity in prostate cancer. *Nat. Rev. Urol.* **2009**, *6*, 454–460. [CrossRef] [PubMed]
7. Good, D.M.; Thongboonkerd, V.; Novak, J.; Bascands, J.L.; Schanstra, J.P.; Coon, J.J.; Dominiczak, A.; Mischak, H. Body fluid proteomics for biomarker discovery: Lessons from the past hold the key to success in the future. *J. Proteome Res.* **2007**, *6*, 4549–4555. [CrossRef] [PubMed]
8. Neuhaus, J.; Schiffer, E.; von Wilcke, P.; Bauer, H.W.; Leung, H.; Siwy, J.; Ulrici, W.; Paasch, U.; Horn, L.-C.; Stolzenburg, J.U. Seminal Plasma as a Source of Prostate Cancer Peptide Biomarker Candidates for Detection of Indolent and Advanced Disease. *PLoS ONE* **2013**, *8*, e67514. [CrossRef] [PubMed]
9. Batruch, I.; Lecker, I.; Kagedan, D.; Smith, C.R.; Mullen, B.J.; Grober, E.; Lo, K.C.; Diamandis, E.P.; Jarvi, K.A. Proteomic analysis of seminal plasma from normal volunteers and post-vasectomy patients identifies over 2000 proteins and candidate biomarkers of the urogenital system. *J. Proteome Res.* **2011**, *10*, 941–953. [CrossRef] [PubMed]
10. Drake, R.R.; Elschenbroich, S.; Lopez-Perez, O.; Kim, Y.; Ignatchenko, V.; Ignatchenko, A.; Nyalwidhe, J.O.; Basu, G.; Wilkins, C.E.; Gjurich, B.; et al. In-depth proteomic analyses of direct expressed prostatic secretions. *J. Proteome Res.* **2010**, *9*, 2109–2116. [CrossRef] [PubMed]
11. Pilch, B.; Mann, M. Large-scale and high-confidence proteomic analysis of human seminal plasma. *Genome Biol.* **2006**. [CrossRef] [PubMed]
12. Emami, N.; Deperthes, D.; Malm, J.; Diamandis, E.P. Major role of human KLK14 in seminal clot liquefaction. *J. Biol. Chem.* **2008**, *283*, 19561–19569. [CrossRef] [PubMed]
13. Mason, S.D.; Joyce, J.A. Proteolytic networks in cancer. *Trends Cell. Biol.* **2011**, *21*, 228–237. [CrossRef] [PubMed]
14. Murphy, G. Tissue inhibitors of metalloproteinases. *Genome Biol.* **2011**. [CrossRef] [PubMed]
15. Wood, M.; Fudge, K.; Mohler, J.L.; Frost, A.R.; Garcia, F.; Wang, M.; Stearns, M.E. In situ hybridization studies of metalloproteinases 2 and 9 and TIMP-1 and TIMP-2 expression in human prostate cancer. *Clin. Exp. Metastasis* **1997**, *15*, 246–258. [CrossRef] [PubMed]
16. Gong, Y.; Chippada-Venkata, U.D.; Oh, W.K. Roles of matrix metalloproteinases and their natural inhibitors in prostate cancer progression. *Cancers* **2014**, *6*, 1298–1327. [CrossRef] [PubMed]
17. Kessenbrock, K.; Plaks, V.; Werb, Z. Matrix metalloproteinases: Regulators of the tumor microenvironment. *Cell* **2010**, *141*, 52–67. [CrossRef] [PubMed]
18. Taylor, R.A.; Toivanen, R.; Frydenberg, M.; Pedersen, J.; Harewood, L.; Australian, P.C.B.; Collins, A.T.; Maitland, N.J.; Risbridger, G.P. Human epithelial basal cells are cells of origin of prostate cancer, independent of CD133 status. *Stem Cells* **2012**, *30*, 1087–1096. [CrossRef] [PubMed]
19. Varambally, S.; Yu, J.; Laxman, B.; Rhodes, D.R.; Mehra, R.; Tomlins, S.A.; Shah, R.B.; Chandran, U.; Monzon, F.A.; Becich, M.J.; et al. Integrative genomic and proteomic analysis of prostate cancer reveals signatures of metastatic progression. *Cancer Cell* **2005**, *8*, 393–406. [CrossRef] [PubMed]
20. Toth, M.; Chvyrkova, I.; Bernardo, M.M.; Hernandez-Barrantes, S.; Fridman, R. Pro-MMP-9 activation by the MT1-MMP/MMP-2 axis and MMP-3: Role of TIMP-2 and plasma membranes. *Biochem. Biophys. Res. Commun.* **2003**, *308*, 386–395. [CrossRef]
21. Arumugam, S.; Van Doren, S.R. Global orientation of bound MMP-3 and N-TIMP-1 in solution via residual dipolar couplings. *Biochemistry* **2003**, *42*, 7950–7958. [CrossRef] [PubMed]
22. Fritz, H. Human mucus proteinase inhibitor (human MPI). Human seminal inhibitor I (HUSI-I), antileukoprotease (ALP), secretory leukocyte protease inhibitor (SLPI). *Biol. Chem. Hoppe Seyler.* **1988**, *369*, 79–82. [PubMed]
23. Ohlsson, K.; Bjartell, A.; Lilja, H. Secretory leucocyte protease inhibitor in the male genital tract: PSA-induced proteolytic processing in human semen and tissue localization. *J. Androl.* **1995**, *16*, 64–74. [PubMed]

24. Caughey, G.H.; Schaumberg, T.H.; Zerweck, E.H.; Butterfield, J.H.; Hanson, R.D.; Silverman, G.A.; Ley, T.J. The human mast cell chymase gene (*CMA1*): Mapping to the cathepsin G/granzyme gene cluster and lineage-restricted expression. *Genomics* **1993**, *15*, 614–620. [CrossRef] [PubMed]
25. Korkmaz, B.; Horwitz, M.S.; Jenne, D.E.; Gauthier, F. Neutrophil elastase, proteinase 3, and cathepsin G as therapeutic targets in human diseases. *Pharmacol. Rev.* **2010**, *62*, 726–759. [CrossRef] [PubMed]
26. McCauley, T.C.; Zhang, H.M.; Bellin, M.E.; Ax, R.L. Identification of a heparin-binding protein in bovine seminal fluid as tissue inhibitor of metalloproteinases-2. *Mol. Reprod. Dev.* **2001**, *58*, 336–341. [CrossRef]
27. Mannello, F.; Gazzanelli, G. Tissue inhibitors of metalloproteinases and programmed cell death: Conundrums, controversies and potential implications. *Apoptosis* **2001**, *6*, 479–482. [CrossRef] [PubMed]
28. Sinno, M.; Biagioni, S.; Ajmone-Cat, M.A.; Pafumi, I.; Caramanica, P.; Medda, V.; Tonti, G.; Minghetti, L.; Mannello, F.; Cacci, E. The matrix metalloproteinase inhibitor marimastat promotes neural progenitor cell differentiation into neurons by gelatinase-independent TIMP-2-dependent mechanisms. *Stem Cells Dev.* **2013**, *22*, 345–358. [CrossRef] [PubMed]
29. Baumgart, E.; Lenk, S.V.; Loening, S.A.; Jung, K. Tissue inhibitors of metalloproteinases 1 and 2 in human seminal plasma and their association with spermatozoa. *Int. J. Androl.* **2002**, *25*, 369–371. [CrossRef] [PubMed]
30. Shimokawa, K.; Katayama, M.; Matsuda, Y.; Takahashi, H.; Hara, I.; Sato, H. Complexes of gelatinases and tissue inhibitor of metalloproteinases in human seminal plasma. *J. Androl.* **2003**, *24*, 73–77. [PubMed]
31. McVary, K.T. BPH: Epidemiology and comorbidities. *Am. J. Manag. Care* **2006**, *12*, S122–S128. [PubMed]
32. Szarvas, T.; Becker, M.; Vom Dorp, F.; Meschede, J.; Scherag, A.; Bankfalvi, A.; Reis, H.; Schmid, K.W.; Romics, I.; Rubben, H.; et al. Elevated serum matrix metalloproteinase 7 levels predict poor prognosis after radical prostatectomy. *Int. J. Cancer* **2011**, *128*, 1486–1492. [CrossRef] [PubMed]
33. Babichenko, I.I.; Pul'bere, S.A.; Motin, P.I.; Loktev, A.V.; Abud, M. Significance of matrix metalloproteinase-9, tissue inhibitor of metalloproteinase and protein Ki-67 in prostate tumors. *Urologiia.* **2014**, *5*, 82–86.
34. Reis, S.T.; Viana, N.I.; Iscaife, A.; Pontes-Junior, J.; Dip, N.; Antunes, A.A.; Guimarães, V.R.; Santana, I.; Nahas, W.C.; Srougi, M.; et al. Loss of TIMP-1 immune expression and tumor recurrence in localized prostate cancer. *Int. Braz. J. Urol.* **2015**, *41*, 1088–1095. [CrossRef] [PubMed]
35. Livak, K.J.; Schmittgen, T.D. Analysis of relative gene expression data using real-time quantitative PCR and the $2^{-\Delta\Delta Ct}$ Method. *Methods* **2001**, *25*, 402–408. [CrossRef] [PubMed]

10

A Panel of MicroRNAs as Diagnostic Biomarkers for the Identification of Prostate Cancer

Rhonda Daniel [1,†], Qianni Wu [1,†], Vernell Williams [2], Gene Clark [1], Georgi Guruli [3] and Zendra Zehner [1,*]

1 Department of Biochemistry and Molecular Biology, VCU Medical Center and the Massey Cancer Center, Virginia Commonwealth University, Richmond, VA 23298-0614, USA; danielr@vcu.edu (R.D.); wuq3@vcu.edu (Q.W.); clarkgc@mymail.vcu.edu (G.C.)
2 Molecular Diagnostic Laboratory, Department of Pathology, VCU Health System, Virginia Commonwealth University, Richmond, VA 23298-0248, USA; Vernell.Williamson@vcuhealth.org
3 Division of Urology, VCU Medical Center and the Massey Cancer Center, Virginia Commonwealth University, Richmond, VA 23298-0037, USA; Georgi.guruli@vcuhealth.org
* Correspondence: zendra.zehner@vcuhealth.org
† These authors contributed equally to this work.

Abstract: Prostate cancer is the most common non-cutaneous cancer among men; yet, current diagnostic methods are insufficient, and more reliable diagnostic markers need to be developed. One answer that can bridge this gap may lie in microRNAs. These small RNA molecules impact protein expression at the translational level, regulating important cellular pathways, the dysregulation of which can exert tumorigenic effects contributing to cancer. In this study, high throughput sequencing of small RNAs extracted from blood from 28 prostate cancer patients at initial stages of diagnosis and prior to treatment was used to identify microRNAs that could be utilized as diagnostic biomarkers for prostate cancer compared to 12 healthy controls. In addition, a group of four microRNAs (miR-1468-3p, miR-146a-5p, miR-1538 and miR-197-3p) was identified as normalization standards for subsequent qRT-PCR confirmation. qRT-PCR analysis corroborated microRNA sequencing results for the seven top dysregulated microRNAs. The abundance of four microRNAs (miR-127-3p, miR-204-5p, miR-329-3p and miR-487b-3p) was upregulated in blood, whereas the levels of three microRNAs (miR-32-5p, miR-20a-5p and miR-454-3p) were downregulated. Data analysis of the receiver operating curves for these selected microRNAs exhibited a better correlation with prostate cancer than PSA (prostate-specific antigen), the current gold standard for prostate cancer detection. In summary, a panel of seven microRNAs is proposed, many of which have prostate-specific targets, which may represent a significant improvement over current testing methods.

Keywords: microRNA; high throughput RNA sequencing; small RNA sequencing; qRT-PCR; prostate cancer; PSA

---

1. Introduction

Prostate Cancer (PCa) is the most common non-cutaneous cancer among men, yet current diagnostic methods are insufficient at detecting this disease, and more reliable biomarkers need to be developed. Currently, the prostate-specific antigen (PSA) is used as a diagnostic marker for PCa; however, many factors have been found to elevate PSA levels. Age, infection, trauma, ejaculation, urinary retention, instrumentation, certain medications and even bike riding can lead to false positive diagnoses, generating unnecessary concern and over-treatment with dire outcomes for the patient [1–4]. Even worse are the chances of false negative diagnoses, which result in PCa remaining undetected until its later stages. Therefore, although the use of the PSA level has had its clinical advantages, it has failed to sufficiently bridge the gap to accurately diagnose disease or distinguish indolent from aggressive disease. One answer that might close this gap and enable more efficient diagnoses may lie in microRNAs (miRs) [5].

Small RNAs play an extremely important role in gene regulation. Their function in the suppression of unwanted genetic materials is vital to the proper operation of the cell. Small RNAs fall into three classifications: microRNAs, siRNA and PIWI-interacting RNAs (piRNA), the most dominating of which are microRNAs [6]. MicroRNAs are small non-coding RNA molecules (18–22 nts in length) that are evolutionarily conserved and associated with the Argonaute family of proteins. These microRNAs function at the translational level through silencing mechanisms to regulate gene expression.

MicroRNAs have been shown to be significantly altered throughout the course of disease progression [7]. This is especially true in cancer where abnormal cell growth and angiogenesis are critical for tumorigenesis to occur. The loss of microRNAs that suppress the translation of oncogenes, termed tumor suppressors, has been shown to contribute to the development and progression of many cancers [7]. These microRNAs are primarily responsible for controlling apoptotic pathways and cell cycle checkpoints [7].

Since the discovery of microRNAs, many research groups have analyzed blood in hopes of establishing a correlation to disease. Mitchell et al. first reported that PCa cells released microRNAs into the bloodstream in protective capsules, the content of which could be monitored by PCR-based methods [8]. Schultz et al. studied whole blood for the identification of microRNAs that could be used as biomarkers for the detection of pancreatic cancer [9]. By confirmatory qRT-PCR, they found 38 microRNAs dysregulated and were able to identify two diagnostic microRNA panels that could distinguish between patients with pancreatic cancer from healthy controls [9]. Another study compared microRNA levels between plasma and serum from PCa patients by measuring four microRNAs: hsa-miR-15b, hsa-miR-16, hsa-miR-19b and hsa-miR-24. Interestingly, they found a strong correlation in the microRNA content of these two types of body fluids supporting either serum or plasma as a sufficient source of material for disease studies [8]. Using qRT-PCR, Cochetti et al. suggested a panel of serum microRNAs that could distinguish PCa from benign prostatic hyperplasia in age-matched patients with elevated PSA levels [10]. Thus, the use of blood, serum or plasma as a worthwhile source of material to diagnose disease is well documented [8–10].

To date, a number of studies have used PCR technology to identify microRNAs that could be used as relevant biomarkers to diagnose PCa [11,12]. Certainly, these are important studies, but for the most part, they have used preformed panels of microRNA arrays or focused qRT-PCR assays for specific microRNAs suggested from studying a wide range of different cancers and then applied to PCa. By this approach, only predetermined, known microRNAs are being evaluated. In an effort to widen the scope of microRNA candidates, high throughput sequencing (HTS), also referred to as deep sequencing or RNA sequencing, would better evaluate all possible microRNAs, as well as permitting the discovery of new, novel microRNAs. Keller et al. used HTS of whole blood samples collected with PAXgene blood tubes to study microRNA profiles in lung cancer patients [13]. However, in this case, samples were pooled prior to sequencing, thereby preventing an analysis of microRNA dysregulation across individual samples. To our knowledge, only two reports have used HTS to identify microRNAs diagnostic for PCa. In one case, HTS was used to compare the microRNA content of prostate tumors to adjacent tumor-free margins with the discovery of a loss of miR-143 and miR-145 expression in tumor tissues [14]. A second report applied HTS to exosomal material isolated from blood and found miR-1290 and miR-375 as prognostic markers for castration-resistant prostate cancer (CRPC) [15]. However, in this case, these microRNAs would be useful for identifying late stage prostate cancers.

To better define microRNAs that could be used to more accurately predict PCa at early, not later stages of disease, in this pilot study, we have used HTS of blood from PCa patients at initial stages of diagnosis and before undergoing treatment compared to healthy controls. Moreover, samples were analyzed individually rather than as a pool so that variability between patients or control samples could be followed. RNA sequencing results were also analyzed to identify normalization microRNAs that could be used as endogenous controls for subsequent qRT-PCR analyses. Confirmatory qRT-PCR was then used to corroborate HTS results for the top seven dysregulated microRNAs. Data analysis of the area under the curve (AUC) of the receiver operating curves (ROC) for these selected microRNAs exhibited a better correlation with prostate cancer (AUC range = 0.819–0.950) than the reported value for PSA (AUC 0.678 comparing PCa to non-cancer) [16]. In summary, a panel of seven microRNAs is proposed, many of which have prostate-specific targets, which upon follow-up confirmatory studies could represent a significant improvement over current testing methods.

2. Results

2.1. High Throughput Sequencing Results

A summary of the characteristics and pathological data for patients (n = 28) and controls (n = 12) selected for this study is compared in Table 1. Data for each individual can be found in Appendix A Table A1. Blood was retrieved from patients at early stages of diagnosis and prior to treatment. For most cases, age, ethnicity, PSA and Gleason scores obtained from biopsy were reported. The Gleason score was obtained by microscopic analysis by a trained pathologist and is the combined score of the most common and second most abundant cell type based on cell morphology. When the Gleason score or PSA were not available, it is designated as unknown. Although some mix of ethnicity was obtained, Caucasian was most prevalent with no ethnicity or age recorded for nine individuals. Low Gleason scores of G6 and G7 and PSA values ranging from 3.4–22 predominated, since samples were taken from patients at early stages of diagnosis. Although Gleason scores were not reported for four patients, elevated PSA levels including the high of 22 was found within this group supporting their inclusion to analyze as many samples as possible in this pilot study. Every effort was made to select a control group that had no evidence of PCa either for the individual or within the family. PCa being predominately a disease of the elderly, the average age of the patient group did exceed that of the controls, but since all data were analyzed as individuals, we could subsequently evaluate differences within each group. In this case, we did not find notable discrepancies in data within either the patient or control group due to age or the group of four with elevated PSA values, but unknown Gleason scores, further supporting their inclusion in this study.

Table 1. Characteristics and pathological data of patients and controls involved in the study.

Characteristics	PCa (n = 28)	Controls (n = 12)
AGE (years)		
Range Age	55–92 (n = 19)	23–91 (n = 12)
Mean Age	65.9	50
Unknown	9	0
ETHINICITY (race)		
Caucasian	12	9
African American	6	1
Asian/Hawaiian	1	1
Unknown	9	0
PSA (Prostate Specificity Antigen)		
Range	3.2–22 (n = 19)	–
Mean	7.39	–
Elevated	n = 3	–
Unknown	n = 6	–
PATHOLOGY (Gleason Score)		
G6	n = 9	–
G7	n = 11	–
G8	n = 2	–
G9	n = 2	–
Unknown	n = 4	–

Blood was collected and small RNAs extracted from individual patient and control samples as described in the Materials and Methods. The HTS data revealed that among the 2588 microRNAs present in the miRBase (mature 21 June 2014) [17], about 550 were found at detectable levels in the samples tested. To better refine this list of potential candidates, *p*-values were adjusted using the Benjamini-Hochberg method to yield a False Detection Rate, or FDR value. The FDR value indicates the possible false detection rate using a generalized linearization model. This method is considered a Type 1 error expansion multiple comparison model that reduces the risk of rejecting a true null hypothesis. In order to include as many positive hits as possible in the HTS screening, a cutoff FDR value of <0.2 was selected. An FDR value of 0.2 would mean that 20% of selected microRNAs may be false positives. Since all HTS results would be subsequently confirmed by qRT-PCR, it was felt that lowering the stringency to include more potential microRNA candidates for future confirmation was acceptable at this initial stage. In fact, lowering the stringency of this selection generated a list of 10 possible dysregulated microRNAs for future study (Table 2). Subsequently, miR-5582-3p and miR-543 were dropped because there were no manufactured primers readily available in the market, and their abundance was low. In addition, miR-500b-3p was also dropped due to its low abundance. Thus, seven microRNAs were chosen for future analysis.

Table 2. HTS differential expression analysis the top 10 dysregulated miRNA candidates.

MicroRNA	LogCPM	LogFC	*p*-Value	FDR
miR-5582-3p	0.861	−2.477	2.36×10^{-6}	0.001
miR-32-5p	2.436	−2.036	1.23×10^{-5}	0.003
miR-500b-3p	1.141	2.035	5.77×10^{-4}	0.105
miR-329-3p	1.760	2.096	1.11×10^{-3}	0.132
miR-487b-3p	0.854	2.596	1.20×10^{-3}	0.132
miR-454-3p	5.239	−0.933	1.50×10^{-3}	0.138
miR-204-5p	1.646	1.781	1.93×10^{-3}	0.151
miR-20a-5p	9.049	−1.085	2.97×10^{-3}	0.167
miR-127-3p	4.337	1.433	3.16×10^{-3}	0.167
miR-543	3.353	1.359	3.48×10^{-3}	0.167

LogFC = Log2 comparing patients to controls. FDR = false detection rate.

During the bioinformatics analysis, the HTS total reads for patients and controls were not significantly different from each other, suggesting that blood from normal and patient groups contained similar amounts of total microRNA (Figure 1). This similarity increased the confidence of dysregulation, as it could be confirmed that the differential expression of certain microRNAs was not due to differences in library size.

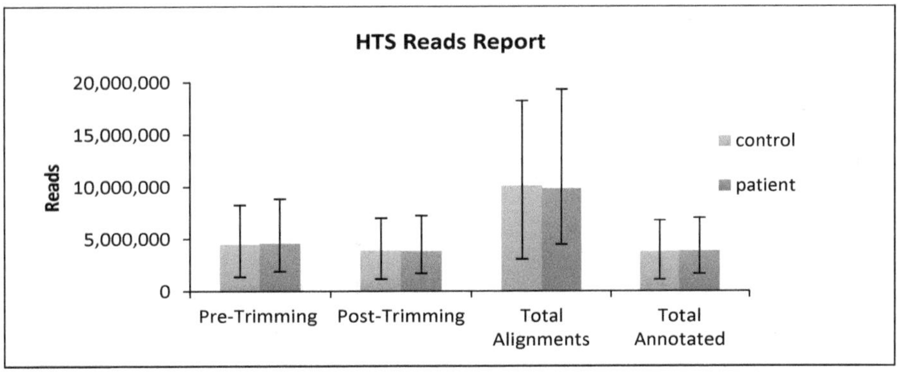

Figure 1. Analysis of HTS reads in blood from PCa patients and controls. HTS was performed on a total number of 40 samples (28 patients and 12 controls) with an RNA concentration of 100 ng/μL. Total reads are shown before and after the Partek Flow® (St. Louis, MO, USA) process.

Processed raw reads were further normalized using the Trimmed Mean of M-values (TMM) method provided by the Edge R program [18]. Based on the hypothesis that most genes are not differentially expressed, the TMM method generates a scaling factor applied to library sizes, which attempts to minimize the intra-group variation in gene expression. This normalization method can further minimize the effect of technical variations caused by sequencing depth and batch variation. The TMM method is a very powerful method when varying library size, and high-count genes can exist [19]. Compared to the commonly-used normalization methods of Total Counts (TC) or Reads Per Kilobase per Million mapped reads (RPKM), the TMM method is more reliable, because it not only normalizes the library size, but also takes into account the effect of RNA composition [18]. The effectiveness of the TMM method in normalizing the microRNA sequencing results was later confirmed via qRT-PCR.

The seven dysregulated microRNAs indicated by HTS differential expression analysis showed great differences in normalized reads between control and patient groups (Figure 2a–g). According to the HTS data, four microRNAs were upregulated (miR-127-3p, miR-204-5p, miR-329-3p and miR-487b-3p) in patients' blood samples (Figure 2a–d), while three microRNAs (miR-32-5p, miR-20a-5p and miR-454-3p) were downregulated (Figure 2e–g).

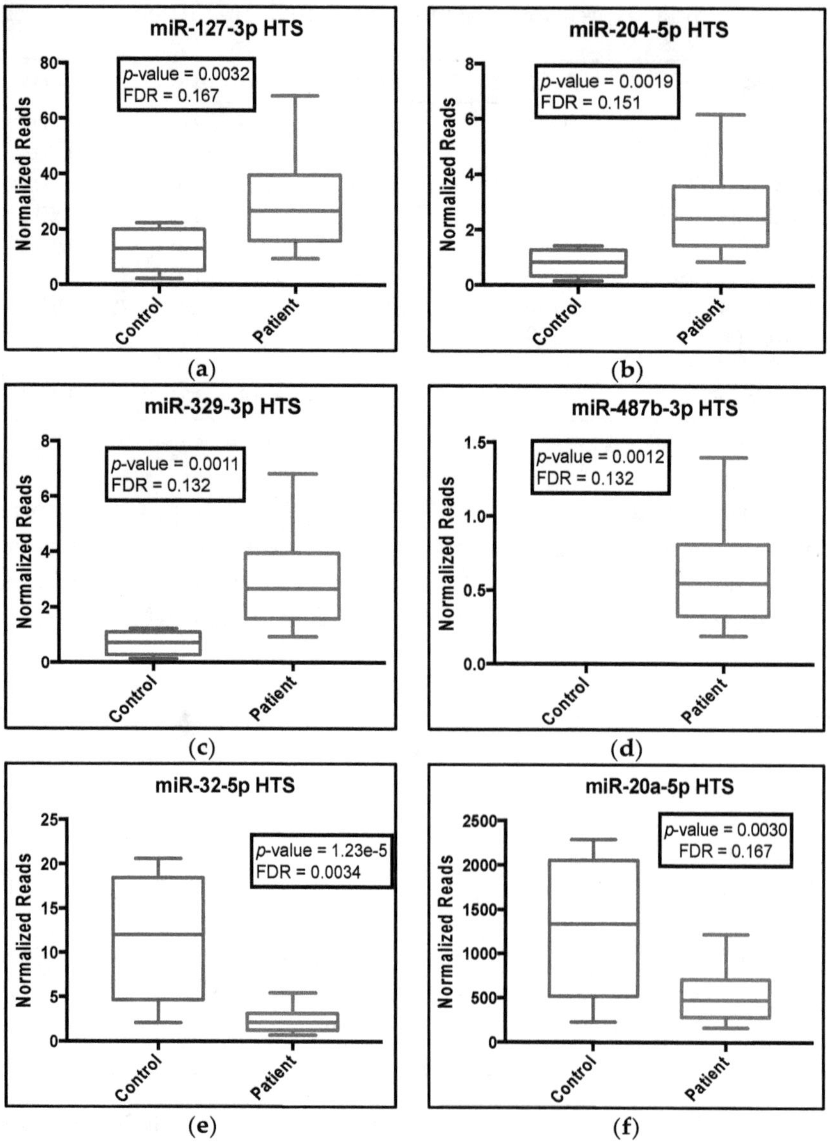

Figure 2. *Cont.*

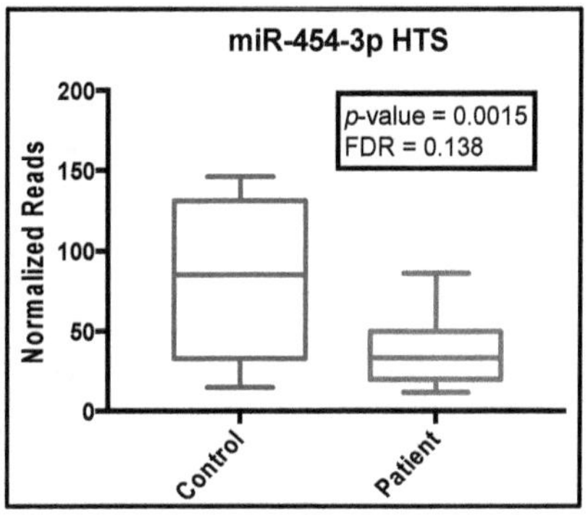

(g)

Figure 2. HTS data show dysregulation of seven microRNAs in blood from PCa patients (red) compared to controls (blue). (**a–g**) Box plots of the top seven dysregulated microRNAs as indicated on each panel are based on Edge R differential expression analysis. *p*-Values and FDR values were generated by Edge R using the generalized linear method. Box-and-whiskers graphs were plotted using Prism. The minimum, the 25th percentile, the median, the 75th percentile and the maximum are shown on each box plot as the bottom to the top lines, respectively. An FDR < 0.2 was considered significant.

2.2. *Identification of MicroRNAs as Normalization Standards for qRT-PCR*

In order to confirm HTS data by qRT-PCR, a normalization method needed to be developed to ensure that microRNA dysregulation was due to true biological variation and not technical error. Ideally, microRNA normalizers should exhibit small standard deviations and display similar expression levels to the dysregulated microRNAs under study. To this end, the concentration of small RNAs in each sample was determined from bioanalyzer results, set to a constant amount, and the Cq value determined by qRT-PCR. Results were analyzed using the NormFinder program, which scrutinizes intra- and inter-group variations to determine which microRNA candidates are best suited for normalization using an algorithm to calculate a stability value for each microRNA, i.e., the lower the value, the lower the variation.

The NormFinder program selected eight microRNAs as exhibiting stable expression patterns; miR-146a-5p, miR-1538, miR-197-3p, miR-1468-3p, miR-26b-5p, miR-296-5p, miR-1248 and miR-23a-3p (Figure 3a; raw data Appendix A Table 2). Due to limiting amounts of material, the search for potential microRNA normalizers was initially monitored in a subset of samples, i.e., eight patients and eight controls. Of these, the first four candidates, which exhibited the closest stability values (ranging from 0.009–0.0016) with minimal differences in expression between control and patient samples, were subsequently analyzed in a fuller spectrum of samples (26 patients and 10 controls). Unfortunately, two samples from each group of HTS data had to be dropped from further analysis due to a lack of material (Figure 3b; raw data Appendix A Table 3). NormFinder suggested that the single best candidate was miR-146a-5p. However, when there is no obvious single, outstanding normalization candidate, NormFinder suggests using a combination of microRNAs to increase reliability and produce less intra- and inter-group variability. Since the top four microRNAs (miR-146a-5p, miR-1538, miR-197-3p, miR-1468-3p) all showed very close stability values, the Cq value of each was compared to each other, as well as the geometric mean of the top two candidates (miR-146-5p and miR-1538) or all four top candidates together (Figure 3b). The top two candidates showed decreased intra-group variation, especially for the patient group (Figure 3b). However, the geometric mean of all four candidates together showed even smaller intra- and inter-variations within and between both control and patient groups (Figure 3b). Therefore, these four microRNAs were selected as a group of normalizers to be used for downstream qRT-PCR analyses.

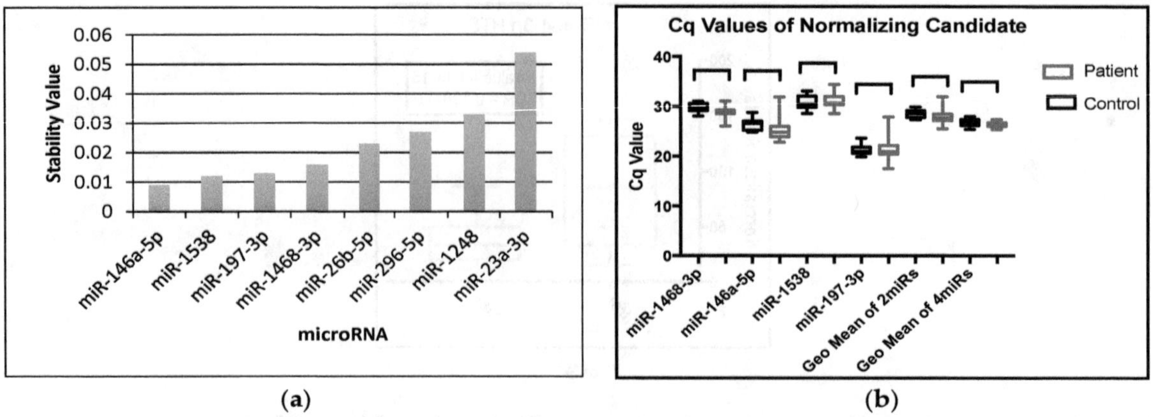

Figure 3. Analysis by the NormFinder program identified four microRNAs as the best normalization candidates for qRT-PCR studies. (**a**) Eight stably-expressed microRNAs (miR-146a-5p, miR-1538, miR-197-3p, miR-1468-3p, miR-26b-5p, miR-296-5p, miR-1248 and miR-23a-3p) suggested by HTS data were confirmed by qRT-PCR in triplicate (eight controls and eight patients). The small RNA concentration for each sample was normalized to roughly 0.012 ng/µL in each reaction. A stability value was generated for each candidate by the NormFinder program, where the lower the value, the better; (**b**) The Cq value of the top four microRNA candidates (miR-1468-3p, miR-146a-5p, miR-1538, miR-197-3p) was subsequently evaluated in 26 patients and 10 controls and plotted individually as box plots versus the geometric (Geo) mean of two candidates (miR-146a-5p and miR-1538) or four candidates (miR-146a-5p, miR-1538, miR-197-3p and miR-1468-3p) as analyzed in triplicate by qRT-PCR.

2.3. Validation of HTS Data by qRT-PCR Analysis

The elucidation of valid microRNA normalizers permitted further analysis of HTS results via qRT-PCR. The individual dot plots of dCq (ΔCq) values are shown for the seven dysregulated miRs suggested by HTS data (Figure 4). According to the qRT-PCR results, miR-127-3p, miR-204-5p, miR-329-3p and miR-487b-3p were all upregulated in patients compared to controls (Figure 4a–d), while miR-32-5p, miR-20a-5p and miR-454-3p were downregulated (Figure 4e–g) The differences in expression in control versus patient samples was calculated for each microRNA as the –ddCq (Log2 fold change) and shown in Figure 4h. Raw and normalized Cq values for controls and patients are included in Appendix A Tables 3 and 4, respectively. Thus, the qRT PCR results agreed with the HTS data, confirming that all seven microRNAs were dysregulated in PCa patients.

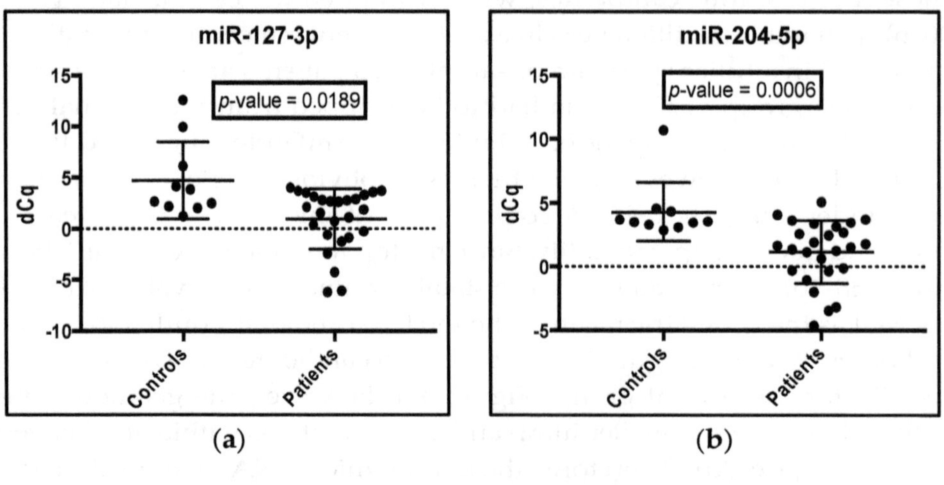

Figure 4. *Cont.*

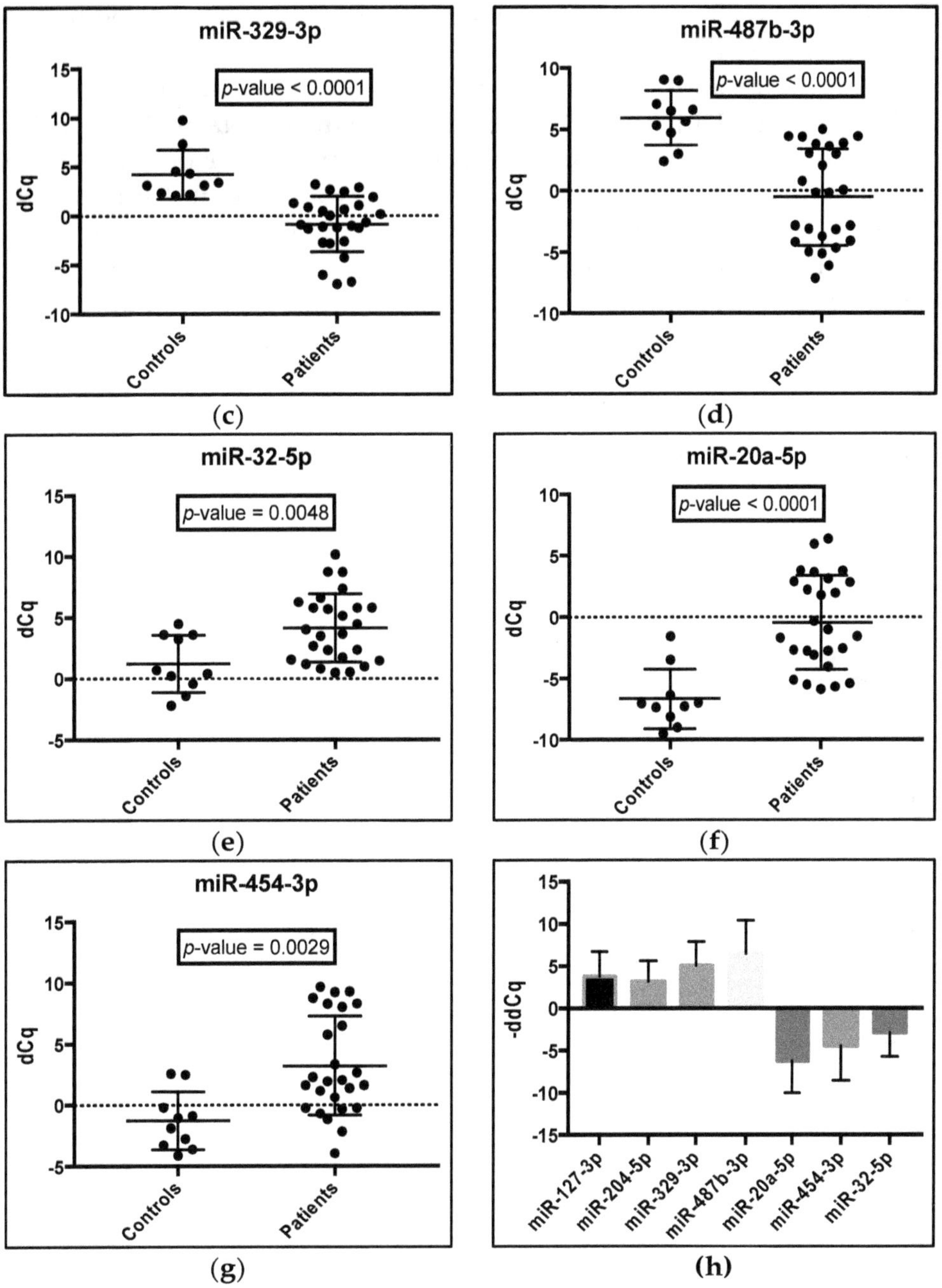

Figure 4. Confirmatory qRT-PCR results for dysregulated miRNA candidates suggested by HTS data. (**a**–**g**) A comparison between normalized Cq values (dCq) from qRT-PCR analysis of blood from patients and controls and plotted as dot blots. qRT-PCR was performed on 36 samples (10 controls and 26 patients) in triplicate. Samples were adjusted to the same small RNA concentration (0.012 ng/μL) per reaction. Raw Cq values were normalized by subtracting the geometric mean Cq value of the top four normalization candidates (miR-146a-5p, miR-1538, miR-197-3p and miR-1468-3p) suggested by the NormFinder program from individual Cq values to generate dCq. A *p*-value was obtained using the Mann–Whitney nonparametric test assuming that data do not follow a Gaussian distribution. A *p*-value < 0.05 was considered significant. The minimum, median and maximum values are shown as respective lines from the bottom to the top; (**h**) The −ddCq values of the seven dysregulated microRNAs are shown. The −ddCq for each candidate was obtained by taking the mean of the normalized dCq of all controls minus the normalized dCq of each patient sample. This value equals the fold change on a Log2 scale.

In order to further assess whether the seven microRNAs could serve as good biomarkers, Receiver Operator Curves (ROC) were drawn based on the qRT-PCR data. ROC analysis demonstrates the trade-off between sensitivity and specificity where a good biomarker should display both high sensitivity and high specificity [20]. The ROC curve for each microRNA is shown in Figure 5. In ROC analysis, the Area Under the Curve (AUC) quantifies the biomarker potential for each candidate where the higher the AUC value, the better a candidate microRNA is at distinguishing PCa patients from controls. Via ROC analysis, the currently used PCa biomarker, PSA, has a reported AUC value of 0.678 for distinguishing PCa from no cancer [16]. The seven microRNAs identified in our study exhibited a respectable range of AUC values from 0.7538 for miR-127-3p up to 0.9462 for miR-329-3p, all significantly better than that reported for PSA, with p-values ranging from 1.9435×10^{-6} to 0.0094 (Figure 5a–g).

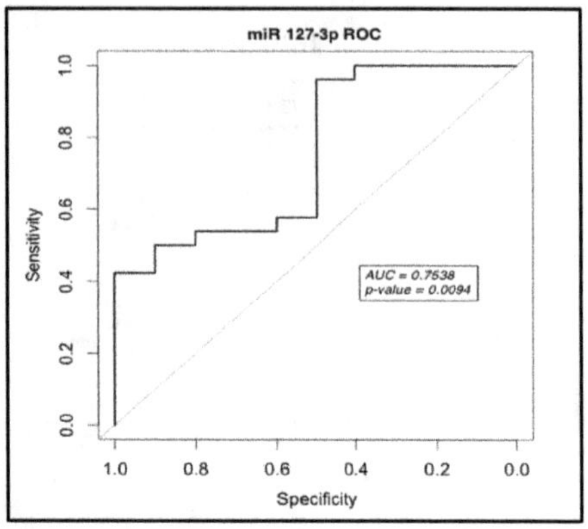

(a)

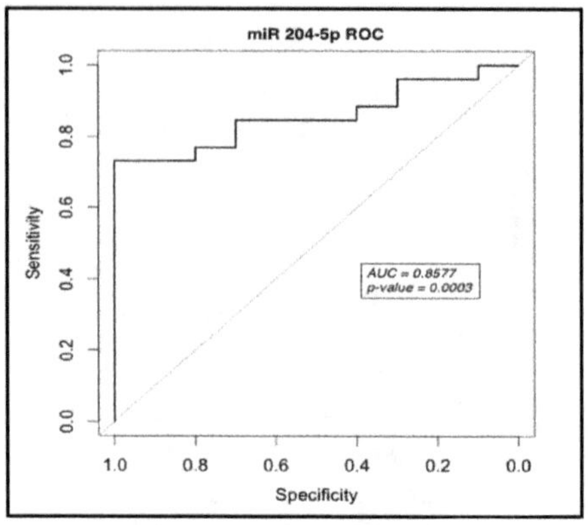

(b)

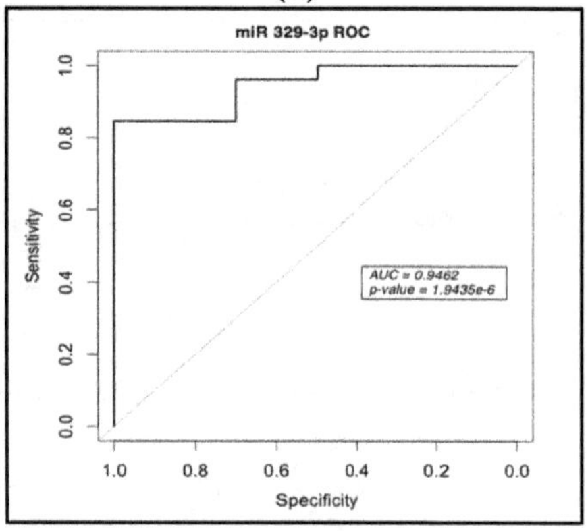

(c)

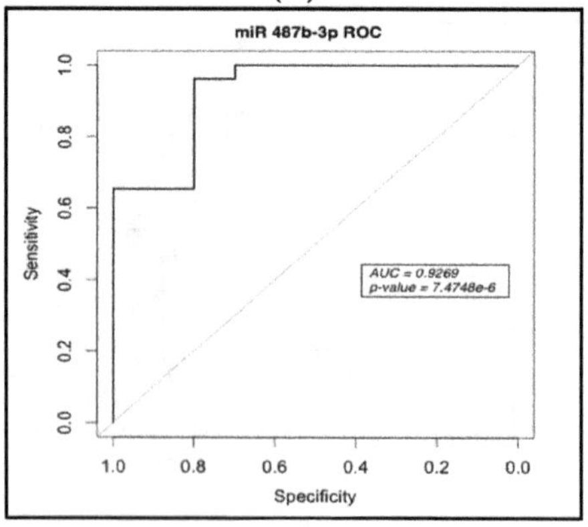

(d)

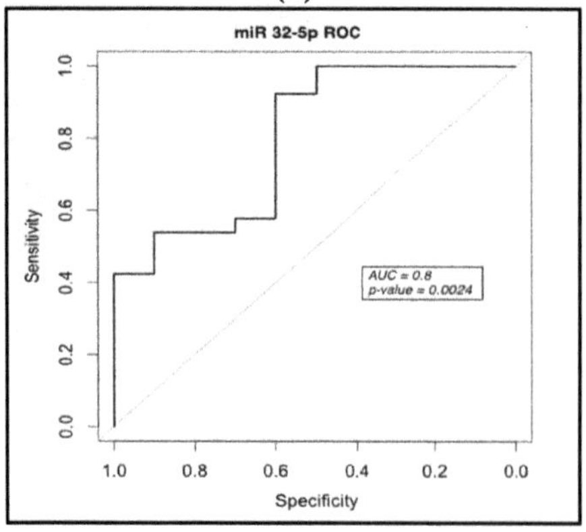

(e)

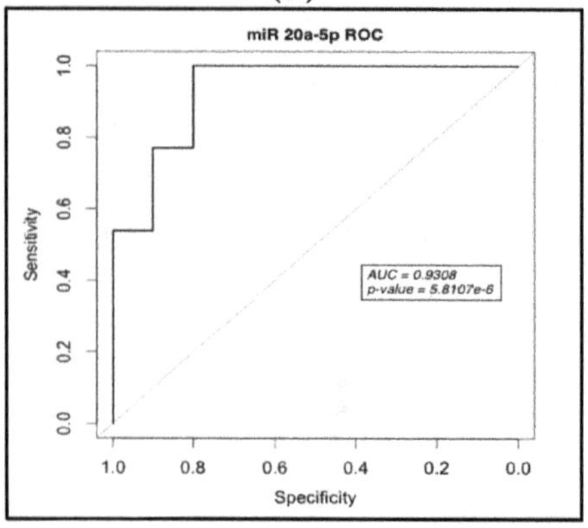

(f)

Figure 5. *Cont.*

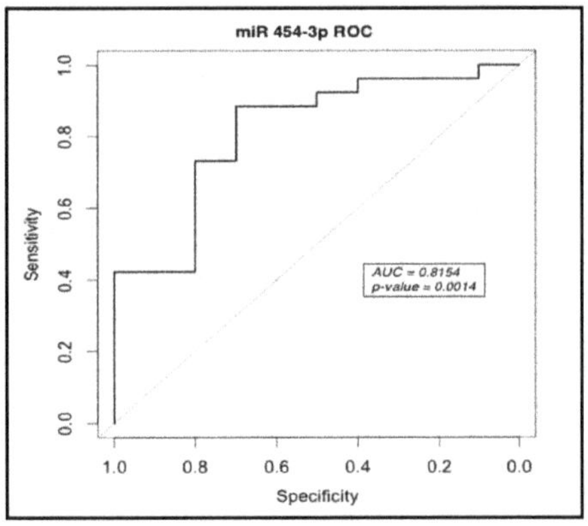

(g)

Figure 5. Receiver operator curves for dysregulated microRNAs. (**a**–**g**) Analysis was performed based on the qRT-PCR results in triplicate of individual microRNAs as indicated on each graph and plotted as sensitivity versus specificity. An AUC > 0.5 is considered significant.

2.4. Comparison of Blood Results to TCGA Database

The expression of our panel of blood microRNAs was compared to expression levels in tumor tissue by our analysis of data in The Cancer Genome Atlas (TCGA) database. Although the TCGA microRNA sequencing data were annotated with the stem-loop transcripts instead of the mature strands, all seven microRNAs from our study derive from the major expressed mature strand of their stem-loop precursor based on data in miRBase [17]. Therefore, the expression of these seven mature microRNAs is directly proportional to the abundance of their stem-loop precursors. The mature miR-127-3p, miR-204-5p, miR-487b-3p, miR-32-5p, miR-20a-5p and miR-454-3p are derived from precursors miR-127, miR-204, miR-487b, miR-32, miR-20a and miR-454, respectively. The mature miR-329-3p was derived from two precursors, miR-329-1 and miR-329-2.

The expression of each precursor in PCa tissues compared to their disease-free matched margins showed significant dysregulation, and the direction of dysregulation agreed with the literature results (Figure 6). However, the pattern of dysregulation for each microRNA in tumor tissue was opposite to that pattern observed in our blood samples. For example, miR-127, miR-204, miR-329-1, miR-329-2 and miR-487b were all upregulated in PCa tissue, which suggested that their major mature strands (miR-127-3p, miR-204-5p, miR-329-3p and miR-487b-3p) were also upregulated. However, these four microRNAs were shown to be downregulated in our blood samples. The inverse correlation was observed for the three microRNAs (miR-32-5p, miR-20a-5p and miR-454-3p) that are downregulated in blood. Again, their precursor transcripts and presumably major, mature microRNA products were upregulated in the TCGA tissue data. A comparison of the fold changes between our HTS blood data versus that from the TCGA database are included in the Appendix A (Table 5).

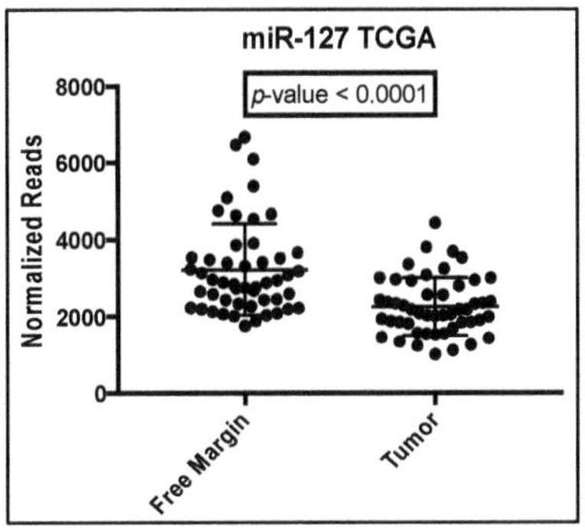

(a)

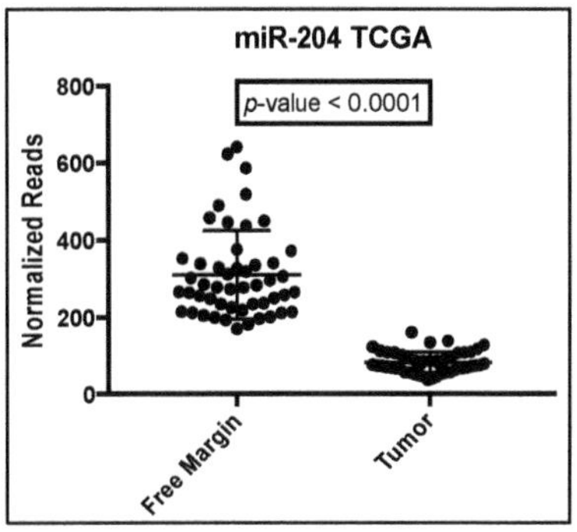

(b)

Figure 6. *Cont.*

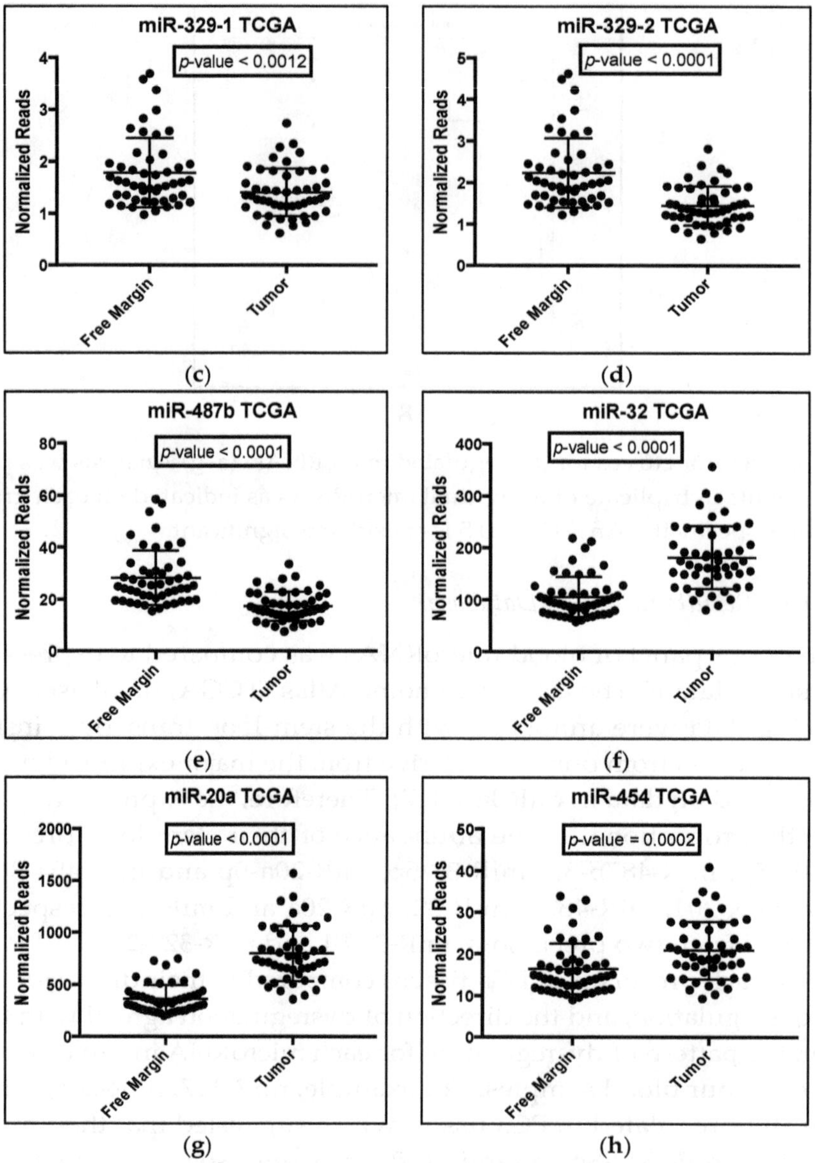

Figure 6. An analysis of microRNA sequencing results from the TGCA matched tissue database for the seven microRNA candidates. (**a–h**) Reads for each microRNA candidate as indicated were normalized using the Edge R TMM method and plotted as a dot blot with a line (bottom to top, respectively) representing the minimum, median (or mean) and maximum value for the tumor versus the disease-free matched tissue (free-margin) from PCa patients. A *p*-value was obtained using the Mann–Whitney nonparametric test assuming that that data do not follow a Gaussian distribution. A $p < 0.05$ was considered significant. TCGA, The Cancer Genome Atlas.

3. Discussion

Analysis of HTS sequencing results suggested a panel of seven microRNAs that could be useful in diagnosing PCa in blood. Previously, the lack of reliable microRNA standards for normalization across different samples had been detrimental to subsequent qRT-PCR validation studies. In some studies, snRNAs have been used for this purpose, but since these are not normally secreted and are not produced by pathways that correlate with microRNA synthesis, their use as normalizers for complex body fluids such as blood is questionable. A review of our HTS data selected four microRNAs (miR-197-3p or -5p, miR-1538, miR-1468-3p and miR-146a-5p) that were consistently expressed across all patient and control samples and could be used as reliable normalization standards for future qRT-PCR studies. Kirschner et al. also found miR-146a to be stably expressed in plasma and serum, not affected by hemolysis, in agreement with our results in blood [21]. Moreover, the enhanced geometric mean of these microRNAs was shown to be significantly better than any single microRNA alone.

With a proven group of normalization standards, it was important to confirm HTS results via qRT-PCR. Significantly, results from these two very different methodologies agreed well, further supporting the validity of our approach. All of the microRNAs with low *p*- and FDR-values via HTS data showed significant *p*-values with qRT-PCR and notable AUC values upon ROC analysis. This agreement was encouraging because thus far, investigators had been determining diagnostic microRNAs by screening of pre-selected microRNA arrays, which represented only a small subset of microRNAs from the database of >2580 total microRNAs [17]. This approach is limited to analyzing only those microRNAs that have already been shown to be dysregulated in some disease and then selected for analyzing PCa. However, HTS permits the identification of all possible diagnostic miRNAs, both known and perhaps novel, expanding the spectrum of microRNA candidates evaluated. Interestingly, a few novel microRNA species were identified, but these always turned out to be a single report; thus, their relevance as a "new" molecule warranting further verification was hard to justify in this pilot study due to their low abundance. More importantly, HTS results were validated by qRT-PCR for all seven candidates generating ROC curves with individual AUC values better than PSA (AUC = 0.678), the current gold standard for diagnosing PCa [16].

Another value of our suggested panel is that four microRNAs are upregulated in blood, whereas three are downregulated. This result means that each group can serve as an additional internal control for each other, thereby further serving to verify the accuracy of results, i.e., they do not all go up or all go down. Constructing a diagnostic panel with only downregulated microRNAs is always hard to justify; however, by pairing the loss of three microRNAs with an increase in the other four allows for greater diagnostic confidence.

In some previous studies, PCa samples were pooled in order to obtain sufficient material for subsequent analysis [22,23]. This approach prevents an analysis of variability across individual samples and blocks any correlation to the stage of disease when Gleason scores are available. Not only is it important to diagnose PCa, but eventually to identify biomarkers that could serve to stage disease and, more importantly, discern indolent from aggressive disease, thereby impacting subsequent treatment options. Thus, the fact that valid HTS data could be acquired from individual samples without requiring pooling might enable a correlation between microRNA and tumor stage in future studies. Samples analyzed here were predominately from lower Gleason-scored patients (Table 1: 9 or 11 patients with a G6 or G7 score respectively with only 2 samples scored as G8 or G9). Thus, our panel is more diagnostic for early detection and, if these patients could be followed, might elucidate microRNAs useful for separating indolent from more aggressive disease. In any case, more patient samples are needed particularly with higher Gleason scores to determine microRNAs that could identify later stages of disease as proposed for miR-1290 and miR-375 in CRPC [15].

3.1. Literature Review of Diagnostic Panel of Dysregulated MicroRNAs in Cancer

A brief review of these diagnostic seven microRNAs, their Chromosomal (Chr) location and known targets was carried out to determine if their dysregulation might support a functional role in prostate tumorigenesis.

3.1.1. miR-127-3p, miR-204-5p, miR-329-3p and miR-487b-3p as Tumor Suppressors

miR-127-3p (Chr 14) is situated near a cluster of microRNAs (has-miR-431, hsa-miR-433, hsa-miR-432 and hsa-miR-136) susceptible to epigenetic silencing [24]. It has been shown to target BCL6 and is downregulated in breast cancer tissue where overexpression of miR-127-3p or depletion of BCL6 supported its role as a tumor suppressor [25]. In addition, BCL6 plays an important role in cell proliferation by suppressing transcription of the anti-apoptotic *BCL-XL* gene and the adhesion molecule VCAM [26,27].

miR-204-5p (Chr 9) is highly downregulated in many tumor types including breast, kidney and prostate [28]. The absence of miR-204-5p led to a decrease in Kir7.1 proteins, which connect TGF-BR2 and maintain potassium homeostasis, thereby playing a crucial role in maintaining epithelial barrier function and cell physiology [28]. miR-204-5p has been shown to suppress the growth, migration and invasion of endometrial carcinomas by binding to TrkB mRNA and interfering with JAK2 and STAT3 phosphorylation [29].

miR-329-3p (Chr14) is part of an extensive microRNA cluster containing over 40 microRNAs. Yang et al. found miR-329-3p to be downregulated in metastatic, neuroblastoma tumor tissue compared to the primary tumor [30]. One promising target for miR-329-3p is KDM1A, which has been shown to be significantly upregulated in the androgen-dependent LnCaP prostate cell line [30,31]. Upon depletion of KDMA1 using siRNA, VEGF-A expression was also decreased, which in turn blocked androgen-induced VEGF-A, PSA and Tmprss2 expression, suggesting a role for miR-329-3p as a tumor suppressor.

miR-487-3p (Chr 14 within the same microRNA cluster as miR-329) has been found to be downregulated in neuroblastomas and in PCa [32,33]. Moreover, 10 microRNAs from this cluster were found to be significantly downregulated in PCa as Gleason scores increased, thereby playing an important role in regulating proliferation, apoptosis, migration and invasion in metastatic PCa cells [32]. An interesting predicted target for miR-487b-3p is ALDH1A3, aldehyde dehydrogenase 1A3, an enzyme known to be upregulated four-fold in the LnCaP PCa cell lines [34] when exposed to the androgen Dihydrotestosterone (DHT).

3.1.2. miR-32-5p, miR-20a-5p and miR-454-3p as OncomiRs

miR-32-5p (Chr 9) has been found to be an androgen-regulated microRNA that targets BTG2 [35]. Its overexpression has been shown to block apoptosis and promote PCa in CRPC. Furthermore, this microRNA was discovered to be regulated by DHT and displays putative upstream androgen receptor-binding sites (ARBS).

miR-20a-5p (Chr 13) is part of the miR-17–92 cluster, which plays an important role in cell cycle progression, proliferation, apoptosis and other cellular processes [36]. One of the most studied targets of miR-20a is the E2F family, particularly E2F2 and E2F3 [37]. The overexpression of miR-20a-5p in the PC3 PCa cell line was shown to regulate the cell cycle via targeting of E2F2 and E2F3 mRNAs [36]. In addition, this microRNA also targets several cyclin-dependent kinases, including p21 and p57, which halt cell cycle progression. Finally, another notable target is FasI, which promotes cell death [37]. Thus, the major targets of miR-20a-5p promote tumorigenesis and angiogenesis by blocking cell cycle checkpoints [36].

miR-454-3p is located on Chr 17 in the first intronic region of its host gene *SKA2* (Spindle and Kinetochore-Associated Complex Subunit 2). SKA2 is essential for proper chromosome segregation. During the cell cycle, both SKA2 and miR-454-3p have been shown to be upregulated. miR-454-3p targets the tumor suppressor gene, *BTG1* (B cell Translocation Gene 1), which plays an important role in cell cycle progression and is involved in the stress response [38]. This anti-proliferative gene is expressed at its highest concentration during the G0/G1 phases of the cell cycle and is then downregulated when the cell progresses through the G1 phase. In renal carcinoma cells, an increase in miR-454-3p displayed a marked decrease in BTG1 via a direct interaction with the 3′-UTR of BTG1 mRNA [38].

3.1.3. Summary of the Literature Review for Targets of Panel MicroRNAs

A summary of these results is shown in Table 3. The four upregulated microRNAs in patient blood (miR-127-3p, miR-329-3p, miR-487b-3p and miR-204-5p) cumulatively target BCL6, TrkB, KDM1A and ALDH1A3, all of which have been shown to be important regulators in PCa [24–34]. Since these proteins exert oncogenic effects in prostate tissue, their regulators are viewed as tumor suppressors, the loss of which could contribute to tumorigenesis. On the other hand, the three downregulated microRNAs in patient blood (miR-20a-5p, miR-32-5p and miR-454-3p) have been shown to target the tumor suppressor proteins E2F2/3, BTG2 and BTG1, respectively [35–38]. Although they were downregulated in our patient blood samples, they have been shown to be oncomiRs in tumor tissue, the retention of which could promote tumor progression. A review of this literature supports how these microRNAs could play a role in PCa progression.

Table 3. Summary of targets and their role in prostate cancer for the miRNA panel.

MicroRNA	Validated Target	Possible Role in Cancer
miR-127-3p	BCL6 [24–27]	Tumor suppressor
miR-204-5p	TrkB [28,29]	Tumor suppressor
miR-329-3p	KDMA1 [30,31]	Tumor suppressor
miR-487b-3p	ALDH1A3 [32–34] *	Tumor suppressor
miR-32-5p	BTG2 [35]	OncomiR
miR-20a-5p	E2F family, P21, p57 [36,37]	OncomiR
miR-454-3p	BTG1 [38]	OncomiR

* A predicted target.

Interestingly, three of the microRNAs in our panel belong to the same mega cluster on Chr 14. A post-review of our data did note differential expression for several additional members from this cluster. However, due to their low abundance, slightly higher FDR values and limited budget, they were not included in subsequent qRT-PCR confirmatory studies. Analysis of the HTS data showed that five mega cluster members (miR-654-5p, miR 654-3p, miR-493-3p, miR-493-5p and 433-5p) were present in the top 50 dysregulated microRNAs ranking 17th–59th from the top (Appendix A Table 6). A review of the TGCA data showed that all were downregulated to different degrees in tumor tissue, fitting with their loss as tumor suppressors. Interestingly, one of these microRNAs, miR-433-3p, has been shown to target CREB (cAMP Response Element Binding protein), a nuclear transcription factor shown to be involved in tumor initiation, progression and metastasis [39]. Sun et al. showed that overexpression of miR-433-3p could counteract the effects of CREB. Studies have shown that the microRNAs in this Chr 14 cluster are downregulated through unknown mechanisms. If increases in these microRNAs are found in blood, it is possible to hypothesize that the expression of these microRNAs is not just being turned off at the transcriptional level, but that they are being shuttled out of the tumor cell and into the blood as a survival and growth mechanism for the developing tumor.

3.2. *Relevance of Comparing Blood HTS and qRT-PCR Data to the TCGA Database*

An unanticipated discovery from this study was the inverse relationship between blood and tumor microRNA expression levels (Figures 2 and 4 compared to Figure 6). Since all of our blood microRNAs displayed an inverse expression level with our analysis of data from the TCGA database, we propose that it is possible that tumors are retaining oncomiRs for the purpose of driving tumorigenesis and angiogenesis, and therefore, less of these oncomiRs are released into the blood (Figure 7). Conversely, tumor suppressors block tumor growth and may need to be disposed of to enhance tumorigenesis and ultimately metastasis; hence, the increase in blood levels of these microRNAs. If this were the case for only one or two members of our diagnostic panel of seven microRNAs, perhaps not, but the recurrence for all seven candidates lends credibility to this hypothesis. Moreover, a review of their known targets and the roles they could play in PCa further supports this idea (Table 3).

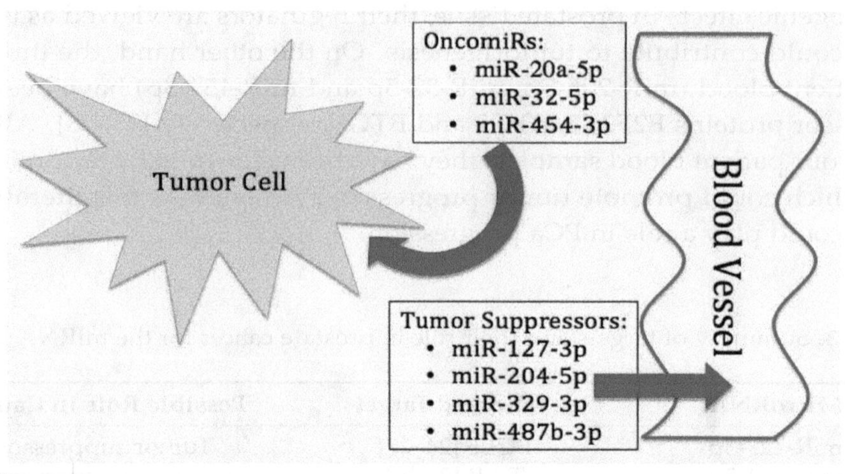

Figure 7. Relationship between microRNA content in prostate tumor cell derived from the TCGA database versus our analysis of blood in prostate cancer patients. The tumor cell retains oncomiRs, but disposes of tumor suppressors to enhance tumorigenesis.

It has been shown that cancer cells secrete vesicles containing not only mature microRNAs to modify their environment for future metastasis, but the entire processing machinery (dicer, RISC with premiR) to ensure that once taken up by the target cell, the microRNA is efficiently processed and actively moved into the translational silencing mechanism of target mRNAs [40]. It is proposed that if only the mature microRNA were delivered to a secondary site, it might not be as efficient in modifying translation within the target cell. Thus, the preferential cellular export of certain microRNAs as "hormomirs" may function to modulate gene expression at secondary sites, thereby affecting disease pathology [41,42]. With this in mind, it is not much of a stretch to propose a developing tumor wants to dispose of compromising microRNAs that could restrict its growth; thus, excluding tumor suppressor microRNAs. Concomitantly, holding onto an oncomiR to quickly modulate the proteome is fast and efficient, faster than modifying gene expression at the transcriptional level. In support of this hypothesis, Selth et al. found a similar inverse relationship between the loss of miR-146b-3p expression in the prostate tumor with a concomitant increase in circulation [41]. Conversely, in the same study, a direct correlation between increased expression of miR-194 in the tumor and in circulation was noted, suggesting that microRNAs may vary in their expression and patterns of secretion. Since overexpression of miR-194 blocks cell proliferation, induces apoptosis, caspase-3/-9 activities and p53/p21 signaling while suppressing PI3K/AKT/FoxO3a signaling, it is difficult to understand how a tumor could tolerate an increase in the expression of this microRNA, which was not discussed [43]. Another study found miR-194 to be decreased in prostate tumors, befitting its function as a tumor suppressor [44]. On the other hand, miR-1 and miR-133a have been shown to be increased in serum in response to acute myocardial infarction where the levels of both are reduced in the infarcted myocardial tissue [45]. Thus, some evidence for an inverse correlation between tissue expression and microRNAs in circulation exists, but at this time, additional studies in PCa with more patient samples and expansion to other cancers and disease states need to be completed to determine the overall merits of this hypothesis.

3.3. Comparison of HTS Data to Screens of MicroRNA Panels and qRT-PCR Analysis

To date, the elucidation of microRNAs to identify PCa has been mostly generated from screens of preformed microRNA panels or qRT-PCR assays for microRNAs already shown to be involved in cancer. In both cases, the decision as to what microRNAs should be surveyed has already been made rather than using a technology like HTS, which uses no preselection and permits the identification of any potential microRNA. Cochetti et al. chose 23 microRNAs from an in silico survey of predicted target genes to analyze serum from PCa patients [10]. A review of a variety of such studies using serum or plasma has suggested miR-141, -21, -200b, -375, -221, -26a, -195, -15b, -16, -19b, -24, -451 or let-7i as biomarkers to distinguish PCa patients from healthy individuals [5,8,14,41,42]. Some of these microRNAs have also been proposed as biomarkers for other cancers not being unique to PCa (miR-141, -21, -16, -451) or are heavily influenced by hemolysis (miR-15b, -16, -451), making their utility for PCa diagnosis debatable [8,42]. Interestingly, we did not find any of these microRNAs to be significantly altered in our HTS data. In part, this could be due to differences in analyzing serum or plasma versus blood, a very different source of body fluid, as well as the use of HTS data as the starting point for investigation.

HTS has been applied to a very limited number of studies for identifying microRNAs diagnostic for PCa. Szczyrba et al. looked at microRNA profiles of prostate carcinoma compared to normal tissue and cell lines [14]. Here, the loss of miR-143 and miR-145 targeting myosin VI (MYO6) was suggested as a diagnostic marker for prostate carcinoma. However, we did not find these two microRNAs to be dysregulated in blood. Of more significance to our study was the reported HTS data of blood exosomal material isolated from CRPC patients [15]. Here, as well, a group of normalizing RNAs (miR-301a/e-5p, miR-99a-5p, let-7c, miR-125a-5p, miR-16-5 and RNU6B) was proposed for subsequent qRT-PCR analysis. Since RNU6B is not a secreted microRNA, it is doubtful that it should have been included in this analysis, but discounting this snRNA, the rest would be useful normalizers for exosomal material. Interestingly, we found a completely different group of normalizing microRNAs with no overlap of this group, supporting how different an exosomal pool might be to the blood samples analyzed here. Upon normalization, these authors proposed miR-1290 and miR-375 as prognostic markers for CRPC. Since this was only for CRPC patients, perhaps it is not surprising that we did not find these two microRNAs in our analysis, since we are not focused on CRPC. Perhaps our panel of seven microRNAs would be better suited for identifying early stages of prostate cancer, rather than this later stage. Again, additional studies for CRPC versus patients that have not progressed to later stage disease are needed to clarify this hypothesis.

3.4. Limitations to This Pilot Study

This study was meant as a pilot study and, as such, suffers from some limitations, which should be addressed. First, to obtain sufficient material for HTS analysis, blood was used as the initial source of small RNAs. Thus, small RNAs will be contaminated with cellular microRNAs, not just circulating microRNAs. However, circulating microRNAs can come in many forms as exosomes, microvesicles, apoptotic bodies or bound to HDL, argonaute 2 or RNA-binding proteins, such as nucleophosmin 1 [42]. At this time, it is not clear which of these forms or combinations thereof would be the most diagnostic as biomarkers for PCa. Thus, focusing on some particles (exosomes or microvesicles) at the exclusion of the others might not be the most relevant source. Isolation of small RNAs from whole blood rather than purification of a subset of these particles seemed like a more inclusive starting point. More importantly, it was assumed that control samples will contain the same contaminates as patient samples, and thus, contaminating cellular microRNAs should cancel out and not be found amongst the dysregulated microRNAs, if samples are handled consistently. In support of this premise, it was reassuring that microRNAs known to reflect WBC (miRs-15- and -230), RBCs affected by hemolysis (miR-16-485-3p, -532-3p, -15b, -16 and -451), RBCs not-affected by hemolysis (miR-1274b, -142-3p and 146a), myeloid (miR-7a, -223, -197 and 574-3p) or lymphoid (miR-150) cells were not found in our panel of dysregulated microRNAs [21,41,42,46]. Our final panel of seven microRNAs was unique amongst those proposed in the literature, perhaps due to the fact that they were compiled from HTS data rather than screens of predetermined miR array panels or primer sets. Second, PSA values were not reported for control samples, making it impossible to obtain an AUC value for this cohort. Thus, an AUC value for PSA was taken from the literature [16], and it could be higher for our control group with its younger age, a problem encountered by other such studies [42]. However, all seven panel members yielded individual AUC values considerably better than the reported value for PSA, which when used as a panel should be stronger than any single microRNA. In fact, in a review by Selth, it was proposed that "no single analyte is likely to achieve the desired level of diagnostic or prognostic accuracy for PCa ... requiring a signature of multiple microRNAs rather than a single miR", as proposed here [42]. Third, validation of HTS results by qRT-PCR was on the same cohort of samples analyzed by HTS. In a future study, a third larger cohort should be evaluated independently to better validate panel members as relevant biomarkers. Finally, these samples did not span the spectrum of higher Gleason scores, but reflect earlier stages of PCa. Thus, at this time, they are not useful for staging or separating indolent from aggressive disease, an important future correlate. Nevertheless, it is proposed that despite these limitations, this initial pilot study does present new novel microRNAs that have not been previously suggested, which warrant inclusion in future studies sampling larger cohorts.

Here, we have proposed a panel of seven microRNAs generated from HTS data rather than pre-judged screens of microRNA arrays proposed from other cancers with unknown relevance to PCa. The same criticism exists for data generated by qRT-PCR studies, since again, only a subset of chosen total microRNAs is being investigated. We propose that HTS data confirmed by qRT-PCR analysis are a worthwhile approach for deducing biomarkers for PCa. Certainly, our ROC curves and AUC values appear superior compared to the current PSA gold standard [16]. As a group, the value of a panel of diagnostic microRNAs is substantial. However, additional studies with more extensive patient sampling are required to determine their future usefulness in not only identifying PCa, but ultimately staging prostate cancer and separating indolent versus aggressive disease. This will require sampling, preferably individually, of a vast number of patient and control samples, but our initial study certainly justifies the merits of future investigation.

4. Materials and Methods

4.1. Sample Extraction and HTS Sequencing

Whole blood samples from patients and controls were obtained from the Nelson Urology Clinic, VCU (Virginia Commonwealth University) Medical Center and Mcguire Veterans Hospital following approval by the ethics committee (IRB Panel D Approval #HM14344). All patients provided written consent. Blood samples were taken prior to treatment, radiotherapy or prostatectomy. In most cases, age, ethnicity, PSA values and Gleason scores from biopsies were provided (Table 1). Controls were carefully selected to not have any history of PCa either as an individual or within the family, and written consent was obtained. A complete analysis of information provided to us for each individual is included in Appendix A Table A1. Samples were collected in PAXgene blood tubes (PreAnalytiX, Qiagen/BD, Franklin Lakes, NJ, USA), which contain a manufacture's additive to stabilize RNA. The total RNA, including microRNAs in each sample, was extracted using a corresponding PAXgene blood miRNA kit following the manufacture's protocol, which removes DNA and results in the purification of pure RNA. The quality and concentration of small RNAs ranging from 10–40 nts were measured using the small RNA Chip Assay (Agilent) based on the manufacturer's instructions. A total number of 40 samples (12 controls and 28 patients) with a small RNA concentration >100 ng/μL was selected for HTS microRNA sequencing using the Illumina® TruSeq Small RNA Library Preparation kit (New England Biolabs, Ipswich, MA, USA) and HiSeq 2500 system (Illumina, San Diego CA, USA) according to the manufacturer's protocol.

4.2. Bioinformatics Analysis

The raw deep sequencing data were processed using Flow® v 3.0 (Partek Incorporated, St. Louis, MO, USA). The adapter sequence "AGATCGGAAGAGCACACGTCT" (TruSeq Adapter, Index 7), frequently detected from all reads, was removed from both the 5′- and 3′-ends. A second trimming was performed to further eliminate bases at both ends with a Phred quality score lower than the average 35, indicating a probability that every 1 in 5000 bases was incorrect; accuracy of 99.95%. The minimum read length detected by the program was changed from 25 to 16 nts in order to include all possible microRNA reads in a suitable range. The trimmed data were aligned to the human genome (GRCh38) with only 1 seed mismatch allowed. The three best alignments satisfying such criteria were reported for each read using Bowtie 1.0. The parameters used by Bowtie while performing the alignment were as follows: alignment mod = quality limit, seed mismatch limit = 1, seed length = 28 and quality limit = 70, both strand alignment and alignments reported per read = 3. The aligned reads were annotated with miRBase (mature 21, Version 2). The differential expression analysis was conducted on the annotated sequencing reads exported from Partek Flow® using Edge R (Version 3.12) (Roswell Park Cancer Institute, Buffalo, NY, USA) [18,47]. The reads were normalized using the default "Trimmed Mean of M values" (TMM method) algorithm, which aims at minimizing the effect of sequencing depth and RNA composition [47].

4.3. Quantitative Real Time-Polymerase Chain Reaction

The search for microRNA candidates serving as good qRT-PCR endogenous controls was attempted using NormFinder software [48]. The microRNAs showing a relative high abundance and minimal intergroup variation suggested by the HTS data were selected for exploratory qRT-PCR on 16 samples (8 controls, 8 patients) in triplicate (Appendix A Table 2). Each RNA sample (3 ngs) was converted to cDNA (final volume 20 µL) using the qScript™ synthesis kit (Quanta Biosciences Inc., Gaithersburg, MD, USA) following the manufacturer's protocol and qPCR conducted as previously described [49]. Briefly, the cDNA was diluted with RNase-free water 1:1 (*v*/*v*), and 2 µL were used for each PCR reaction run in triplicate. Each PCR reaction was scaled down to 6.25 µL SYBR® Green Master Mix, 0.25 µL primer, 4.0 µL RNase-free H_2O for the purpose of saving reagents without compromising the results. qRT-PCR was conducted in an Applied Biosystems 7500 real-time PCR instrument (Life Technologies, Foster City, CA, USA) using the following conditions: 50 °C for 2 min, followed by 40 cycles at 95 °C for 15 s, 60 °C for 15 s and 70 °C for 30 s. Data were collected at 70 °C and analyzed using SDS software v1.3.1 (Life Technologies), using automatic threshold and baseline settings. Negative amplification controls and DNase-treated controls were routinely included for each microRNA and did not impact analysis. PCR efficiency for each microRNA primer set was tested and found to be within the acceptable range (80–110%). The Cq values of each candidate microRNA were imported into the NormFinder program, which generated stability values for each candidate after evaluating both intra- and inter-group variations. Lower stability values suggested higher consistency of a microRNA across different samples and groups. A combination of the four microRNAs with the lowest stability values showed a greater stability and consistency. Therefore, a normalization factor for each plate was determined by taking the geometric mean of the Cq values of the four microRNAs.

Next qRT-PCR was performed on dysregulated candidate microRNAs using 10 controls and 26 patients (raw and normalized values in Appendix A Tables 3 and 4, respectively) analyzed in triplicate ($SD < 0.2$). Unfortunately, material from two patient and control samples evaluated by HTS was found to be insufficient for confirmatory qRT-PCR analysis. For all other samples, the protocol was the same as described above. Raw Cq values were normalized by subtracting the geometric mean Cq value of the top four normalization candidates (miR-146a-5p, miR-1538, miR-197-3p and miR-1468-3p) from individual Cq values to generate dCq. A *p*-value was obtained using the Mann–Whitney nonparametric test assuming that data do not follow a Gaussian distribution. A p-value <0.05 was considered significant. The −ddCq value for each candidate was obtained by taking the mean of the normalized dCq for all controls minus the normalized dCq of each patient sample. The −ddCq values were equivalent to Log2 fold change, as the fold change was calculated by $2^{-\mathrm{ddCq}}$.

4.4. The Cancer Genome Atlas Tissue Data Analysis

Illumina HiSeq level 3 miRNA sequencing data of 50 prostate tumor tissue samples and their matched normal margins were selected and downloaded from The Cancer Genome Atlas database (TCGA database) for analysis. The reads were annotated with stem-loop transcripts of each microRNA [50]. The raw reads were normalized in the same way as described above using the Edge R software [18].

4.5. Statistical Analysis

Differential expression analysis was conducted on the normalized next generation sequencing reads for both blood samples and TCGA tissue data using EdgeR [18]. As the distribution of microRNA sequencing reads remains unclear, the dispersion of reads was estimated via the Cox–Reid profile adjusted likelihood method default in Edge R [51]. The reads matrix was fitted to a generalized linear model and a likelihood ratio test was performed on the fitted data. The *p*-value was adjusted to the number of comparisons (equal to total number of microRNAs detected in the sequencing) using the Benjamini–Hochberg method, which yields a False Discovery Rate (FDR) to minimize Type I error [52]. In order to maximize the screening results, a FDR value smaller than 0.2 was considered significant in this experiment.

For dysregulated microRNA PCR results, the normalized dCq values of each candidate between control and patient groups were compared using the Mann–Whitney nonparametric test assuming that the data do not follow a Gaussian distribution on Prism (GraphPad Software Inc., Version 6, 2015). A *p*-value lower than 0.05 was considered significant. ROC curves were generated for candidate microRNAs showing a statistically-significant difference between two groups [20]. The ROC was obtained by plotting sensitivity against specificity using the pROC package (Version 1.8). An area greater than 0.5 under the curve (AUC) suggests the diagnostic potential of each microRNA candidate.

5. Conclusions

In summary, we propose a group of four microRNAs (miR-146a-5p, miR-1538, miR197-3p and miR-1468-5p) that could be used as normalization standards for the comparative analysis of blood samples at least for PCa and perhaps other cancers, as well. In addition, a panel of seven microRNAs (miR-127-3p, miR-204-5p, miR-329-3p, miR-487b-3p, miR-32-5p, miR-20a-5p and miR-454-3p) might be useful for diagnosing PCa dependent on further validation. Individual members of this panel display better diagnostic capabilities than PSA alone and as a group are superior.

Acknowledgments: The authors acknowledge the VCU Urology Clinic and Mcguire Veterans Administration Hospital for providing patient samples utilized in this research. In addition, we are grateful to the Massey Cancer Center for supplying funds for this pilot project. No funds were reserved for covering the costs to publish in open access from this source. HTS data have been submitted to the GEO Database as submission GSE97901.

Author Contributions: Rhonda Daniel, Qianni Wu, Gene Clark, Georgi Guruli and Zendra Zehner conceived of and designed the experiments. Rhonda Daniel performed the experiments. Rhonda Daniel, Qianni Wu, Vernell Williams, Gene Clark and Zendra Zehner analyzed the data. Georgi Guruli and Vernell Williams contributed reagents, materials and analysis tools. Rhonda Daniel, Qianni.Wu, Vernell Williams and Zendra Zehner wrote the manuscript. All authors reviewed and approved of the final manuscript.

Abbreviations

ALDH1A3	Aldehyde Dehydrogenase 1A3
ARBS	Androgen Receptor-Binging Sites
AUC	Area Under the Curve
BCL6	B-Cell Lymphoma 6 Protein
BCL-XL	B-Cell Lymphoma-Extra Large
BTG1	B Cell Translocation Gene 1
Chr	Chromosome
CPM	Counts Per Million
CREB	Cyclic-AMP Response Element Binding Protein
CRPC	Castration-Resistant Prostate Cancer
Cq	Quantification Cycle
FC	Fold Change
FDR	False Detection Rate
hsa	A Human microRNA
HTS	High Throughput Sequencing
JAK2	Janus Kinase 2
KDM1A	Lysine Demethylase 1A
LnCaP	Androgen-Sensitive Human Prostate Adenocarcinoma Cells derived from the left supraclavicular lymph node metastasis from a 50-year old caucasian male
miR	MicroRNA
PIWI	P-Element-Induced Wimpy Testis
PSA	Prostate-Stimulating Antigen
PCa	Cancer of the Prostate
qRT-PCR	Quantitative Reverse Transcription Polymerase Chain Reaction
RPKM	Reads Per Kilobase of transcript per Million mapped reads
SKA2	Spindle and Kinetochore-Associated Complex Subunit 2
siRNA	Small interfering RNA
snRNA	Small nuclear RNA
STAT3	Signal Transducer and Activator of Transcription 3
TGF-BR2	Transforming Growth Factor Beta Receptor, Type II
TC	Total Counts
TCGA	The Cancer Genome Atlas
TMM	Trim Mean of M values
Tmprss2	Transmembrane protease, serine 2
TRKB	Tropomyosin Receptor Kinase B
UTR	Untranslated Region
VEGF-A	Vascular Endothelial Growth Factor A
VCAM	Vascular Cell Adhesion Protein

Appendix A

Table A1. Characteristics and pathological data of individual patients and controls involved in the study.

Sample Name	Sample Type	Gleason Score	Age	PSA	Race/Ethnicity	HTS Sample	Confirmatory PCR Sample	NormFinder Sample	Number in Appendix
Z1B-SEQ 1	Patient	G9	92	–	Caucasian	yes	yes		Sample 36
Z2B-SEQ 1	Patient	G7	–	–	–	yes	yes		Sample 26
Z3B-SEQ 1	Patient	G7	–	–	–	yes	yes		Sample 27
Z4B-SEQ 1	Patient	G7	–	–	–	yes	yes		Sample 28
Z5B-SEQ 1	Patient	G9	–	–	–	yes	yes		Sample 35
Z6B-SEQ 1	Patient	–	–	Elevated	–	yes	yes		Sample 11
Z7B-SEQ 1	Patient	–	–	22		yes	yes		sample 12
Z8B-SEQ 1	Patient	–	–	Elevated		yes	yes		Sample 13
091714-SEQ 2	Control	Control	51	–	Caucasian	yes	no		–
Case100-SEQ 2	Patient	G7	61	7.78	African American	yes	yes	yes	Sample 24
10212014FAM-SEQ 2	Control	Control	62	–	–	yes	yes	yes	Sample 10
12172014a-SEQ 2	Patient	G7	–	–	–	yes	no		–
12172014b-SEQ 2	Patient	–	–	Elevated	–	yes	no		–
12192014-SEQ 2	Control	Control	51	–	Caucasian	yes	yes	yes	Sample 8
Case18-SEQ 2	Patient	G6	68	6.8	African American	yes	yes	yes	Sample 14
Case20-SEQ 2	Patient	G6	64	4.15	African American	yes	yes		Sample 18
Case31-SEQ 2	Patient	G6	67	12.47	Caucasian	yes	yes	yes	Sample 15
Case33-SEQ 2	Patient	G6	63	3.2	Caucasian	yes	yes		Sample 21
Case36-SEQ 2	Patient	G6	55	10.73	Caucasian	yes	yes	yes	Sample 22
Case40-SEQ 2	Patient	G7	66	3.42	Caucasian	yes	yes		Sample 29
Case56-SEQ 2	Patient	G7	68	4.57	Caucasian	yes	yes		Sample 30
Case72-SEQ 2	Patient	G8	63	4.77	Caucasian	yes	yes		Sample 34
Case85-SEQ 2	Patient	G7	65	6.1	Caucasian	yes	yes	yes	Sample 23
Case9-SEQ 2	Patient	G6	55	8.82	Asian/Hawaiian	yes	yes		Sample 20
Z9B-SEQ 2	Control	Control	54	–	Caucasian	yes	yes	yes	Sample 7
Z10B-SEQ 2	Control	Control	39	–	African American	yes	yes		Sample 6
03242015-SEQ 3	Control	Control	46	–	Caucasian	yes	yes	yes	Sample 4
03262015-SEQ 3	Control	Control	43	–	Caucasian	yes	yes	yes	Sample 3
04062015-SEQ 3	Control	Control	91	–	Caucasian	yes	yes	yes	Sample 9
04242015-SEQ 3	Control	Control	59	–	Caucasian	yes	yes	yes	Sample 5
04282015-SEQ 3	Control	Control	55	–	Asian/Hawaiian	yes	no		–
Case16-SEQ 3	Patient	G8	76	7.99	Caucasian	yes	yes	yes	Sample 33
Case51-SEQ 3	Patient	G7	64	6.06	Caucasian	yes	yes	yes	Sample 25
Case 6-SEQ 3	Patient	G6	58	11	African American	yes	yes	yes	Sample 16
Case82-SEQ 3	Patient	G7	62	8.36	African American	yes	yes		Sample 31
Case83-SEQ 3	Patient	G6	66	4.21	Caucasian	yes	yes		Sample 19
Case89-SEQ 3	Patient	G7	66	3.5	Caucasian	yes	yes		Sample 32
Case8-SEQ 3	Patient	G6	73	4.4	African American	yes	yes		Sample 17
Z11B-SEQ 3	Control	Control	24	–	Caucasian	yes	yes		Sample 2
Z12B-SEQ 3	Control	Control	23	–	Caucasian	yes	yes	yes	Sample 1

Table 2. Raw Cq values of exploratory qRT-PCR analysis of blood samples from controls (n = 8) and patients (n = 8) to identify normalizer microRNAs for confirmatory qRT-PCR analysis. Cq values are the average of triplicates (SD $\leq$ 0.2).

Sample	Sample Type	miR197-3p	miR26b-5p	miR296-5p	miR23a-3p	miR146a-5p	miR 1248	miR1468-3p	miR1538
7	Control	22.74829	21.628092	26.089388	18.800253	27.064646	19.802492	30.705496	31.02948
10	Control	21.136293	25.414007	32.061626	18.889477	26.500956	16.915016	30.051926	29.690506
1	Control	22.46137	19.360636	24.926224	17.68174	25.192787	17.260515	29.683975	30.3445345
8	Control	29.555853	27.222218	31.271189	19.254599	29.127176	21.902388	33.016678	32.38471
5	Control	20.826368	23.358286	28.328314	19.247988	26.861567	16.149588	26.136414	28.535395
9	Control	22.516693	23.018911	27.688248	21.737234	28.745064	18.812151	29.16825	29.95835
3	Control	22.004297	21.192694	26.759714	17.74209	25.819382	15.312261	26.210001	29.330034
4	Control	20.42111	21.1323	27.237703	29.127176	26.609123	16.747427	26.76587	28.660437
22	Patient	21.886065	23.961235	30.295868	17.754295	26.563072	16.856455	28.191488	29.235413
14	Patient	28.050713	27.764153	32.219086	21.700003	28.97425	22.934767	33.360752	32.80031
23	Patient	20.232058	20.535894	28.087671	15.586144	25.002638	20.58262	27.846542	28.899343
24	Patient	20.934057	20.589144	26.781439	16.453804	24.992987	15.296409	28.57466	29.60646
15	Patient	20.324524	21.27265	28.345781	23.688972	31.2935	16.856455	31.182531	32.48879
25	Patient	22.465195	22.984718	26.560272	21.267275	27.856596	20.140722	28.645343	30.621424
16	Patient	21.8991	23.907438	28.562735	21.182196	27.760199	18.519064	27.570486	30.55234
33	Patient	19.746403	22.80751	28.66214	18.871817	27.803125	17.341208	27.578966	28.894281

Table 3. Raw Cq values of confirmatory qRT-PCR analysis of blood samples from controls ($n = 10$) and patients ($n = 26$). Cq values are the average of triplicates (SD $\leq$ 0.2).

Number	Sample Type	miR127-3p	miR1468-3p	miR146a-5p	miR1538	miR197-3p	miR204-5p	miR20a-5p	miR32-5p	miR329-3p	miR454-3p	miR487b-3p
1	Control	36.908432	30.543045	25.765848	32.149563	20.931528	30.270754	17.96527	25.546413	36.75606	22.844046	36.028534
2	Control	37.981623	28.062347	24.830622	30.136032	19.910437	36.117193	15.91111	23.228275	32.757341	22.673447	34.425587
3	Control	28.144186	28.446253	25.333971	30.515898	20.662188	30.312696	18.96527	29.557442	29.08623	25.073465	31.28196
4	Control	28.527613	29.671013	26.744165	30.476606	20.475235	30.221922	19.232796	29.752726	29.638098	26.315996	32.190907
5	Control	30.057663	29.518211	26.824263	28.535395	20.943573	30.793854	22.753603	26.935396	30.549356	28.72201	33.296204
6	Control	30.720682	29.358604	24.906527	31.398394	21.780424	29.43325	20.239492	30.17968	29.987643	25.529074	33.19684
7	Control	30.600016	31.048105	27.055967	33.107254	21.905685	31.476599	20.894003	27.493944	30.090225	24.6573	32.67403
8	Control	33.510212	30.512245	28.752623	29.60646	21.71274	30.86007	19.256899	31.885645	29.467866	23.78831	30.392588
9	Control	29.977875	29.733969	27.0654	29.95835	23.657553	30.979445	20.109362	27.893682	32.036114	25.58172	29.871424
10	Control	28.420685	30.848099	26.421408	32.04854	20.955032	30.269693	25.617834	27.432236	29.530313	29.78074	33.72329
11	Patient	25.514578	28.478271	23.705612	30.452873	22.588583	27.87504	23.345776	28.470451	23.393488	25.4003	25.936775
12	Patient	28.76194	28.892448	24.489096	31.246782	21.041815	29.743967	23.559605	27.84227	26.779068	27.28158	29.112656
13	Patient	28.005022	28.854507	23.039087	32.001001	21.060934	28.308046	23.194078	26.389101	27.779022	27.499535	29.67564
14	Patient	23.12572	30.165638	25.97425	34.46028	20.858582	23.945423	24.633371	33.6321	24.79482	28.784933	31.840466
15	Patient	25.970835	28.054586	22.90155	32.48879	26.455523	27.135048	25.562134	35.949183	27.743675	23.302767	29.316404
16	Patient	30.06621	31.15792	24.450277	31.151573	21.628485	23.59674	20.898695	32.535934	26.933802	28.414148	23.654408
17	Patient	29.233658	29.118433	24.842314	31.093117	22.109777	29.91673	28.335602	27.745428	29.466345	24.386953	30.998627
18	Patient	24.328703	28.683714	29.701113	30.66745	19.658997	25.6975	29.903137	30.435247	25.765816	26.52373	29.824835
19	Patient	21.014902	29.878317	31.95202	32.125797	17.540724	25.09019	26.061022	34.43073	22.8402	32.833908	26.911285
20	Patient	26.311941	28.65756	22.998682	32.747137	25.313272	26.886536	26.856186	27.684212	24.394753	33.664633	20.06597
21	Patient	26.961014	26.03805	22.823648	28.527018	27.915817	25.870775	30.0119	29.701286	26.257238	25.049133	20.115797
22	Patient	27.535292	28.895426	26.545149	30.66663	20.694304	29.86962	24.83243	35.122456	27.294931	29.74388	21.432922
23	Patient	29.402014	29.05626	25.683632	28.899343	20.198837	28.838037	22.598902	32.26222	28.878447	27.629982	22.840466
24	Patient	26.196487	29.45417	24.96972	32.38471	20.566633	29.10848	20.786528	28.78074	29.102547	35.674986	22.73802
25	Patient	29.829214	29.245398	25.854036	30.621424	20.477509	27.870811	29.884722	27.046827	20.211077	34.532679	23.396152
26	Patient	29.333616	29.284616	25.595312	30.323542	20.69581	29.889395	29.074312	27.739935	28.65606	34.9503	31.2132
27	Patient	26.915873	28.553482	24.359283	29.934687	23.699072	28.018053	28.724783	29.167513	25.274988	35.780039	27.273096
28	Patient	29.36677	29.126135	25.857595	31.09918	20.901865	27.674309	29.272202	27.905403	25.156372	34.727425	30.325487
29	Patient	30.076767	27.860743	24.468689	32.051258	21.122679	27.960495	20.559242	31.840103	25.185661	25.716452	21.408869
30	Patient	29.482193	28.605219	24.295252	30.460472	21.434538	21.330612	29.717953	29.96257	25.31598	25.70342	21.854279
31	Patient	29.213333	29.811007	26.022947	30.650206	20.445127	27.530617	21.284222	31.529474	25.304756	28.699488	30.818052
32	Patient	27.923819	28.06331	22.805868	29.62851	25.487047	30.44813	28.31951	27.352371	25.182838	34.379427	29.983652
33	Patient	29.104956	30.537256	28.080553	31.083038	20.618134	27.849699	21.825888	33.01379	20.256021	27.8463	23.03477
34	Patient	29.28003	28.26641	24.822348	30.753214	19.842566	26.921324	21.533236	30.028503	26.876923	35.232162	25.622961
35	Patient	28.177826	28.581133	23.973612	30.277636	20.03753	27.943693	31.369062	35.510693	26.46978	28.047266	20.259644
36	Patient	20.407839	28.817247	26.935812	30.680155	21.042847	31.687258	33.005196	32.28391	19.864021	28.640589	23.454853

Table 4. Normalized Cq values for confirmatory qRT-PCR analysis of blood samples from controls (n = 10) and patients (n = 26). Cq values are the average of triplicates (SD $\leq$ 0.2).

Number	Sample Type	miR127-3p	miR204-5p	miR20a-5p	miR32-5p	miR329-3p	miR454-3p	miR487b-3p
1	Control	9.932081552	3.294403552	−9.011080448	−1.429937448	9.779709552	−4.132304448	9.052183552
2	Control	12.55318916	10.68875916	−9.51732384	−2.20015884	7.32890716	−2.75498684	8.99715316
3	Control	2.181017005	4.349527005	−6.997898995	3.594273005	3.123061005	−0.889703995	5.318791005
4	Control	2.000546379	3.694855379	−7.294270621	3.225659379	3.111031379	−0.211070621	5.663840379
5	Control	3.829786882	4.565977882	−3.474273118	0.707519882	4.321479882	2.494133882	7.068327882
6	Control	4.128401402	2.840969402	−6.352788598	3.587399402	3.395362402	−1.063206598	6.604559402
7	Control	2.662065759	3.538648759	−7.043947241	-0.444006241	2.152274759	−3.280650241	4.736079759
8	Control	6.106260714	3.456118714	−8.147052286	4.481693714	2.063914714	−3.615641286	2.988636714
9	Control	2.496480815	3.498050815	−7.372032185	0.412287815	4.554719815	−1.899674185	2.390029815
10	Control	1.220601618	3.069609618	−1.582249382	0.232152618	2.330229618	2.580656618	6.523206618
11	Patient	−0.590230547	1.770231453	−2.759032547	2.365642453	−2.711320547	−0.704508547	−0.168033547
12	Patient	2.645655116	3.627682116	−2.556679884	1.725985116	0.662783116	1.165295116	2.996371116
13	Patient	2.133020459	2.436044459	−2.677923541	0.517099459	1.907020459	1.627533459	3.803638459
14	Patient	−4.268868334	−3.449165334	−2.761217334	6.237511666	−2.599768334	1.390344666	4.445877666
15	Patient	−1.289403891	−0.125190891	−1.698104891	8.688944109	0.483436109	−3.957471891	2.056165109
16	Patient	3.299833617	−3.169636383	−5.867681383	5.769557617	0.167425617	1.647771617	−3.111968383
17	Patient	2.67829958	3.36137158	1.78024358	1.19006958	2.91098658	−2.16840542	4.44326858
18	Patient	−2.442123688	−1.073326688	3.132310312	3.664420312	−1.005010688	−0.247096688	3.054008312
19	Patient	−6.067611542	−1.992323542	−1.021491542	7.348216458	−4.242313542	5.751394458	−0.171228542
20	Patient	−0.875350601	−0.300755601	−0.331105601	0.496920399	−2.792538601	6.477341399	−7.121321601
21	Patient	0.732417073	−0.357821927	3.783303073	3.472689073	0.028641073	−1.179463927	−6.112799927
22	Patient	1.121376344	3.455704344	−1.581485656	8.708540344	0.881015344	3.329964344	−4.980993656
23	Patient	3.711214401	3.147237401	−3.091897599	6.571420401	3.187647401	1.939182401	−2.850333599
24	Patient	−0.259009595	2.652983405	−5.668968595	2.325243405	2.647050405	9.219489405	−3.717476595
25	Patient	3.588714461	1.630311461	3.644222461	0.806327461	−6.029422539	8.292179461	−2.844347539
26	Patient	3.144817167	3.700596167	2.885513167	1.551136167	2.467261167	8.761501167	5.024401167
27	Patient	0.412117905	1.514297905	2.221027905	2.663757905	−1.228767095	9.276283905	0.769340905
28	Patient	2.915212989	1.222751989	2.820644989	1.453845989	−1.295185011	8.275867989	3.873929989
29	Patient	4.012268775	1.895996775	−5.505256225	5.775604775	−0.878837225	−0.348046225	−4.655629225
30	Patient	3.528189418	−4.623391582	3.763949418	4.008566418	−0.638023582	−0.250583582	−4.099724582
31	Patient	2.808155968	1.125439968	−5.120955032	5.124296968	−1.100421032	2.294310968	4.412874968
32	Patient	1.55724467	4.08155567	1.95293567	0.98579667	−1.18373633	8.01285267	3.61707767
33	Patient	1.877809959	0.622552959	−5.401258041	5.786643959	−6.971125041	0.619153959	−4.192376041
34	Patient	3.700034457	1.341328457	−4.046759543	4.448507457	1.296927457	9.652166457	0.042965457
35	Patient	2.785951344	2.551818344	5.977187344	10.11881834	1.077905344	2.655391344	−5.132230656
36	Patient	−6.198563209	5.080855791	6.398793791	5.677507791	−6.742381209	2.034186791	−3.151549209

Table 5. Comparison of fold change in blood HTS data to tissue HTS data from the TCGA database. Fold change was calculated in the same method as panel members using the Edge R program.

MicroRNA	Fold Change in Blood *	Fold Change in TCGA **
hsa-miR-32-5p	−4.11	1.71
hsa-miR-329-3p	4.29	−1.27
hsa-miR-487b-3p	6.06	−1.66
hsa-miR-454-3p	−1.91	1.26
hsa-miR-204-5p	3.43	−3.81
hsa-miR-20a-5p	−2.11	2.19
hsa-miR-127-3p	2.69	−1.43

* FDR < 0.2; ** FDR < 0.05.

Table 6. Chromosome 14 q32.31 dysregulated microRNAs in our analysis of blood samples compared to data from the TCGA tissue database. In addition to our proposed panel members (miR-329-3p, miR-487b-3p and miR-127-3p), subsequent analysis of HTS data uncovered five other microRNAs from this locus (miR-654-5p, miR-654-3p, miR-493-3p, miR-493-5p and miR-433-3p) to be upregulated in blood. Since these microRNAs were not within the top ten potential candidates, they were not carried forth for qRT-PCR confirmation. However, analysis of the TCGA database did confirm these microRNAs to be tumor suppressors lost in tumor tissue compared to matched tumor-free margins, fitting with our model that tumors may strive to get rid of tumor suppressors in order to progress. Fold change is shown in a Log2 scale and was calculated with the same method as panel members using the edge R program.

miRNA	Dysregulation Ranking in Blood	Log Fold Change in Blood	Log Fold Change in TCGA
miR-329-3p	4	2.10	−0.34
miR-487b-3p	5	2.60	−0.73
miR-127-3p	9	1.43	−0.52
miR-654-5p	17	1.96	−0.61
miR-654-3p	36	1.08	−0.61
miR-493-3p	37	1.74	−0.58
miR-493-5p	59	1.29	−0.58
miR-433-3p	43	1.30	−0.16

References

1. Barry, M.J. Clinical practice. Prostate-specific-antigen testing for early diagnosis of prostate cancer. *N. Engl. J. Med.* **2001**, *344*, 1373–1377. [CrossRef] [PubMed]
2. Tchetgen, M.-B.; Song, J.T.; Strawderman, M.; Jacobsen, S.J.; Oesterling, J.E. Ejaculation increases the serum prostate-specific antigen concentration. *Urology* **1996**, *47*, 511–516. [CrossRef]
3. Herschman, J.D.; Smith, D.S.; Catalona, W.J. Effect of ejaculation on serum total and free prostate-specific antigen concentrations. *Urology* **1997**, *50*, 239–243. [CrossRef]
4. Nadler, R.B.; Humphrey, P.A.; Smith, D.S.; Catalona, W.J.; Ratliff, T.L. Effect of inflammation and benign prostatic hyperplasia on elevated serum prostate specific antigen levels. *J. Urol.* **1995**, *154*, 407–413. [CrossRef]
5. Endzeliņš, E.; Melne, V.; Kalniņa, Z.; Lietuvietiss, V.; Riekstia, U.; Llorente, A.; Line, A. Diagnostic, prognostic and predictive value of cell-free miRNAs in prostate cancer: A systematic review. *Mol. Cancer* **2016**, *15*, 41–54. [CrossRef] [PubMed]
6. Ha, M.; Kim, V.N. Regulation of microRNA biogenesis. *Nat. Rev. Mol. Cell Biol.* **2014**, *15*, 509–524. [CrossRef] [PubMed]
7. O'Donnell, K.A.; Mendell, J.T. Dysregulation of microRNAs in human malignancy. In *MicroRNAs: From Basic Science to Disease Biology*, 1st ed.; Krishnarao, A., Ed.; Cambridge University Press: Cambridge, UK; New York, NY, USA, 2008; pp. 295–306.
8. Mitchell, P.S.; Parkin, R.K.; Kroh, E.M.; Fritz, B.R.; Wyman, S.K.; Pogosova-Agadjanyan, E.L.; Peterson, A.; Noteboom, J.; O'Briant, K.C.; Allen, A.; et al. Circulating microRNAs as stable blood-based markers for cancer detection. *Proc. Natl. Acad. Sci. USA* **2008**, *105*, 10513–10518. [CrossRef] [PubMed]

9. Schultz, N.A.; Dehlendorff, C.; Jensen, B.V.; Bjerregaard, J.K.; Nielsen, K.R.; Bojesen, S.E.; Calatayud, D.; Nielsen, S.E.; Yilmaz, M.; Hollander, N.H.; et al. MicroRNA biomarkers in whole blood for detection of pancreatic cancer. *JAMA* **2014**, *311*, 392–404. [CrossRef] [PubMed]
10. Cochetti, G.; Pol, G.; Guelfi, G.; Boni, A.; Egidi, M.G.; Mearini, E. Different levels of serum microRNAs in prostate cancer and benign prostatic hyperplasia: Evaluation of potential diagnostic and prognostic role. *OncoTargets Ther.* **2016**, *9*, 7545–7553. [CrossRef] [PubMed]
11. Lodes, M.J.; Caraballo, M.; Suciu, D.; Munro, S.; Kumar, A.; Anderson, B. Detection of cancer with serum miRNAs on an oligonucleotide microarray. *PLoS ONE* **2009**, *4*, e6229. [CrossRef] [PubMed]
12. Roberts, M.J.; Richards, R.S.; Chow, C.W.; Doi, S.A.; Schirra, H.J.; Buck, M.; Samaratunga, H.; Perry-Keene, J.; Payton, A.; Yaxley, J.; et al. Prostate-based biofluids for the detection of prostate cancer: A comparative study of the diagnostic performance of cell-sourced RNA biomarkers. *Prostate Int.* **2016**, *4*, 97–102. [CrossRef] [PubMed]
13. Keller, A.; Leidinger, P.; Messe, E.; Haas, J.; Backes, C.; Rasche, L.; Behrens, J.R.; Pfuhl, C.; Wakonig, K.; GieB, R.M.; et al. Next-generation sequencing identifies altered whole blood microRNAs in neuromyelitis optica spectrum disorder which may permit discrimination from multiple sclerosis. *J. Neuroinflamm.* **2015**, *12*, 196–208. [CrossRef] [PubMed]
14. Szczyrba, J.; Löprich, E.; Wach, S.; Jung, V.; Unteregger, G.; Barth, S.; Grobholz, R.; Wieland, W.; Stohr, R.; Hartmann, A.; et al. The MicroRNA profile of prostate carcinoma obtained by deep sequencing. *Mol. Cancer Res.* **2010**, *8*, 529–538. [CrossRef] [PubMed]
15. Huang, X.; Yuan, T.; Liang, M.; Du, M.; Xia, S.; Dittmar, R.; Wang, D.; See, W.; Costello, B.A.; Quevedo, F.; et al. Exosomal miR-1290 and miR-375 as prognostic markers in castration-resistant prostate cancer. *Eur. Urol.* **2015**, *67*, 33–41. [CrossRef] [PubMed]
16. Thompson, I.M.; Ankerst, D.P.; Chi, C.; Lucia, M.S.; Goodman, P.J.; Crowley, J.J.; Parnes, H.L.; Coltman, C.A. Operating characteristics of prostate-specific antigen in men with an initial PSA level of 3.0 ng/mL or lower. *JAMA* **2005**, *294*, 66–70. [CrossRef] [PubMed]
17. Sam, G.; Russell, J.G.; Stijn, D.; Alex, B.; Anton, J.E. MiRBase: MicroRNA sequences, targets and gene nomenclature. *Nucleic Acids Res.* **2006**, *34* (Suppl. S1), D140–D144. [CrossRef]
18. Chen, Y.; McCarthy, D.; Robinson, M.; Smyth, G. *EdgeR: Differential Expression Analysis of Digital Gene Expression User's Guide*; Bioconductor, Roswell Park Cancer Institute: Buffalo, NY, USA, 2014.
19. Dillies, M.-A.; Rau, A.; Aubert, J.; Hennequet-Antier, C.; Jeanmougin, M.; Servant, N.; Keime, C.; Marot, G.; Castel, D.; Estelle, J.; et al. A comprehensive evaluation of normalization methods for Illumina high-throughput RNA sequencing data analysis. *Brief Bioinform.* **2012**. [CrossRef]
20. Centor, R.M. Signal detectability: The use of ROC curves and their analyses. *Med. Decis. Mak.* **1991**, *11*, 102–106. [CrossRef] [PubMed]
21. Kirschner, M.B.; Edelman, J.J.B.; Kao, S.C.-H.; Vallely, M.P.; van Zandwijk, N.; Reid, G. The impact of hemolysis on cell-free microRNA biomarkers. *Front. Genet.* **2013**, *4*, 1–13. [CrossRef] [PubMed]
22. Watahiki, A.; Macfarlane, R.J.; Gleave, M.E.; Crea, F.; Wang, Y.; Helgason, C.D. Plasma miRNAs as biomarkers to identify patients with castration-resistant metastatic prostate cancer. *Int. J. Mol. Sci.* **2013**, *14*, 7757–7770. [CrossRef] [PubMed]
23. Cheng, H.H.; Mitchell, P.S.; Kroh, E.M.; Dowell, A.E.; Chery, L.; Siddiqui, J.; Nelson, P.S.; Vessella, R.L.; Knudsen, B.S.; Chinnaiyan, A.M.; et al. Circulating microRNA profiling identifies a subset of metastatic prostate cancer patients with evidence of cancer-associated hypoxia. *PLoS ONE* **2013**, *8*, e69239. [CrossRef] [PubMed]
24. Lopez-Serra, P.; Esteller, M. DNA methylation-associated silencing of tumor-suppressor microRNAs in cancer. *Oncogene* **2012**, *31*, 1609–1622. [CrossRef] [PubMed]
25. Chen, J.; Wang, M.; Guo, M.; Xie, Y.; Cong, Y.-S. MiR-127 Regulates Cell Proliferation and Senescence by Targeting BCL6. *PLoS ONE* **2013**, *8*, e80266. [CrossRef]
26. Tang, T.T.; Dowbenko, D.; Jackson, A.; Toney, L.; Lewin, D.A.; Dent, A.L.; Lasky, L.A. The Forkhead transcription factor AFX activates apoptosis by induction of the Bcl-6 transcriptional repressor. *J. Biol. Chem.* **2002**, *277*, 14255–14265. [CrossRef] [PubMed]
27. Mencarelli, A.; Renga, B.; Distrutti, E.; Fiorucci, S. Antiatherosclerotic effect of farnesoid X receptor. *Am. J. Physiol. Heart Circ. Physiol.* **2009**, *296*, 272–281. [CrossRef] [PubMed]

28. Wang, F.E.; Zhang, C.; Maminishkis, A.; Dong, L.; Zhi, C.; Li, R.; Zhao, J.; Majerciak, V.; Gaur, A.B.; Chen, S.; et al. MicroRNA-204/211 alters epithelial physiology. *FASEB J.* **2010**, *24*, 1552–1571. [CrossRef] [PubMed]
29. Bao, W.; Wang, H.H.; Tian, F.J.; He, X.Y.; Wang, J.Y.; Zhang, H.J.; Wang, L.H.; Wan, X.P. A TrkB-STAT3-miR-204–5p regulatory circuitry controls proliferation and invasion of endometrial carcinoma cells. *Mol. Cancer* **2013**, *12*, 155. [CrossRef] [PubMed]
30. Yang, H.; Li, Q.; Zhao, W.; Yian, D.; Zhao, H.; Zhou, Y. MiR-329 suppresses the growth and motility of neuroblastoma by targeting KDM1A. *FEBS Lett.* **2014**, *588*, 192–197. [CrossRef] [PubMed]
31. Kashyap, V.; Ahmad, S.; Nilsson, E.M.; Helczynski, L.; Kenna, S.; Persson, J.L.; Gudas, L.J.; Mongan, N.P. The lysine specific demethylase-1 (LSD1/KDM1A) regulates VEGF-A expression in prostate cancer. *Mol. Oncol.* **2013**, *7*, 555–566. [CrossRef] [PubMed]
32. Formosa, A.; Markert, E.K.; Lena, A.M.; Italiano, D.; Finazzi-Ago, E.; Levine, A.J.; Dernardini, S.; Garabadgiu, A.V.; Melino, G.; Candi, E. MicroRNAs, miR-154, miR-299-5p, miR-376a, miR-376c, miR-377, miR-381, miR-487b, miR-485-3p, miR-495 and miR-654-3p, mapped to the 14q32.31 locus, regulate proliferation, apoptosis, migration and invasion in metastatic prostate cancer cells. *Oncogene* **2014**, *33*, 5173–5182. [CrossRef] [PubMed]
33. Gattolliat, C.H.; Thomas, L.; Ciafrè, S.A.; Meurice, G.; Le Teuff, G.; Job, B.; Richon, C.; Combaret, B.; Dessen, P.; Valteau-Couanet, D.; et al. Expression of miR-487b and miR-410 encoded by 14q32.31 locus is a prognostic marker in neuroblastoma. *Br. J. Cancer* **2011**, *105*, 1352–1361. [CrossRef] [PubMed]
34. Le Magnen, C.; Bubendorf, L.; Rentsch, C.A.; Mengus, C.; Gsponer, J.; Zellweger, T.; Rieken, M.; Thaimann, G.N.; Cecchini, M.G.; Germann, M.; et al. Characterization and clinical relevance of ALDH bright populations in prostate cancer. *Clin. Cancer Res.* **2013**, *19*, 5361–5371. [CrossRef] [PubMed]
35. Jalava, S.E.; Urbanucci, A.; Latonen, L.; Waltering, K.K.; Sahu, B.; Janne, O.A.; Seppaia, J.; Lahdesmaki, H.; Tammela, T.L.; Visakorpi, T. Androgen-regulated miR-32 targets BTG2 and is overexpressed in castration-resistant prostate cancer. *Oncogene* **2012**, *31*, 4460–4471. [CrossRef] [PubMed]
36. Mogilyansky, E.; Rigoutsos, I. The miR-17/92 cluster: A comprehensive update on its genomics, genetics, functions and increasingly important and numerous roles in health and disease. *Cell Death Differ.* **2013**, *20*, 1603–1614. [CrossRef] [PubMed]
37. Pesta, M.; Klecka, J.; Kulda, V.; Topolcan, O.; Hora, M.; Eret, V.; Ludvikova, M.; Babjuk, M.; Novak, K.; Stoiz, J.; et al. Importance of miR-20a expression in prostate cancer tissue. *Anticancer Res.* **2010**, *30*, 3579–3583. [PubMed]
38. Wu, X.; Ding, N.; Hu, W.; He, J.; Xu, S.; Pei, H.; Hua, J.; Zhou, G.; Wang, J. Down-regulation of BTG1 by miR-454-3p enhances cellular radiosensitivity in renal carcinoma cells. *Radiat. Oncol.* **2014**, *9*, 179. [CrossRef] [PubMed]
39. Sun, S.; Wang, S.; Xu, X.; Di, H.; Du, J.; Xu, B.; Qang, W.; Wang, J. MiR-433-3p suppresses cell growth and enhances chemosensitivity by targeting CREB in human glioma. *Oncotarget* **2017**, *8*, 5057–5068. [CrossRef] [PubMed]
40. Melo, S.A.; Sugimoto, H.; O'Connell, J.T. Cancer Exosomes perform cell-independent microRNA biogenesis and promote tumorgenesis. *Cancer Cell* **2014**, *26*, 707–721. [CrossRef] [PubMed]
41. Selth, L.A.; Townley, S.L.; Bert, A.G.; Stricker, P.D.; Sutherland, P.D.; Horvath, L.G.; Goodall, G.J.; Butler, L.M.; Tilley, W.D. Circulating microRNAs predict biochemical recurrence in prostate cancer patients. *Br. J. Cancer* **2013**, *109*, 641–650. [CrossRef] [PubMed]
42. Selth, L.A.; Tilley, W.D.; Butler, W.D. Circulating microRNAs: Macro-utility as markers of prostate cancer? *Endocr. Relat. Cancer* **2012**, *19*, R99–R113. [CrossRef] [PubMed]
43. Bai, M.; Zhang, M.; Long, F.; Yu, N.; Zeng, A.; Zhao, R. Circulating microRNA-194 regulates human melanoma cells via PI3K/AKT/FoxO3a and p53/p21 signaling pathways. *Oncol. Rep.* **2017**, *37*, 2702–2710. [CrossRef] [PubMed]
44. Volinia, S.; Calin, G.A.; Liu, C.G.; Ambs, S.; Cimmino, A.J.; Petrocca, F.; Visone, R.; Lanza, G.; Scarpa, A.; Vecchione, A.; et al. A microRNA expression signature of human solid tumors defines cancer gene targets. *Proc. Natl. Acad. Sci. USA* **2006**, *103*, 2257–2261. [CrossRef] [PubMed]
45. Kuwabara, Y.; Ono, K.; Horie, T.; Nishi, H.; Nagao, K.; Kinoshita, M.; Watanabe, S.; Baba, O.; Kojima, Y.; Shizuta, S.; et al. Increased microRNA-1 and microRNA-133a levels in serum of patients with cardiovascular disease indicate myocardial damage. *Circ. Cardiovasc. Genet.* **2011**, *4*, 446–454. [CrossRef] [PubMed]

46. Pritchard, C.C.; Kroh, E.; Wood, B.; Arroyo, J.D.; Dougherty, K.J.; Miyaji, M.M.; Tait, J.F.; Tewari, M. Blood cell origin of circulating microRNAs; a cautionary note for cancer biomarker studies. *Cancer Prev. Res.* **2012**, *5*, 492–497. [CrossRef] [PubMed]
47. Robinson, M.D.; Oshlack, A. A scaling normalization method for differential expression analysis of RNA-seq data. *Genome Biol.* **2010**, *11*, R25. [CrossRef] [PubMed]
48. Andersen, C.L.; Ledet-Jensen, J.; Ørntoft, T. Normalization of real-time quantitative RT-PCR data: A model based variance estimation approach to identify genes suited for normalization—Applied to bladder—And colon-cancer data-sets. *Cancer Res.* **2004**, *64*, 5245–5250. [CrossRef] [PubMed]
49. Seashols-Williams, S.; Lewis, C.; Calloway, C.; Peace, N.; Harrison, A.; Hayes-Nash, C.; Fleming, S.; Wu, Q.; Zehner, Z.E. High-throughput miRNA sequencing and identification of biomarkers for forensically relevant biological fluids. *Electrophoresis* **2016**, *37*, 2780–2788. [CrossRef] [PubMed]
50. Chu, A.; Robertson, G.; Brooks, D.; Mungall, A.J.; Birol, I.; Coope, R.; Marra, M.A. Large-scale profiling of microRNAs for The Cancer Genome Atlas. *Nucleic Acids Res.* **2016**, *44*, e3. [CrossRef] [PubMed]
51. McCarthy, D.J.; Chen, Y.; Smyth, G.K. Differential expression analysis of multifactor RNA-Seq experiments with respect to biological variation. *Nucleic Acids Res.* **2012**, *40*, 4288–4297. [CrossRef] [PubMed]
52. Benjamini, Y.; Hochberg, Y. Controlling the false discovery rate: A practical and powerful approach to multiple testing. *J. R. Statist. Soc.* **1995**, *57*, 289–300.

11

Fasting Enhances the Contrast of Bone Metastatic Lesions in ^{18}F-Fluciclovine-PET: Preclinical Study Using a Rat Model of Mixed Osteolytic/Osteoblastic Bone Metastases

Shuntaro Oka [1,*], Masaru Kanagawa [1], Yoshihiro Doi [1], David M. Schuster [2], Mark M. Goodman [2] and Hirokatsu Yoshimura [1]

1 Research Center, Nihon Medi-Physics Co., Ltd., 3-1 Kitasode, Sodegaura, Chiba 299-0266, Japan; masaru_kanagawa@nmp.co.jp (M.K.); yoshihiro_doi@nmp.co.jp (Y.D.); hirokatsu_yoshimura@nmp.co.jp (H.Y.)

2 Division of Nuclear Medicine and Molecular Imaging, Department of Radiology and Imaging Sciences, Emory University, Atlanta, GA 30329, USA; dschust@emory.edu (D.M.S.); mgoodma@emory.edu (M.M.G.)

* Correspondence: shuntaro_oka@nmp.co.jp

Academic Editor: Carsten Stephan

Abstract: ^{18}F-fluciclovine (*trans*-1-amino-3-^{18}F-fluorocyclobutanecarboxylic acid) is an amino acid positron emission tomography (PET) tracer used for cancer staging (e.g., prostate and breast). Patients scheduled to undergo amino acid-PET are usually required to fast before PET tracer administration. However, there have been no reports addressing whether fasting improves fluciclovine-PET imaging. In this study, the authors investigated the influence of fasting on fluciclovine-PET using triple-tracer autoradiography with ^{14}C-fluciclovine, [5,6-^{3}H]-2-fluoro-2-deoxy-D-glucose (^{3}H-FDG), and ^{99m}Tc-hydroxymethylene diphosphonate (^{99m}Tc-HMDP) in a rat breast cancer model of mixed osteolytic/osteoblastic bone metastases in which the animals fasted overnight. Lesion accumulation of each tracer was evaluated using the target-to-background (muscle) ratio. The mean ratios of ^{14}C-fluciclovine in osteolytic lesions were 4.6 $\pm$ 0.8 and 2.8 $\pm$ 0.6, respectively, with and without fasting, while those for ^{3}H-FDG were 6.9 $\pm$ 2.5 and 5.1 $\pm$ 2.0, respectively. In the peri-tumor bone formation regions (osteoblastic), where ^{99m}Tc-HMDP accumulated, the ratios of ^{14}C-fluciclovine were 4.3 $\pm$ 1.4 and 2.4 $\pm$ 0.7, respectively, and those of ^{3}H-FDG were 6.2 $\pm$ 3.8 and 3.3 $\pm$ 2.2, respectively, with and without fasting. These results suggest that fasting before ^{18}F-fluciclovine-PET improves the contrast between osteolytic and osteoblastic bone metastatic lesions and background, as well as ^{18}F-FDG-PET.

Keywords: bone metastasis; breast cancer; FACBC; fluciclovine; FDG; positron emission tomography; prostate cancer

---

1. Introduction

The most used positron emission tomography (PET) tracer for cancer imaging is 2-deoxy-2-^{18}F-fluoro-D-glucose (^{18}F-FDG), which is an analogue of D-glucose. Cancer cells take up this PET tracer because ^{18}F-FDG shares its transport routes (i.e., glucose transporters) with D-glucose. High concentrations of plasma glucose may compete with ^{18}F-FDG at glucose transporters in cancer cells and elevates plasma insulin which unfavorably alters the biodistribution to the radiotracer [1]. Thus, patients scheduled to undergo ^{18}F-FDG-PET are required to fast for 4 h to 6 h to lower plasma glucose concentration before PET imaging.

Several amino acid (AA) PET tracers, including ^{11}C-methionine, have been used for diagnostic purposes in cancer patients [2]. Although studied previously, issues regarding the necessity of fasting in clinical PET with AA tracers [3] have yet to be resolved. Fasting is routinely recommended for patients undergoing AA-PET as well as ^{18}F-FDG-PET. There have been few studies investigating the influence of fasting or food intake before AA-PET. The authors of one study investigating ^{11}C-methionine-PET for head and neck cancer concluded that food ingestion may decrease ^{11}C-methionine uptake in tumors, although the image quality remained satisfactory after food ingestion [4].

^{18}F-fluciclovine, also known as *trans*-1-amino-3-^{18}F-fluorocyclobutanecarboxylic acid (FACBC; code name: NMK36, Nihon Medi-Physics; brand name: Axumin, Blue Earth Diagnostics, Burlington, MA, USA), is an AA-PET tracer, and has been approved by the United States Food and Drug Administration for the detection of prostate cancer (PCa) recurrence since 2016. Even in ^{18}F-fluciclovine-PET imaging, patients usually fast for $\geq$4 h before tracer administration without any conclusive evidence supporting the influence of fasting for ^{18}F-fluciclovine uptake in tumors [5]. Although one clinical research study involving non-fasted breast cancer (BCa) patients has been published, PET imaging was performed for the chest only and no comparison was made to control fasted subjects [6]. Thus, it is not known whether fasting influences tumor uptake of ^{18}F-fluciclovine in PCa and BCa patients.

Most patients with advanced PCa and BCa present with mixed osteolytic and osteoblastic bone metastases [7]. To investigate the influence of fasting on ^{18}F-fluciclovine accumulation in bone metastatic lesions, we established a rat bone metastatic model, which forms both osteolytic and osteoblastic lesions in the tibia and/or femur, by intra-arterial injection of MRMT-1 cells, a rat BCa cell line with a 100% success rate for skeletal metastases. Using this animal model, triple-tracer autoradiography was performed using *trans*-1-amino-3-fluoro[1-^{14}C]cyclobutanecarboxylic acid (^{14}C-fluciclovine), [5,6-^{3}H]-2-Fluoro-2-deoxy-d-glucose (^{3}H-FDG), and ^{99m}Tc-hydroxymethylene diphosphonate (^{99m}Tc-HMDP) to compare the tracers' accumulation at identical bony lesions. Our findings suggest that overnight fasting influenced the uptake of ^{18}F-fluciclovine in the bony lesions, and that the tumor-to-muscle uptake ratios in osteolytic and osteoblastic lesions were higher in the fasted condition compared with the fed condition.

2. Results

2.1. In Vitro Experiments

^{14}C-fluciclovine is a synthetic AA and is transported by AA transporters (AATs). To investigate which transport system mediates the transport of this tracer in MRMT-1 cells, in vitro uptake inhibition experiments were performed. As shown in Figure 1a, the uptake of ^{14}C-fluciclovine decreased to 38.4% in choline buffer compared with sodium buffer, corresponding to contributions of the Na^+-dependent and -independent carriers for ^{14}C-fluciclovine transport in MRMT-1 cells of 61.6% and 38.4%, respectively. To narrow the subtypes of AATs involved in ^{14}C-fluciclovine transport in MRMT-1 cells, competitive uptake experiments were performed in the absence or presence of several synthetic and naturally-occurring AAs as inhibitors. As shown in Figure 1b, small neutral AAs, such as glutamine and serine, showed strong inhibitory effects for ^{14}C-fluciclovine uptake (82.4% and 77.0% decreases vs. control, respectively), while phenylalanine, a branched-chain AA, and 2-amino-bicyclo[2,2,1]heptane-2-carboxylic acid (BCH) demonstrated smaller inhibitory effects (33.3% and 37.6% decreases, respectively, vs. control) in the presence of sodium ion. In contrast, phenylalanine and BCH inhibited ^{14}C-fluciclovine transport by more than 90% versus control in the absence of sodium ion. Proline, 2-(methylamino)-isobutyric acid (MeAIB), arginine, and glutamate had no statistically-significant inhibitory effect on ^{14}C-fluciclovine transport into MRMT-1 cells. These results suggest that the strong inhibitory effects of glutamine and serine in the presence of sodium ion mean that the alanine-serine-cysteine (ASC) system, especially the ASC transporter 2 (ASCT2), is the primary carrier in Na^+-dependent AATs. On the other hand, the intense inhibitory effects of phenylalanine and BCH in the absence of sodium ion suggest that system L, especially the L-type AA transporter (LAT1), is the primary carrier in Na^+-independent AATs for the transport of ^{14}C-fluciclovine in MRMT-1 cells.

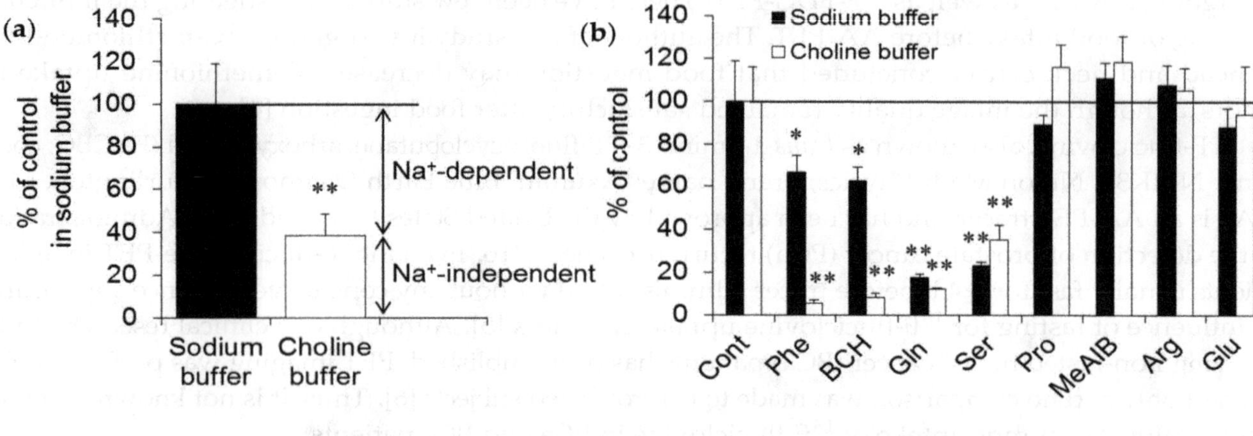

Figure 1. Characteristics of ^{14}C-fluciclovine transport in MRMT-1 cells. (**a**) Contributions of Na^+-dependent and -independent carriers on the uptake of ^{14}C-fluciclovine. The transport of ^{14}C-fluciclovine in sodium buffer was normalized to 100%. (**b**) Competitive inhibition of 10 μmol/L ^{14}C-fluciclovine transport by naturally-occurring and synthetic amino acids (2.0 mmol/L). The control transport (absence of inhibitors) of ^{14}C-fluciclovine in sodium and choline buffer was normalized to 100%. Each bar represents the mean ± standard deviation (SD) ($n = 6$). * $p < 0.05$, ** $p < 0.01$. Arg: arginine, BCH: 2-amino-bicyclo[2,2,1]heptane-2-carboxylic acid, Cont: control, Gln: glutamine, Glu: glutamate, MeAIB: 2-(methylamino)-isobutyric acid, Phe: phenylalanine, Pro: proline, Ser: serine.

2.2. *In Vivo Experiments*

The distribution patterns of ^{14}C-fluciclovine in the tibia and/or femur were basically similar to ^{3}H-FDG in both fasted and fed conditions, as shown in Figure 2. Visualization of the tumor mass in bone marrow cavities was clearer with ^{3}H-FDG because the physiological accumulation of ^{14}C-fluciclovine in bone marrow was higher than ^{3}H-FDG. Although ^{14}C-fluciclovine and ^{3}H-FDG accumulated at the peri-tumor bone formation (pTBF) in osteoblastic lesions, characterized by ^{99m}Tc-HMDP accumulation, the images were obscure compared with the tumor parenchyma (Figure 2).

Figure 3 shows the results of histological examination in osteolytic and osteoblastic bone metastasis lesions in a representative rat that was fed. In the osteolytic lesion (black frame on the toluidine blue (TB) image in Figure 3b), the absorption pits with tartrate-resistant acid phosphatase (TRAP) activity indicating osteoclast infiltration was observed. Hematoxylin and eosin (H&E) staining revealed many osteoclasts, characterized by multiple nuclei on the surface of cortical bone in the pits (Figure 3c). On the other hand, the osteoblastic lesions (the yellow frame on the TB image in Figure 3b) revealed alkaline phosphatase (ALP) activity and pTBF, indicating the appearance of osteoblasts and osteoids, respectively, between tumor mass and the surface of cortical bone (H&E and TB images in Figure 3c). Almost all of the tumor cells in the osteolytic lesion were positive for ASCT2 (upper row in Figure 3c). On the other hand, ASCT2 expression in intra-tumoral cells was scant compared with that in the peripheral cells of the tumor mass and osteoblasts on the bone surface in the osteoblastic lesion (lower row in Figure 3c). LAT1-positive cells were scattered in all of the tumor tissues from both osteolytic and osteoblastic lesions (Figure 3c). No obvious differences were observed in the expression of ASCT2 and LAT1 between the fasted and fed rats (supplementary Figure S1). These results demonstrate that ^{14}C-fluciclovine and ^{3}H-FDG accumulated in histologically confirmed osteolytic and osteoblastic bone metastasis lesions.

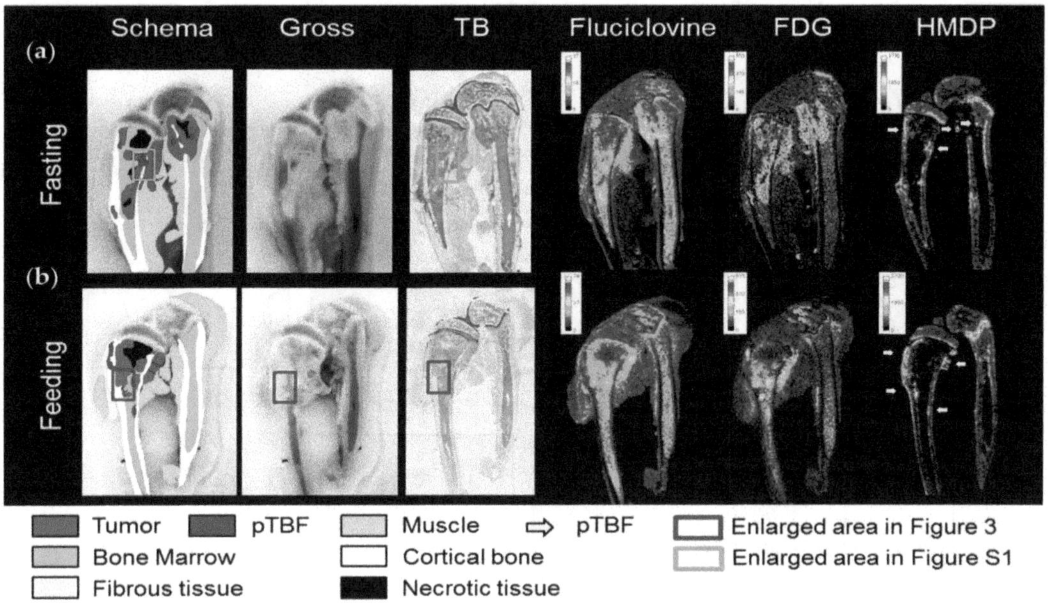

Figure 2. Triple-tracer autoradiography using ^{14}C-fluciclovine, 2-deoxy-2-^{18}F-fluoro-d-glucose (^{3}H-FDG), and ^{99m}Tc-hydroxymethylene diphosphonate (^{99m}Tc-HMDP) in breast cancer bone metastasis model rats. Macroscopic images (schema, gross, toluidine blue (TB) staining) and autoradiograms of each tracer in (**a**) fasting and (**b**) fed rats are shown. Each image was adjusted for optimal contrast and color scale bars on each autoradiogram represent Bq range for each tracer. The high-power microscopic fields of typical osteolytic and osteoblastic lesions corresponding to the blue and green frames on the macroscopic images in Figure 2a,b are shown in Figure 3 and supplementary Figure S1, respectively. The lesions correspond to ^{99m}Tc-HMDP-positive areas, except for physiological accumulation in growth plates, which were considered peri-tumor bone formation (pTBF) in osteoblastic lesions (yellow arrows).

Semi-quantitative analyses were used to evaluate tumor-to-muscle accumulation ratios of ^{14}C-fluciclovine and ^{3}H-FDG are shown in Figure 4 and Table 1. The target$_{mean}$ (metastatic lesion)-to-background$_{mean}$ (muscle) (T/BG) ratio of both tracers were statistically higher in the fasting condition than in the fed condition in osteolytic and pTBF lesions ($p < 0.01$). Comparing tracers, the ratios of ^{3}H-FDG were statistically higher than ^{14}C-fluciclovine in osteolytic lesions ($p < 0.01$), but not in pTBF lesions, under fasting and fed conditions. The distributions of T/BG ratios of ^{3}H-FDG in both lesions were wider than that of ^{14}C-fluciclovine, as shown in Figure 4 and Table 1.

Table 1. Summary of the distributions of T/BG ratios of ^{3}H-FDG and ^{14}C-fluciclovine in the osteolytic lesions and pTBF in osteoblastic lesions of breast cancer bone metastasis model rat with and without overnight fasting.

Lesion	Tracer	Diet	Min.	Max.	Median	1st Qu.	3rd Qu.	Mean ± S.D.
OL	^{3}H-FDG	Fasting	2.9	13.2	6.2	5.5	7.0	6.9 ± 2.5
		Feeding	1.6	10.7	5.0	3.7	6.1	5.1 ± 2.0
	^{14}C-fluciclovine	Fasting	3.1	6.8	4.4	3.9	5.1	4.6 ± 0.8
		Feeding	1.4	5.9	2.7	2.4	3.1	2.8 ± 0.6
pTBF	^{3}H-FDG	Fasting	1.6	12.8	5.6	3.7	10.5	6.6 ± 3.8
		Feeding	0.6	8.2	2.8	1.7	4.3	3.3 ± 2.2
	^{14}C-fluciclovine	Fasting	2.6	7.6	4.1	3.8	4.9	4.5 ± 1.4
		Feeding	1.0	3.9	2.5	1.8	2.9	2.4 ± 0.7

1st Qu.: first quartile, 3rd Qu.: third quartile, ^{3}H-FDG: 2-deoxy-2-^{18}F-fluoro-d-glucose, Max.: maximum value of T/BG ratios, Min.: minimum value of T/BG ratios, pTBF: peri tumor bone formation, OL: osteolytic, S.D.: standard deviation, T/BG: target$_{mean}$ (metastatic lesion)-to-background$_{mean}$ (muscle).

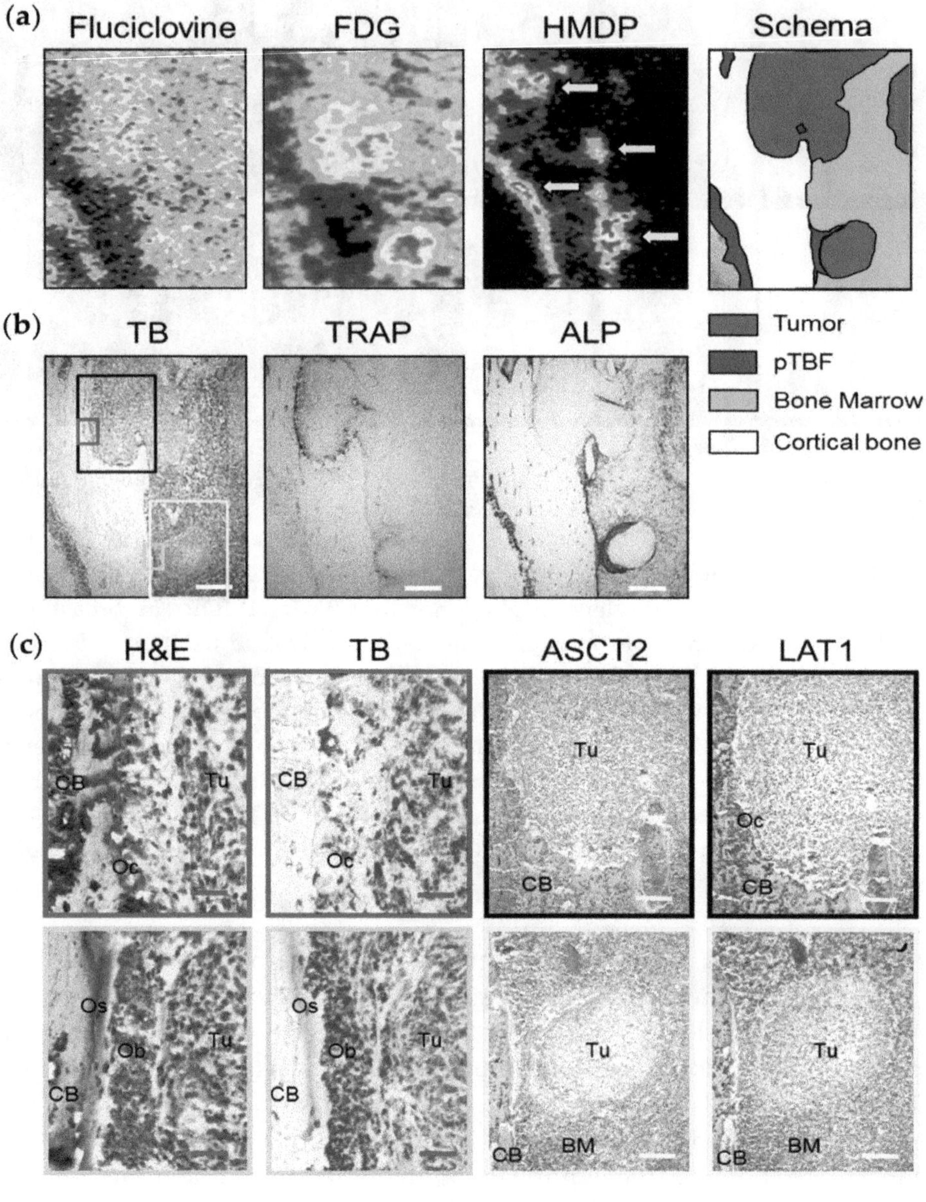

Figure 3. Comparison of the tracer accumulations of ^{14}C-fluciclovine, 2-deoxy-2-^{18}F-fluoro-d-glucose (^{3}H-FDG) and ^{99m}Tc-hydroxymethylene diphosphonate (^{99m}Tc-HMDP), and the histological characteristics of typical osteolytic and osteoblastic lesions in a representative breast cancer bone metastasis model rat that was fed. (**a**) The enlarged autoradiograms and the schema and (**b**) the histological images (toluidine blue (TB), tartrate-resistant acid phosphatase (TRAP), alkaline phosphatase (ALP)) correspond to the blue frame on the schema in Figure 2b are represented. The lesions corresponding to ^{99m}Tc-HMDP-positve were considered peri-tumor bone formation (pTBF) in osteoblastic lesions (yellow arrows). (**c**) The high-power microscopic fields (hematoxylin and eosin (H&E), TB, alanine-serine-cysteine transporter 2 (ASCT2), L-type amino acid transporter 1 (LAT1)) correspond to the black, red, yellow, and cyan frames on the TB image in Figure 3b are shown. The red, yellow, and white scale bars on each panel correspond to 50 μm, 200 μm, and 500 μm, respectively. BM: bone marrow, CB: cortical bone, Ob: osteoblasts, Oc: osteoclasts, Os: osteoids, Tu: tumor.

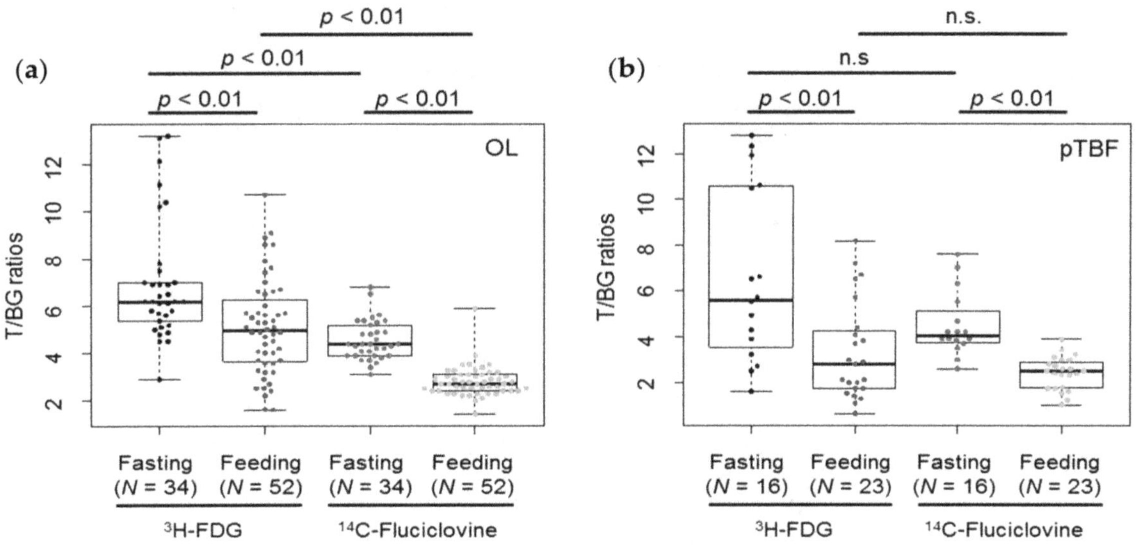

Figure 4. Beeswarm and box plots showing the distributions of $target_{mean}$ (metastatic lesion)-to-$background_{mean}$ (muscle) (T/BG) ratios of 2-deoxy-2-^{18}F-fluoro-D-glucose (^{3}H-FDG) and ^{14}C-fluciclovine in (**a**) osteolytic lesions (OL), and (**b**) peri-tumor bone formation (pTBF) in osteoblastic lesions in breast cancer bone metastasis model rats, with and without overnight fasting. The numbers under each box indicate the number of lesions. n.s.: not significant.

3. Discussion

We aimed to determine whether fasting before ^{18}F-fluciclovine-PET imaging improved visualization of bone metastasis lesions using a rat BCa bone metastasis model exhibiting osteolytic and osteoblastic lesions. Our findings suggest that fasting before fluciclovine-PET imaging improves the background contrast between osteolytic/osteoblastic bony lesions and muscle.

First, we investigated the AATs involved in the uptake of ^{14}C-fluciclovine in MRMT-1 cells, a rat BCa cell line. We confirmed that ASCT2 and LAT1 were the primary AATs for ^{14}C-fluciclovine transport in MRMT-1 cells, as well as prostate and brain cancer cell lines [8–12]. Second, we designed a bone metastasis model and injected MRMT-1 cells into the saphenous artery of the hind legs of rats. In this model, the mixed lesions of osteolytic and osteoblastic metastases, closely mimicking clinical findings [7], were formed in the tibia and/or femur.

Using this animal model, we performed triple-tracer autoradiography with ^{14}C-fluciclovine/^{3}H-FDG/^{99m}Tc-HMDP and evaluated the accumulation of each tracer in identical bony lesions. Comparing the T/BG ratios of ^{14}C-fluciclovine accumulation in rats that were fasted overnight with those in rats fed ad libitum, the ratios were higher in both osteolytic and osteoblastic lesions under the fasted condition than in the fed condition. It has been reported that the sum concentration of all plasma AAs decrease by 10% in rats fasted for one day, although the decreases do not involve drastic changes, unlike blood glucose (−35%) [13]. Among the AAs, proline (−48.9%), alanine (−21.8%), histidine (−18.2%), and glutamine (−13.1%), which are substrates of the ASC or L systems, demonstrated relatively high reduction rates in this experiment [13]. Thus, we expected that the concentration of these neutral AAs in rat plasma would be decreased by fasting before the injection of ^{14}C-fluciclovine and, consequently, that the autoradiography images of tumor lesions would be improved by increased ^{14}C-fluciclovine transport into the cancer cells. The T/BG ratios of ^{14}C-fluciclovine were, in fact, statistically higher under the fasted condition compared with the fed condition. Thus, we believe that it is reasonable to prescribe fasting to PCa patients before fluciclovine-PET, not only to decrease plasma AA concentration, but to force the AA concentration toward favoring fluciclovine transport, thus achieving a more quantitative fluciclovine-PET scan.

There have been some reports describing the influence of meal or plasma AAs on AA-tracer accumulation in tumors. Lindholm et al. [4] performed an intra-individual clinical study to investigate whether the ingestion of a liquid meal influenced the accumulation of ^{11}C-methionine, which is transported by LAT1 [10,11], in patients with head and neck cancer. In that study, initial PET imaging was performed after an overnight fast; the second PET imaging was then performed after ingesting the liquid meal containing L-methionine and branched-chain AAs 6 to 7 days after the first PET imaging. PET imaging was initiated 45 min after ingestion. The standard uptake values of ^{11}C-methionine in the tumor after ingestion decreased to a statistically lower level than that in tumors after fasting, although the tracer entering rate (i.e., K_1) into the tumor was not changed substantially [4]. Additionally, ^{11}C-methionine uptake in gliomas and normal brain tissue, while the patient received an intravenous infusion of branched-chain AAs, decreased [14]. Similar results were observed in glioma patients injected with 3-^{123}I-Iodo-L-α-methyltyrosine (^{123}I-3-IMT), which is known to be transported by LAT1, with intravenous infusion of a mixture of naturally-occurring L-AAs during imaging [15]. The decreasing level of tracer accumulation in tumors observed in these three studies was believed to be caused by competitive inhibition between the exogenous AAs and tracers on LAT1. Thus, it is believed that ingesting food containing abundant AAs before, or intravenous infusion of AAs during, fluciclovine-PET imaging decreases the tumor accumulation of ^{18}F-fluciclovine in PCa patients because ^{18}F-fluciclovine is also transported by LAT1.

ASCT2 and LAT1 are obligatory AA exchangers with a 1:1 stoichiometry. If cancer cells are preloaded with AAs, which can trans-stimulate the influx of extracellular AAs (trans-stimulators), the velocity of AA transport through the AA exchangers is accelerated [8]. Thus, the preinjection of trans-stimulators into cancer patients would be expected to accelerate the uptake of PET tracers into cancer cells. Based on this hypothesis, Lahoutte et al. investigated the effect of intraperitoneal preinjection (30 min before tracer injection) of each naturally-occurring AA (arginine, aspartate, glutamate, phenylalanine, proline, tryptophan) on the uptake of ^{123}I-3-IMT into the subcutaneous tumor of Rhabdomyosarcoma (R1M) tumor-bearing rats fasted for 4 h [16]. They found that the strongest effect was observed with the preinjection of tryptophan, which is a substrate of LAT1, although all AAs used in the study accelerated the uptake of ^{123}I-3-IMT into the tumor. This increase of ^{123}I-3-IMT transport into the subcutaneous tumor is explainable and based on trans-stimulation by preloaded tryptophan via LAT1. Accordingly, it is believed that ^{18}F-fluciclovine transport also would be accelerated by the preinjection of trans-stimulators because this PET tracer is also recognized by ASCT2 and LAT1. On the other hand, Lahoutte's findings are discrepant with findings involving ^{11}C-methionine reported by Lindholm et al. [4]. The reason for the discrepancy may be the result of differences in experimental protocols between the studies: the injected substance (liquid meal vs. AA), the injection route (oral vs. intravenous), the species (rats vs. human), and fasting duration before tracer injection (4 h vs. non-fasting). Although fasting and preloading AAs appear to be conflicting treatments, there is a possibility that both may improve the visualization of PCa on fluciclovine-PET. Sophisticated, non-clinical studies are needed to determine the optimal imaging conditions for fluciclovine-PET, including variables such as fasting duration, type and dose of trans-stimulators, and timing of ^{18}F-fluciclovine administration after fasting, or preinjection of trans-stimulators, because the metabolism of AAs in rats differs from that in humans.

We demonstrated that the T (tumor)/BG (muscle) ratios of ^{14}C-fluciclovine in osteolytic and osteoblastic lesions in fasted rats were higher than in rats that were fed. We believe that the increased rate of ^{14}C-fluciclovine uptake in cancer cells was greater than in muscular cells under experimental starvation. Our hypothesis for these findings is as follows: the most abundant and important neutral AA for mammalian cells is glutamine, which is transported by ASCT2 and sodium-dependent neutral amino acid transporter 2 (SNAT2) [17]. In muscle, SNAT2 is abundantly expressed compared with ASCT2 [18], and regulates intramuscular glutamine concentration [19–21]. A portion of intracellular glutamine is used for transport exchange with extracellular leucine via LAT1, and leucine regulates the production and degradation of protein in muscle as an activator for the mammalian target of rapamycin complex 1 (mTORC1), a key player in cellular functions such as protein and lipid synthesis, glycolysis, autophagy, etc. [22,23]. Decreases in intramuscular leucine represses mTORC1 signaling under fasting conditions, followed by the activation of the autophagic pathway, protein degradation, and the production of AAs [24]. The AAs are released from muscle and delivered to the liver and used for glycogenesis [25]. Thus, the efflux of AAs from muscular cells is facilitated under the starvation condition.

On the other hand, many types of cancers co-express ASCT2 and LAT1 on the cell surface [26], and these AATs function as key players for AA transport including glutamine and leucine in cancer cells [17]. In fact, many studies have reported that the co-expression of ASCT2 and LAT1 correlates with malignancy and prognosis in several types of cancer [27–33]. Although cancer cells can also actuate an autophagic process during starvation, the AAs produced by protein degradation in cancer cells are used for cancer-cell survival [34]. Instead, cancer facilitates the autophagic process in muscle tissue [35]. Thus, it is believed that cancer cells accelerate the influx of AAs rather than efflux, unlike muscle under fasting conditions. Because ASCT2 and LAT1 are the primary AATs mediating ^{14}C-fluciclovine transport, we speculate that the increased rate of ^{14}C-fluciclovine uptake in cancer cells is greater than in muscle cells under conditions of starvation. Therefore, the T/BG ratios of ^{14}C-fluciclovine in the bone metastatic lesions in fasted rats were higher than in rats that were fed.

As mentioned, AA metabolism is a complex process, and different in humans and rats. The duration of fasting for fluciclovine-PET (4 to 6 h) scans in clinical settings and our animal experiment (17 to 18 h) is quite different. Thus, there is a possibility that the influence of fasting on ^{18}F-fluciclovine accumulation in cancer tissue is reduced in clinical practice compared with the influence observed in our animal experiments. Additionally, the imaging time in the current study was 30 min, which falls within the plateau phase of ^{18}F-fluciclovine uptake in orthotopic transplanted PCa of a previously described animal model [36]. On the other hand, imaging results at 30 min correspond to the late phase of a clinical fluciclovine-PET scan (typically 5 to 30 min); by that time, ^{18}F-fluciclovine uptake decreases in prostate, lymph node, and bone lesions [37,38]. Consequently, uptake may have been underestimated in the current animal experiment. Further in vitro and in vivo studies are needed to extrapolate our findings to humans. Furthermore, intra-individual clinical studies are required to elucidate whether fasting and/or preloading trans-stimulators before fluciclovine-PET influences tumor accumulation of ^{18}F-fluciclovine and improves fluciclovine-PET imaging in cancer patients.

4. Materials and Methods

4.1. Reagents

All reagents were purchased from Life Technologies (Carlsbad, CA, USA), Sigma-Aldrich (St. Louis, MO, USA), Nacalai Tesque (Kyoto, Japan), and Wako Pure Chemical Industries (Osaka, Japan), unless otherwise indicated. ^{14}C-labeled fluciclovine (^{14}C-fluciclovine) and ^{3}H-labeled FDG (^{3}H-FDG) were used instead of ^{18}F-labeled tracers because their long half-lives make them more suitable for experiments than tracers labeled with ^{18}F ($t\,\frac{1}{2}$ = 110 min). ^{14}C-Fluciclovine (specific activity, 2.08 GBq/mmol; radiochemical purity (RCP) >98%), which has the same chemical structure as ^{18}F-fluciclovine, with the exception of the position of the radioisotope, was commercially synthesized by Nemoto Science (Tokyo, Japan), as described previously [8]. ^{3}H-FDG (specific actvity 2.22 TBq/mmol; RCP, >99%) was purchased from American Radiolabeled Chemicals (St. Louis, MO, USA). The authors' company, Nihon Medi-Physics (Tokyo, Japan), produced ^{99m}Tc-HMDP (740 MBq/vial; RCP, >95%). All AAs used in this study were the L-form.

4.2. Cell Culture

A rat BCa cell line, MRMT-1, was procured from RIKEN BioResource Center (Tsukuba, Japan; obtained in January 2014) and maintained in RPMI 1640 medium supplemented with 10% fetal bovine serum (American Type Culture Collection, Rockville, MD, USA), 100 μg/mL streptomycin, and 100 U/mL penicillin.

4.3. Competitive Inhibition Assay

The contributions of Na^+-dependent and -independent AATs to ^{14}C-fluciclovine transport was estimated using competitive inhibition assays between ^{14}C-fluciclovine and naturally-occurring or synthetic AAs, as described in a previous report [8]. Briefly, MRMT-1 cells were cultured in 24-well, flat-bottom tissue culture plates, and culture medium was replaced with sodium buffer (140 mmol/L NaCl, 5 mmol/L KCl, 5.6 mmol/L glucose, 0.9 mmol/L $CaCl_2$, 1.0 mmol/L $MgCl_2$ and 10 mmol/L HEPES (pH 7.3)) or choline buffer (NaCl of the sodium buffer was preplaced with 140 mmol/L choline chloride) containing 10 μmol/L ^{14}C-fluciclovine in the presence or absence of 2.0 mmol/L inhibitor. Cells were placed in an incubator at 37 °C for 5 min, and radioactivity was measured using a liquid scintillation counter (Tri-Carb 2910TR, Perkin Elmer, Waltham, MA, USA). Protein concentrations of cell lysates were determined using the BCA Protein Assay Kit (Thermo Fisher Scientific, Waltham, MA, USA). Tracer uptake was calculated as pmol/mg protein and the control transport (absence of inhibitors) of ^{14}C-fluciclovine in sodium/choline buffer was normalized to 100%. In this study, the following synthetic and naturally-occurring AAs were used as inhibitors: BCH, MeAIB, phenylalanine, proline, glutamine, serine, arginine, and glutamate; the specificity of each AA to AATs have been described in a previous report [8].

4.4. Animal Handling

All animal handling procedures and experimental protocols were conducted in accordance with Japanese laws as stipulated in the Act on Welfare and Management of Animals, and approved by the Institutional Animal Care and Use Committee of Nihon Medi-Physics (No. 142-019) on 24 October 2014. Male Sprague-Dawley rats (9–12 weeks old; CLEA Japan, Tokyo, Japan) were used for all experiments. Rats were housed in a 12 h light-dark cycle and were maintained on a standard laboratory diet, Labo MR Stock (Nosan Corporation, Kanagawa, Japan) containing approximately 9.2% water, 18.8% crude protein, 3.9% crude fat, 6.6% crude fiber, 6.9% crude ash, 54.7% of nitrogenous compounds, amino acids (1.09% arginine, 0.46% histidine, 0.67% isoleucine, 1.36%, leucine, 0.89%, lysine, 0.26% methionine, 0.84% phenylalanine, 0.64% threonine, 0.21% tryptophan, 0.79% valine, 0.28% cystein), and drinking water. All animals were anesthetized using 1% isoflurane (Pfizer Japan, Tokyo, Japan). In the surgical procedures, 0.5% meloxicam (Boehringer Ingelheim Vetmedica, Tokyo, Japan) was injected subcutaneously to relieve pain.

4.5. BCa Bone Metastatic Model

A BCa bone metastatic model, described previously [39], was used. Briefly, 100 mL of a cell suspension containing 2.5×10^4 MRMT-1 cells in Hank's Balanced Salt Solution without Ca^{2+} and Mg^{2+} was injected into the saphenous artery of the right hind legs. Development of osteolytic lesions was monitored using a microfocus X-ray imaging system (μFX-1000; FUJIFILM Corporation, Tokyo, Japan) or a preclinical imaging system (FX3000 CT, TriFoil Imaging, Chatsworth, CA, USA) and triple-tracer autoradiography was performed 12 ± 1 days after the cell injection. Osteolytic lesions were induced in the tibia and/or femur of the experimental rats.

4.6. Triple-Tracer Autoradiography

To compare the distribution of each tracer visually in identical lesions, triple-tracer autoradiography was performed using ^{14}C-fluciclovine, ^3H-FDG, and ^{99m}Tc-HMDP in the BCa osteolytic model as described in the supplementary material. Briefly, rats with (n = 5) or without (n = 6) fasting overnight (17 h to 18 h) were injected (tail vein) with three tracers (^{14}C-fluciclovine: 2.75 MBq/kg, ^3H-FDG: 18.5 MBq/kg, ^{99m}Tc-HMDP: 74 MBq/kg). ^{14}C-Fluciclovine and ^3H-FDG were allowed to remain in circulation for 30 min; ^{99m}Tc-HMDP was allowed to remain for 2 h before euthanizing the animal. The tibiae and femora were removed and frozen in isopentane/dry ice; the frozen bone was then embedded in Super Cryoembedding Medium (SCEM) (Section-Lab, Hiroshima, Japan), followed by freezing again in isopentane/dry ice until the SCEM set. The frozen samples were sectioned using a CM3050S cryostat (Leica Microsystems, Tokyo, Japan) at −20 °C with an adhesive film (Cryofilm Type 2C(9), Section-Lab) using Kawamoto's film method (5 µm slices and 10 µm slices for the histological and autoradiography specimens, respectively) [40]. The frozen samples were provided for triple-tracer autoradiography and each ^{14}C-, ^{3}H-, and ^{99m}Tc-image was created as described in the supplementary materials. The regions-of-interest (ROIs) were manually drawn around each lesion while referring to the histological images from H&E and TB staining. In the ^{14}C-fluciclovine and ^{3}H-FDG images, tumor lesions with bone absorption were defined as OL (typical osteolytic lesions) and the lesions corresponding to ^{99m}Tc-HMDP accumulation were defined as peri-tumor bone formation (pTBF) in the osteoblastic lesions (typical osteoblastic lesions). Furthermore, three ROIs of random size were manually positioned on the normal regions of muscle surrounding tibiae and/or femora and the average ROI count from the three ROIs was calculated as the background radioactivity. The target$_{mean}$ (metastatic lesion)-to-background$_{mean}$ (muscle) (T/BG) ratios were then calculated and lesion-based analyses were performed.

4.7. Histological Analysis

The following procedures for each histological stain were performed on 5 µm serial sections using general methods: H&E and TB staining for histological changes at the lesion sites; ALP for osteoblast and fibroblast activity; and TRAP staining for osteoclast-activity. Anti-ASCT2 (J-25) polyclonal antibody (1:40; Santa Cruz Biotechnology, Dallas, TX, USA) and anti-LAT1 (H-75) polyclonal antibody (1:200; Santa Cruz Biotechnology) for the amino acid transporters were used in the immunohistochemical assessments with EnVision+ System HR-labeled polymer anti-rabbit (Dako Japan, Tokyo, Japan) and Liquid DAB+ Substrate Chromogen System (Dako Japan). A BZ-9000 HS all-in-one fluorescence microscope (Keyence Corporation, Osaka, Japan) was used for pathological examinations.

4.8. Statistical Analysis

Data are presented as mean ± the standard deviation. To create beeswarm plots with box plots, R version 3.3.2 (R Foundation, Vienna, Austria) for Windows (Microsoft Corporation, Redmond, WA, USA) was used. In these plots, each dot represents a T/BG ratio in each lesion and the center lines in the boxes represent the medians; box limits indicate the 25th and 75th percentiles; whiskers extend 1.5 times the interquartile range from the 25th and 75th percentiles. All statistical analyses were performed using SAS version 9.4 (SAS Institute, Cary, NC, USA). The two groups were compared using Wilcoxon rank-sum tests for non-normal distribution datasets, or the F-test, followed by two-tailed unpaired Student's *t*-test or Welch's *t*-test for datasets with normal distribution. In all analyses, $p < 0.05$ was considered to be statistically significant.

5. Conclusions

Our findings suggest that fasting influences the uptake of ^{18}F-fluciclovine in osteolytic and osteoblastic bone metastasis lesions, and can facilitate clearer visualization of lesions in fluciclovine-PET imaging. However, because AA metabolism is a complex process, further animal and clinical studies are required to confirm our findings.

Acknowledgments: The authors thank Masahiro Ono for his assistance with the histological examinations; Sachiko Naito for her assistance in the daily maintenance of the cell cultures; and Shiro Yoshida for his assistance in the daily maintenance of the animals. We thank Editage for English language editing.

Author Contributions: Shuntaro Oka conceived and designed the experiments; Shuntaro Oka, Masaru Kanagawa, and Yoshihiro Doi performed the experiments; Shuntaro Oka and Masaru Kanagawa analyzed the data; Yoshihiro Doi contributed analysis tools; All authors wrote, reviewed, and revised the manuscript.

Abbreviations

AA	amino acid
AAT	amino acid transporter
ALP	alkaline phosphatase
ASC	alanine-serine-cysteine
ASCT2	alanine-serine-cysteine transporter 2
BCa	breast cancer
BM	bone marrow
^{11}C	carbon-11
^{14}C	carbon-14
CB	cortical bone
^{18}F	fluorine-18
FDG	2-deoxy-2-fluoro-D-glucose
^{3}H	tritium-3
H&E	hematoxylin-eosin
HMDP	hydroxymethylene diphosphonate
LAT1	L-type amino acid transporter 1
mTORC1	mammalian target of rapamycin complex 1
^{99m}Tc	technetium-99m
Ob	osteoblasts
Oc	osteoclasts
Os	osteoids
PET	positron emission tomography
PCa	prostate cancer
pTBF	peri-tumor bone formation
RCP	radiochemical purity
ROI	region-of-interest
SCEM	Super Cryoembedding Medium
SNAT2	sodium-dependent neutral amino acid transporter 2
TB	toluidine blue
T/BG	$target_{mean}$ (metastatic leion)-to-$background_{mean}$ (muscle)
TRAP	tartrate-resistant acid phosphatase

References

1. Lindholm, P.; Minn, H.; Leskinen-Kallio, S.; Bergman, J.; Ruotsalainen, U.; Joensuu, H. Influence of the blood glucose concentration on FDG uptake in cancer—A PET study. *J. Nucl. Med.* **1993**, *34*, 1–6. [PubMed]
2. Lewis, D.Y.; Soloviev, D.; Brindle, K.M. Imaging tumor metabolism using positron emission tomography. *Cancer J.* **2015**, *21*, 129–136. [CrossRef] [PubMed]
3. Jager, P.L. Improving amino acid imaging: Hungry or stuffed? *J. Nucl. Med.* **2002**, *43*, 1207–1209. [PubMed]
4. Lindholm, P.; Leskinen-Kallio, S.; Kirvelä, O.; Någren, K.; Lehikoinen, P.; Pulkki, K.; Peltola, O.; Ruotsalainen, U.; Teräs, M.; Joensuu, H. Head and neck cancer: Effect of food ingestion on uptake of C-11 methionine. *Radiology* **1994**, *190*, 863–867. [CrossRef] [PubMed]
5. Schuster, D.M.; Nanni, C.; Fanti, S.; Oka, S.; Okudaira, H.; Inoue, Y.; Sörensen, J.; Owenius, R.; Choyke, P.; Turkbey, B.; et al. Anti-1-amino-3-^{18}F-fluorocyclobutane-1-carboxylic acid: Physiologic uptake patterns, incidental findings, and variants that may simulate disease. *J. Nucl. Med.* **2014**, *55*, 1986–1992. [CrossRef] [PubMed]

6. Ulaner, G.A.; Goldman, D.A.; Gönen, M.; Pham, H.; Castillo, R.; Lyashchenko, S.K.; Lewis, J.S.; Dang, C. Initial Results of a Prospective Clinical Trial of ^{18}F-Fluciclovine PET/CT in Newly Diagnosed Invasive Ductal and Invasive Lobular Breast Cancers. *J. Nucl. Med.* **2016**, *57*, 1350–1356. [CrossRef] [PubMed]
7. Rahim, F.; Hajizamani, S.; Mortaz, E.; Ahmadzadeh, A.; Shahjahani, M.; Shahrabi, S.; Saki, N. Molecular regulation of bone marrow metastasis in prostate and breast cancer. *Bone Marrow Res.* **2014**, *2014*, 405920. [CrossRef] [PubMed]
8. Oka, S.; Okudaira, H.; Yoshida, Y.; Schuster, D.M.; Goodman, M.M.; Shirakami, Y. Transport mechanisms of *trans*-1-amino-3-fluoro[1-(14)C]cyclobutanecarboxylic acid in prostate cancer cells. *Nucl. Med. Biol.* **2012**, *39*, 109–119. [CrossRef] [PubMed]
9. Okudaira, H.; Nakanishi, T.; Oka, S.; Kobayashi, M.; Tamagami, H.; Schuster, D.M.; Goodman, M.M.; Shirakami, Y.; Tamai, I.; Kawai, K. Kinetic analyses of *trans*-1-amino-3-[^{18}F]fluorocyclobutanecarboxylic acid transport in *Xenopus laevis* oocytes expressing human ASCT2 and SNAT2. *Nucl. Med. Biol.* **2013**, *40*, 670–675. [CrossRef] [PubMed]
10. Ono, M.; Oka, S.; Okudaira, H.; Schuster, D.M.; Goodman, M.M.; Kawai, K.; Shirakami, Y. Comparative evaluation of transport mechanisms of *trans*-1-amino-3-[^{18}F]fluorocyclobutanecarboxylic acid and l-[methyl-^{11}C]methionine in human glioma cell lines. *Brain Res.* **2013**, *1535*, 24–37. [CrossRef] [PubMed]
11. Oka, S.; Okudaira, H.; Ono, M.; Schuster, D.M.; Goodman, M.M.; Kawai, K.; Shirakami, Y. Differences in transport mechanisms of *trans*-1-amino-3-[^{18}F]fluorocyclobutanecarboxylic acid in inflammation, prostate cancer, and glioma cells: Comparison with L-[methyl-^{11}C]methionine and 2-deoxy-2-[^{18}F]fluoro-D-glucose. *Mol. Imaging Biol.* **2014**, *16*, 322–329. [CrossRef] [PubMed]
12. Liang, Z.; Cho, H.T.; Williams, L.; Zhu, A.; Liang, K.; Huang, K.; Wu, H.; Jiang, C.; Hong, S.; Crowe, R.; et al. Potential Biomarker of L-type Amino Acid Transporter 1 in Breast Cancer Progression. *Nucl. Med. Mol. Imaging* **2011**, *45*, 93–102. [CrossRef] [PubMed]
13. Holecek, M.; Kovarik, M. Alterations in protein metabolism and amino acid concentrations in rats fed by a high-protein (casein-enriched) diet—Effect of starvation. *Food Chem. Toxicol.* **2011**, *49*, 3336–3342. [CrossRef] [PubMed]
14. Bergström, M.; Ericson, K.; Hagenfeldt, L.; Mosskin, M.; von Holst, H.; Norén, G.; Eriksson, L.; Ehrin, E.; Johnström, P. PET study of methionine accumulation in glioma and normal brain tissue: Competition with branched chain amino acids. *J. Comput. Assist. Tomogr.* **1987**, *11*, 208–213. [CrossRef] [PubMed]
15. Langen, K.J.; Roosen, N.; Coenen, H.H.; Kuikka, J.T.; Kuwert, T.; Herzog, H.; Stöcklin, G.; Feinendegen, L.E. Brain and brain tumor uptake of L-3-[^{123}I]iodo-α-methyl tyrosine: Competition with natural L-amino acids. *J. Nucl. Med.* **1991**, *32*, 1225–1229. [PubMed]
16. Lahoutte, T.; Caveliers, V.; Franken, P.R.; Bossuyt, A.; Mertens, J.; Everaert, H. Increased tumor uptake of 3-(123)I-Iodo-L-α-methyltyrosine after preloading with amino acids: An in vivo animal imaging study. *J. Nucl. Med.* **2002**, *43*, 1201–1206. [PubMed]
17. Pochini, L.; Scalise, M.; Galluccio, M.; Indiveri, C. Membrane transporters for the special amino acid glutamine: Structure/function relationships and relevance to human health. *Front. Chem.* **2014**, *2*, 61. [CrossRef] [PubMed]
18. Nishimura, M.; Naito, S. Tissue-specific mRNA expression profiles of human ATP-binding cassette and solute carrier transporter superfamilies. *Drug Metab. Pharmacokinet.* **2005**, *20*, 452–477. [CrossRef] [PubMed]
19. Bevington, A.; Brown, J.; Butler, H.; Govindji, S.; M-Khalid, K.; Sheridan, K.; Walls, J. Impaired system A amino acid transport mimics the catabolic effects of acid in L6 cells. *Eur. J. Clin. Investig.* **2002**, *32*, 590–602.
20. Evans, K.; Nasim, Z.; Brown, J.; Butler, H.; Kauser, S.; Varoqui, H.; Erickson, J.D.; Herbert, T.P.; Bevington, A. Acidosis-sensing glutamine pump SNAT2 determines amino acid levels and mammalian target of rapamycin signalling to protein synthesis in L6 muscle cells. *J. Am. Soc. Nephrol.* **2007**, *18*, 1426–1436.
21. Hyde, R.; Hajduch, E.; Powell, D.J.; Taylor, P.M.; Hundal, H.S. Ceramide down-regulates System A amino acid transport and protein synthesis in rat skeletal muscle cells. *FASEB J.* **2005**, *19*, 461–463. [CrossRef] [PubMed]
22. Drummond, M.J.; Glynn, E.L.; Fry, C.S.; Timmerman, K.L.; Volpi, E.; Rasmussen, B.B. An increase in essential amino acid availability upregulates amino acid transporter expression in human skeletal muscle. *Am. J. Physiol. Endocrinol. Metab.* **2010**, *298*, E1011–E1018. [CrossRef] [PubMed]
23. Dodd, K.M.; Tee, A.R. Leucine and mTORC1: A complex relationship. *Am. J. Physiol. Endocrinol. Metab.* **2012**, *302*, E1329–E1342. [CrossRef] [PubMed]

24. Sancak, Y.; Peterson, T.R.; Shaul, Y.D.; Lindquist, R.A.; Thoreen, C.C.; Bar-Peled, L. The Rag GTPases bind raptor and mediate amino acid signaling to mTORC1. *Science* **2008**, *320*, 1496–1501. [CrossRef] [PubMed]
25. Sandri, M. Signaling in muscle atrophy and hypertrophy. *Physiology* **2008**, *23*, 160–170. [CrossRef] [PubMed]
26. Fuchs, B.C.; Bode, B.P. Amino acid transporters ASCT2 and LAT1 in cancer: Partners in crime? *Semin. Cancer Biol.* **2005**, *15*, 254–266. [CrossRef] [PubMed]
27. Wang, Q.; Tiffen, J.; Bailey, C.G.; Lehman, M.L.; Ritchie, W.; Fazli, L. Targeting amino acid transport in metastatic castration-resistant prostate cancer: Effects on cell cycle, cell growth, and tumor development. *J. Natl. Cancer Inst.* **2013**, *105*, 1463–1473. [CrossRef] [PubMed]
28. Toyoda, M.; Kaira, K.; Ohshima, Y.; Ishioka, N.S.; Shino, M.; Sakakura, K.; Takayasu, Y.; Takahashi, K.; Tominaga, H.; Oriuchi, N.; et al. Prognostic significance of amino-acid transporter expression (LAT1, ASCT2, and xCT) in surgically resected tongue cancer. *Br. J. Cancer* **2014**, *110*, 2506–2513. [CrossRef] [PubMed]
29. Namikawa, M.; Kakizaki, S.; Kaira, K.; Tojima, H.; Yamazaki, Y.; Horiguchi, N.; Sato, K.; Oriuchi, N.; Tominaga, H.; Sunose, Y.; et al. Expression of amino acid transporters (LAT1, ASCT2 and xCT) as clinical significance in hepatocellular carcinoma. *Hepatol. Res.* **2014**. [CrossRef] [PubMed]
30. Kaira, K.; Arakawa, K.; Shimizu, K.; Oriuchi, N.; Nagamori, S.; Kanai, Y.; Oyama, T.; Takeyoshi, I. Relationship between CD147 and expression of amino acid transporters (LAT1 and ASCT2) in patients with pancreatic cancer. *Am. J. Transl. Res.* **2015**, *7*, 356–363. [PubMed]
31. Nikkuni, O.; Kaira, K.; Toyoda, M.; Shino, M.; Sakakura, K.; Takahashi, K.; Tominaga, H.; Oriuchi, N.; Suzuki, M.; Iijima, M.; et al. Expression of Amino Acid Transporters (LAT1 and ASCT2) in Patients with Stage III/IV Laryngeal Squamous Cell Carcinoma. *Pathol. Oncol. Res.* **2015**, *21*, 1175–1181.
32. Kaira, K.; Nakamura, K.; Hirakawa, T.; Imai, H.; Tominaga, H.; Oriuchi, N.; Nagamori, S.; Kanai, Y.; Tsukamoto, N.; Oyama, T.; et al. Prognostic significance of L-type amino acid transporter 1 (LAT1) expression in patients with ovarian tumors. *Am. J. Transl. Res.* **2015**, *7*, 1161–1171. [PubMed]
33. Honjo, H.; Kaira, K.; Miyazaki, T.; Yokobori, T.; Kanai, Y.; Nagamori, S.; Oyama, T.; Asao, T.; Kuwano, H. Clinicopathological significance of LAT1 and ASCT2 in patients with surgically resected esophageal squamous cell carcinoma. *J. Surg. Oncol.* **2016**, *113*, 381–389. [CrossRef] [PubMed]
34. Sato, K.; Tsuchihara, K.; Fujii, S.; Sugiyama, M.; Goya, T.; Atomi, Y.; Ueno, T.; Ochiai, A.; Esumi, H. Autophagy is activated in colorectal cancer cells and contributes to the tolerance to nutrient deprivation. *Cancer Res.* **2007**, *67*, 9677–9684. [CrossRef] [PubMed]
35. Luo, Y.; Yoneda, J.; Ohmori, H.; Sasaki, T.; Shimbo, K.; Eto, S.; Kato, Y.; Miyano, H.; Kobayashi, T.; Sasahira, T.; et al. Cancer usurps skeletal muscle as an energy repository. *Cancer Res.* **2014**, *74*, 330–340.
36. Oka, S.; Hattori, R.; Kurosaki, F.; Toyama, M.; Williams, L.A.; Yu, W.; Votaw, J.R.; Yoshida, Y.; Goodman, M.M.; Ito, O. A preliminary study of anti-1-amino-3-^{18}F-fluorocyclobutyl-1-carboxylic acid for the detection of prostate cancer. *J. Nucl. Med.* **2007**, *48*, 46–55. [PubMed]
37. Schuster, D.M.; Votaw, J.R.; Nieh, P.T.; Yu, W.; Nye, J.A.; Master, V.; Bowman, F.D.; Issa, M.M.; Goodman, M.M. Initial experience with the radiotracer anti-1-amino-3-^{18}F-fluorocyclobutane-1-carboxylic acid with PET/CT in prostate carcinoma. *J. Nucl. Med.* **2007**, *48*, 56–63. [PubMed]
38. Inoue, Y.; Asano, Y.; Satoh, T.; Tabata, K.; Kikuchi, K.; Woodhams, R.; Baba, S.; Hayakawa, K. Phase IIa Clinical Trial of Trans-1-Amino-3-^{18}F-Fluoro-Cyclobutane carboxylic acid in metastatic prostate cancer. *Asia Ocean J. Nucl. Med. Biol.* **2014**, *2*, 87–94. [PubMed]
39. Zepp, M.; Bauerle, T.J.; Elazar, V.; Peterschmitt, J.; Lifshitz-Shovali, R.; Adwan, H.; Armbruster, F.P.; Golomb, G.; Berger, M.R. Treatment of breast cancer lytic skeletal metastasis using a model in nude rats. In *Breast Cancer—Current and Alternative Therapeutic Modalities*; Gunduz, E., Ed.; InTech: Rijeka, Croatia, 2011; Available online: http://www.intechopen.com/books/breast-cancer-current-and-alternative-therapeutic-modalities/treatment-of-breast-cancer-lytic-skeletal-metastasis-using-a-model-in-nude-rats (accessed on 28 April 2017).
40. Kawamoto, T. Use of a new adhesive film for the preparation of multi-purpose fresh-frozen sections from hard tissues, whole-animals, insects and plants. *Arch. Histol. Cytol.* **2003**, *66*, 123–413. [CrossRef] [PubMed]

12

Perioperative Search for Circulating Tumor Cells in Patients Undergoing Prostate Brachytherapy for Clinically Nonmetastatic Prostate Cancer

Hideyasu Tsumura [1,*], Takefumi Satoh [1], Hiromichi Ishiyama [2], Ken-ichi Tabata [1], Kouji Takenaka [2], Akane Sekiguchi [2], Masaki Nakamura [3], Masashi Kitano [2], Kazushige Hayakawa [2] and Masatsugu Iwamura [1]

1 Department of Urology, Kitasato University School of Medicine, Sagamihara 252-0374, Japan; tsatoh@kitasato-u.ac.jp (T.S.); ktabata@med.kitasato-u.ac.jp (K.T.); miwamura@med.kitasato-u.ac.jp (M.I.)
2 Department of Radiology and Radiation Oncology, Kitasato University School of Medicine, Sagamihara 252-0374, Japan; hishiyam@kitasato-u.ac.jp (H.I.); takenaka@kitasato-u.ac.jp (K.T.); akane.o.enaka@gmail.com (A.S.); m-kitano@jcom.home.ne.jp (M.K.); hayakazu@med.kitasato-u.ac.jp (K.H.)
3 Department of Microbiology, Kitasato University School of Allied Health Sciences, Kanagawa 252-0373, Japan; nakamu7@mac.com
* Correspondence: tsumura@med.kitasato-u.ac.jp

Academic Editor: Carsten Stephan

Abstract: Despite the absence of local prostate cancer recurrence, some patients develop distant metastases after prostate brachytherapy. We evaluate whether prostate brachytherapy procedures have a potential risk for hematogenous spillage of prostate cancer cells. Fifty-nine patients who were undergoing high-dose-rate (HDR) or low-dose-rate (LDR) brachytherapy participated in this prospective study. Thirty patients with high-risk or locally advanced cancer were treated with HDR brachytherapy after neoadjuvant androgen deprivation therapy (ADT). Twenty-nine patients with clinically localized cancer were treated with LDR brachytherapy without neoadjuvant ADT. Samples of peripheral blood were drawn in the operating room before insertion of needles (preoperative) and again immediately after the surgical manipulation (intraoperative). Blood samples of 7.5 mL were analyzed for circulating tumor cells (CTCs) using the CellSearch System. While no preoperative samples showed CTCs (0%), they were detected in intraoperative samples in 7 of the 59 patients (11.8%; preoperative vs. intraoperative, $p = 0.012$). Positive CTC status did not correlate with perioperative variables, including prostate-specific antigen (PSA) at diagnosis, use of neoadjuvant ADT, type of brachytherapy, Gleason score, and biopsy positive core rate. We detected CTCs from samples immediately after the surgical manipulation. Further study is needed to evaluate whether those CTCs actually can survive and proliferate at distant sites.

Keywords: prostate cancer; brachytherapy; circulating tumor cell

---

1. Introduction

Brachytherapy approaches have been accepted as a useful method to control localized and locally advanced prostate cancers [1–5]. One of the most appealing reasons for selecting this treatment is favorable long-term outcome with a low degree of toxicity [6]. Low-dose-rate (LDR) brachytherapy provides superior outcomes in patients with low- and intermediate-risk diseases [1,2]. The combination of high-dose-rate (HDR) brachytherapy and external irradiation is an effective treatment for delivering radiation doses more precisely in prostate cancer, even if patients have extracapsular invasion and seminal vesicle invasion [3–5]. Technical modifications for prostate brachytherapy are being developed to obtain the better treatment outcome [2,7–10]. However, approximately 5%–20% of those patients, as it now stands, show recurrence within 5 years after brachytherapy [1,2,5,11,12].

When patients are suspected to have treatment failure, evaluation—including abdominal computed tomography scan, pelvic magnetic resonance imaging, a bone scan, and prostate biopsy—are usually conducted to identify the site of relapse. Some patients develop distant metastases despite the absence of local recurrence. In those cases, micrometastasis that was not detected by radiographic images may have been present at initial diagnosis. Another possibility is that surgical manipulation that involves needles being inserted into prostate tissue may pose a potential risk for hematogenous spillage of prostate cancer cells and play a role in distant metastases in patients undergoing prostate brachytherapy. A no-touch isolation technique, in which vascular control is achieved prior to tumor manipulation, is generally considered to reduce cancer dissemination and subsequently reduce future disease recurrence in various cancer-related surgeries [13–17]. However, this technique is not used during brachytherapy procedures. In addition, needles being inserted into prostate tissue directly penetrate the cancer lesions at a certain rate.

Elucidating the mechanism and causes of relapse is a key challenge for the enhancement of treatment outcome [18,19]. We suspect that iatrogenic circulating tumor cell (CTC) spillage can convert a nonmetastatic cancer to a systemic one. In this study, we evaluated whether brachytherapy procedures can provoke hematogenous spillage of prostate cancer cells. We detected perioperative CTCs using the CellSearch System and compared preoperative CTC counts with intraoperative ones. We analyzed whether intraoperative CTC increases were associated with perioperative clinicopathological features.

2. Results

Characteristics of the 59 patients are shown in Table 1. As shown in Figure 1, no CTCs were detected in preoperative samples. CTCs were detected from samples collected immediately after insertion of needles in 7 of 59 patients (11.8%). Intraoperative CTC detection rates were significantly higher than preoperative ones (11.8% vs. 0%, $p = 0.012$).

Table 1. Patient characteristics ($n = 59$).

Factors	HDR ($n = 30$)		LDR ($n = 29$)		Total ($n = 59$)	
	Median	**(Range)**	**Median**	**(Range)**	**Median**	**(Range)**
Age (year)	71.5	(58–82)	70	(51–77)	71	(51–82)
PSA at diagnosis (ng/mL)	26.8	(4.5–396)	6.5	(4.2–14.1)	10.1	(4.2–396)
Prostate volume (cc) *	14.4	(4.6–29.7)	30.7	(20.3–58.4)	22.2	(4.6–58.4)
Number of needles	18	(18–18)	21	(17–29)	–	–
Duration of NHT (months)	16	(7–25)	0	(0)	–	–
	n	**(%)**	n	**(%)**	n	**(%)**
Gleason Score						
≤6	0	(0)	8	(28)	8	(14)
7	7	(23)	19	(65)	26	(44)
8 to 10	23	(77)	2	(7)	25	(42)
Clinical T Stage						
1c–2a	6	(20)	20	(69)	26	(44)
2b–2c	6	(20)	9	(31)	15	(25)
3a	11	(37)	0	(0)	11	(19)
3b	6	(20)	0	(0)	6	(10)
4	1	(3)	0	(0)	1	(2)

Table 1. *Cont.*

Factors	HDR (n = 30)		LDR (n = 29)		Total (n = 59)	
	Median	(Range)	Median	(Range)	Median	(Range)
	n	(%)	n	(%)	n	(%)
Biopsy Positive Core Rate						
<34%	8	(27)	21	(73)	29	(49)
34%–67%	12	(40)	7	(24)	19	(32)
>67%	10	(33)	1	(3)	11	(19)
NCCN Risk Criteria (2015)						
Low	0	(0)	6	(21)	6	(10)
Intermediate	0	(0)	21	(72)	21	(36)
High	20	(67)	2	(7)	22	(37)
Very high	10	(33)	0	(0)	10	(17)

* Prostate volume was measured by transrectal ultrasound sonography immediately before insertion of needles. HDR: high-dose-rate brachytherapy; LDR: low-dose-rate brachytherapy; PSA: prostate-specific antigen; NHT: neoadjuvant hormonal therapy; NCCN: National Comprehensive Cancer Network.

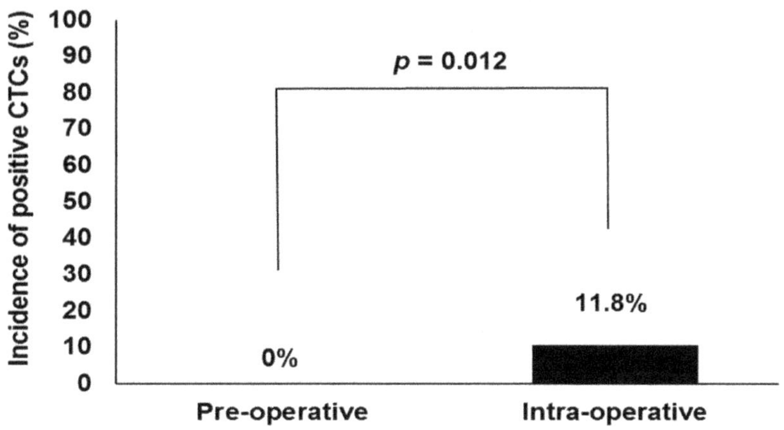

Figure 1. Comparison of circulating tumor cell (CTC) detection rates between pre- and intraoperative blood specimens in all patients undergoing high-dose-rate or low-dose-rate brachytherapy (n = 59).

Figure 2A,B showed perioperative CTC detection rates in patients undergoing HDR and LDR brachytherapy, respectively. Intraoperative CTCs were detected in 4 of 30 (13.3%) patients and 3 of 29 (10.5%) patients with HDR and LDR brachytherapy, respectively. While intraoperative CTC detection rates were relatively high when compared with preoperative ones in each group, according to a Fisher's exact test, the differences did not reach statistical significance in the HDR brachytherapy group (p = 0.112) or in the LDR brachytherapy group (p = 0.236).

Table 2 lists the characteristics of the 7 patients who became positive for CTCs intraoperatively. The intraoperative CTC count was 1 CTC in 3 patients and 2 CTCs in 1 patient treated with HDR brachytherapy, and 1 CTC was detected in 3 patients who underwent LDR brachytherapy.

To investigate the secondary outcome measures, patients were divided into two groups according to positive or negative status for intraoperative CTCs. Positive status did not correlate with clinicopathological and perioperative variables, including use of neoadjuvant hormonal therapy, type of brachytherapy, age, prostate-specific antigen (PSA) at diagnosis, Gleason score, clinical stage, biopsy positive core rates, prostate volume at brachytherapy, or National Comprehensive Cancer Network (NCCN) risk criteria 2015 (Table 3). Neither patients with positive status nor those with negative status for intraoperative CTCs had postoperative clinical progression, with a median follow-up of 18 months (range, 15–24 months).

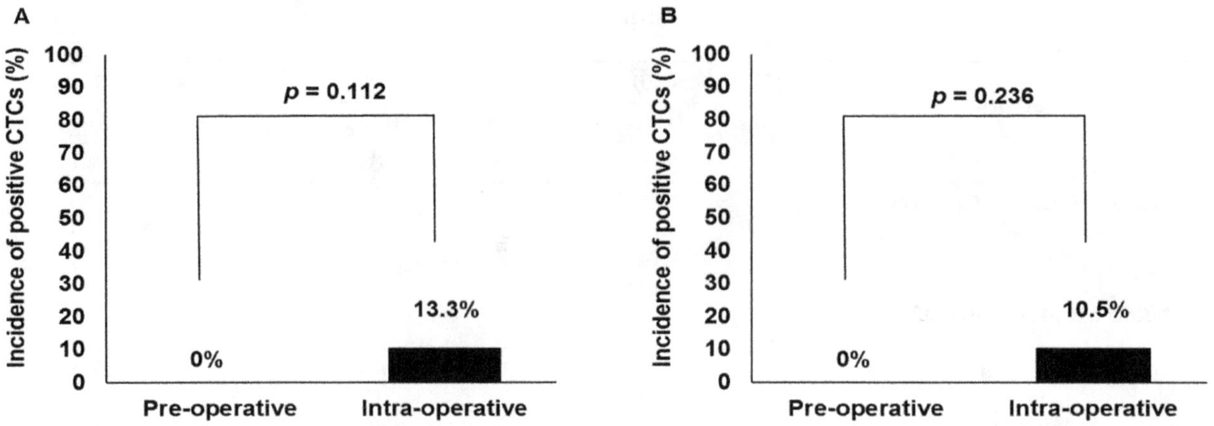

Figure 2. Comparison of circulating tumor cell (CTC) detection rates between pre- and intraoperative blood specimens in patients undergoing high-dose-rate (**A**, $n = 30$) and low-dose-rate (**B**, $n = 29$) brachytherapy.

Table 2. Characteristics of seven patients who changed to positive status for intraoperative circulating tumor cells (CTCs).

Type of Brachytherapy	HDR	HDR	HDR	HDR	LDR	LDR	LDR
Case number	9	26	34	36	8	19	43
Number of CTC counts (/7.5 mL)	2	1	1	1	1	1	1
Age (years)	71	75	65	75	58	65	67
Duration of NHT (months)	17	16	16	17	0	0	0
PSA nadir during NHT (ng/mL)	0.014	<0.008	<0.008	0.14	–	–	–
PSA at diagnosis (ng/mL)	31	13.5	17.6	66.7	8.6	4.6	14.1
Prostate volume (cc) *	7	29.7	21.3	13.9	26.1	38.4	37
Number of needles	18	18	18	18	24	28	18
Gleason score	8	8	7	9	6	7	7
Clinical T stage	1c	3a	3b	2c	2a	2a	2c
Biopsy positive core rate (%)	75	50	25	100	10	16.6	33.3
NCCN risk criteria 2015	H	H	VH	H	L	I	I

* Prostate volume was measured by transrectal ultrasound sonography immediately before insertion of needles; HDR: high-dose-rate brachytherapy; LDR: low-dose-rate brachytherapy; NHT: neoadjuvant hormonal therapy; PSA: prostate-specific antigen; NCCN: National Comprehensive Cancer Network; H: high risk; VH: very high risk; L: low risk; I: intermediate risk.

Table 3. Association of positive status for intraoperative circulating tumor cells (CTCs) with perioperative features ($n = 59$).

Factors	CTC Positive Rates	(n)	p
Age (>70 vs. ≤70 years)	8.8% vs. 16.0%	(3/34 vs. 4/25)	0.442
Type of brachytherapy (HDR vs. LDR)	13.3% vs. 10.3%	(4/30 vs. 3/29)	>0.999
NHT (yes vs. no)	13.3% vs. 10.3%	(4/30 vs. 3/29)	>0.999
PSA at diagnosis (≥10 vs. <10 ng/mL)	16.1% vs. 7.1%	(5/31 vs. 2/28)	0.424
Prostate volume (cc)	14.8% vs. 9.3%	(4/27 vs. 3/32)	0.691
Prostate volume/number of needle (≥1 vs. <1 cc/needle)	14.2% vs. 8.3%	(5/35 vs. 2/24)	0.689
Gleason score (≥8 vs. <8)	12.0% vs. 11.7%	(3/25 vs. 4/34)	>0.999
Clinical T stage (≥3a vs. ≤2c)	11.7% vs. 11.9%	(2/17 vs. 5/42)	>0.999
Biopsy positive core rate (>34% vs. ≤34%)	10.0% vs. 13.7%	(3/30 vs. 4/29)	0.706
NCCN risk criteria 2015 (H or VH vs. I or L)	12.5% vs. 11.1%	(4/32 vs. 3/27)	>0.999

3. Discussion

In this study of clinically nonmetastatic prostate cancer patients, we detected CTCs from samples immediately after insertion of needles in patients undergoing prostate brachytherapy. Intraoperative

CTC detection rates were significantly higher than preoperative ones. Our results may support a potential risk for hematogenous spread of cancer cells during the procedure.

Historically, transurethral resection of prostate (TURP) was generally performed to relieve the urinary tract obstruction caused by prostate cancer. In 1986, Levine et al. reported the possibility that cancer cells might be disseminated during TURP in patients with clinically evident cancer confined to the prostate [13]. They noted that the 5-year survival rate in those patients undergoing TURP was significantly lower than those not undergoing the procedure ($p = 0.02$). Several investigators then measured perioperative CTCs and reported the possibility of hematogenous spillage of cancer cells during radical prostatectomy in clinically nonmetastatic cancer patients [20–24]. Eschwege et al. investigated the dissemination of malignant prostatic cells during open radical prostatectomy [20], and they confirmed prostate-specific membrane antigen (PSMA) using reverse-transcription nested PCR for CTC detection. The incidence of positive CTC status increased from 21% before the surgery to 86% immediately afterward, supporting the possibility of intraoperative hematogenous dissemination during the open radical prostatectomy. They concluded that surgeons should minimize prostate manipulation to avoid seeding from the gland for the prevention of metastatic disease.

Prostate needle biopsy is one of the most similar procedures to prostate brachytherapy in that needles being inserted into prostate tissue directly penetrate the cancer lesions. Hara et al. examined PSA-mRNA-bearing cells in peripheral blood of the 108 patients before and after prostate biopsy [25]. Of 46 patients who were diagnosed with prostate cancer, the incidence of positive PSA-mRNA-bearing cells increased from 3% before the biopsy to 45% immediately afterward. In addition, the incidence of positive PSA-mRNA status after prostate biopsy in patients diagnosed with prostate cancer were higher than those without prostate cancer (45% vs. 25%, $p < 0.001$). This study supported the possibility of tumor spreading by prostate biopsy.

While we detected intraoperative hematogenous spillage of prostate cancer cells during brachytherapy procedures, it is still controversial whether the CTCs spilled iatrogenically into circulation have the biological capability to implant into distant sites and subsequently develop metastatic foci. Most studies—including the present study that detected the intraoperative CTC increase during radical treatment for primary lesion and prostate biopsy—had a small sample size and lacked a long follow-up period. Thus, the clinical significance of intraoperative CTC increase remains unclear, and we still have the question of whether this kind of iatrogenic CTC is clinically metastable. Eschwege et al. evaluated the cancer-cell seeding impact on recurrence-free survival [23]. Hematogenous spread of prostate cells was assessed by a dual PSA/PSMA PCR assay using very specific PSMA and PSA primers. Ninety-eight patients with negative status for preoperative CTC were divided into two groups according to status for intraoperative CTC: 53 (54%) remained negative and 45 (46%) became positive. Median biological and clinical recurrence-free time did not significantly differ between the two groups (69.6 vs. 65 months). The authors concluded that intraoperative hematogenous spillage of prostate cancer cells does not have a statistically significant adverse effect on recurrence. Their results seem to exclude tumor surgical management as a major cause of metastatic development. Some studies demonstrated that a primary tumor contains subpopulations of metastatic and nonmetastatic cancer cells. Only a restricted fraction of the cells in a primary tumor are considered to be highly metastatic [26,27]. Mareel et al. reported that 0.1% of CTC is responsible for the formation of metastatic foci [28]. When intraoperative hematogenous spillage of prostate cancer cells occurs during surgical procedures, we suspect that it may provoke distant metastases. However, the possibility of metastatic foci formation caused by the iatrogenic CTC spillage from a primary tumor may occur fairly infrequently.

We could not find any association of intraoperative CTC increases with perioperative clinicopathological features in the present study. This may reflect the fact that all patients undergoing brachytherapy have a risk of intraoperative hematogenous spillage of prostate cancer cells, irrespective of use of neoadjuvant hormonal therapy, type of brachytherapy, age, PSA at diagnosis, Gleason score, clinical stage, and biopsy positive core rates. In our regiment of HDR brachytherapy for high-risk and locally advanced cancers, we administered at least 6 months of neoadjuvant androgen deprivation therapy (ADT). Nonetheless, intraoperative CTCs were detected in 13.3% of patients in that group. Although the use of neoadjuvant ADT may reduce the cellular viability of iatrogenic CTCs enough to prevent implantation into distant sites, this could not completely eliminate the hematogenous spillage of CTCs during the procedure.

Several potential limitations of this study must be considered. The sample size for the present study was not calculated to detect a statistical difference in clinical progression between patients with intraoperative CTC increases and those without increases. A large-scale study involving more patients is needed to clarify whether intraoperative CTC increases actually affect the postoperative progression. Second, samples for CTC detection were not drawn before neoadjuvant ADT in patients treated with HDR brachytherapy. These patients were classified with clinically high-risk or locally advanced cancer and were more likely to have occult distant metastasis than lower-risk patients. Some of these patients may have had positive status for CTC before neoadjuvant ADT [29]. In addition, samples for CTC detection were not drawn a few days or months after the brachytherapy procedures in patients with positive status for intraoperative CTCs [20]. Longer detection of CTCs may have a higher risk of later metastases than others. Third, the CellSearch System may lack sensitivity in nonmetastatic cancer patients and consequently underestimates the incidence of perioperative CTCs. In addition, this system only detects the epithelial cancer cells and does not detect the mesenchymal ones. In metastatic formation from primary epithelial cancers, epithelial–mesenchymal transition at primary sites is considered to be important for cancer metastasis [30,31]. This cellular transition allows epithelial cancer cells to acquire the more invasive characteristics. The mesenchymal cancer cells may have a higher metastatic potential than the epithelial ones. In future clinical series, the detection of such highly metastatic potential cells may be helpful in assessing the possibility of metastatic diseases caused by iatrogenic CTCs during prostate brachytherapy procedures.

4. Materials and Methods

4.1. Patient Selection

From October 2014 to July 2015, 59 patients with clinically nonmetastatic prostate cancer who underwent HDR or LDR brachytherapy participated in this prospective study. Thirty patients with high-risk or locally advanced prostate cancer were treated with HDR brachytherapy. Twenty-nine patients with clinically localized prostate cancer were treated with LDR brachytherapy. Samples of peripheral blood were drawn before insertion of needles (preoperative) and again immediately after the surgical manipulation (intraoperative) in each patient. Pretreatment evaluation included clinical history, physical examination, blood laboratory findings, pelvic computed tomography, pelvic magnetic resonance imaging, and a bone scan. Exclusion criteria were a history of cancer, previous surgery for benign prostatic hyperplasia, or concomitant active urinary tract infection. Patients who had a suspicious lesion of cancer other than prostate cancer on the pretreatment evaluation were also excluded. Patients were removed from the study if they wished to discontinue. All biopsy slides were reviewed by our institutional pathologists. Approval was granted by the ethics committee of our institution (B14-20), and all patients signed written informed consent.

4.2. HDR Brachytherapy and Blood Sample Collection

The protocol and procedure for HDR brachytherapy and hormonal therapy in high-risk or locally advanced prostate cancer were reported previously [5,32]. All patients underwent $\geq$6 months of neoadjuvant ADT, which combined nonsteroidal anti-androgen agents with luteinizing hormone-releasing hormone agonist injections. Either flutamide (375 mg/day) or bicalutamide (80 mg/day) were prescribed as the nonsteroidal anti-androgen agents. Either goserelin (10.8 mg/3 months or 3.6 mg/month) or leuprorelin (11.25 mg/3 months or 3.75 mg/month) were administrated as luteinizing hormone-releasing hormone agonist therapy.

In the operating room, preoperative samples of peripheral blood were drawn in a supine position before epidural anesthesia. Patients were then placed in a lithotomy position. Metallic marker seeds were placed transperineally into the base and apex for the purpose of image-guided external beam radiotherapy following HDR brachytherapy. Treatment was started using placement of a closed transperineal hollow needle under transrectal ultrasound guidance. Multiple 25 cm long, closed-end, 15-G plastic hollow needles were inserted transperineally using a 15-G Prostate Template (Best Medical International Inc., Springfield, VA, USA). Eighteen needles were routinely implanted. Flexible cystoscopy was conducted to check that the urethra had not been penetrated by the implanted needles. The needle tips were left within the urinary bladder, 15 mm above the sonographically or cystoscopically defined base of the prostate. Immediately after all of these procedures had been completed, intraoperative samples of peripheral blood were drawn from each patient again.

4.3. LDR Brachytherapy and Blood Sample Collection

The protocol and procedure for LDR brachytherapy were performed as previously reported [8]. No patients were treated with ADT and external beam radiation therapy before and after LDR brachytherapy.

In the operating room, preoperative samples of peripheral blood were drawn in a supine position before spinal anesthesia. Patients were then placed in a lithotomy position. Results of transrectal ultrasonography in the axial plane were imported into the VariSeed brachytherapy planning system (Varian Medical Systems, Palo Alto, CA, USA). The prostate, urethra, and rectal wall were contoured by radiation oncologists. Seed number and location for both peripheral and centrally located needles were determined manually. The prescribed dose was set at 145 Gy. Dose–volume histograms and isodose lines were evaluated based on predetermined dosimetric parameters. Needle insertion and implantation were done by urologists. As needed, modifications to the plan can be made, and the software recalculates the dose–volume histograms and isodose lines by using a real-time intraoperative dosimetry technique [7]. Patients were assigned to receive loose or intraoperatively built custom-linked (IBCL) seed brachytherapy based on the week of the month, with loose or IBCL seeds used during alternate weeks. In the present study, 14 and 15 patients were implanted with loose and IBCL seeds, respectively. Loose seeds were implanted using a Mick applicator (Mick Radio Nuclear Instruments, Mount Vernon, NY, USA). IBCL seeds were constructed using a Quicklink device (CR Bard, Covington, GA, USA) and implanted. Zauls et al. described the detailed mechanisms of constructing IBCL seeds [33], and we applied the same devices in our study. Immediately after all seeds had been implanted, intraoperative samples of peripheral blood were drawn from each patient.

4.4. CTC Detection

Twenty milliliters of peripheral blood was collected into 10 mL CellSave Preservation Tubes (Immunicon, Hatboro, PA, USA), which contained ethylenediaminetetraacetic acid (EDTA) as an anticoagulant and a cellular preservative. Samples were maintained at room temperature and processed within 72 h of collection. Blood samples of 7.5 mL were analyzed for CTCs.

The CellSearch system was used for the isolation and enumeration of CTCs. This system consists of the CellTracks AutoPrep and the CellTracks Analyzer II unit (Veridex LLC, Raritan, NJ, USA). The AutoPrep is a semiautomated sample preparation for the isolation of CTCs. The procedure enriches the sample for cells expressing epithelial cell adhesion molecule (EpCAM) using antibody-coated magnetic beads. After the magnetic separation, these cells were stained with the fluorescent nucleic acid dye 4′,6-diamidino-2-phenylindole (DAPI) and fluorescently labeled with anticytokeratin 8,18,19-phycoerythrin peridinin and anti-CD45 chlorophyll protein to distinguish epithelial cells from leukocytes. The stained and fluorescently labeled cells were analyzed for the identification of CTCs using the Analyzer II (Veridex LLC). The criteria for CTC included positive staining for DAPI and the cytokeratin and negative staining for the CD45. A CTC must show round or oval morphology.

4.5. Statistical Analysis

The primary outcome measures were changes in CTC detection rates from preoperative to intraoperative blood samples. As secondary outcome measures, incidence of increase in the intraoperative CTC count relative to the preoperative one was tested for association with clinicopathological and perioperative variables. For the purpose of analysis, clinicopathological and perioperative variables including age (>70 vs. ≤70), PSA at diagnosis (≥10 ng/mL vs. <10 ng/mL), Gleason score (≥8 vs. ≤7), clinical T stage (T1c–2c vs. T3a–4), biopsy positive core rates (>34% vs. ≤34%), prostate volume at brachytherapy (>25 cc vs. ≤25 cc), and NCCN risk criteria 2015 (high/very high vs. intermediate/low) were evaluated as dichotomous variables. A Fisher's exact test was used to evaluate the primary and secondary outcome measures.

Sample size calculations determined that 60 patients would be needed to detect a 15% rise from preoperative to intraoperative CTC detection rates with α equal to 0.05 and power equal to 80%. A rise from preoperative to intraoperative CTC detection rates was estimated from the first 30 cases in this study.

Differences were regarded as statistically significant at the $p < 0.05$ level. Analyses were performed using SPSS, version 11.0 for Windows (SPSS, Inc., Chicago, IL, USA) and Microsoft Excel (Microsoft, Redmond, WA, USA).

5. Conclusions

We detected CTCs from samples immediately after insertion of needles in patients undergoing prostate brachytherapy for clinically nonmetastatic prostate cancer. Further research is needed to assess whether those cancer cells actually can survive and proliferate at distant sites. Although the brachytherapy approaches have demonstrated favorable long-term outcomes [6], understanding the mechanism of relapse should lead to the better treatment outcomes in patients undergoing prostate brachytherapy.

Acknowledgments: This work was supported by JSPS KAKENHI Grant Number 26861293 and The Japanese Foundation of Prostate Research.

Author Contributions: Hideyasu Tsumura was mainly collecting data and samples, writing the manuscript and performing the treatment as urologist; Takefumi Satoh was conceived of and designed the experiments; Ken-ichi Tabata was mainly involved in performance of statistics and performing the treatment as urologist; Hiromichi Ishiyama, Kouji Takenaka, Akane Sekiguchi and Masashi Kitano were performing the treatment as radio-oncologists and collecting data; Masaki Nakamura was supervisor of performing the experiments; Kazushige Hayakawa and Masatsugu Iwamura were supervisor of writing the manuscript.

Abbreviations

LDR	low-dose-rate
HDR	high-dose-rate
CTC	circulating tumor cell
PSA	prostate-specific antigen
NCCN	National Comprehensive Cancer Network
TURP	transurethral resection of prostate
PSMA	prostate-specific membrane antigen
ADT	androgen deprivation therapy
IBCL	intraoperatively built custom-linked
EpCAM	expressing epithelial cell adhesion molecule
DAPI	4′,6-diamidino-2-phenylindole

References

1. Zelefsky, M.J.; Kuban, D.A.; Levy, L.B.; Potters, L.; Beyer, D.C.; Blasko, J.C.; Moran, B.J.; Ciezki, J.P.; Zietman, A.L.; Pisansky, T.M.; et al. Multi-institutional analysis of long-term outcome for stages T1-T2 prostate cancer treated with permanent seed implantation. *Int. J. Radiat. Oncol. Biol. Phys.* **2007**, *67*, 327–333. [CrossRef] [PubMed]
2. Stone, N.N.; Stock, R.G.; Cesaretti, J.A.; Unger, P. Local control following permanent prostate brachytherapy: Effect of high biologically effective dose on biopsy results and oncologic outcomes. *Int. J. Radiat. Oncol. Biol. Phys.* **2010**, *76*, 355–360. [CrossRef] [PubMed]
3. Hoskin, P.J.; Rojas, A.M.; Bownes, P.J.; Lowe, G.J.; Ostler, P.J.; Bryant, L. Randomised trial of external beam radiotherapy alone or combined with high-dose-rate brachytherapy boost for localised prostate cancer. *Radiother. Oncol.* **2012**, *103*, 217–222. [CrossRef] [PubMed]
4. Prada, P.J.; Gonzalez, H.; Fernandez, J.; Jimenez, I.; Iglesias, A.; Romo, I. Biochemical outcome after high-dose-rate intensity modulated brachytherapy with external beam radiotherapy: 12 Years of experience. *BJU Int.* **2012**, *109*, 1787–1793. [CrossRef] [PubMed]
5. Ishiyama, H.; Satoh, T.; Kitano, M.; Tabata, K.; Komori, S.; Ikeda, M.; Soda, I.; Kurosaka, S.; Sekiguchi, A.; Kimura, M.; et al. High-dose-rate brachytherapy and hypofractionated external beam radiotherapy combined with long-term hormonal therapy for high-risk and very high-risk prostate cancer: Outcomes after 5-year follow-up. *J. Radiat. Res.* **2014**, *55*, 509–517. [CrossRef] [PubMed]
6. Grimm, P.; Billiet, I.; Bostwick, D.; Dicker, A.P.; Frank, S.; Immerzeel, J.; Keyes, M.; Kupelian, P.; Lee, W.R.; Machtens, S.; et al. Comparative analysis of prostate-specific antigen free survival outcomes for patients with low, intermediate and high risk prostate cancer treatment by radical therapy: Results from the prostate cancer results study group. *BJU Int.* **2012**, *109*, 22–29. [CrossRef] [PubMed]
7. Stock, R.G.; Stone, N.N.; Wesson, M.F.; DeWyngaert, J.K. A modified technique allowing interactive ultrasound-guided three-dimensional transperineal prostate implantation. *Int. J. Radiat. Oncol. Biol. Phys.* **1995**, *32*, 219–225. [CrossRef]
8. Ishiyama, H.; Satoh, T.; Kawakami, S.; Tsumura, H.; Komori, S.; Tabata, K.; Sekiguchi, A.; Takahashi, R.; Soda, I.; Takenaka, K.; et al. A prospective quasi-randomized comparison of intraoperatively built custom-linked seeds versus loose seeds for prostate brachytherapy. *Int. J. Radiat. Oncol. Biol. Phys.* **2014**, *90*, 134–139. [CrossRef] [PubMed]
9. Yoshioka, Y.; Suzuki, O.; Otani, Y.; Yoshida, K.; Nose, T.; Ogawa, K. High-dose-rate brachytherapy as monotherapy for prostate cancer: Technique, rationale and perspective. *J. Contemp. Brachytherapy* **2014**, *6*, 91–98. [CrossRef] [PubMed]
10. Morton, G.C. High-dose-rate brachytherapy boost for prostate cancer: Rationale and technique. *J. Contemp. Brachytherapy* **2014**, *6*, 323–330. [CrossRef] [PubMed]
11. Sekiguchi, A.; Ishiyama, H.; Satoh, T.; Tabata, K.; Komori, S.; Tsumura, H.; Kawakami, S.; Soda, I.; Iwamura, M.; Hayakawa, K. 125Iodine monotherapy for Japanese men with low- and intermediate-risk prostate cancer: Outcomes after 5 years of follow-up. *J. Radiat. Res.* **2014**, *55*, 328–333. [CrossRef] [PubMed]
12. Aoki, M.; Miki, K.; Kido, M.; Sasaki, H.; Nakamura, W.; Kijima, Y.; Kobayashi, M.; Egawa, S.; Kanehira, C. Analysis of prognostic factors in localized high-risk prostate cancer patients treated with HDR brachytherapy, hypofractionated 3D-CRT and neoadjuvant/adjuvant androgen deprivation therapy (trimodality therapy). *J. Radiat. Res.* **2014**, *55*, 527–532. [CrossRef] [PubMed]
13. Levine, E.S.; Cisek, V.J.; Mulvihill, M.N.; Cohen, E.L. Role of transurethral resection in dissemination of cancer of prostate. *Urology* **1986**, *28*, 179–183. [CrossRef]
14. Hayashi, N.; Egami, H.; Kai, M.; Kurusu, Y.; Takano, S.; Ogawa, M. No-touch isolation technique reduces intraoperative shedding of tumor cells into the portal vein during resection of colorectal cancer. *Surgery* **1999**, *125*, 369–374. [CrossRef]
15. Wiggers, T.; Jeekel, J.; Arends, J.W.; Brinkhorst, A.P.; Kluck, H.M.; Luyk, C.I.; Munting, J.D.; Povel, J.A.; Rutten, A.P.; Volovics, A.; et al. No-touch isolation technique in colon cancer: A controlled prospective trial. *Br. J. Surg.* **1988**, *75*, 409–415. [CrossRef] [PubMed]
16. Liu, C.L.; Fan, S.T.; Lo, C.M.; Tung-Ping Poon, R.; Wong, J. Anterior approach for major right hepatic resection for large hepatocellular carcinoma. *Ann. Surg.* **2000**, *232*, 25–31. [CrossRef] [PubMed]

17. Gall, T.M.; Jacob, J.; Frampton, A.E.; Krell, J.; Kyriakides, C.; Castellano, L.; Stebbing, J.; Jiao, L.R. Reduced dissemination of circulating tumor cells with no-touch isolation surgical technique in patients with pancreatic cancer. *JAMA Surg.* **2014**, *149*, 482–485. [CrossRef] [PubMed]
18. Giesing, M.; Suchy, B.; Driesel, G.; Molitor, D. Clinical utility of antioxidant gene expression levels in circulating cancer cell clusters for the detection of prostate cancer in patients with prostate-specific antigen levels of 4–10 ng/mL and disease prognostication after radical prostatectomy. *BJU Int.* **2010**, *105*, 1000–1010. [CrossRef] [PubMed]
19. Forsythe, K.; Burri, R.; Stone, N.; Stock, R.G. Predictors of metastatic disease after prostate brachytherapy. *Int. J. Radiat. Oncol. Biol. Phys.* **2012**, *83*, 645–652. [CrossRef] [PubMed]
20. Eschwege, P.; Dumas, F.; Blanchet, P.; le Maire, V.; Benoit, G.; Jardin, A.; Lacour, B.; Loric, S. Haematogenous dissemination of prostatic epithelial cells during radical prostatectomy. *Lancet* **1995**, *346*, 1528–1530. [CrossRef]
21. Badwe, R.A.; Vaidya, J.S. Haematogenous dissemination of prostate epithelial cells during surgery. *Lancet* **1996**, *347*, 325–326. [PubMed]
22. Davis, J.W.; Nakanishi, H.; Kumar, V.S.; Bhadkamkar, V.A.; McCormack, R.; Fritsche, H.A.; Handy, B.; Gornet, T.; Babaian, R.J. Circulating tumor cells in peripheral blood samples from patients with increased serum prostate specific antigen: Initial results in early prostate cancer. *J. Urol.* **2008**, *179*, 2187–2191. [CrossRef] [PubMed]
23. Eschwege, P.; Moutereau, S.; Droupy, S.; Douard, R.; Gala, J.L.; Benoit, G.; Conti, M.; Manivet, P.; Loric, S. Prognostic value of prostate circulating cells detection in prostate cancer patients: A prospective study. *Br. J. Cancer* **2009**, *100*, 608–610. [CrossRef] [PubMed]
24. Kauffman, E.C.; Lee, M.J.; Alarcon, S.V.; Lee, S.; Hoang, A.N.; Walton Diaz, A.; Chelluri, R.; Vourganti, S.; Trepel, J.B.; Pinto, P.A. Lack of impact of robotic-assisted laparoscopic radical prostatectomy on intraoperative levels of prostate cancer circulating tumor cells. *J. Urol.* **2015**, *195*, 1936–1942. [CrossRef] [PubMed]
25. Hara, N.; Kasahara, T.; Kawasaki, T.; Bilim, V.; Tomita, Y.; Obara, K.; Takahashi, K. Frequency of PSA-mRNA-bearing cells in the peripheral blood of patients after prostate biopsy. *Br. J. Cancer* **2001**, *85*, 557–562. [CrossRef] [PubMed]
26. Fidler, I.J. Selection of successive tumour lines for metastasis. *Nat. New Biol.* **1973**, *242*, 148–149. [CrossRef] [PubMed]
27. Yokota, J. Tumor progression and metastasis. *Carcinogenesis* **2000**, *21*, 497–503. [CrossRef] [PubMed]
28. Mareel, M.M.; van Roy, F.M.; Bracke, M.E. How and when do tumor cells metastasize? *Crit. Rev. Oncog.* **1993**, *4*, 559–594. [PubMed]
29. Meyer, C.P.; Pantel, K.; Tennstedt, P.; Stroelin, P.; Schlomm, T.; Heinzer, H.; Riethdorf, S.; Steuber, T. Limited prognostic value of preoperative circulating tumor cells for early biochemical recurrence in patients with localized prostate cancer. *Urol. Oncol.* **2016**, *34*, 211–236. [CrossRef] [PubMed]
30. Tsai, J.H.; Donaher, J.L.; Murphy, D.A.; Chau, S.; Yang, J. Spatiotemporal regulation of epithelial-mesenchymal transition is essential for squamous cell carcinoma metastasis. *Cancer Cell* **2012**, *22*, 725–736. [CrossRef] [PubMed]
31. Sethi, S.; Macoska, J.; Chen, W.; Sarkar, F.H. Molecular signature of epithelial-mesenchymal transition (EMT) in human prostate cancer bone metastasis. *Am. J. Transl. Res.* **2010**, *3*, 90–99. [PubMed]
32. Tsumura, H.; Satoh, T.; Ishiyama, H.; Tabata, K.; Komori, S.; Sekiguchi, A.; Ikeda, M.; Kurosaka, S.; Fujita, T.; Kitano, M.; et al. Prostate-specific antigen nadir after high-dose-rate brachytherapy predicts long-term survival outcomes in high-risk prostate cancer. *J. Contemp. Brachytherapy* **2016**, *8*, 95–103. [CrossRef] [PubMed]
33. Zauls, A.J.; Ashenafi, M.S.; Onicescu, G.; Clarke, H.S.; Marshall, D.T. Comparison of intraoperatively built custom linked seeds versus loose seed gun applicator technique using real-time intraoperative planning for permanent prostate brachytherapy. *Int. J. Radiat. Oncol. Biol. Phys.* **2011**, *81*, 1010–1016. [CrossRef] [PubMed]

13

Sensitivity of HOXB13 as a Diagnostic Immunohistochemical Marker of Prostatic Origin in Prostate Cancer Metastases: Comparison to PSA, Prostein, Androgen Receptor, *ERG*, *NKX3.1*, PSAP and PSMA

Ilka Kristiansen [1], Carsten Stephan [2], Klaus Jung [3], Manfred Dietel [4], Anja Rieger [4], Yuri Tolkach [1,†] and Glen Kristiansen [1,*,†]

1 Institute of Pathology, University Hospital Bonn, 53127 Bonn, Germany; ilka.kristiansen@gmx.de (I.K.); Yuri.tolkach@ukbonn.de (Y.T.)
2 Department of Urology, Charité-Universitätsmedizin Berlin, 10117 Berlin, Germany; carsten.stephan@charite.de
3 Berlin Institute of Urologic Research, 10117 Berlin, Germany; klaus.jung@charite.de
4 Institute of Pathology, Charité-Universitätsmedizin Berlin, 10117 Berlin, Germany; Manfred.dietel@charite.de (M.D.); Anja.rieger@charite.de (A.R.)
* Correspondence: glen.kristiansen@ukbonn.de
† These authors contributed equally to this work.

Academic Editor: William Chi-shing Cho

Abstract: Aims: Determining the origin of metastases is an important task of pathologists to allow for the initiation of a tumor-specific therapy. Recently, homeobox protein Hox-B13 (HOXB13) has been suggested as a new marker for the detection of prostatic origin. The aim of this study was to evaluate the diagnostic sensitivity of HOXB13 in comparison to commonly used immunohistochemical markers for prostate cancer. Materials and methods: Histologically confirmed prostate cancer lymph node metastases from 64 cases were used to test the diagnostic value of immunohistochemical markers: prostate specific antigen (PSA), Prostatic acid phosphatase (PSAP), prostate specific membrane antigen (PSMA), homeobox gene *NKX3.1*, prostein, androgen receptor (AR), HOXB13, and ETS-related gene (ERG). All markers were evaluated semi-quantitatively using Remmele's immune reactive score. Results: The detection rate of prostate origin of metastasis for single markers was 100% for NKX3.1, 98.1% for AR, 84.3% for PSMA, 80.8% for PSA, 66% for PSAP, 60.4% for HOXB13, 59.6% for prostein, and 50.0% for ERG. Conclusions: Our data suggest that HOXB13 on its own lacks sensitivity for the detection of prostatic origin. Therefore, this marker should be only used in conjunction with other markers, preferably the highly specific PSA. The combination of PSA with NKX3.1 shows a higher sensitivity and thus appears preferable in this setting.

Keywords: prostate cancer; metastasis; immunohistochemistry; detection; PSA; PSAP; PSMA; NKX3.1; prostein; HOXB13; ERG; AR

1. Introduction

Determining the origin of the primary tumor in metastases is an important task of pathologists to allow for the initiation of a tumor-specific therapy. Since its description in the 1970s, prostate specific antigen (PSA) has in due course become the dominant prostate marker in serum [1,2]. PSA could be detected by immunohistochemistry in tissue and was quickly adopted by pathologists as a diagnostic marker [3,4]. PSA is still regarded as a highly specific marker of prostatic origin, but due to its decreased or even lost expression in higher grade or metastatic tumors, which was already noted in initial studies, its sensitivity is clearly limited, which necessitates the use of additional markers in PSA negative cases [5]. Prostein, coded by the *SLC45A3* gene and identified by transcript profiling studies of prostate cancer, was found to be highly specific for prostatic origin and displays a characteristic Golgi-type cytoplasmic staining pattern [6,7]. As seen with PSA, prostein expression also shows a slightly diminished expression with tumor progression, but in combination with PSA it proved to be a valuable tool to identify prostatic origin [8,9]. An alternative marker for prostatic origin was the protein coded by the homeobox gene *NKX3.1*, which shows nuclear staining on immunohistochemistry and which was also found to be highly though not exclusively specific for prostate tissues [10,11]. At the 2014 consensus conference of the International Society of Urological Pathology (ISUP), it was recommended to use immunohistochemistry for PSA, NKX3.1 and prostein to ascertain a prostatic origin in doubtful cases [5].

Another diagnostic candidate marker that was not considered at that conference was homeobox protein Hox-B13 (HOXB13), which was characterized as a marker for prostate cancer by Edwards et al. [12]. HOXB13 also has a nuclear staining pattern and has been recommended by several studies as a prostate specific marker [13–16]. To date, the diagnostic value and especially the performance of HOXB13 immunohistochemistry as a marker of prostatic origin in direct comparison to the commonly used prostate markers (PSA, prostein, ERG, the androgen receptor (AR), NKX3.1, Prostatic acid phosphatase (PSAP) and prostate specific membrane antigen (PSMA)) in metastases has not been evaluated, which was therefore the aim of this study.

2. Results

2.1. Immunohistochemical Staining Patterns

All markers showed the expected patterns of immunoreactivity in metastatic prostate cancer. Prostate specific antigen (PSA) and prostatic phosphatase (PSAP) displayed diffuse cytoplasmic staining (Figure 1A,C), where prostein showed the characteristic Golgi-type staining (Figure 1B). Prostate specific membrane antigen (PSMA, Figure 1D) showed a predominantly membranous but also cytoplasmic immunoreactivity. Nuclear staining was seen for the androgen receptor (AR), ERG, NKX3.1, and HOXB13 (Figure 1E–H).

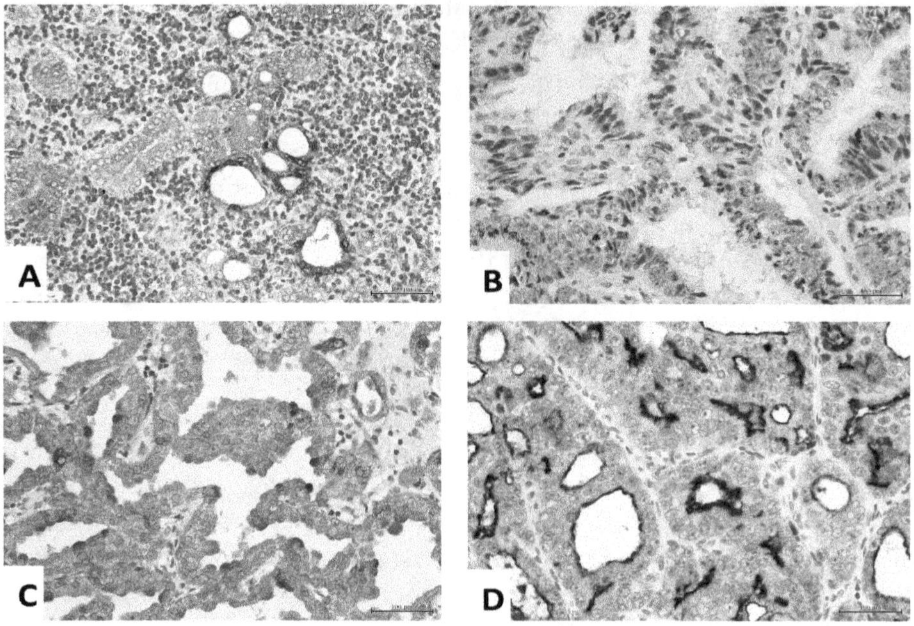

Figure 1. *Cont.*

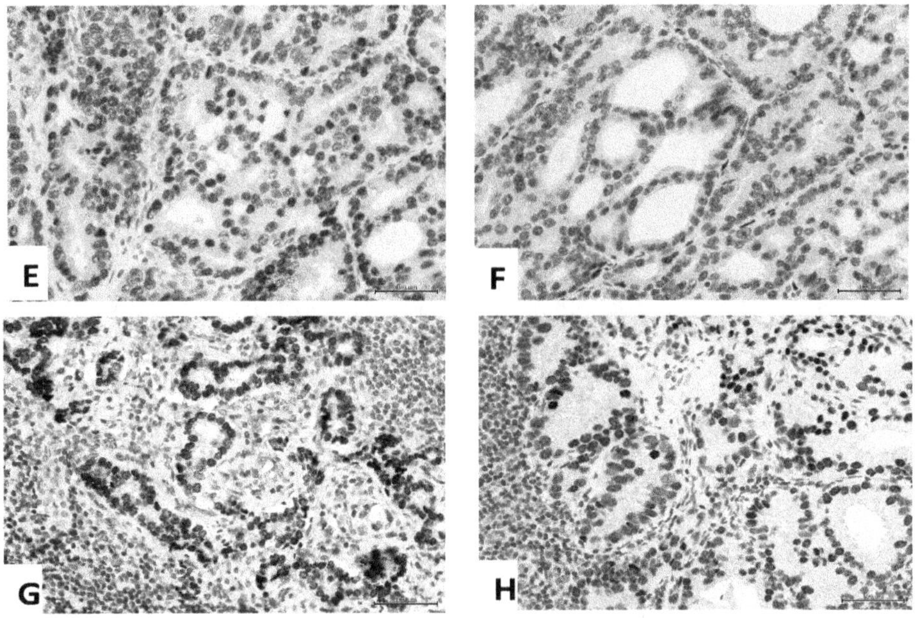

Figure 1. Immunohistochemistry of candidate diagnostic prostate markers. (**A**) Prostate specific antigen (PSA) shows diffuse cytoplasmic staining with a higher degree of heterogeneity in this case. (**B**) Prostein immunoreactivity is restricted to the Golgi apparatus area. (**C**) Prostate specific alkaline phosphatase (PSAP) also displays a diffuse cytoplasmic staining pattern. (**D**) Prostate specific membrane antigen (PSMA) has characteristic cytoplasmic but also membranous staining. (**E**) Androgen receptor shows epithelial nuclear staining. (**F**) ERG is also located in the nucleus and has a higher degree of heterogeneity, as seen here. (**G**) Homeobox gene *NKX3.1* commonly displays strong nuclear staining. (**H**) Homeobox protein HOXB3 is also seen in nuclei, however, the staining intensity is weaker. All images are taken in 400×.

2.2. Statistical Evaluation of Prostate Markers

The highest detection rate was seen with NKX3.1 followed by the androgen receptor and PSMA. PSA, as the most commonly used antibody to specifically recognize prostate cancer, correctly detected nearly 81% of cases. ERG labeled, as expected, only 50% of prostate cancer metastases. Prostein, PSAP, and HOXB13 were only slightly superior, detecting approximately two thirds of cases (Table 1).

Table 1. Detection rates of prostate markers in prostate cancer metastases.

Marker	Detection Rate (%)	Mean IRS	Number of Cases
PSA	80.8	6.3	52
PSAP	66.0	3.5	53
PSMA	84.3	6.0	51
Prostein	59.6	4.2	52
Androgen receptor (AR)	98.1	6.7	53
ERG	50.0	2.6	52
NKX3.1	100.0	8.0	50
HOXB13	60.4	4.7	53

Abbreviations: IRS = immunoreactive Score according to Remmele.

A Spearman rank correlation analysis of IRS values of these markers revealed the following significant associations: AR and HOXB13 (correlation coefficient (CC) = 0.358, $p = 0.009$), AR and NKX3.1 (CC = 0.505, $p = 0.001$), AR and PSAP (CC = −0.277, $p = 0.047$), ERG and HOXB13 (CC = 0.283, $p = 0.044$), PSA and Prostein (CC = 0.367, $p = 0.008$), PSA and PSAP (CC = 0.623, $p = 0.001$), PSA and PSMA (CC = 0.350, $p = 0.012$), prostein and PSAP (CC = 0.277, $p = 0.049$), and prostein and HOXB13 (CC = −0.296, $p = 0.035$).

We then investigated which combination of prostate markers would achieve the highest detection rate by combining the most commonly used marker PSA with the other markers in cross tables. PSAP recognized 10% of PSA negative cases, which did not add significant information. PSMA performed slightly better, labelling 50% of PSA negative cases. HOXB13 correctly recognized 70%, and finally *NKX3.1* correctly detected all PSA negative cases, leading to a detection rate (of the combination of PSA and *NKX3.1*) of 100% in this dataset. Prostein and PSA correctly detected 82% of cases, HOXB13 and PSA labeled 94.2% of cases correctly, AR and PSA detected 100% of cases, and ERG and PSA recognized 88% of prostate cancer metastases.

In a direct analysis of HOXB13 and NKX3.1 expression, both markers together recognized 100%, as NKX3.1 labeled 100% of HOXB13 negative cases. NKX3.1 combined with AR also achieved a detection rate of 100%.

3. Material and Methods

3.1. Case Selection and Construction of Tissue Microarray

First, prostate cancer patients who underwent radical prostatectomy (RP) and lymphadenectomy and who were diagnosed at the Institute of Pathology, Charité–Universitätsmedizin Berlin between 1998 and 2005 were identified. Histologically confirmed metastases from 64 cases were used for tissue microarray construction with one spot per case and a punch size of 1 mm. The tissue microarray comprised of two blocks. The metastases consisted of 57 local lymph node metastases and seven systemic metastases (4× bone, 1× penis, 1× oral mucosa, 1× cervical lymph node). Lymph nodes were submitted to frozen section analysis prior to RP, which was usually not performed in case of a positive node. Only 13 RPs were performed. Therefore, histopathological RP data on the primary tumor was not available for the majority of cases. For the thirteen RP cases that were completed, the Gleason scores (GS) were: GS7-2, GS8-4, GS9-4, GS10-3. The pT categories (according to Union for International Cancer Control (UICC) TNM classification of malignant tumors, 8th edition) were: pT2-2, pT3a-1, pT3b-10. Positive margins were seen in 11 cases. The bilateral lymphonodectomy specimens ($n = 57$) contained a median of 12 lymph nodes (range 1 to 23). Twenty-nine cases had a single positive lymph node, 15 cases had two metastases, seven cases had three metastases and six cases had four or more positive nodes (maximum 11). The use of this tissue was approved by the Charité University Ethics Committee (EA1/06/2004). No animals were involved in this study.

3.2. Immunohistochemistry

Immunohistochemistry was conducted using semi-automated platforms (Benchmark Ultra, Roche, and Autostainer, Medac) with protocols that are in routine use at the Institute of Pathology, University of Bonn (Table 2).

Table 2. Antibodies used for immunohistochemistry in this study.

Antigen	Clone	Provider	Dilution	Platform	Protocol
PSA	Polyclonal, rabbit	DAKO	1:20,000	Autostainer	No pretreatment
PSAP	PASE/4LJ	Cell Marque	1:6000	Autostainer	HIER (pH 6, 20 s 98 °C)
PSMA	3E6	DAKO	1:500	Benchmark	CC1 (pH 8), ultraview
Prostein	10E3	DAKO	1:100	Benchmark	CC1 (pH 8), ultraview
Androgen Receptor (AR)	AR441	DAKO	1:400	Autostainer	HIER (pH 6, 20 s 98 °C)
ERG	EPR3864	Biologo	1:100	Autostainer	HIER (pH 6, 20 s 98 °C)
NKX3.1	EP356	Cell Marque	1:200	Benchmark	CC1 (pH 8), ultraview
HOXB13	F-9	Santa Cruz	1:50	Benchmark	CC1 (pH 8), optiview

Abbreviations: HIER-Heat Induced Epitope Retrieval.

3.3. Evaluation of Immunohistochemistry

All markers were evaluated semi-quantitatively using the immune reactive score (IRS), which gives the product of categorized percentage of stained cells (0: negative, 1: 1–10%, 2: 11–50%, 3:

51–80%, and 4: >80%) and staining intensity (ranging from negative (0) to strong (3)), and hence has a range from 0 to 12. For statistical evaluation, an IRS below 3 was considered a negative test and higher values were considered as positive, as suggested by Remmele and Stegner in their original proposal of the IRS scoring system [17]. The evaluation was carried out under the immediate supervision of a Genito–Urinary pathologist with broad expertise in immunohistochemistry (Glen Kristiansen).

3.4. Statistics

All data were processed using SPSS (IBM SPSS Statistics for Macintosh, Version 22.0, IBM Corp., Armonk, NY, USA). Spearman Rank correlations were used to analyze the associations among markers.

4. Discussion

This study evaluates the sensitivity of prostate markers to detect lymph node and distant metastases of prostate cancer. It confirms that PSA, as the most commonly used antibody for routine purposes, has a relatively high detection rate of nearly 81%. The value of PSA is its high specificity, as apart from prostate cancer only breast cancer may be PSA positive, but this is usually not in the closer differential diagnosis [18]. The loss of PSA expression with tumor dedifferentiation and progression is long known and constitutes the necessity to use other markers in a combination.

As prostate cancer is an androgen-driven disease, the high rates of androgen receptor expression found in primary and metastatic prostate tumors are not surprising, and again this study confirms that metastases retain their AR expression well. The disadvantage of AR is the relative lack of specificity, as other neoplasms including urothelial carcinoma or salivary gland tumors may also be AR positive [19,20].

The overexpression of ERG, often resulting from the Transmembrane protease, serine 2-erythroblast transformation-specific-related gene TMPRSS2-ERG translocation which is found in nearly half of primary prostate cancer cases, is therefore typical of prostate cancer, but with a detection rate of 50% it clearly lacks sensitivity [21]. It is less well known that even though the genomic translocation is highly specific for prostate cancer, ERG protein expression is seen in a variety of other tumors, too. This includes, apart from vascular tumors, round cell sarcomas and leukemias, the more common differential diagnosis of urothelial carcinoma and, according to the human protein atlas (hppt://www.proteinatlas.org), also melanoma, testicular, and gastrointestinal tumors [22–24].

Prostein was described and characterized by Xu et al. as a prostate specific protein, which was quickly used by surgical pathologists for the differential diagnosis of prostate cancer, especially to rule out urothelial carcinoma, which is almost consistently prostein-negative [6,7,9,25,26]. Prostein also has the advantage of a distinctive Golgi-type staining pattern, which can be reassuring in cases with only weak positivity. In primary prostate cancer, prostein expression is inversely correlated with Gleason scores and is a prognostic marker of disease progression [27]. As our study confirms, the sensitivity of prostein in metastases is fairly limited with a detection rate of 59%, and even in conjunction with PSA only 82% of cases can be confirmed as prostatic in origin, which equals the detection rate of PSA alone in our cohort. As we found that both markers correlated, this redundancy of diagnostic information is not surprising. The same holds true for PSAP, which we found strongly and highly positively correlated to PSA, and this did not add significant information as only 10% of PSA negative cases were picked up by PSAP. A larger cohort may be necessary to demonstrate the additional diagnostic value of prostein or PSAP to PSA.

Prostate specific membrane antigen (PSMA) is overexpressed during tumor progression, and Bostwick et al. found 82% positivity rates in primary prostate cancer [28]. However, despite its name it is not prostate specific at all, but is also seen in a wide variety of tumors including colon, bladder, and renal cancer, so its use as a marker for prostatic differentiation is now discouraged [29].

NKX3.1 is a homeobox gene that shows a prostate and testis specific expression pattern, but may also be found in breast cancer. Its crisp nuclear staining pattern and its high rate of positivity in metastases (98.6%, Gurel et al. [30]), which this study confirms, have made it a popular diagnostic marker that is already endorsed by ISUP in their recommendations on diagnostic markers for genito–urinary pathology [11,30–33]. In particular, its combination with PSA is promising, as the high detection rate of 100% found in this study witnesses.

HOXB13 is another, so far less acknowledged diagnostic marker candidate, which has been recommended lately as a prostate specific marker [12,13,15,16]. Barresi et al. analyzed 15 prostate cancer metastases and found all of them strongly positive (in >75% of tumor cells) which equates a sensitivity of 100% [15]. Minimally lower rates were reported by Varinot et al., who analyzed 74 cases of lymph node metastases and 15 additional bone metastases. They found HOXB13 positivity in 33% of bone metastases and 93% of lymph node metastases. Interestingly, the expression of HOXB13 was also found as an independent prognostic marker in primary prostate cancer and to correlate with AR expression [14]. While our study confirms the significant association with AR, the diagnostic value of HOBX13 appears less convincing, as only 60.4% of prostate cancer metastases were positively stained. Of course, besides aspects of cohort composition that may influence the tumor biology, technical issues of the immunohistochemistry protocol or the tissue micro array construction may also explain this rather significant discrepancy. This detection rate increased markedly to 94.2% if combined with PSA, but it remains inferior to the combination of PSA with NKX3.1. HOXB13 is also expressed in other carcinomas including endometrial cancer, which in itself does not limit its diagnostic value, but also in pancreatic cancer and hepatocellular carcinoma [34–36]. In light of these data, we do not recommend HOXB13 as a sole marker to detect a prostatic origin in a metastasis, but rather prefer PSA in conjunction with NKX3.1. However, prostein or HOXB13 may well be considered as third line markers in doubtful cases, and here combinations are advisable and often necessary [5,37].

This study has several weaknesses. The number of cases is relatively small, which precludes a more detailed analysis of combinational subgroups. Still, the cohort size is large enough to confirm the known expression rates of the markers under question and it is the first study to critically analyze HOXB13 in direct comparison to these other markers in prostate cancer metastases. This study is restricted to the correct detection of prostate markers in known prostate metastases and hence only evaluates the sensitivity of these markers. Also, this study lacks data on the Gleason scores of biopsies of primary tumors, which precludes further correlation analyses of biomarker expression. Finally, we did not aim to verify the specificity of our candidate biomarkers, which would have necessitated an additional large analysis of non-prostatic neoplasms [38].

In summary, our data suggest that the novel marker candidate HOXB13 alone is not a good diagnostic marker for the detection of prostatic origin. Only in combination with PSA does it achieve satisfactory detection rates. Alternatively, the combination of PSA with the already well-established marker NKX3.1 shows an even higher sensitivity and is therefore recommended in this setting.

Acknowledgments: We are greatly indebted to the Sonnenfeldstiftung, Berlin, who funded the tissue microarrayer. We thank Britta Beyer for excellent technical support and Alfred E. Neumann for his enduring sense of humour and constructive discussions.

Author Contributions: Ilka Kristiansen collected data, prepared the statistics and wrote the paper; Carsten Stephan and Klaus Jung provided clinical information, supervised the statistics and revised the paper; Manfred Dietel and Anja Rieger provided tissues and clinico-pathological data, constructed the tissue micro array (TMA) and revised the paper; Yuri Tolkach and Glen Kristiansen conceived the study, conducted the central review of tissues on the TMA, performed the statistics and supervised writing of the paper and its revision.

References

1. Ablin, R.J.; Bronson, P.; Soanes, W.A.; Witebsky, E. Tissue- and species-specific antigens of normal human prostatic tissue. *J. Immunol.* **1970**, *104*, 1329–1339. [PubMed]
2. Frankel, A.E.; Rouse, R.V.; Wang, M.C.; Chu, T.M.; Herzenberg, L.A. Monoclonal antibodies to a human prostate antigen. *Cancer Res.* **1982**, *42*, 3714–3718. [PubMed]
3. Steffens, J.; Friedmann, W.; Lobeck, H. Immunohistochemical diagnosis of the metastasizing prostatic carcinoma. *Eur. Urol.* **1985**, *11*, 91–94. [PubMed]

4. Stein, B.S.; Vangore, S.; Petersen, R.O.; Kendall, A.R. Immunoperoxidase localization of prostate-specific antigen. *Am. J. Surg. Pathol.* **1982**, *6*, 553–557. [CrossRef] [PubMed]
5. Epstein, J.I.; Egevad, L.; Humphrey, P.A.; Montironi, R.; Members of the ISUP Immunohistochemistry in Diagnostic Urologic Pathology Group. Best practices recommendations in the application of immunohistochemistry in the prostate: Report from the international society of urologic pathology consensus conference. *Am. J. Surg. Pathol.* **2014**, *38*, e6–e19. [PubMed]
6. Kalos, M.; Askaa, J.; Hylander, B.L.; Repasky, E.A.; Cai, F.; Vedvick, T.; Reed, S.G.; Wright, G.L., Jr.; Fanger, G.R. Prostein expression is highly restricted to normal and malignant prostate tissues. *Prostate* **2004**, *60*, 246–256. [CrossRef] [PubMed]
7. Xu, J.; Kalos, M.; Stolk, J.A.; Zasloff, E.J.; Zhang, X.; Houghton, R.L.; Filho, A.M.; Nolasco, M.; Badaro, R.; Reed, S.G. Identification and characterization of prostein, a novel prostate-specific protein. *Cancer Res.* **2001**, *61*, 1563–1568. [PubMed]
8. Yin, M.; Dhir, R.; Parwani, A.V. Diagnostic utility of p501s (prostein) in comparison to prostate specific antigen (PSA) for the detection of metastatic prostatic adenocarcinoma. *Diagn. Pathol.* **2007**, *2*, 41. [CrossRef] [PubMed]
9. Sheridan, T.; Herawi, M.; Epstein, J.I.; Illei, P.B. The role of p501s and PSA in the diagnosis of metastatic adenocarcinoma of the prostate. *Am. J. Surg. Pathol.* **2007**, *31*, 1351–1355. [CrossRef] [PubMed]
10. He, W.W.; Sciavolino, P.J.; Wing, J.; Augustus, M.; Hudson, P.; Meissner, P.S.; Curtis, R.T.; Shell, B.K.; Bostwick, D.G.; Tindall, D.J.; et al. A novel human prostate-specific, androgen-regulated homeobox gene (*NKX3.1*) that maps to 8p21, a region frequently deleted in prostate cancer. *Genomics* **1997**, *43*, 69–77. [CrossRef] [PubMed]
11. Bowen, C.; Bubendorf, L.; Voeller, H.J.; Slack, R.; Willi, N.; Sauter, G.; Gasser, T.C.; Koivisto, P.; Lack, E.E.; Kononen, J.; et al. Loss of NKX3.1 expression in human prostate cancers correlates with tumor progression. *Cancer Res.* **2000**, *60*, 6111–6115. [PubMed]
12. Edwards, S.; Campbell, C.; Flohr, P.; Shipley, J.; Giddings, I.; Te-Poele, R.; Dodson, A.; Foster, C.; Clark, J.; Jhavar, S.; et al. Expression analysis onto microarrays of randomly selected cDNA clones highlights HOXB13 as a marker of human prostate cancer. *Br. J. Cancer* **2005**, *92*, 376–381. [CrossRef] [PubMed]
13. Varinot, J.; Cussenot, O.; Roupret, M.; Conort, P.; Bitker, M.O.; Chartier-Kastler, E.; Cheng, L.; Comperat, E. HOXB13 is a sensitive and specific marker of prostate cells, useful in distinguishing between carcinomas of prostatic and urothelial origin. *Virchows Arch.* **2013**, *463*, 803–809. [CrossRef] [PubMed]
14. Zabalza, C.V.; Adam, M.; Burdelski, C.; Wilczak, W.; Wittmer, C.; Kraft, S.; Krech, T.; Steurer, S.; Koop, C.; Hube-Magg, C.; et al. HOXB13 overexpression is an independent predictor of early PSA recurrence in prostate cancer treated by radical prostatectomy. *Oncotarget* **2015**, *6*, 12822–12834. [CrossRef] [PubMed]
15. Barresi, V.; Ieni, A.; Cardia, R.; Licata, L.; Vitarelli, E.; Reggiani Bonetti, L.; Tuccari, G. HOXB13 as an immunohistochemical marker of prostatic origin in metastatic tumors. *APMIS* **2016**, *124*, 188–193. [CrossRef] [PubMed]
16. Varinot, J.; Furudoi, A.; Drouin, S.; Phe, V.; Penna, R.R.; Roupret, M.; Bitker, M.O.; Cussenot, O.; Comperat, E. HOXB13 protein expression in metastatic lesions is a promising marker for prostate origin. *Virchows Arch.* **2016**, *468*, 619–622. [CrossRef] [PubMed]
17. Remmele, W.; Stegner, H.E. Recommendation for uniform definition of an immunoreactive score (IRS) for immunohistochemical estrogen receptor detection (ER-ICA) in breast cancer tissue. *Der. Pathol.* **1987**, *8*, 138–140.
18. Howarth, D.J.; Aronson, I.B.; Diamandis, E.P. Immunohistochemical localization of prostate-specific antigen in benign and malignant breast tissues. *Br. J. Cancer* **1997**, *75*, 1646–1651. [CrossRef] [PubMed]
19. Ide, H.; Inoue, S.; Miyamoto, H. Histopathological and prognostic significance of the expression of sex hormone receptors in bladder cancer: A meta-analysis of immunohistochemical studies. *PLoS ONE* **2017**, *12*, e0174746. [CrossRef] [PubMed]
20. Udager, A.M.; Chiosea, S.I. Salivary duct carcinoma: An update on morphologic mimics and diagnostic use of androgen receptor immunohistochemistry. *Head Neck Pathol.* **2017**. [CrossRef] [PubMed]
21. van Leenders, G.J.; Boormans, J.L.; Vissers, C.J.; Hoogland, A.M.; Bressers, A.A.; Furusato, B.; Trapman, J. Antibody EPR3864 is specific for *ERG* genomic fusions in prostate cancer: Implications for pathological practice. *Mod. Pathol.* **2011**, *24*, 1128–1138. [CrossRef] [PubMed]

22. Miettinen, M.; Wang, Z.F.; Paetau, A.; Tan, S.H.; Dobi, A.; Srivastava, S.; Sesterhenn, I. ERG transcription factor as an immunohistochemical marker for vascular endothelial tumors and prostatic carcinoma. *Am. J. Surg. Pathol.* **2011**, *35*, 432–441. [CrossRef] [PubMed]
23. Yamada, Y.; Kuda, M.; Kohashi, K.; Yamamoto, H.; Takemoto, J.; Ishii, T.; Iura, K.; Maekawa, A.; Bekki, H.; Ito, T.; et al. Histological and immunohistochemical characteristics of undifferentiated small round cell sarcomas associated with *CIC-DUX4* and *BCOR-CCNB3* fusion genes. *Virchows Arch.* **2017**, *470*, 373–380. [CrossRef] [PubMed]
24. Xu, B.; Naughton, D.; Busam, K.; Pulitzer, M. ERG is a useful immunohistochemical marker to distinguish leukemia cutis from nonneoplastic leukocytic infiltrates in the skin. *Am. J. Dermatopathol.* **2016**, *38*, 672–677. [CrossRef] [PubMed]
25. Chuang, A.Y.; DeMarzo, A.M.; Veltri, R.W.; Sharma, R.B.; Bieberich, C.J.; Epstein, J.I. Immunohistochemical differentiation of high-grade prostate carcinoma from urothelial carcinoma. *Am. J. Surg. Pathol.* **2007**, *31*, 1246–1255. [CrossRef] [PubMed]
26. Srinivasan, M.; Parwani, A.V. Diagnostic utility of p63/P501S double sequential immunohistochemical staining in differentiating urothelial carcinoma from prostate carcinoma. *Diagn. Pathol.* **2011**, *6*, 67. [CrossRef] [PubMed]
27. Perner, S.; Rupp, N.J.; Braun, M.; Rubin, M.A.; Moch, H.; Dietel, M.; Wernert, N.; Jung, K.; Stephan, C.; Kristiansen, G. Loss of SLC45A3 protein (prostein) expression in prostate cancer is associated with *SLC45A3-ERG* gene rearrangement and an unfavorable clinical course. *Int. J. Cancer* **2013**, *132*, 807–812. [CrossRef] [PubMed]
28. Bostwick, D.G.; Pacelli, A.; Blute, M.; Roche, P.; Murphy, G.P. Prostate specific membrane antigen expression in prostatic intraepithelial neoplasia and adenocarcinoma: A study of 184 cases. *Cancer* **1998**, *82*, 2256–2261. [CrossRef]
29. Silver, D.A.; Pellicer, I.; Fair, W.R.; Heston, W.D.; Cordon-Cardo, C. Prostate-specific membrane antigen expression in normal and malignant human tissues. *Clin. Cancer Res.* **1997**, *3*, 81–85. [PubMed]
30. Gurel, B.; Ali, T.Z.; Montgomery, E.A.; Begum, S.; Hicks, J.; Goggins, M.; Eberhart, C.G.; Clark, D.P.; Bieberich, C.J.; Epstein, J.I.; et al. *NKX3.1* as a marker of prostatic origin in metastatic tumors. *Am. J. Surg. Pathol.* **2010**, *34*, 1097–1105. [CrossRef] [PubMed]
31. Gelmann, E.P.; Bowen, C.; Bubendorf, L. Expression of *NKX3.1* in normal and malignant tissues. *Prostate* **2003**, *55*, 111–117. [CrossRef] [PubMed]
32. Skotheim, R.I.; Korkmaz, K.S.; Klokk, T.I.; Abeler, V.M.; Korkmaz, C.G.; Nesland, J.M.; Fossa, S.D.; Lothe, R.A.; Saatcioglu, F. NKX3.1 expression is lost in testicular germ cell tumors. *Am. J. Pathol.* **2003**, *163*, 2149–2154. [CrossRef]
33. Conner, J.R.; Hornick, J.L. Metastatic carcinoma of unknown primary: Diagnostic approach using immunohistochemistry. *Adv. Anat. Pathol.* **2015**, *22*, 149–167. [CrossRef] [PubMed]
34. Tong, H.; Ke, J.Q.; Jiang, F.Z.; Wang, X.J.; Wang, F.Y.; Li, Y.R.; Lu, W.; Wan, X.P. Tumor-associated macrophage-derived CXCL8 could induce ERα suppression via HOXB13 in endometrial cancer. *Cancer lette.* **2016**, *376*, 127–136. [CrossRef] [PubMed]
35. Zhu, J.Y.; Sun, Q.K.; Wang, W.; Jia, W.D. High-level expression OF HOXB13 Is closely associated with tumor angiogenesis and poor prognosis of hepatocellular carcinoma. *Int. J. Clin. Exp. Pathol.* **2014**, *7*, 2925–2933. [PubMed]
36. Zhai, L.L.; Wu, Y.; Cai, C.Y.; Tang, Z.G. Overexpression of homeobox B-13 correlates with angiogenesis, aberrant expression of emt markers, aggressive characteristics and poor prognosis in pancreatic carcinoma. *Int. J. Clin. Exp. Pathol.* **2015**, *8*, 6919–6927. [PubMed]
37. Queisser, A.; Hagedorn, S.A.; Braun, M.; Vogel, W.; Duensing, S.; Perner, S. Comparison of different prostatic markers in lymph node and distant metastases of prostate cancer. *Mod. Pathol.* **2015**, *28*, 138–145. [CrossRef] [PubMed]
38. Gown, A.M. Diagnostic immunohistochemistry: What can go wrong and how to prevent it. *Arch. Pathol. Lab. Med.* **2016**, *140*, 893–898. [CrossRef] [PubMed]

14

CTC-mRNA (AR-V7) Analysis from Blood Samples—Impact of Blood Collection Tube and Storage Time

Alison W. S. Luk [1], Yafeng Ma [1], Pei N. Ding [1,2,3], Francis P. Young [1,4], Wei Chua [2], Bavanthi Balakrishnar [2], Daniel T. Dransfield [5,†], Paul de Souza [1,2,3,4] and Therese M. Becker [1,3,4,*]

1 Centre for Circulating Tumour Cell Diagnostics and Research, Ingham Institute for Applied Medical Research, 1 Campbell St., Liverpool, NSW 2170, Australia; alisonluk@gmail.com (A.W.S.L.); yafeng.ma@unsw.edu.au (Y.M.); Pei.Ding@sswahs.nsw.gov.au (P.N.D.); francis.young@student.unsw.edu.au (F.P.Y.); P.DeSouza@westernsydney.ed u.au (P.d.S.)
2 Department of Medical Oncology, Liverpool Hospital, Elizabeth St & Goulburn St, Liverpool, NSW 2170, Australia; Wei.Chua2@sswahs.nsw.gov.au (W.C.); Bavanthi.Balakrishnar@sswahs.nsw.gov.au (B.B.)
3 Western Sydney University Clinical School, Elizabeth St, Liverpool, NSW 2170, Australia
4 South Western Clinical School, University of New South Wales, Goulburn St., Liverpool, NSW 2170, Australia
5 Tokai Pharmaceuticals, Inc., 255 State Street, 6th Floor, Boston, MA 02109, USA; dan@siamab.com
* Correspondence: t.becker@unsw.edu.au
† Current address: Siamab Therapeutics, 90 Bridge Street, Suite 100, Newton, MA 02458, USA.

Academic Editor: Carsten Stephan

Abstract: Circulating tumour cells (CTCs) are an emerging resource for monitoring cancer biomarkers. New technologies for CTC isolation and biomarker detection are increasingly sensitive, however, the ideal blood storage conditions to preserve CTC-specific mRNA biomarkers remains undetermined. Here we tested the preservation of tumour cells and CTC-mRNA over time in common anticoagulant ethylene-diamine-tetra-acetic acid (EDTA) and acid citrate dextrose solution B (Citrate) blood tubes compared to preservative-containing blood tubes. Blood samples spiked with prostate cancer cells were processed after 0, 24, 30, and 48 h storage at room temperature. The tumour cell isolation efficiency and the mRNA levels of the prostate cancer biomarkers androgen receptor variant 7 (AR-V7) and total AR, as well as epithelial cell adhesion molecule (EpCAM) were measured. Spiked cells were recovered across all storage tube types and times. Surprisingly, tumour mRNA biomarkers were readily detectable after 48 h storage in EDTA and Citrate tubes, but not in preservative-containing tubes. Notably, AR-V7 expression was detected in prostate cancer patient blood samples after 48 h storage in EDTA tubes at room temperature. This important finding presents opportunities for measuring AR-V7 expression from clinical trial patient samples processed within 48 h—a much more feasible timeframe compared to previous recommendations.

Keywords: circulating tumour cell; biomarker; androgen receptor; AR-V7; droplet digital polymerase chain reaction (ddPCR); blood storage tube

1. Introduction

Circulating tumour cells (CTCs) are cells shed from tumours into the peripheral blood, and are believed to be the mechanism for metastasis [1,2]. The enumeration of CTCs has great prognostic value, and further molecular profiling of CTCs has great potential in providing insights on cancer progression, identifying CTC specific molecular therapeutic targets, determining prognostic and relapse indicators, and allowing longitudinal monitoring of disease response to treatments [3,4].

Therefore, relatively simple, non-invasive CTC analysis has exciting potential to investigate changes in tumour biomarkers during a cancer patient's disease progression. In prostate cancer, CTC counts have been associated with prognosis and importantly, isolated CTCs can function as a surrogate tumour samples to detect therapy-determining biomarkers, including the mRNA based androgen receptor variant AR-V7 in CTCs [5–8]. However, CTC analysis is still a rapidly-evolving field due to the complexities of isolation and detection of true CTCs. While it is estimated that 10^6 CTCs are shed per 1 g of tumour tissue per day, CTCs are thought to have a short half-life of less than 3 h in the bloodstream [9–12]. Hence, a major technical challenge for CTC analysis has been efficient recovery of rare CTCs from a background of approximately 10^9 erythrocytes and 10^7 leukocytes per mL of blood, and this has spurred the development of improved technologies for CTC isolation [13–15]. Despite these advances, feasible CTC analysis for clinical trials involving multiple sites are particularly challenging, due to strict requirements for pre-analytical conditions of blood samples in transport and storage, and time restrictions to ensure CTC integrity and biomarker detectability is maintained. Parameters, such as blood tube composition, storage or shipping temperature, sample agitation, and delays in sample processing in a large-throughput laboratory need to be considered before such measurements are conducted for clinical trials. Ideally, CTCs should be protected from apoptosis or cell lysis and, importantly, preserve relevant tumour biomarkers, an issue that is considered especially challenging for mRNA-based biomarkers.

Ethylene-diamine-tetra-acetic acid (EDTA) and acid citrate dextrose solution B (Citrate) are commonly used as anticoagulants in blood tubes for pathology blood tests. These tubes are compatible with downstream polymerase chain reaction (PCR) analysis [16,17] and have also been used for CTC isolation. However, as these tubes do not contain fixatives, early studies recommended that blood should be processed within 24 h, and ideally within 5 h, as it was thought that CTCs rapidly enter apoptosis [18]. To target this problem, new blood tubes have been designed with preservatives intended to extend time before sample processing. Cell-free DNA blood collection tubes (DNA BCT) and Cell-free RNA blood collection tubes (RNA BCT) (Streck, Omaha, NE, USA) are proposed to stabilise nucleated blood cells, preventing the release of cellular DNA and RNA into the plasma, and also inhibiting degradation of cell-free DNA and RNA [19,20]. Therefore, these tubes might be advantageous for CTC sample analysis. Additionally, Cyto-Chex blood collection tubes (Cyto-Chex BCT) were originally designed to preserve cell surface antigens for white blood cell immunophenotyping [21] which may allow improved CTC recovery by immunomagnetic isolation.

There have been previous reports suggesting the added preservatives in BCTs indeed aids CTC stability [22,23]. However, the preservative effects on actionable mRNA-based tumour biomarkers, such as AR-V7 has, to our knowledge, not been tested thoroughly in CTCs isolated from any blood collection tube type. We have previously reported a very sensitive method to detect AR-V7, an emerging RNA-based prostate cancer biomarker in prostate cancer patient CTC samples, showing that AR-V7 is not expressed in residual blood cells, and is expressed heterogeneously in CTCs [7]. In this study, we compare the effects of preservative-containing BCTs to commonly used EDTA and Citrate blood tubes on tumour cell isolation and detection of AR-V7 using our sensitive method.

2. Results

2.1. *Spiked Cell Recovery*

To test CTC preservation and recovery from the five different blood tubes, CTCs were modelled by spiking defined cell numbers of the 22Rv1 prostate cancer cell line into healthy female donor blood. At 0, 24, 30, and 48 h after spiking, tumour cells were enriched and enumerated. Three experiments were performed using 192 mL blood each from three healthy donors. The mean recovery of spiked cells ranged from 13% to 44% across all time points. All blood tubes showed preservation of spiked cells up to 48 h, with mean recovery between 24% and 39% (Figure 1a). The mean recovery of all blood tubes at each time point was compared against recovery at 0 h. Processing samples at 24 and 30 h resulted in significantly lower recovery than when processed at 0 h ($p < 0.05$). Within each time point, the recovery of each blood tube was compared to EDTA. No blood tube had significantly different recovery from EDTA, but the mean recovery of RNA BCT exceeded EDTA at each time point ($p < 0.05$).

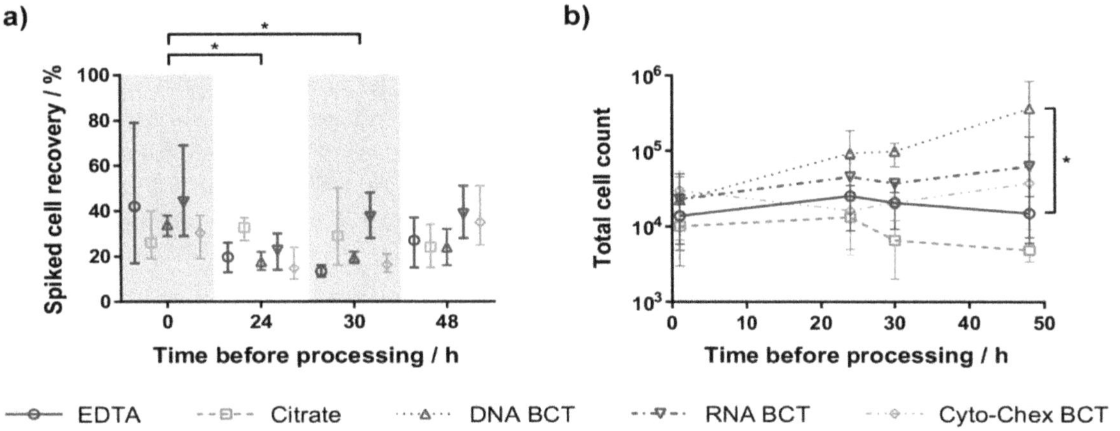

Figure 1. (**a**) Recovery of spiked 22Rv1 cells after tumour cell enrichment. The mean recovery at 24 h and 30 h was significantly different from recovery at 0 h (* $p < 0.05$). (**b**) Total cell count (recovered spiked cells and residual leukocytes after cell enrichment) from samples processed 0 h, 24 h, 30 h, and 48 h after spiking. At 48 h, DNA blood collection tubes (DNA BCT) cell count was significantly different from ethylene-diamine-tetra-acetic acid (EDTA) (* $p < 0.05$). For both (**a**,**b**), symbols represent the mean from three independent experiments, and whiskers represent the range.

2.2. Leukocyte Contamination

DNA BCT and RNA BCT generally had increased total cell counts (tumour cells plus residual co-purified leucocytes) when samples were processed later (Figure 1b). In comparison, EDTA, Citrate and Cyto-Chex BCT cell counts remained similar across all time points. When compared to EDTA tubes, DNA BCT and RNA BCT had higher mean cell counts at each time point, whereas Citrate tubes gave lower cell counts. A two-way ANOVA of each blood tube compared to EDTA at the same time point indicated that for samples processed at 48 h, DNA BCT total cell counts were significantly higher than for EDTA tubes ($p < 0.05$).

2.3. Cellular RNA Recovery

To evaluate the ability of each blood tube in preserving cellular RNA, tumour cell-specific gene expression (AR-V7, total AR and epithelial cell adhesion molecule (EpCAM)) was measured by droplet digital PCR (ddPCR) for each blood tube at each tumour cell enrichment time point (Figure 2). Cells from EDTA and Citrate tubes generally showed decreased mRNA detection the longer the sample storage time, with mRNA biomarkers still readily detectable even after 48 h. In all BCT samples, gene expression was low when processed immediately and undetectable after any storage duration. Thus, while mRNA detection from Citrate and EDTA blood tube samples was similar, BCT samples showed a striking loss in detectable gene expression compared to EDTA tube samples ($p < 0.01$).

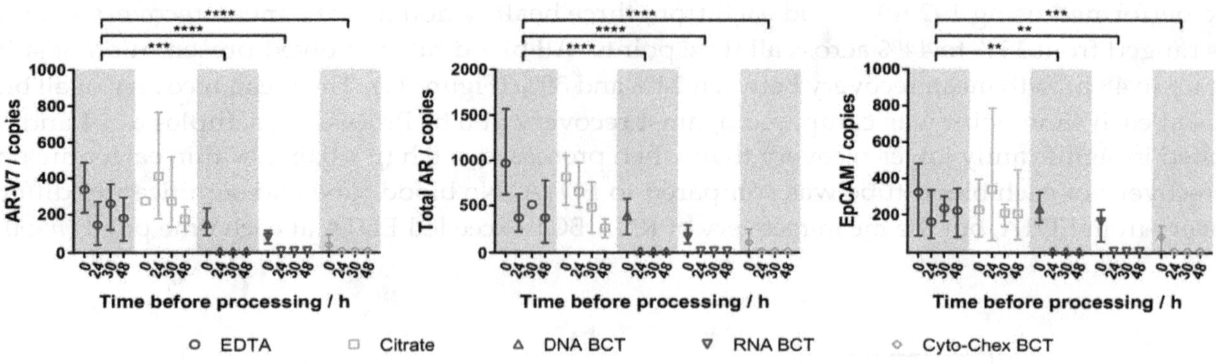

Figure 2. Expression of spiked tumour cell specific genes in samples processed 0 h, 24 h, 30 h, and 48 h after spiking. Symbols represent mean expression from three independent experiments, whiskers represent the range, and are not shown when smaller than the data symbol. The mean gene expression in DNA BCT, RNA BCT, and Cyto-Chex BCT were significantly different from EDTA (** $p < 0.01$, *** $p < 0.001$, **** $p < 0.0001$). AR-V7: androgen receptor variant 7; AR: androgen receptor.

2.4. Increased Proteinase K Treatment

We also investigated the effect of increased proteinase K digestion on the cellular RNA recovery as per manufacturer's suggestions for the BCTs. 22Rv1 cells were spiked into a new set of blood tubes (EDTA, Citrate, DNA BCT, and RNA BCT), followed by enrichment after 48 h of storage. RNA was extracted with and without additional 2 h proteinase K treatment, and gene expression was measured in RNA samples from two independent experiments. In EDTA and Citrate blood tubes, increased proteinase K digestion did not aid RNA recovery but decreased the number of measured copies of all three genes (Figure 3). In DNA BCT and RNA BCT, there was no detectable AR-V7, total AR or EpCAM with standard RNA extraction, and with increased digestion there was a small, but statistically insignificant, increase in the detection of total AR and AR-V7 in DNA BCT and RNA BCT, respectively.

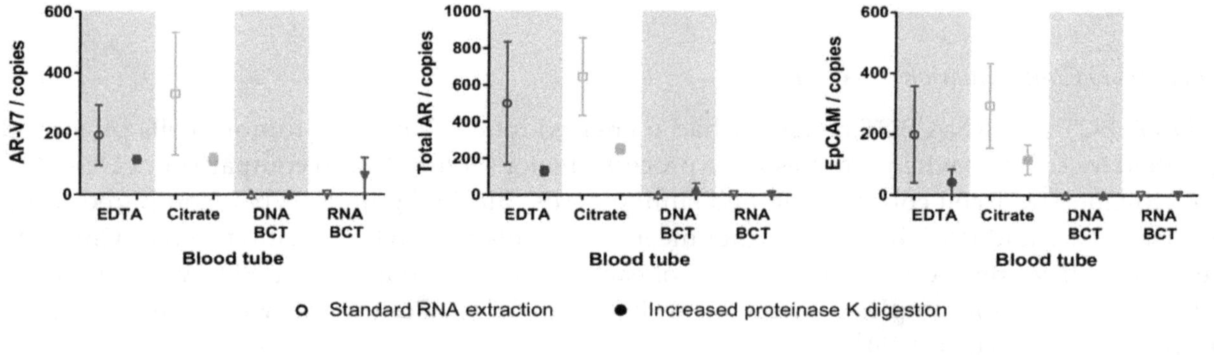

Figure 3. Effect of increased proteinase K treatment on the detection of spiked cell specific genes in samples processed 48 h after spiking. Symbols represent the mean expression from two independent experiments, whiskers represent the range, and are not shown when smaller than the data symbol. EpCAM: epithelial cell adhesion molecule.

2.5. Patient CTC Cellular RNA Detection

Given that spiked cell-specific gene expression was detectable even in samples processed 48 h following spiking of 22Rv1 cells into fresh blood in EDTA and Citrate tubes, we wished to confirm that AR-V7 also remains detectable that long in patient-derived CTCs. Common EDTA tube blood samples from three prostate cancer patients were processed at 4, 24, and 48 h after collection. After CTC enrichment, all patient samples had detectable AR-V7, total AR and EpCAM at all time points (Figure 4). AR-V7 expression varied between the three patients, while being comparable to the expression detected for these patients in a sample collected previously (Table 1). The AR-V7 and total AR detected in patient samples decreased with longer time before processing, but the decrease was not statistically significant.

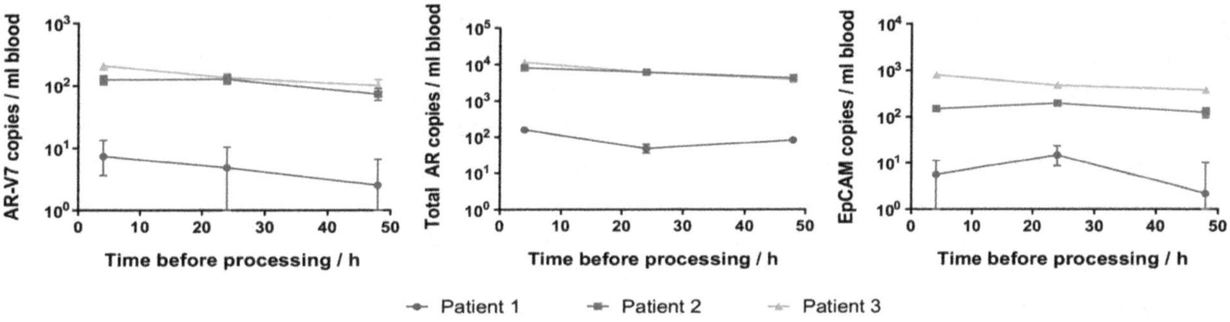

Figure 4. Detection of gene expression in prostate cancer patient circulating tumour cells (CTCs) isolated 4, 24, and 48 h after blood collection in EDTA tubes. Error bars represent 95% confidence intervals of droplet digital polymerase chain reaction (ddPCR) measurements, and error bars smaller than the data symbols are not shown.

Table 1. Androgen receptor variant 7 (AR-V7) and total AR expression in prostate cancer patient blood samples.

Patient	Hormone Sensitivity Status [1]	CTC Count/mL Blood	AR-V7 Copies/mL Blood				Total AR Copies/mL Blood			
		<4 h *	<4 h *	4 h	24 h	48 h	<4 h *	4 h	24 h	48 h
1	CRPC	9 *	2 *	7	5	3	96 *	155	49	84
2	CRPC	2 *	110 *	126	128	74	19,140 *	7963	6083	4191
3	CRPC	6 *	45 *	210	135	102	2610 *	11,392	5994	3848

[1] CRPC = castrate resistant prostate cancer. Patients who had 7–9 month previously high AR-V7 levels detected [7] were chosen for this study (* for comparison previous data are presented; note in the previous study CTC isolation was performed using a different instrument (IsoFlux, Fluxion, San Francisco, CA, USA), CTC counts are normalized per mL blood). New AR-V7 and total AR expression data of the same patients are presented.

3. Discussion

3.1. *Tumour Cell Preservation*

New blood tubes such as DNA BCT, RNA BCT, and Cyto-Chex BCT contain formaldehyde-free fixatives in addition to traditionally used anticoagulants in blood tubes [19–21]. As these BCTs were previously shown to preserve leukocytes and prevent the release of cellular RNA into plasma, even after over three days of storage at room temperature [20,24,25], our study compared commonly-used EDTA and Citrate tubes with BCTs in terms of the ability to preserve modelled CTCs (spiked cultured tumour cells) and of greater interest, cellular RNA.

From our study, the total cell count by Hoechst staining showed that leukocyte retention after tumour cell enrichment increased over time in DNA BCT compared to other blood tubes. Since BCTs were designed for analysis of plasma cell-free nucleic acids, this has not previously been a concern. However, downstream analysis of CTCs can be adversely affected by contaminating leukocytes, such as for single CTC isolation or CTC nucleic acid analysis. Disregarding background leukocytes, intact tumour cells were visible under bright field microscopy from all blood tubes after 48 h (data not shown), and enumeration of cell tracker-stained cells indicated that the recovery of spiked tumour cells was not significantly different across all blood tube types within each time point. Furthermore, although spiked cell recovery generally decreased with longer storage time before processing, there was no significant difference between recovery at 0 and 48 h, with a mean recovery of 35% and 30%, respectively. Our results are in agreement with a previous study which found that CTC yields from lung cancer patients did not decline significantly when processed after 24, 48, or 72 h storage in EDTA tubes [26]. We suggest that the observed variation in spiked cell recovery in our data can be mostly attributed to the difficulties of spiking exact cell numbers of the 22Rv1 cell line, which shows a very strong tendency towards cell clustering. Nevertheless, this line was chosen due to its high AR-V7 expression, and cell strainers were used to keep the effects of cell aggregates to a minimum. Conversely, our results differ from a recent study which reported that the recovery of 2000 spiked MCF-7 breast cancer cells from DNA BCT after one day and four days was very similar at 60% and 58%, respectively, while the recovery decreased from 32% to 16% for EDTA tubes [23]. The discrepancies between the results may be attributed to the difference in the spiked cell line, spiked cell numbers, method of tumour cell isolation, and detection and blood storage time. Importantly, the observed differences in the limited number of studies in this area highlights the need for more research to further compare and improve methods of CTC isolation after blood storage.

Despite common recommendations to process blood samples as soon as possible to reduce cell lysis, our data indicates that cell fixation is not necessary for the recovery of tumour cells, and common EDTA or Citrate tubes are sufficient for tumour cell detection within 48 h.

3.2. Cellular RNA Preservation

Analysis of gene expression from CTCs can provide valuable information on CTC activity and cancer progression, but is particularly challenging as delays in blood sample processing may cause alterations in CTC gene expression, and existing mRNAs may have a short half-life. DNA BCT and RNA BCT were designed to preserve cellular DNA and RNA, respectively, from being released and, hence, were expected to perform better than commonly-used EDTA and Citrate tubes, which only contain anticoagulants. We used our previously-reported, highly-sensitive and specific ddPCR assay to screen for AR-V7, total AR, and EpCAM; this assay has shown before that AR-V7 and total AR were highly expressed in the 22Rv1 cell line or patient CTCs while having no, or negligible, expression in healthy control peripheral lymphocytes [7]. We were surprised to find AR-V7, total AR, and EpCAM readily detectable after 48 h in common EDTA and Citrate tubes. The data suggest that mRNAs encoding these genes have relatively long half-life and/or are continuously expressed by viable tumour cells during storage in a blood sample. Additionally, the detection of mRNA confirms that cells remain intact in the blood sample as it is well established that any released free RNA will be quickly degraded by RNases in the blood [27]. Since cultured 22Rv1 cells are potentially more robust and survive extended storage in blood samples better than CTCs, we confirmed that AR-V7 detection after 48 h storage was translatable to patient CTC samples by testing three patients previously shown to have high CTC AR-V7 expression [7]. Although a small decrease in AR-V7 levels after 48 h was detected in these patient samples, the decrease was marginal in this time frame and even in patient blood with low AR-V7, CTC derived AR-V7 was still detectable after 48 h blood storage at room temperature. AR-V7 expression was comparable to the previous testing of the same patients [7].

In contrast to our data from blood storage in common blood tubes, the BCT samples processed immediately produced much lower detectable tumour cell specific mRNA, and any storage of spiked blood samples in these tubes prevented detection of gene expression completely. We propose that the preservative in the tubes renders RNA inaccessible, likely due to RNA cross-linking with proteins and DNA, which would be incomplete when samples are processed immediately, explaining the limited gene expression detected for our 0 h samples. This interpretation is supported by a report that spiked breast cancer cells could be retrieved from DNA BCTs after up to 72 h storage and had accessible DNA, however, whole genome amplification (WGA) yielded consistently significantly less DNA than WGA from EDTA tubes [22]. Alternatively, RNA could have degraded in the BCTs in our study, however, mRNA was reported detectable by in situ hybridisation from spiked tumour cells isolated from blood stored for four days at room temperature in DNA BCTs [23], suggesting that RNA remains intact but possibly cross-linked, which would interfere less with in situ hybridisation than RNA extraction. While, according to the manufacturers guidelines, RNA should be extractable from samples stored in BCTs, an extended protein K digest is recommended, which might help to reverse cross-linking effects.

We, therefore, investigated whether increased proteinase K treatment during RNA extraction would allow relevant gene expression detection for samples stored for 48 h. However, increased proteinase K digest failed to produce relevant effects and decreased RNA detectability in EDTA and Citrate tubes.

Previous studies showed BCTs to preserve leukocyte cellular RNA, and prevent cellular RNA contamination of cell-free RNA [20,24]. Additionally, the detection of cellular GAPDH, c-Fos and p53 RNA was reported to show variation in expression in neutrophils from blood samples stored over three days in EDTA tubes, whereas there was no change when stored in RNA BCT [25]. While the reasons for the difference to our data are not completely clear, it stands out that all genes tested in that study are abundantly-expressed genes in common blood cells, which might be easier to detect. We have not extended testing past 48 h, as blood samples from within Australia can be processed in this time frame in our facility; however, it is an area of interest for future studies to determine the maximum storage time for EDTA and Citrate tubes.

From our data, it is evident that CTC-derived AR-V7 can be detected from blood stored in commonly-used EDTA and Citrate tubes for up to 48 h, while blood tubes with preservatives (DNA BCT, RNA BCT, and Cyto-Chex BCT) should not be used for CTC isolation if downstream RNA analysis by PCR is intended.

4. Materials and Methods

4.1. Blood Collection

Prostate cancer patients ($n = 3$) and healthy female blood donors ($n = 4$) provided written informed consent to participate in the study. The study was approved by the South Western Sydney Local Healthy District Ethics Committee, Australia (HREC/13/LPOOL/158; 02/09/2013). Peripheral blood was drawn by venipuncture into blood tubes with the initial 3 mL discarded to prevent keratinocyte contamination and false positive CTCs being present. For the main comparison experiment, a total of 192 mL blood from each healthy donor ($n = 3$) was drawn into a total of 24 blood tubes including: 4 × 9 mL K_3EDTA tube (Greiner Bio-One, Kremsmünster, Austria), 4 × 9 mL acid citrate dextrose-B tube (Greiner Bio-One, Kremsmünster, Austria), 4 × 10 mL Cell-free DNA BCT (Streck, Omaha, NE, USA), 4 × 10 mL Cell-free RNA BCT (Streck, Omaha, NE, USA), and 4 × 2 × 5 mL Cyto-Chex BCT (Streck, Omaha, NE, USA). In the follow-up experiment to test increased proteinase K treatment, 38 mL blood from two healthy donors was drawn into one set of EDTA, Citrate, and DNA BCT and RNA BCT tubes. In the experiment with prostate cancer patients, blood was drawn into 3 × 6 mL K_2EDTA tubes (BD, Franklin Lakes, NJ, USA) available in the clinic.

4.2. Cell Spiking

The human prostate cancer cell line 22Rv1 was purchased from the American Type Culture Collection (In Vitro Technologies, Melbourne, Australia). Cells were routinely passaged in Roswell Park Memorial Institute culture medium (RPMI 1640) (Lonza, Basel, Switzerland) supplemented with 10% fetal bovine serum (FBS) (Invitrogen, Carlsbad, CA, USA) in a humidified incubator with 5% CO_2 at 37 °C. For spiking experiments, 22Rv1 cells, cultured for two days after passaging, were gently detached with accutase (Sigma-Aldrich, St. Louis, MO, USA), washed with phosphate buffered saline (PBS), and passed through a 20 µm pre-separation filter "cell strainer" (Miltenyi Biotec, Bergisch Gladbach, Germany) to remove cell aggregates. Cells were then incubated with 15 µM CellTracker Green CMFDA (Life Technologies, Carlsbad, CA, USA) in 100 µL serum-free RPMI media at 37 °C for 1 h. Stained 22Rv1 cells were washed with PBS and a known number (100–200 cells) were spiked into blood tubes. The spiked input cell numbers were verified by aliquoting the same volume onto glass slides in between inoculating blood samples, Hoechst staining, and enumeration by fluorescent microscopy.

4.3. Tumour Cell Enrichment from Whole Blood

Spiked blood samples were enriched for tumour cells after storage (dark, room temperature) for 0, 24, 30, and 48 h. The peripheral blood mononuclear cell (PBMC) layer was extracted using 50 mL SepMate tubes and Lymphoprep according to the manufacturer's instructions (Stemcell Technologies, Vancouver, BC, Canada). PBMCs were washed with separation buffer (PBS with 0.5% FBS and 2 mM EDTA), then incubated at 4 °C for 30 min with 50 μL FcR blocking reagent (Miltenyi Biotec, Bergisch Gladbach, Germany), 50 μL EpCAM conjugated immunomagnetic microbeads (Miltenyi Biotec, Bergisch Gladbach, Germany), 1 μL 50× Hoechst (Fluxion, San Francisco, CA, USA), and made up to a total volume of 500 μL with separation buffer. Cell separation was performed with the Posselds program on the AutoMACS Pro Separator (Miltenyi Biotec, Bergisch Gladbach, Germany). After separation, the positive selected fraction was separated into two aliquots: one was kept on ice until enumeration on the same day, while the other was centrifuged at 400× *g* for 10 min, and the pellet frozen at −80 °C until RNA extraction. For testing of extended proteinase K treatment, samples were enriched after 48 h, with both aliquots frozen at −80 °C until RNA extraction. For prostate cancer patient samples, one blood tube from each patient was processed within 4 h of blood draw, and the other two blood tubes were processed after 24 and 48 h of storage, respectively, before freezing at −80 °C until RNA extraction. Supplementary Figure S1 illustrates the different work flows.

4.4. Cell Enumeration

The enriched enumeration sample was mounted onto slides coated with 2% bovine serum albumine (BSA), then visualised and scanned at 20× magnification with a CellCelector microscope (ALS GmbH, Jena, Thüringen, Germany). The exposure times for the instrument's DAPI and FITC channels were 50 ms and 100 ms, respectively. Scanned images were analysed with ALS CellCelector software v3.0 (ALS GmbH). Nucleated (Hoechst-positive) cells were detected for total cell counts, while cells positive for both Hoechst and CellTracker were considered recovered spiked cells.

To calculate the percentage recovery of spiked cells, the number of cells enumerated after tumour cell enrichment was multiplied by two (to account for CTCs being enumerated in half of the sample while the other half was processed for RNA) and then divided by the original number of spiked cells as determined from input controls.

4.5. Cellular RNA Extraction

Total RNA was extracted from the second enriched sample or from CTC-enriched patient samples with the Total RNA Purification Micro Kit (Norgen Biotek Corp., Thorold, ON, Canada). RNA was double-eluted in 20 μL followed by 10 μL molecular-grade H_2O. For complementary DNA (cDNA) synthesis, 15 μL of eluted RNA was added to form a total volume of 20 μL with the SensiFAST cDNA Synthesis Kit (Bioline, London, UK). For testing increased proteinase K digestion, 0.5 mg of DNAase and RNAase free proteinase K (Bioline) was added with buffer RL at the cell lysate preparation step, and the sample was incubated for 2 h at 60 °C before the addition of ethanol.

4.6. Digital Droplet PCR

Quantification by ddPCR was performed for three tumour cell specific genes. Total androgen receptor (total AR), androgen receptor splice variant 7 (AR-V7), and epithelial cell adhesion molecule (EpCAM) using primers and probes shown in Table 2. In brief, 20 μL ddPCR reactions contained 10 μL ddPCR Supermix for Probes (No dUTP) (Bio-Rad, Hercules, CA, USA), 500 nM of each relevant primer and 250 nM probe Fluorescein (6-FAM) or HEX. Total AR and AR-V7 reactions were multiplexed as previously-described [7]. Droplets were generated with 70 μL oil using a QX200 droplet generator (Bio-Rad). Amplification was performed at 95 °C for 10 min, followed by 40 cycles of 94 °C for 30 s and 55 °C for 1 min using a C1000 Touch Thermo Cycler (Bio-Rad). After amplification, the droplets were read with a QX200 Droplet Reader (Bio-Rad) and analysed with QuantaSoft software v1.7.4.

The fluorescence thresholds used were 6-FAM 2000 for AR-V7, HEX 2500 for total AR, and HEX 1500 for EpCAM. Readings with ≥5 droplets were considered positive. The total error calculated by the software was used as the 95% confidence intervals of ddPCR measurements.

Table 2. Primers and probes.

Gene	Primers (5′→3′)	Probes (5′→3′)
Total AR	F: GGA ATT CCT GTG CAT GAA AGC R: CGA TCG AGT TCC TTG ATG TAG TTC	[HEX] CTT CAG CAT TAT TCC AGT G [BHQ1]
AR-V7	F: CGG AAA TGT TAT GAA GCA GGG ATG A R: CTG GTC ATT TTG AGA TGC TTG CAA T	[6FAM] TCT GGG AGA AAA ATT CCG [BHQ1]
EpCAM	F: CGT CAA TGC CAG TGT ACT TCA R: TTT CTG CCT TCA TCA CCA AA	[HEX] TAC TGT CAT TTG CTC AAA GC [BHQ1]

AR: androgen receptor; AR-V7: androgen receptor variant 7; EpCAM: epithelial cell adhesion molecule; 6FAM: Fluorescein; BHQ1:black hole quencher 1. F: Forward, R: Reverse.

4.7. Statistical Analysis

Analysis of cell and RNA recovery was performed by two-way Analysis of Variance (ANOVA), using GraphPad Prism software v6.07 (GraphPad Software Inc., San Diego, CA, USA).

5. Conclusions

While spiked cell recovery was not affected by the blood tube type even after 48 h of storage, tumour cell-specific RNA was undetectable by ddPCR in CTCs from stored blood samples containing preservatives, likely due to crosslinking effects suppressing RNA accessibility. Surprisingly, AR-V7 was readily detectable in patient CTCs enriched from common EDTA blood tubes after up to 48 h. Although BCTs have been thoroughly tested for circulating tumour nucleic acid detection [28–33], and some initial studies of blood storage in BCTs for tumour cell analysis were also encouraging when using image-based cell analysis involving fluorescent probing for proteins or nucleic acids [23], our data suggests that RNA extraction and downstream analysis by PCR-based methods is severely impeded by the preservatives.

Acknowledgments: This work was supported by the Cancer Institute New South Wales through the Centre for Oncology Education and Research Translation (CONCERT) and the National Breast Cancer Foundation (NBCF). Research was also funded by TOKAI Pharmaceuticals, Boston MA, USA. Francis P. Young is recipient of an Ingham Institute's Honours Scholarship. Human ethics approval, HREC/13/LPOOL/158, was obtained and managed by the CONCERT Biobank.

Author Contributions: Alison W. S. Luk, Therese M. Becker, Daniel T. Dransfield, and Paul de Souza conceived and designed the experiments; Alison W. S. Luk, Yafeng Ma, Pei N. Ding, and Francis P. Young performed the experiments; Alison W. S. Luk analysed the data; Paul de Souza, Wei Chua, Bavanthi Balakrishna, and Daniel T. Dransfield contributed reagents and materials, and coordinated patient recruitment; Alison W. S. Luk and Therese M. Becker wrote the paper and all authors have agreed on the final manuscript version.

References

1. Caixeiro, N.J.; Kienzle, N.; Lim, S.H.; Spring, K.J.; Tognela, A.; Scott, K.F.; Souza, P.D.; Becker, T.M. Circulating tumour cells—A bona fide cause of metastatic cancer. *Cancer Metastasis Rev.* **2014**, *33*, 747–756. [CrossRef] [PubMed]
2. Joosse, S.A.; Gorges, T.M.; Pantel, K. Biology, detection, and clinical implications of circulating tumor cells. *EMBO Mol. Med.* **2015**, *7*, 1–11. [CrossRef] [PubMed]
3. Becker, T.M.; Caixeiro, N.J.; Lim, S.H.; Tognela, A.; Kienzle, N.; Scott, K.F.; Spring, K.J.; de Souza, P. New frontiers in circulating tumor cell analysis: A reference guide for biomolecular profiling toward translational clinical use. *Int. J. Cancer* **2014**, *134*, 2523–2533. [CrossRef] [PubMed]

4. Krebs, M.G.; Metcalf, R.L.; Carter, L.; Brady, G.; Blackhall, F.H.; Dive, C. Molecular analysis of circulating tumour cells—Biology and biomarkers. *Nat. Rev. Clin. Oncol.* **2014**, *11*, 129–144. [CrossRef] [PubMed]
5. De Bono, J.S.; Scher, H.I.; Montgomery, R.B.; Parker, C.; Miller, M.C.; Tissing, H.; Doyle, G.V.; Terstappen, L.W.W.M.; Pienta, K.J.; Raghavan, D. Circulating tumor cells predict survival benefit from treatment in metastatic castration-resistant prostate cancer. *Clin. Cancer Res.* **2008**, *14*, 6302–6309. [CrossRef] [PubMed]
6. Antonarakis, E.S.; Lu, C.; Luber, B.; Wang, H.; Chen, Y.; Nakazawa, M.; Nadal, R.; Paller, C.J.; Denmeade, S.R.; Carducci, M.A.; et al. Androgen receptor splice variant 7 and efficacy of taxane chemotherapy in patients with metastatic castration-resistant prostate cancer. *JAMA Oncol.* **2015**, *1*, 582–591. [CrossRef] [PubMed]
7. Ma, Y.; Luk, A.; Young, F.P.; Lynch, D.; Chua, W.; Balakrishnar, B.; de Souza, P.; Becker, T.M. Droplet digital PCR based androgen receptor variant 7 (AR-V7) detection from prostate cancer patient blood biopsies. *Int. J. Mol. Sci.* **2016**, *17*, 1264. [CrossRef] [PubMed]
8. Antonarakis, E.S.; Lu, C.; Luber, B.; Wang, H.; Chen, Y.; Zhu, Y.; Silberstein, J.L.; Taylor, M.N.; Maughan, B.L.; Denmeade, S.R.; et al. Clinical significance of androgen receptor splice variant-7 mRNA detection in circulating tumor cells of men with metastatic castration-resistant prostate cancer treated with first- and second-line abiraterone and enzalutamide. *J. Clin. Oncol.* **2017**. [CrossRef] [PubMed]
9. Liotta, L.A.; Kleinerman, J.; Saidel, G.M. Quantitative relationships of intravascular tumor cells, tumor vessels, and pulmonary metastases following tumor implantation. *Cancer Res.* **1974**, *34*, 997–1004. [PubMed]
10. Butler, T.P.; Gullino, P.M. Quantitation of cell shedding into efferent blood of mammary adenocarcinoma. *Cancer Res.* **1975**, *35*, 512–516. [PubMed]
11. Chang, Y.S.; Tomaso, E.D.; McDonald, D.M.; Jones, R.; Jain, R.K.; Munn, L.L. Mosaic blood vessels in tumors: Frequency of cancer cells in contact with flowing blood. *Proc. Natl. Acad. Sci. USA* **2000**, *97*, 14608–14613. [CrossRef] [PubMed]
12. Meng, S.; Tripathy, D.; Frenkel, E.P.; Shete, S.; Naftalis, E.Z.; Huth, J.F.; Beitsch, P.D.; Leitch, M.; Hoover, S.; Euhus, D.; et al. Circulating tumor cells in patients with breast cancer dormancy. *Clin. Cancer Res.* **2004**, *10*, 8152–8162. [CrossRef] [PubMed]
13. Sun, Y.; Yang, X.; Zhou, J.; Qiu, S.; Fan, J.; Xu, Y. Circulating tumor cells: Advances in detection methods, biological issues, and clinical relevance. *J. Cancer Res. Clin. Oncol.* **2011**, *137*, 1151–1173. [CrossRef] [PubMed]
14. Yu, M.; Stott, S.; Toner, M.; Maheswaran, S.; Haber, D.A. Circulating tumor cells: Approaches to isolation and characterization. *J. Cell Biol.* **2011**, *192*, 373–382. [CrossRef] [PubMed]
15. Alix-Panabières, C.; Pantel, K. Challenges in circulating tumour cell research. *Nat. Rev. Cancer* **2014**, *14*, 623–631. [CrossRef] [PubMed]
16. Lam, N.Y.L.; Rainer, T.H.; Chiu, R.W.K.; Lo, Y.M.D. EDTA is a better anticoagulant than heparin or citrate for delayed blood processing for plasma DNA analysis. *Clin. Chem.* **2004**, *50*, 256–257. [CrossRef] [PubMed]
17. Palmirotta, R.; Ludovici, G.; de Marchis, M.L.; Savonarola, A.; Leone, B.; Spila, A.; de Angelis, F.; Morte, D.D.; Ferroni, P.; Guadagni, F. Preanalytical procedures for DNA studies: The experience of the interinstitutional multidisciplinary BioBank (BioBIM). *Biopreserv. Biobank.* **2011**, *9*, 35–45. [CrossRef] [PubMed]
18. Fehm, T.; Solomayer, E.F.; Meng, S.; Tucker, T.; Lane, N.; Wang, J.; Gebauer, G. Methods for isolating circulating epithelial cells and criteria for their classification as carcinoma cells. *Cytotherapy* **2005**, *7*, 171–185. [CrossRef] [PubMed]
19. Fernando, M.R.; Chen, K.; Norton, S.; Krzyzanowski, G.; Bourne, D.; Hunsley, B.; Ryan, W.L.; Bassett, C. A new methodology to preserve the original proportion and integrity of cell-free fetal DNA in maternal plasma during sample processing and storage. *Prenat. Diagn.* **2010**, *30*, 418–424. [CrossRef] [PubMed]
20. Fernando, M.R.; Norton, S.E.; Luna, K.K.; Lechner, J.M.; Qin, J. Stabilization of cell-free RNA in blood samples using a new collection device. *Clin. Biochem.* **2012**, *45*, 1497–1502. [CrossRef] [PubMed]
21. Warrino, D.E.; DeGennaro, L.J.; Hanson, M.; Swindells, S.; Pirruccello, S.J.; Ryan, W.L. Stabilization of white blood cells and immunologic markers for extended analysis using flow cytometry. *J. Immunol. Methods* **2005**, *305*, 107–119. [CrossRef] [PubMed]
22. Yee, S.S.; Lieberman, D.B.; Blanchard, T.; Rader, J.; Zhao, J.; Troxel, A.B.; DeSloover, D.; Fox, A.J.; Daber, R.D.; Kakrecha, B.; et al. A Novel approach for next-generation sequencing of circulating tumor cells. *Mol. Genet. Genom. Med.* **2016**, *4*, 395–406. [CrossRef] [PubMed]

23. Qin, J.; Alt, J.R.; Hunsley, B.A.; Williams, T.L.; Fernando, M.R. Stabilization of circulating tumor cells in blood using a collection device with a preservative reagent. *Cancer Cell Int.* **2014**, *14*, 23. [CrossRef] [PubMed]
24. Qin, J.; Williams, T.L.; Fernando, M.R. A novel blood collection device stabilizes cell-free RNA in blood during sample shipping and storage. *BMC Res. Notes* **2013**, *6*, 380. [CrossRef] [PubMed]
25. Das, K.; Norton, S.E.; Alt, J.R.; Krzyzanowski, G.D.; Williams, T.L.; Fernando, M.R. Stabilization of cellular RNA in blood during storage at room temperature: A comparison of cell-free RNA BCT with K3EDTA tubes. *Mol. Diagn. Ther.* **2014**, *18*, 647–653. [CrossRef] [PubMed]
26. Flores, L.M.; Kindelberger, D.W.; Ligon, A.H.; Capelletti, M.; Fiorentino, M.; Loda, M.; Cibas, E.S.; Jänne, P.A.; Krop, I.E. Improving the yield of circulating tumour cells facilitates molecular characterisation and recognition of discordant HER2 amplification in breast cancer. *Br. J. Cancer* **2010**, *102*, 1495–1502. [CrossRef] [PubMed]
27. Tsui, N.B.Y.; Ng, E.K.O.; Lo, Y.M.D. Stability of endogenous and added RNA in blood specimens, serum, and plasma. *Clin. Chem.* **2002**, *48*, 1647. [PubMed]
28. Denis, M.G.; Knol, A.; Théoleyre, S.; Vallée, A.; Dréno, B. Efficient detection of BRAF mutation in plasma of patients after long-term storage of blood in cell-free DNA blood collection tubes. *Clin. Chem.* **2015**, *61*, 886–888. [CrossRef] [PubMed]
29. Schiavon, G.; Hrebien, S.; Garcia-Murillas, I.; Cutts, R.J.; Pearson, A.; Tarazona, N.; Fenwick, K.; Kozarewa, I.; Lopez-Knowles, E.; Ribas, R.; et al. Analysis of ESR1 mutation in circulating tumor DNA demonstrates evolution during therapy for metastatic breast cancer. *Sci. Transl. Med.* **2015**, *7*, 313ra182. [CrossRef] [PubMed]
30. Toro, P.V.; Erlanger, B.; Beaver, J.A.; Cochran, R.L.; VanDenBerg, D.A.; Yakim, E.; Cravero, K.; Chu, D.; Zabransky, D.J.; Wong, H.Y.; et al. Comparison of cell stabilizing blood collection tubes for circulating plasma tumor DNA. *Clin. Biochem.* **2015**, *48*, 993–998. [CrossRef] [PubMed]
31. Diaz, I.M.; Nocon, A.; Mehnert, D.H.; Fredebohm, J.; Diehl, F.; Holtrup, F. Performance of streck cfDNA blood collection tubes for liquid biopsy testing. *PLoS ONE* **2016**, *11*, e0166354.
32. Kang, Q.; Henry, N.L.; Paoletti, C.; Jiang, H.; Vats, P.; Chinnaiyan, A.M.; Hayes, D.F.; Merajver, S.D.; Rae, J.M.; Tewari, M. Comparative analysis of circulating tumor DNA stability in K3EDTA, Streck, and CellSave blood collection tubes. *Clin. Biochem.* **2016**, *49*, 1354–1360. [CrossRef] [PubMed]
33. Sherwood, J.L.; Corcoran, C.; Brown, H.; Sharpe, A.D.; Musilova, M.; Kohlmann, A. Optimised pre-analytical methods improve KRAS mutation detection in circulating tumour DNA (ctDNA) from patients with non-small cell lung cancer (NSCLC). *PLoS ONE* **2016**, *11*, e0150197. [CrossRef] [PubMed]

Permissions

All chapters in this book were first published by MDPI; hereby published with permission under the Creative Commons Attribution License or equivalent. Every chapter published in this book has been scrutinized by our experts. Their significance has been extensively debated. The topics covered herein carry significant findings which will fuel the growth of the discipline. They may even be implemented as practical applications or may be referred to as a beginning point for another development.

The contributors of this book come from diverse backgrounds, making this book a truly international effort. This book will bring forth new frontiers with its revolutionizing research information and detailed analysis of the nascent developments around the world.

We would like to thank all the contributing authors for lending their expertise to make the book truly unique. They have played a crucial role in the development of this book. Without their invaluable contributions this book wouldn't have been possible. They have made vital efforts to compile up to date information on the varied aspects of this subject to make this book a valuable addition to the collection of many professionals and students.

This book was conceptualized with the vision of imparting up-to-date information and advanced data in this field. To ensure the same, a matchless editorial board was set up. Every individual on the board went through rigorous rounds of assessment to prove their worth. After which they invested a large part of their time researching and compiling the most relevant data for our readers.

The editorial board has been involved in producing this book since its inception. They have spent rigorous hours researching and exploring the diverse topics which have resulted in the successful publishing of this book. They have passed on their knowledge of decades through this book. To expedite this challenging task, the publisher supported the team at every step. A small team of assistant editors was also appointed to further simplify the editing procedure and attain best results for the readers.

Apart from the editorial board, the designing team has also invested a significant amount of their time in understanding the subject and creating the most relevant covers. They scrutinized every image to scout for the most suitable representation of the subject and create an appropriate cover for the book.

The publishing team has been an ardent support to the editorial, designing and production team. Their endless efforts to recruit the best for this project, has resulted in the accomplishment of this book. They are a veteran in the field of academics and their pool of knowledge is as vast as their experience in printing. Their expertise and guidance has proved useful at every step. Their uncompromising quality standards have made this book an exceptional effort. Their encouragement from time to time has been an inspiration for everyone.

The publisher and the editorial board hope that this book will prove to be a valuable piece of knowledge for researchers, students, practitioners and scholars across the globe.

List of Contributors

Monika Jung, Sabine Weickmann, Bernhard Ralla and Antonia Franz
Department of Urology, Charité-Universitätsmedizin Berlin, 10117 Berlin, Germany

Hannah Rochow, Carsten Stephan and Klaus Jung
Department of Urology, Charité-Universitätsmedizin Berlin, 10117 Berlin, Germany
Berlin Institute for Urologic Research, 10115 Berlin, Germany

Sefer Elezkurtaj
Institute of Pathology, Charité-Universitätsmedizin Berlin, 10117 Berlin, Germany

Ergin Kilic
Institute of Pathology, Charité-Universitätsmedizin Berlin, 10117 Berlin, Germany
Institute of Pathology, Hospital Leverkusen, 51375 Leverkusen, Germany

Zhongwei Zhao
Department of Urology, Charité-Universitätsmedizin Berlin, 10117 Berlin, Germany
Department of Urology, Qilu Hospital of Shandong University, Jinan 250012, China

Annika Fendler
Department of Urology, Charité-Universitätsmedizin Berlin, 10117 Berlin, Germany
Max Delbrueck Center for Molecular Medicine in the Helmholtz Association, Cancer Research Program, 13125 Berlin, Germany
Cancer Dynamics Laboratory, The Francis Crick Institute, 1 Midland Road, London NW1 1AT, UK

Matteo Bauckneht
Nuclear Medicine, IRCCS Ospedale Policlinico San Martino, 16132 Genova, Italy

Sara Elena Rebuzzi, Veronica Murianni, Roberto Borea, Alessandra Damassi, Fabio Catalano, Valentino Martelli and Giuseppe Fornarini
Medical Oncology Unit 1, IRCCS Ospedale Policlinico San Martino, 16132 Genova, Italy

Alessio Signori, Maria Isabella Donegani, Alberto Miceli, Stefano Raffa and Marta Ponzano
Department of Health Sciences (DISSAL), University of Genova, Largo R. Benzi 10, 16132 Genova, Italy

Silvia Morbelli and Gianmario Sambuceti
Nuclear Medicine, IRCCS Ospedale Policlinico San Martino, 16132 Genova, Italy
Department of Health Sciences (DISSAL), University of Genova, Largo R. Benzi 10, 16132 Genova, Italy

Cecilia Marini
Nuclear Medicine, IRCCS Ospedale Policlinico San Martino, 16132 Genova, Italy
CNR Institute of Molecular Bioimaging and Physiology (IBFM), 20090 Segrate (MI), Italy

Francesco Boccardo
Academic Unit of Medical Oncology, IRCCS Ospedale Policlinico San Martino, 16132 Genova, Italy
Department of Internal Medicine and Medical Specialties (DiMI), School of Medicine, University of Genova, 16132 Genova, Italy

Jörgen Elgqvist
Department of Medical Physics and Biomedical Engineering, Sahlgrenska University Hospital, 413 45 Gothenburg, Sweden
Department of Physics, University of Gothenburg, 412 96 Gothenburg, Sweden

Shukui Zhou, Qingsong Zou and Qiang Fu
The Department of Urology, Affiliated Sixth People's Hospital, Shanghai JiaoTong University, Shanghai 200233, China

Weixin Zhao
Wake Forest Institute for Regenerative Medicine, Winston-Salem, NC 27101, USA

Kaile Zhang
The Department of Urology, Affiliated Sixth People's Hospital, Shanghai JiaoTong University, Shanghai 200233, China
Wake Forest Institute for Regenerative Medicine, Winston-Salem, NC 27101, USA

Leilei Wang
VIP Department of Beijing Hospital, Beijing 100730, China

Jianlong Wang
Urology Department of Beijing Hospital, Beijing 100730, China

Xiaolan Fang
Department of Cancer Biology, Wake Forest University School of Medicine, Wake Forest Institute for Regenerative Medicine, Winston-Salem, NC 27101, USA

Montserrat Ferrer-Batallé and Esther Llop
Biochemistry and Molecular Biology Unit, Department of Biology, University of Girona, 17003 Girona, Spain
Girona Biomedical Research Institute (IDIBGI), 17190 Salt (Girona), Spain

Manel Ramírez, Rosa Núria Aleixandre and Josep Comet
Girona Biomedical Research Institute (IDIBGI), 17190 Salt (Girona), Spain
Catalan Health Institute, University Hospital of Girona Dr. Josep Trueta, 17007 Girona, Spain

Rafael de Llorens and Rosa Peracaula
Biochemistry and Molecular Biology Unit, Department of Biology, University of Girona, 17003 Girona, Spain
Catalan Health Institute, University Hospital of Girona Dr. Josep Trueta, 17007 Girona, Spain

Marc Saez
Research Group on Statistics, Econometrics and Health (GRECS), University of Girona, 17003 Girona, Spain
CIBER of Epidemiology and Public Health (CIBERESP), 28029 Madrid, Spain

Rhonda Daniel, Qianni Wu, Gene Clark and Zendra Zehner
Department of Biochemistry and Molecular Biology, VCU Medical Center and the Massey Cancer Center, Virginia Commonwealth University, Richmond, VA 23298-0614, USA

Vernell Williams
Molecular Diagnostic Laboratory, Department of Pathology, VCU Health System, Virginia Commonwealth University, Richmond, VA 23298-0248, USA

Georgi Guruli
Division of Urology, VCU Medical Center and the Massey Cancer Center, Virginia Commonwealth University, Richmond, VA 23298-0037, USA

Chi-Long Chen
Graduate Institute of Clinical Medicine, College of Medicine, Taipei Medical University, Taipei 110, Taiwan
Department of Pathology, School of Medicine, College of Medicine, Taipei Medical University, Taipei 110, Taiwan

Wei-Yu Chen
Graduate Institute of Clinical Medicine, College of Medicine, Taipei Medical University, Taipei 110, Taiwan
Department of Pathology, School of Medicine, College of Medicine, Taipei Medical University, Taipei 110, Taiwan
Department of Pathology, Wan Fang Hospital, Taipei Medical University, Taipei 116, Taiwan

Kuo-Tai Hua
Graduate Institute of Toxicology, College of Medicine, National Taiwan University, Taipei 100, Taiwan

Ming-Hsien Chien
Graduate Institute of Clinical Medicine, College of Medicine, Taipei Medical University, Taipei 110, Taiwan
Department of Medical Education and Research, Wan Fang Hospital, Taipei Medical University, Taipei 116, Taiwan

Wei-Jiunn Lee
Department of Medical Education and Research, Wan Fang Hospital, Taipei Medical University, Taipei 116, Taiwan
Department of Urology, School of Medicine, College of Medicine, Taipei Medical University, Taipei 110, Taiwan

Yu-Ching Wen
Department of Urology, School of Medicine, College of Medicine, Taipei Medical University, Taipei 110, Taiwan
Department of Urology, Wan Fang Hospital, Taipei Medical University, Taipei 116, Taiwan

Yung-Wei Lin
Department of Urology, Wan Fang Hospital, Taipei Medical University, Taipei 116, Taiwan

Yen-Nien Liu
Graduate Institute of Cancer Biology and Drug Discovery, College of Medical Science and Technology, Taipei Medical University, Taipei 110, Taiwan

Thorsten H. Ecke and Steffen Hallmann
Department of Urology, HELIOS Hospital, D-15526 Bad Saarow, Germany

Hui-Juan Huang-Tiel
Department of Neurology/Emergency Unit, Vivantes Hospital Spandau, D-13585 Berlin, Germany

Klaus Golka, Silvia Selinski and Berit Christine Geis
Leibniz Research Centre for Working Environment and Human Factors IfADo, D-44139 Dortmund, Germany

Stephan Koswig and Katrin Bathe
Department of Radio-Oncology, HELIOS Hospital, D-15525 Bad Saarow, Germany

Holger Gerullis
School of Medicine and Health Sciences Carl von Ossietzky, University Oldenburg, D-26133 Oldenburg, Germany

Hideyasu Tsumura, Takefumi Satoh, Ken-ichi Tabata and Masatsugu Iwamura
Department of Urology, Kitasato University School of Medicine, Sagamihara 252-0374, Japan

Hiromichi Ishiyama, Kouji Takenaka, Akane Sekiguchi, Masashi Kitano and Kazushige Hayakawa
Department of Radiology and Radiation Oncology, Kitasato University School of Medicine, Sagamihara 252-0374, Japan

Masaki Nakamura
Department of Microbiology, Kitasato University School of Allied Health Sciences, Kanagawa 252-0373, Japan

Vera Genitsch, Inti Zlobec and Achim Fleischmann
Institute of Pathology, University of Bern, Bern 3008, Switzerland

Roland Seiler and George N. Thalmann
Department of Urology, University of Bern, Bern 3010, Switzerland

Ilka Kristiansen, Yuri Tolkach and Glen Kristiansen
Institute of Pathology, University Hospital Bonn, 53127 Bonn, Germany

Carsten Stephan
Department of Urology, Charité-Universitätsmedizin Berlin, 10117 Berlin, Germany

Klaus Jung
Berlin Institute of Urologic Research, 10117 Berlin, Germany

Manfred Dietel and Anja Rieger
Institute of Pathology, Charité-Universitätsmedizin Berlin, 10117 Berlin, Germany

Jochen Neuhaus
Department of Urology, Research Laboratory, University of Leipzig, Liebigstraße 19, 04103 Leipzig, Germany

Eric Schiffer
Numares AG, Regensburg, Am BioPark 9, 93053 Regensburg, Germany

Ferdinando Mannello
Department of Biomolecular Sciences, University "Carlo Bo", Via O. Ubaldini 7, 61029 Urbino (PU), Italy

Lars-Christian Horn
Institute of Pathology, University Hospital Leipzig, Liebigstraße 24, 04103 Leipzig, Germany

Roman Ganzer and Jens-Uwe Stolzenburg
Department of Urology, University Hospital Leipzig, Liebigstraße 20, 04103 Leipzig, Germany

Shuntaro Oka, Masaru Kanagawa, Yoshihiro Doi and Hirokatsu Yoshimura
Research Center, Nihon Medi-Physics Co., Ltd., 3-1 Kitasode, Sodegaura, Chiba 299-0266, Japan

David M. Schuster and Mark M. Goodman
Division of Nuclear Medicine and Molecular Imaging, Department of Radiology and Imaging Sciences, Emory University, Atlanta, GA 30329, USA

Alison W. S. Luk and Yafeng Ma
Centre for Circulating Tumour Cell Diagnostics and Research, Ingham Institute for Applied Medical Research, 1 Campbell St., Liverpool, NSW 2170, Australia

Wei Chua and Bavanthi Balakrishnar
Department of Medical Oncology, Liverpool Hospital, Elizabeth St & Goulburn St, Liverpool, NSW 2170, Australia

Pei N. Ding
Centre for Circulating Tumour Cell Diagnostics and Research, Ingham Institute for Applied Medical Research, 1 Campbell St., Liverpool, NSW 2170, Australia
Department of Medical Oncology, Liverpool Hospital, Elizabeth St & Goulburn St, Liverpool, NSW 2170, Australia
Western Sydney University Clinical School, Elizabeth St, Liverpool, NSW 2170, Australia

Paul de Souza
Centre for Circulating Tumour Cell Diagnostics and Research, Ingham Institute for Applied Medical Research, 1 Campbell St., Liverpool, NSW 2170, Australia
Department of Medical Oncology, Liverpool Hospital, Elizabeth St & Goulburn St, Liverpool, NSW 2170, Australia
Western Sydney University Clinical School, Elizabeth St, Liverpool, NSW 2170, Australia
South Western Clinical School, University of New South Wales, Goulburn St., Liverpool, NSW 2170, Australia

Francis P. Young
Centre for Circulating Tumour Cell Diagnostics and Research, Ingham Institute for Applied Medical Research, 1 Campbell St., Liverpool, NSW 2170, Australia
South Western Clinical School, University of New South Wales, Goulburn St., Liverpool, NSW 2170, Australia

Therese M. Becker
Centre for Circulating Tumour Cell Diagnostics and Research, Ingham Institute for Applied Medical Research, 1 Campbell St., Liverpool, NSW 2170, Australia
Western Sydney University Clinical School, Elizabeth St, Liverpool, NSW 2170, Australia
South Western Clinical School, University of New South Wales, Goulburn St., Liverpool, NSW 2170, Australia

Daniel T. Dransfield
Tokai Pharmaceuticals, Inc., 255 State Street, 6th Floor, Boston, MA 02109, USA

Index